Health Promotion in Nursing

Second Edition

JANICE A. MAVILLE, EdD, MSN, RN
Professor and Coordinator
Master of Science in Nursing Program
Department of Nursing
The University of Texas—Pan American
Edinburg, Texas

CAROLINA G. HUERTA, EdD, MSN, RN
Professor & Chair
Department of Nursing
College of Health Sciences & Human Services
The University of Texas—Pan American
Edinburg, Texas

THOMSON

DELMAR LEARNING

Australia   Brazil   Canada   Mexico   Singapore   Spain   United Kingdom   United States

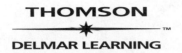

Health Promotion in Nursing, 2nd edition
by Janice A. Maville and Carolina G. Huerta

Vice President, Health Care Business Unit:
William Brottmiller

Director of Learning Solutions:
Matthew Kane

Acquisitions Editor:
Tamara Caruso

Senior Product Manager:
Elisabeth F. Williams

Director of Marketing:
Jennifer McAvey

Marketing Manager:
Michele McTighe

Marketing Coordinator:
Chelsey Iaquinta

Director of Production:
Carolyn Miller

Content Project Manager:
Jessica McNavich

Senior Art Director:
Jack Pendleton

For permission to use material from this text or product, contact us by
Tel (800) 730-2214
Fax (800) 730-2215
www.thomsonrights.com

Library of Congress Cataloging-in-Publication Data
Maville, Janice A.
  Health promotion in nursing/by Janice A. Maville and Carolina G. Huerta. –2nd ed.
    p.; cm.
  Includes bibliographical references and index.
ISBN-13: 978-1-4180-2089-7
ISBN-10: 1-4180-2089-3
  1. Nursing. 2. Health promotion. I. Huerta, Carolina G. II. Title. [DNLM: 1. Nursing Care. 2. Health Promotion. WY 100 M461h 2007]

RT42.M2466 2007
613–dc22   2007016109

Notice to the Reader

Contents

SECTION I CONCEPTUAL FOUNDATIONS AND THEORETICAL APPROACHES

Chapter 1 Health Promotion: Past, Present, and Future

Defining Health Promotion   2
  Health Education   3
  Health Promotion   3
Health Promotion: Past   3
  Ancient Times   3
    Babylonia   4
    Greece   4
    Egypt   4
    Palestine   4
    Rome   5
    China   5
  The Middle Ages, Renaissance,
    and Early America   5
  Health Promotion in the Middle Ages
    (AD 500–1500)   5
  The Renaissance and Early America
    (AD 1500–1800)   6
  The Social Mandate for Health Promotion   6
  The First Movement   7
  The Second Movement   7
  The Third Movement   7
**Sociopolitical Influences for Health
  Promotion in the Twentieth Century**   8
  Health Reform   8
    Federal Government Involvement in Health Care   8
    Medicaid and Medicare   9
**Government Initiatives for Health
  Promotion in the Twentieth Century**   9
  Canadian Influence on Health Promotion   10
  International Goals for Health   10
  The United States and National Goals for Health   10
Health Care Cost Containment   12
  Changes in Nursing Practice   12
  Changes in Nursing Policy   12
Health Promotion: Where Is It Going?   13
  Forces Shaping the Future of Health Promotion   14
  A Framework for Thinking About the Future   14
  Facilitating Your Role in Health Promotion   14
Summary   15

Chapter 2 Nursing Concepts and Health Promotion

**Professional Nursing Practice
  and Health Promotion**   19
Nursing's Metaparadigm   20
Defining Nursing   22

Person, Environment, Health, and Nursing   22
  Person   22
    Maslow's Hierarchy of Needs   23
  Environment   24
  Health   24
    Definitions of Health   25
  Nursing   26
Nursing as a Profession   26
**Nursing Educational Levels
  and Health Promotion**   26
**Integrating Health Promotion Concepts
  into Nursing Practice**   27
  Assumptions   27
Theoretical Foundations   30
  Systems Theory   30
  Adaptation Theory   30
  Needs Theory   31
  Human Becoming Theory and Human
    Care Theory   31
  Transcultural Theory   31
Organizing Nursing Theory   32
  Nursing's Metaparadigm and Nursing Theory   32
Summary   33

Chapter 3 Theoretical Foundations of Health Promotion

Clarifying Terms   40
  Wellness   41
  Disease Prevention and Health Protection   41
  Health Promotion   42
Theoretical Foundations   42
Theories of Human Behavior   42
  Theory of Planned Behavior   42
  Theory of Social Behavior   44
Theories of Human Behavior and Health   44
  Health Belief Model   44
  Protection Motivation Theory   45
  Transtheoretical Model of Behavior Change   45
**Models for Groups, Organizations,
  and Communities**   48
  Consumer Information Processing Model   48
  Diffusion of Innovations Model   48
  PRECEDE-PROCEED Model   49
Health Promotion Models   50
  Pender Model of Health Promotion   50
  O'Donnell Model of Health Promotion Behavior   52
Developing a Health Promotion Plan   53
  Assessment and Data Collection   53
  Planning and Implementation   53
  Evaluation   53
Summary   54

Chapter 4 The Role of the Nurse in Health Promotion

**Domains Fundamental to Nursing Practice
in Health Promotion**   **57**
    Biological Domain   58
    Psychological Domain   58
    Sociological Domain   59
    Environmental Domain   59
    Political Domain   60
    Spiritual Domain   60
    Intellectual Domain   61
    Sexual Domain   61
    Technological Domain   61
Holistic Philosophy   **61**
Holistic Nursing Practice   **62**
Roles of the Nurse in Health Promotion   **62**
    Activist/Proactive Change Agent   62
    Advocate   63
    Educator   63
    Empowering Agent   63
    Communicator   63
    Consultant   63
    Coordinator of Care   63
    Leader/Member of the Profession   64
    Provider of Care/Caregiver   64
    Research User and Health Promotion Models
       Researcher   64
    Role Model   64
Overview of the Nursing Process   **64**
    Assessment (Acquiring Information)   65
    Nursing Diagnosis   65
    Planning   66
    Implementation   67
    Evaluation   67
**Nursing Process and Health Promotion for
the Individual, Families, and Communities**   **67**
    Individual   67
    Family   67
    Community   70
Risk Factors and Health Promotion   **70**
    Environment   70
    Work   70
    Socioeconomic Level   70
    Education   70
    Gender   72
    Cultural and Spiritual Influences   72
**Current Factors Affecting Nursing Roles
in Health Promotion**   **72**
    Health Care System   72
    Nursing Roles   72
    Increasing Technology   72
    Economic Environment   73
    Individual Behavior   73
Summary   **73**

SECTION II   FACTORS INFLUENCING HEALTH PROMOTION

Chapter 5 Communication

Communication and Nursing   **78**
    The Message   79
    Encoding   79
    The Channel   80
    Decoding   80
    Feedback   80
    Context   81
Types of Communication   **81**
    Verbal Communication   81
    Nonverbal Communication   83
       Personal Presentation   83
       Proxemics   84
       Kinesics   85
       Touch   85
       Paralanguage   85
       Vocalizations That Alter the Quality
         of Verbal Messages   85
**Communication and the Therapeutic
Relationship**   **86**
    Communication in Selected Nursing Theories   86
       Peplau   86
       Travelbee   86
       King   86
       Orem   86
    Nurse Characteristics That Promote
       Communication   87
       Unconditional Positive Regard   87
       Empathy   87
       Authenticity and Genuineness   88
       Caring   88
       Active Listening   88
       Specific Techniques That Promote Communication   88
Using Communication for Health Promotion   **88**
    Communication and *Healthy People 2010*   88
    The Health Promotion Model
       and Communication   90
    Empowering Through Communication   91
       What to Teach   91
       How Learners Learn   91
       The Learning Environment   92
Technology and Communication   **93**
Summary   **93**

Chapter 6 Cultural Considerations

The Concept of Culture   **96**
    What Is Culture?   96
    Worldviews   97
    Particular Group   98
       Race   98

Ethnicity	99
Religion	100
Nationality	100
Labels	100
Cultural Pride	101
Cultural Competence	101
Cultural Assessment	**102**
Cultural Assessment Tools	102
Demographics/Individual Profile/Identifying Information	102
Name	103
Gender	103
Religion/Spiritual Faith	103
Race(s)	104
Ethnicity	104
Date of Birth/Age	104
Birthplace/Where Raised	104
Marital Status	104
Generation in the United States	104
Years in the United States	104
Language(s) Spoken, Primary Language, and Preferred Language	104
Education	105
Occupation	105
Cultural Domains	105
General Cultural Life Patterns or Lifestyle	105
Cultural Values, Norms, and Expressions of an Individual or Cultural Group	105
Cultural Taboos and Myths	106
Worldview and Ethnocentric Tendencies	106
Life-Caring Rituals and Rites of Passage	106
Lay, Folk, and Professional Wellness-Illness Cultural Systems	107
Specific Caring Behaviors and Health Care Values, Beliefs, and Practices	108
Cultural Diversities, Similarities, and Variations (Nonfamily)	108
Cultural Changes and Acculturation (Family)	108
Cultural Competence in a Multicultural Society	**109**
Cultural Cataloging	109
Summary	**110**

Chapter 7 Environmental Factors

Problem Identification	**112**
The EPA Model of Risk Assessment	113
The Body's Response to Environmental Influences	**113**
Acute and Chronic Exposure	114
Sources of Pollution Exposure	**114**
Air Pollution	114
Indoor Air	115
Worksite Air Quality Management	119
Outdoor Air	120

Health Promotion and Nursing Interventions for Air Quality	122
Health Promotion and Nursing Interventions for Water and Soil Quality	126
Sound Pollution	126
Health Promotion and Nursing Interventions Related to Sound	128
Light and Health	129
Health Promotion and Nursing Interventions Related to Light	129
Space and Health	130
Health Promotion and Nursing Interventions Related to Space	131
Color and Health	131
Scent and Health	132
Workplace Safety and Health	132
Feng Shui	134
Environmental Disasters	**137**
Natural Disasters	137
Earthquakes	137
Hurricanes	138
Tornadoes	138
Technological Disasters	138
Terror-Related Disasters	139
Posttraumatic Stress Disorder	140
Health Promotion and Nursing Interventions for Environmental Disasters	142
Preparation for Disasters	143
Summary	**144**

Chapter 8 The Mind-Body Connection

The Physiological Basis	**150**
The Nervous System	150
The Neuropeptides	150
The Endocrine System	151
The Immune System	152
Modulation Between the Neuroendocrine and Immune Systems	154
The Role of Stress	**154**
Psychoneuroimmunology Research	**157**
The Effect of Negative Life Stressors	158
Examination Stress	158
Bereavement	158
Chronic Stress	159
Crisis	160
The Effect of Stress on Disease	160
Depression Factors	161
Psychocutaneous Disease	161
Cancer	161
Spirituality and Psychoneuroimmunology	162
Controversies Related to PNI Research	162
Nursing Implications	**163**
Summary	**163**

SECTION III PROMOTING HEALTH THROUGHOUT THE LIFE CYCLE

Chapter 9 The Mother, Infant, and Toddler

The Mother — 171
- Biological Domain — 171
  - Preconception — 171
  - Pregnancy — 173
  - Postpartum — 176
- Psychological and Social Domains — 178
  - Preconception — 178
  - Pregnancy — 178
  - Postpartum — 179
- Political Domain — 180
  - Preconception — 180
  - Pregnancy — 181
  - Postpartum — 181
- Environmental Domain — 181
  - Preconception and Pregnancy — 181
  - Postpartum — 181
- Sexual Domain — 181
  - Preconception — 182
  - Pregnancy — 182
  - Postpartum — 182
- Spiritual Domain — 182

The Infant and Toddler — 182
- Biological Domain — 183
  - Nutrition — 183
  - Elimination — 185
  - Sleep and Activity — 186
  - Immunization — 187
  - Screening — 188
- Psychological Domain — 189
  - Cognitive Development — 189
  - Emotional Development — 189
- Social Domain — 190
  - Family — 190
  - Day Care — 191
  - Child Abuse and Neglect — 191
  - Cultural Influences — 192
- Political Domain — 192
  - WIC Program — 192
  - Safety Legislation — 192
- Environmental Domain — 193
- Sexual Domain — 193
- Spiritual Domain — 193
- **Summary** — 194

Chapter 10 The Child

The Preschool and School-Age Child — 199
- Biological Domain — 199
  - Nutrition — 200
  - Elimination — 202
  - Sleep and Activity — 203
  - Immunization — 204
  - Screening — 205
- Psychological Domain — 209
  - Attention-Deficit/Hyperactivity Disorder — 209
- Social Domain — 210
  - Relationships — 210
  - Television — 210
  - Cultural Influences — 211
- Political Domain — 211
  - Medicaid and the State Children's Health Insurance Program — 211
  - National School Lunch Program — 212
  - The Individuals with Disabilities Education Act — 212
- Environmental Domain — 212
- Sexual Domain — 212
- Spiritual Domain — 213
- **Summary** — 214

Chapter 11 The Adolescent and Young Adult

The Adolescent — 218
- Biological Domain — 218
  - Puberty — 219
  - Nutrition — 221
  - Activity — 222
  - Screening — 222
- Psychological Domain — 226
  - Cognitive Development — 226
  - Emotional Development — 227
- Social Domain — 228
  - Family — 228
  - Peers — 228
  - Abuse — 228
  - Culture — 229
- Political Domain — 229
- Environmental Domain — 230
  - Accidents — 230
  - Violence — 230
- Sexual Domain — 231
  - Adolescent Pregnancy — 232
- Spiritual Domain — 232

The Young Adult — 233
- Biological Domain — 233
  - Nutrition — 233
  - Exercise — 233
  - Skin Cancer Prevention — 234
  - Rest — 234
  - Screening — 234
- Psychological Domain — 236
  - Cognitive Development — 236
  - Emotional Development — 238
- Social Domain — 238
- Political Domain — 240
- Environmental Domain — 241
- Sexual Domain — 241
- Spiritual Domain — 242
- **Summary** — 242

Chapter 12 The Middle-Aged Adult

**Importance of Health Promotion
  in Middle Adulthood** **247**
Current Perspective of Health Promotion
  in Middle-Aged Adults 247
Demographics of Middle Adulthood 248
Middle Adulthood: A Time of Planned Change **249**
Physical Domain 249
Female Climacteric 249
Male Climacteric 251
Psychological Domain 252
Depression 252
Sociological Domain 253
Environmental Domain 253
Sexual/Gender Domain 254
Spiritual Domain 254
Culturally Competent Care **254**
**Guidelines for Health Promotion
  and Screening** **255**
**Strategies for Achieving Lifestyles
  That Promote Health** **255**
Exercise and Nutrition 255
Tobacco Avoidance 257
Immunizations 257
Sleep 258
Dental Health 258
Occupational Safety 259
**Nursing Role in Health Promotion
  and Early Detection** **259**
Educating About Risk Reduction
  and Health-Promoting Activities 259
Assessment of the Middle-Aged Adult **261**
Health Promotion Measures for Major
  Deviations from Health 261
Vision and Hearing 261
Diabetes Mellitus 263
Cancer 263
Osteoporosis 263
Summary **263**

Chapter 13 The Older Adult

Demographic Characteristics of Older Adults 268
Who Are the Older Adults? 268
Population Trends 268
Developmental Domain **270**
Developmental Tasks of Aging 270
Theories Related to Aging 271
Biological Domain **271**
Physical Assessment 271
Nutrition 273
Fitness and Exercise 275
Sleep 276
Sex 276
Socioeconomic Domain **278**
Poverty 278
Education 278
Health Care Expenditures 279

Psychological Domain **279**
Depression 279
Stress 279
Elder Abuse 279
Spiritual Domain **280**
Cultural Domain **282**
Environmental Domain **282**
Safety in Driving 282
Safety at Home 283
Medications and the Elderly 284
Safety and Assisted Living Facilities 284
Summary **288**

SECTION IV HEALTH PROMOTION STRATEGIES AND INTERVENTIONS

Chapter 14 Embracing Proper Nutrition

Importance of Nutrition in Health Promotion **294**
Healthy People Goals and Nutritional Health 297
Domains Influencing Eating Behavior **299**
Biological Domain 299
Psychological Domain 303
Sociocultural, Religious, and Spiritual Domains 304
Environmental Domain 304
Technological Domain 305
**Nutritional Excesses, Deficits, and Fads
  and Health Promotion** **305**
Overnutrition 305
Undernutrition 305
Anorexia Nervosa 306
Bulimia 306
Nutritional Fads 307
Dietary Strategies to Promote a Healthful Diet **307**
Dietary Guidelines for Americans 307
MyPyramid 309
The Exchange System: A Menu Planning Tool 311
Food Labels 311
The Five a Day Program 312
Nutritional Issues and Health
  Promotion Strategies 312
**The Nursing Process in Promoting
  Nutritional Health** **313**
Assessment 313
Nursing Diagnosis 313
Planning 313
Implementation 314
Health Promotion Model and Nutritional Status 315
Evaluation 316
Summary **316**

Chapter 15 Engaging in Physical Fitness

Exercise and Health Promotion **322**
Physical Fitness **322**
Components of Health-Related Fitness **323**
Cardiovascular Fitness 323
Muscular Strength and Endurance 324
Flexibility 324
Body Composition 324

Assessing Health-Related Fitness   **324**
Cardiovascular Fitness   325
Muscular Strength   325
Muscular Endurance   325
Assessing Flexibility   325
Assessing Body Composition   326
Starting a Fitness Training Program:
  Making That Decision   **326**
General Principles of Fitness Training   **327**
Principle of Overload   327
Principle of Specificity   327
Principle of Progression   327
Planning a Fitness Program   **328**
Frequency (F)   328
Intensity (I)   328
Time (T)   328
Type of Training (T)   328
Principles and Concepts of Cardiovascular
  Fitness   **329**
Resting Heart Rate   329
Target Heart Rate   329
A Balanced Fitness Program   **330**
Result Expectations   330
Implementation of Fitness Program: Essential
  Elements of Training   **330**
Frequent Problems Related to Exercise   **331**
Side Stitch   331
Muscle Soreness   331
Strains and Sprains   331
Warm Weather Conditions   331
Exercising in Cold Weather   332
Pollution Problems   332
RICE Concept for Injury Treatment   **332**
Myths About Exercise   **332**
Health Belief and Health Promotion Models   **333**
Utilizing the Nursing Process in Developing
  a Physical Fitness Plan   **334**
Assessments Related to Physical Activity
  and Fitness   334
Nursing Diagnosis Phase   334
Planning the Physical Fitness Program   334
Implementation   335
Evaluation   336
Getting Started and Sticking To It   **336**
Summary   **338**

Chapter 16 Controlling Weight

Consequences of Obesity   **343**
Health Promotion and Weight Control   **345**
Obstacles to Weight Control   **345**
Childhood and Adolescent Obesity   347
Domains Influencing Obesity, Weight
  Control, and Eating Behaviors   **347**
Biological Domain   347
  Theory of Thermogenesis and Weight Control   347
  Theory of Equilibrium Set-Point of Weight Control   348
  Theories of Biochemical Influences and
    Eating Behaviors   348

Environmental Domain   349
  Theories of Environmental Influences   349
Psychological Domain   350
Sociocultural Domain   350
Issues Related to Weight Control   **351**
The Nursing Process   **351**
Assessment (Acquiring Information)   352
Nursing Diagnosis   357
Planning   357
Implementation of Health Promotion Strategies
  to Help Control Weight   358
  Health Promotion Model and Weight Control   359
  Behavior, Attitude, and Weight Control   359
  Shaping and Guided Practice Weight
    Control Techniques   360
Evaluation   360
Summary   **361**

Chapter 17 Avoiding Tobacco, Alcohol, and Substance Abuse

Substance Use and Abuse   **367**
What Are Drugs?   **367**
Sources and Categories of Drugs   **367**
Prescription Drugs   368
Nonprescription Drugs   368
Psychotropic Drugs   368
Drug Mechanics: How They Work   **368**
Drug Misuse, Drug Abuse, and Addiction   **369**
Biological Basis of Addiction   370
  The Effect of Drug Withdrawal   370
Psychosocial Basis of Addiction   370
Commonly Abused Psychotropic Drugs   **371**
Opiates   371
Hallucinogens   372
Household Drugs   372
Stimulants   372
Tobacco Use and Addiction   **373**
Environmental Tobacco Smoke   373
Nicotine   374
Alcohol Use and Addiction   **375**
Why People Drink   375
Alcohol and the Central Nervous System   376
Substance Abuse Patterns   **376**
Gender   376
Age   376
  Adolescents   376
  Elderly   377
Ethnicity   377
Nurses   377
Comorbidity   378
  Mental Health Issues   378
  Physical Health Issues   378
  Spiritual Health Issues   378
Strategies for Health Promotion   **379**
Identification of Risk and Protective Factors   379
Primary Prevention   380
Secondary Prevention   380

Tertiary Prevention 380
  In Control 380
  Out of Control 381
Summary **381**

Chapter 18 Enhancing Holistic Care

What Is Holistic Care? **386**
  What Is Healing? 387
  What Is a Nurse Healer? 387
Holistic Nursing: Past, Present, and Future **388**
  The Past 388
  The Present 388
  The Future 390
The Nurse-Client Relationship **390**
  The Nurse's Attitude About Healing 390
  The Nurse's Attitude About Self 390
  Interaction Between Nurse and Client 391
Holistic Techniques for Health Promotion **392**
  The Teaching and Learning
    of Healing Techniques 392
  Using Energy as a Healing Tool 393
  The Power of Thoughts and Feelings 396
  The Breath 397
  Imagery 398
  Meditation 399
  The Power of Prayer 400
  Light and Color 400
  Sound 402
   Music 403
  Energy-Based Therapies: Therapeutic
    Touch and Healing Touch 404
  Touch Therapies—Reflexology, Massage,
    and Acupressure 404
   Reflexology 405
   Massage 405
   Acupressure 406
  Nurturing the Self 407
   Environment 407
   Sleep 408
   Exercise 408
   Communication 408
   Nutrition 408
   Herbs 408
   Aromatherapy 410
   Love and Healing 410
Summary **411**

SECTION V   HEALTH PROMOTION CONCERNS

Chapter 19 Concerns of the Health Professional

**Change and Its Impact
on the Health Professional** **419**
**Issues Impacting the Health
Care Professional** **419**
Factors Affecting the Nursing Profession **421**
  Nursing Student Characteristics 421
   Nursing Student Stress 421

Professional Nursing Supply 422
  Gender 422
  Age 423
  Ethnicity 423
  Education 424
  Impact of Managed Care on Nursing 424
Health Behavior Patterns **424**
Health Promotion Practices by Domain **426**
  Biological Domain 426
  Psychological Domain 427
  Spiritual Domain 428
  Sociocultural Domain 429
  Environmental Domain 430
  Technological Domain 431
**Nursing Process and Health
Promotion Planning** **431**
Summary **431**

Chapter 20 Economic and Quality Concerns

Factors Driving Costs Up **436**
Efforts to Control Costs **438**
  Medicare and Medicaid 438
   Access to Health Care 438
  Prospective Payment System 439
Consumer Efforts in Cost Containment **439**
Managed Care **440**
  Health Maintenance Organization 440
  Preferred Provider Organization 440
  Exclusive Provider Organization 440
  Capitation 441
Nursing's Role in Managed Care **441**
Quality Measures and Managed Care **442**
  National Committee for Quality Assurance
   (NCQA) 442
  Joint Commission (JC) 442
National Standards and Managed Care **443**
  Nursing Quality Issues 443
**Health Promotion, Health Care Cost,
and Managed Care** **444**
Summary **444**

Chapter 21 Ethical, Legal, and Political Concerns

**Ethical and Legal Issues Influencing
Nursing Care** **448**
Ethical Issues **448**
Ethical Theories **448**
Basic Principles of Ethics **449**
  Principle of Autonomy 449
  Principle of Beneficence 450
  Principle of Nonmaleficence 450
  Principle of Veracity 450
  Principle of Confidentiality 451
  Principle of Justice 451
  Principle of Fidelity 451
  Standard of Best Interest 451
  Principle of Respect for Others 452
Nursing and Ethics **452**

Ethical Decision Making and Personal Values   **452**
   Steps in Values Clarification   452
   Value Conflicts   453
Legal Issues   **453**
Law and Nursing Practice   **453**
Competency Indicators   **454**
   Licensure   454
   Multistate Licensure   455
   Credentialing   455
   Certification   455
   Accreditation   455
   Standards of Care   455
Torts, Negligence, and Breaches in Legal Duty   **456**
Right to Refuse Treatment   **457**

Student Nurse Liability   **457**
**Ethical, Legal, and Political Concerns Related
   to Health Care Cost and Access**   **457**
   Health Care Delivery and Health Care Costs   458
   Health Care Access   458
     Sociological Domain   458
     Cultural Domain   459
Ethical-Legal Concepts and Health Promotion   **459**
Nursing and Health Promotion   **459**
Summary   **461**

GLOSSARY   **465**

INDEX   **475**

Contributors

Chapter 4

Janice Welborn, MSN, RN
Director of Education and Professional Development
Hendrick Medical Center
Abilene, Texas

Chapter 5

Verolyn Barnes Bolander, MS, RN, C
Gwinnett Hospital System
Lawrenceville, Georgia

Chapter 6

M. Sandra (Sandy) Sánchez, PhD, RN
Associate Professor and Coordinator
Bachelor of Science in Nursing Program
Department of Nursing
The University of Texas–Pan American
Edinburg, Texas

Chapter 7

Ruth Tucker Marcott, PhD, RNC
Associate Dean (Retired)
School of Nursing
University of Texas Medical Branch at Galveston
Galveston, Texas

Chapter 8

Cheryl Levine, PhD, FNP-C, RN
School of Nursing
University of Texas Health Science Center–Houston
Houston, Texas

Chapters 9, 10, 11

Barbara A. Tucker, PhD, FNP, APRN-BC
Professor
Department of Nursing
The University of Texas–Pan American
Edinburg, Texas

Chapter 12

Jeanette McNeill, Dr.P.H., AOCN, ANP, RN
Professor
Department of Target Populations, Oncology Division
University of Texas Health Science Center–Houston
Houston, Texas

Chapter 13

Shannon M. Dowdall, MSN, RN
Former Lecturer
Department of Nursing
The University of Texas–Pan American
Edinburg, Texas

Karyn Taplay, MSN, RNC
Former Lecturer
Department of Nursing
The University of Texas–Pan American
Edinburg, Texas

Alma Flores-Vela, MSN, RN
Assistant Professor
Department of Nursing
The University of Texas–Pan American
Edinburg, Texas

Chapter 14

Esperanza R. Briones, PhD, RD, LD
Associate Professor and Coordinator, Retired
Coordinated Program in Dietetics
The University of Texas–Pan American
Edinburg, Texas

Chapter 15

Sue G. Mottinger, PhD
Former Associate Professor
Department of Health and Kinesiology
The University of Texas–Pan American
Edinburg, Texas

Chapter 16

Linda Eanes, EdD, RN
Former Assistant Professor
Department of Nursing
The University of Texas–Pan American
Edinburg, Texas

Chapter 17

Jane A. Newman, PhD
Former Associate Professor
Department of Rehabilitative Services
The University of Texas–Pan American
Edinburg, Texas

Debra Otto, DM, RNP
Assistant Professor
Department of Nursing
The University of Texas–Pan American
Edinburg, Texas

Chapter 18

Marsha Walker, MSN, RMT, HNC, RN
Holistic Health Consultant
Private Practice
Austin, Texas

Chapter 19

Kathie Rickman, LCDC, CARN, DrPh, RN
Psychiatric Clinical Nurse Specialist
Department of Psychiatry
UTMD Anderson
Pearland, Texas

Susan Uecker, CS, MSN, RN
Instructor of Clinical Nursing
University of Texas Health Science Center–Houston
Houston, Texas

Chapter 20

Diane Frazor, EdD, MSN, RN
Bachelor of Science in Nursing Program Director
Wayland Baptist University
San Antonio, Texas

Debra Otto, DM, RNP
Assistant Professor
Department of Nursing
The University of Texas–Pan American
Edinburg, Texas

Chapter 21

Betty Johnson, MSN, RN
Former Assistant Professor
Department of Nursing
The University of Texas–Pan American
Edinburg, Texas

Chapters 1, 3, 5, 7, 8, 13, and 18

Janice A. Maville, EdD, MSN, RN
Professor and Coordinator
Master of Science in Nursing Program
Department of Nursing
The University of Texas–Pan American
Edinburg, Texas

Chapters 2, 3, 4, 14, 15, 16, 19, and 21

Carolina G. Huerta, EdD, MSN, RN
Professor and Department Chair
Department of Nursing
The University of Texas–Pan American
Edinburg, Texas

Reviewers

Preface

The world as we know it has become increasingly chaotic. Many changes have occurred in this millennium resulting in stress and uncertainty for the world in general. The events of September 11, 2001, the wars in the Middle East, and the subsequent constant threat of terrorism have created an unsettling environment that is filled with anxiety and much trepidation. Technological advances have also contributed to the challenges faced today, especially by health care professionals who must focus on extending life while at the same time increasing the quality of life. In view of these multiple challenges, an emphasis on health promotion has become increasingly important. The shift in the delivery of health care, from the hospital to the community, from disease treatment to disease prevention and health promotion, continues. Individual responsibility and community involvement in all areas of health promotion are still essential to the health of our nation. Nurses continue to be on the forefront of this transition and are still the health care professionals best suited to meet the challenges of the health care environment.

In response to the changing needs of society, nursing education today has evolved from an emphasis solely on disease and disease prevention to a focus that includes the maintenance of health and the concept of health promotion. Nurses are taught to address specific community, family, and individual needs. An understanding of concepts related to high-level physical, social, and spiritual wellness and self-care will, without question, positively affect client care. A thorough background in the concepts of wellness and health promotion, therefore, provides an excellent introduction to beginning-level nursing theory and practice.

Health Promotion in Nursing, 2nd edition, was developed from a nursing perspective and examines all aspects of health and wellness, focusing especially on both the community and the individual. This book is designed to prepare the beginning nurse with the basic principles of health promotion found in most health promotion or wellness courses offered at the associate and baccalaureate levels. With more knowledge and information on health promotion, these nurses will be able to successfully confront and manage the challenges of health promotion. To this end, this newly revised edition includes real-life case studies that encourage readers to apply and synthesize the knowledge gleaned from the chapters.

In today's world, a nurse must have an appreciation of the diverse nature of individuals, groups, and differing health practices. Accordingly, *Health Promotion in Nursing*, 2nd edition, places special emphasis on holistic health promotion and the cultural variations inherent in health care. The nurse will also be more effective with others when there is a commitment to incorporate the principles of health promotion into her or his own lifestyle. Several resources as well as opportunities for self-examination and self-reflection are, therefore, included.

ORGANIZATION

Health Promotion in Nursing, 2nd edition, comprises five sections broken down into 21 chapters.

Section I: Conceptual Foundations and Theoretical Approaches

Chapter 1 Health Promotion: Past, Present, and Future

This chapter provides the reader with an introduction to the concept of health promotion and factors influencing its emergence in the United States. Various definitions are examined along with social, economic, environmental, and political forces leading to the dramatic impact of health promotion on contemporary society. The concepts of health promotion and illness prevention are differentiated. *Healthy People 2010* initiatives and leading health indicators are strongly emphasized. The impact of terrorism is introduced.

Chapter 2 Nursing Concepts and Health Promotion

This chapter introduces concepts essential in defining the metaparadigm of nursing practice. Theoretical frameworks as underpinnings of the profession of nursing are included. Nursing educational levels and their relationship to health promotion are discussed. Assumptions basic to the integration of health promotion in nursing practice are emphasized.

Chapter 3 Theoretical Foundations of Health Promotion

This chapter discusses theoretical foundations and planning strategies related to health promotion. Major definitions of health are presented. Numerous theoretical models related to health promotion are detailed, including the Theory of Planned Behavior, Theory of Social Behavior, Protection Motivation Theory, Health Belief Model, Transtheoretical Model of Behavioral Change, Consumer Information Processing Model, Diffusion of Innovations Model, PRECEDE-PROCEED Model, Pender Health Promotion Model, O'Donnell the Model of Health Promotion Behavior. The importance of self-responsibility in health promotion is examined in relation to theoretical concepts of human behavior. Guidelines to develop a health promotion plan are introduced.

Chapter 4 The Role of the Nurse in Health Promotion

This chapter describes the important role of the nurse in health promotion for the individual, family, and community. Domains fundamental to nursing practice in health promotion are described, including a new domain, technology. A collaborative, multidisciplinary approach for client empowerment is discussed. The application of the nursing process in health promotion is specifically addressed. Several classification systems used to support clinical decision making are included. Emphasis is placed on the holistic perspective of nursing practice in health promotion. Nursing diagnoses for health promotion are described and illustrated.

Section II: Factors Influencing Health Promotion

Chapter 5 Communication

This chapter explores the basic concepts of communication and provides an overview of the various models of communication. Topics include types of communication, specific communication techniques, barriers to communication, and the development of a therapeutic relationship to promote health. The influence of technology on communication is addressed. Coverage of the principles and strategies of teaching and learning is included.

Chapter 6 Cultural Considerations

This chapter focuses on the importance of cultural sensitivity in the promotion of health among various cultural groups. Cultural concepts are explained. Cultural competence, cultural awareness, and cultural sensitivity are differentiated. Specific ways of culturally advocating for clients are identified. Instruction on how to do a cultural assessment on self and others is included. Numerous opportunities for critical thinking and self-analysis are presented.

Chapter 7 Environmental Factors

This chapter examines the impact of environmental changes on health, how to prepare for them, and how to respond to them when they do occur. A discussion of global issues related to the environment was been added. Natural disasters, air, water, noise, and waste result in a change in the health of individuals and communities. In addition, readers will be given the opportunity to assess their home and work environments. Terror-related disasters and disaster planning are now specifically addressed.

Chapter 8 The Mind-Body Connection

Psychoneuroimmunology has emerged as a field of science providing increasing evidence of the interrelatedness of psychological, neurological, hormonal, and immunological functions and their connections to health and well-being. This chapter provides an analysis of this concept and describes not only the what but the why of these interrelationships. The controversial nature of psychoneuroimmunology is presented. The link between spirituality/religion and health-related physiological processes is addressed. An emphasis is placed on the effect of stress on the neurological, endocrine, and immune systems.

Section III: Promoting Health Throughout the Life Cycle

Chapter 9 The Mother, Infant, and Toddler

Health promotion is an important aspect in the care of expectant mothers, infants, and toddlers. This new chapter offers a wealth of information that addresses health promotion needs of women, beginning with preconception through pregnancy and postpartum. Special content is devoted to domestic violence and postpartum depression. By detecting health problems early in infants and toddlers, health status can be improved and future problems prevented. Screenings, immunizations, and health promotion risk assessments for infants and toddlers provide a comprehensive look at these age groups.

Chapter 10 The Child

In addition to numerous health screenings for children, regular physical exams and the importance of health education in schools and community centers are emphasized. The importance of immunization against various diseases is presented. Programs for young children and school-age children that focus only on the negative outcomes of unhealthy behavior, but also programs that teach values, build self-esteem, and promote healthy lifestyles are addressed. New coverage of the growing health threat of obesity in childhood and detection of acanthosis nigricans, the pre-diabetes marker, is included.

Chapter 11 The Adolescent and Young Adult

Adolescents and young adults are becoming increasingly interested in health promotion. This chapter focuses on specific topics such as pregnancy, teen pregnancy, smoking cessation, and drug rehabilitation. Information on the role of the nurse in promoting health in the adolescent and the young adult is presented. A health risk assessment tool has been added.

Chapter 12 The Middle-Aged Adult

The middle-aged adult is particularly receptive to the development of health promotion lifestyles. Topics such as general wellness, exercise, identification of personal risk factors, and education on chronic illness are addressed. The role of the nurse in promoting health in the middle-aged adult is presented.

Chapter 13 The Older Adult

Health promotion is an important part of the role of the nurse caring for the older adult. Studies indicate that the elderly are health-conscious and eager to adopt practices that will improve their health. Activities that enable the older adult with chronic illness or disability or both to reach an optimum level of function are given. Physical fitness, nutrition, safety, and stress management are included. A new discussion has been added on health promotion in various settings, such as assisted living, home care, rehab facilities, long-term care, and nursing homes.

Section IV: Health Promotion Strategies and Interventions

Chapter 14 Embracing Proper Nutrition

This chapter presents the concepts of nutrition and the role nutrition plays in maintaining health. The important role of nutrients such as fats, carbohydrates, proteins, and vitamins and minerals is discussed. General guidelines to meet daily nutrient needs are presented, along with charts and tables to depict nutrient needs and food sources. MyPyramid, which has replaced the Food Guide Pyramid, is described. Issues and health promotion strategies related to nutrition are discussed. The importance of cultural sensitivity in nutritional health is emphasized.

Chapter 15 Engaging in Physical Fitness

Physical fitness is an important aspect of health promotion. This chapter examines the relationship between physical fitness and health, benefits of exercise, types of exercise, and the nurse's role in promoting health

through physical fitness. Practical problems related to exercise are now discussed, along with practical tips for increasing activity and incorporating cultural sensitivity into care.

Chapter 16 Controlling Weight

The importance of weight control, theories of obesity, basic principles of weight control, and obstacles encountered in maintaining weight are presented. Recognition of dietary fads and their impact on weight control are newly included. Weight control strategies that incorporate cultural sensitivity and awareness have been added, along with suggestions to overcome obstacles encountered and the role of the nurse in promoting weight control.

Chapter 17 Avoiding Tobacco, Alcohol, and Substance Abuse

This chapter presents an overview of the health risks associated with the use, abuse, and/or addiction to tobacco, alcohol, and other drugs. A discussion of drug effects and the basis of addiction is presented. Identification of risk and protective factors for individuals at risk for substance abuse has been added. The nurse's role in primary, secondary, and tertiary prevention strategies is addressed. A section discussing the nurse with a substance abuse problem is also included.

Chapter 18 Enhancing Holistic Care

Facilitating others in the promotion of their own well-being is essential for nurses involved in supporting the health of individuals, families, and aggregates. This chapter now offers enhanced coverage of complementary and alternative medicine (CAM) and holistic techniques that nurses can incorporate when teaching clients self-care for health promotion. Included in this chapter are breathing and relaxation techniques, pressure and touch therapy, imagery and visualization, music therapy, aromatherapy, meditation, prayer, and other approaches. The effect of light, color, and sound on health is also addressed. Benefits, risks, and cautions for commonly used herbs and essential oils are detailed.

Section V: Health Promotion Concerns

Chapter 19 Concerns of the Health Professional

Those who have chosen careers in the health professions often neglect their own health. This chapter addresses the deleterious effects of such neglect, including physical and psychological illness, burnout, and dropout from educational programs or from the profession. Technology as a source of stress for nurses and other health care professionals is now discussed. Practical strategies for enhancing health are provided for professionals and students.

Chapter 20 Economic and Quality Concerns

Advances in medical technology as well as increased life span have led to the escalation of health care costs. Policies made in the political arena dictate financing of health care by the national and state governments. This chapter includes a new focus on how health promotion and health care costs relate to economic as well as quality issues. The importance of healthy lifestyle practices through health promotion as a means of controlling expenditures is discussed. The American Nurses Association Standards of Care are discussed in terms of safeguarding the quality of care delivered to clients.

Chapter 21 Ethical, Legal, and Political Concerns

Basic principles of ethics will be identified. Students can examine ethical issues pertaining to health care costs, access to health care, and rationing of health care. The involvement by federal and state governments in health care delivery is presented. A new discussion on HIPAA as a national framework for security standards and protection of client confidentiality is included.

OUTSTANDING FEATURES

Several key pedagogical features in *Health Promotion in Nursing,* 2nd edition, make the text user-friendly and draw readers' attention to some of the most critical points that will help them grow in their practice.

Features

- **Nursing Alert:** Highlight serious or life-threatening signs or critical information that needs immediate attention.

- **Research Note:** Emphasize relevant research on a particular issue. This helps readers understand the importance of grounding their practice in evidence-based research.

- **Spotlight On:** Introduce ethical controversies and clinical situations readers are likely to encounter, stimulating critical thinking.

- **Ask Yourself:** Encourage readers to examine their own views on a variety of issues so they may better understand the varying opinions they may soon encounter. These boxes encourage reflection on issues in a personal context and raise awareness.

- **Student Activities:** Stimulating activities for readers to do individually or in groups to enhance content presented in each chapter. Learning Activities, Multiple Choice questions, and True/False questions are included in every chapter for review of information and for self-assessment.

- **Case Studies (newly added to Chapters 8 through 19):** Provide students with the opportunity for critical thinking by featuring a real-life situation that focuses on health promotion issues according to domains.

Support Materials

A new online companion with varying tools and activities supports *Health Promotion in Nursing*, 2nd edition. These resources, complimentary to adopters to the text, support the reader and instructor by offering answers to the Case Studies, Learning Activities, Multiple Choice questions, and True/False questions from the book. Also included on the online companion are PowerPoint slides, a testbank of approximately 650 questions, HIPAA information, and other tools to assist readers in mastering the text content.

SECTION I

CONCEPTUAL FOUNDATIONS AND THEORETICAL APPROACHES

CHAPTER 1

Health Promotion: Past, Present, and Future

CHAPTER 2

Nursing Concepts and Health Promotion

CHAPTER 3

Theoretical Foundations of Health Promotion

CHAPTER 4

The Role of the Nurse in Health Promotion

Chapter 1

HEALTH PROMOTION: PAST, PRESENT, AND FUTURE

Janice A. Maville, EdD, MSN, RN

KEY TERMS

Code of Hammurabi
epidemiology
health education
health promotion

Healthy People 2000
Healthy People 2010
LaLonde Report
Medicaid program

Medicare program
Mosaic Code
Nursing: A Social
   Policy Statement

Social Security Act
yang
yin

OBJECTIVES

Upon completion of this chapter, the reader should be able to:

- Differentiate between health education and health promotion.

- Trace the evolution of health promotion practices and developments from ancient history to the modern-day world.

- Discuss three major movements contributing to the social mandate for health promotion in the nineteenth century.

- Relate scientific, social, economic, environmental, and political forces of the twentieth century contributing to the evolution of health promotion in the United States.

- Describe national, international, and world efforts for health promotion.

- Describe changes in contemporary nursing practice and policy resulting from health care reform.

- Examine the future of nursing in health promotion.

INTRODUCTION

Over the past two decades the explosion of interest and participation in health promotion and wellness activities has resulted in an evolution in health care. Scientific findings, enthusiastic support from health care providers, and strong initiatives for disease prevention and health promotion at local, state, national, and global levels have fueled this evolution. Global and national mandates for promoting health have catapulted health promotion activities to a high level of importance in the health care community and have caught the attention of many policy makers all over the world. Some health care programs focus exclusively on health promotion activities, and there is much hope for health promotion legislation. In the new millennium, collaborative and cooperative efforts for health promotion among individuals, families, communities, health professionals, and government agencies will have dramatic effects upon the health of the United States and of the world.

Nurses have a rich history of practice and advocacy for health promotion. A knowledge of the heritage of health promotion is important to understand its powerful relationship to nursing. This chapter will define health promotion and differentiate this concept from health education. The history of health promotion practices and sociopolitical developments will be explored and related to a vision and a mission for nurses in the emerging collaborative practice paradigm of the future.

DEFINING HEALTH PROMOTION

Nations unite for it, programs are built on it, health professionals prescribe for it, and individuals either practice it or not. Yet, a universally accepted definition of health promotion does not exist. In fact, health promotion is often confused with or used synonymously with health education. The confusion is the result of a change in the way of thinking about, or paradigm shift in, the concept of health (refer to Chapter 2) which has undergone dramatic changes through the decades.

Not having a precise definition for health promotion may not be necessarily bad, though, as it allows for fluidity, flexibility, and diversity. It is important, however, to review pertinent definitions, to highlight the definition guiding this textbook, and to differentiate health promotion from health education. Other related concepts and theories will be explored in greater detail in Chapter 3.

Health Education

The practice of **health education** is a tool or mechanism for health-related learning resulting in increased knowledge, skill development, and change in behavior. Health education, then, is directed toward changing behavior toward preset goals.

Health education can be expanded to include the society in which the individual functions. Knowledge gained to empower individuals and to promote change in the environment, economy, and society for better health is essential for health promotion. In this sense, health education is not the same as, but is part of, the larger concept of health promotion.

Health Promotion

In 1986 the World Health Organization sponsored the first International Conference on Health Promotion in which the Ottawa Charter was developed and adopted by 38 countries, with the object to "achieve Health for All by the Year 2000 and beyond" (Anonymous, 1986; Nutbeam, 1996). Health promotion, as presented in the Ottawa Charter, included enabling people to live healthy lifestyles by building healthy public policy, creating supportive environments, strengthening community action, developing personal skills, and reorienting health services. Furthering these objectives, the United States created *Healthy People 2000,* followed by *Healthy People 2010,* to provide a type of national road map to health for all Americans (U.S. Dept. of Health and Human Services, 2000; U.S. Public Health Service, 1990). Since 1986, health promotion has been described as a theme, an activity, a process, a principle, a strategy, a discipline, a philosophy, an art, and a science. It is no wonder that it has been difficult to arrive at a consensus for a definition.

Although a contextual analysis of the myriad of health promotion definitions is beyond the scope of this chapter, there are four major themes that provide for some unity. These themes relate to *empowerment, lifestyles, health enhancement,* and *well-being.* Imbedded in these themes are issues of ethics, values, personal choice, responsibility, and potential. The definition guiding this textbook encompasses these themes and issues. Basically, **health promotion** is any endeavor directed at enhancing the quality of health and well-being of individuals, families, groups, communities, and/or nations through strategies involving supportive environments, coordination of resources, and respect for personal choice and values. Related concepts, including health education, health protection, and disease prevention, are part of the broader concept of health promotion. The definition that an individual or organization adopts depends upon political, societal, and philosophical viewpoints.

The term "health promotion" was introduced in 1974 by Canadian Health Minister LaLonde (Macdonald & Bunton, 1992) and was not popular until the 1980s

when the World Health Organization began a campaign for global public health. Prior to that, efforts to improve health centered on education.

HEALTH PROMOTION: PAST

An understanding of basic terminology is not enough to fully appreciate health promotion. A knowledge of how health promotion has evolved over time and has been influenced by various cultures and scientific advances helps to gain further perspective. The following sections provide a review of contributions to promoting health from ancient cultures through modern societies.

Ancient Times

As humankind has evolved, so has the practice of promoting health. Earliest attempts at promoting health might be described in terms of basic survival and avoidance of hazardous situations. Over time, connections were made between illness and causation of the illness. Since early humans knew little about the functioning of the body, the causes both of illness and of healing were thought to be magical or part of the supernatural. In some ancient cultures, holes were bored into the heads of diseased individuals to release the evil spirits deemed responsible. This surgical procedure, referred to as trephining, was performed thousand of years ago. This example of combining belief in magic or religion with the use of medical technique suggests a dual or double nature of medical care at a primitive stage. Such dualism can be found in cultures throughout time, and some still exists. In other words, the knowledge of health and health technology of a society, at whatever level, is interwoven with the values, attitudes, and beliefs of the people that make up that society.

Today, society comprises many different cultures whose beliefs unite with, and sometimes conflict with, modern professional health care practice. A contemporary example of the unity of belief and health care can be seen in the practice of drinking herbal teas. Previously thought to be part of folk or cultural beliefs, the benefits of many herbal teas have been confirmed, accepted, and recommended by professional health care providers.

A closer look at major ancient cultures reflects the varied levels of sophistication of health promotion and health care practices as well as their particular values, attitudes, and beliefs. The contributions of the ancient people of Babylonia (Iraq), Greece, Egypt, Rome, and China are significant to our understanding of the rich foundation in which health promotion is rooted.

Babylonia

Although evidence of medical records was discovered in Egypt around 3000 BC (Ellis & Hartley, 2004), the earliest written reference to health is attributed to King Hammurabi of Babylonia (now Iraq), approximately 2000 BC (Clark, 2003). This written reference was called the *Code of Hammurabi,* and it established standards and practices of living for Babylonians. Hammurabi claimed that the gods had instructed him to write these early legal statutes or laws for justice in the land and to uphold the weak so that they may not be oppressed by the strong (*Babylonia,* n.d.).

The regulations or laws in the *Code of Hammurabi* were based on promoting fairness and equality. A portion of this code regulated specific health practices and the conduct of physicians. With an "eye for an eye" premise, some of the regulations seem drastic compared to present day standards. For example, if a surgeon operated on a member of the wealthy upper class and saved the patient's life, the surgeon would be paid ten coins of silver for that service. If the same service was provided for a common person, the surgeon would be given five coins. If the patient was a slave, the surgeon would get two coins of silver. If the doctor made an error in performing the surgery and the patient died, then the surgeon's hand could be cut off (Babylonia, n.d.).

Although the promotion of health was not a primary focus of this document, the laws that were recorded support the understanding that health has always been broadly defined and that the community and individuals have shared responsibilities for health.

Greece

The early Greeks are known for their practice of worshiping gods and goddesses, all of whom were strong, beautiful, and powerful. Apollo was known as the god

of health while his son, Asclepius, was the god of healing. Hygeia, daughter of Asclepius, was the goddess of health, and another daughter, Panacea, was the restorer of health (Stanhope & Lancaster, 2004). In deifying these two goddesses, the Greeks signified their strong belief in keeping healthy. Striving to be more like the mythological gods they worshiped, the Greeks focused on health with an emphasis on personal health and hygiene, exercise, and healthy diets.

Some find it surprising that Hippocrates, the Father of Medicine, came from a culture holding such strong beliefs in mythology and the power of gods. It was Hippocrates, born around 400 BC, who emphasized a natural cause for disease and initiated the scientific method for solving patient problems. He identified the importance of incorporating social, environmental, mental, and physical factors in treating the patient as a whole person (Guisepi, 2001). Hippocrates believed health to be dependent upon equilibrium among the mind, body, and environment rather than the whim of the gods. This belief, known as the holistic approach in health care practice today, continues to guide the practice of health care professionals and is a key element in understanding the concept of health promotion.

Egypt

Ancient Egyptians, around 3000 BC, contributed significantly to health through progress made in disease prevention. The Egyptians are especially known for their efforts in developing practices for hygiene and water sanitation. As citizens of one of the healthiest of ancient cultures, Egyptians developed a sophisticated system to supply pure water and dispose of wastes. They developed stringent regulations related to cleanliness, food, drink, exercise, and sexual relations (Ellis & Hartley, 2004).

Palestine

The Hebrews of Palestine, located next to Egypt, also provided evidence of concern for promoting health. Their greatest contribution was the creation of the **Mosaic Code,** about 1500 BC, reflected in the Old Testament. Developed under the leadership of Moses, the Code contained an organized system for disease prevention (Clark, 2003). The Mosaic Code differentiated clean from unclean and emphasized the segregation of those with communicable diseases. This principle of quarantine was to be of great importance in later history when populations of Europe were besieged with plagues of disease.

Rome

Ancient Romans, unlike the Egyptians, Greeks, and Palestinians, lacked originality for health promotion and disease prevention practices. Medical practices of the Romans were obtained from their conquered regions, and physicians from these countries became slaves to the Roman Empire (Stanhope & Lancaster, 2004). Nonetheless, in a manner similar to the Egyptians, Roman accomplishments were mostly directed at public health with the establishment of regulations for sanitation, street cleaning, building construction, ventilation, and heating among others (Clark, 2003).

From about 500 BC to AD 500, health promotion practices of the ancient Romans, which included exercise, massage, and therapeutic baths, were more geared to those seeking luxury and personal indulgence than to the promotion of health. Elaborate bathhouses were built where the practices of therapeutic baths and massage were perfected.

Another similarity between the Greeks and Romans can be seen in their philosophies regarding health and illness. The Greek physician Hippocrates and the Roman physician Galen both viewed health as an interaction between a person and his or her environment. It is Galen who is credited with formulating the beginnings of a definition of health that emphasized the ability of an individual to carry out the functions of daily life without hindrance or pain (Moore & Williamson, 1984).

China

The Chinese were perhaps the greatest advocates for health promotion of all ancient cultures. They viewed a healthy life as one that stayed in harmony with the uni-

verse by maintaining a perfect balance between the dualistic forces of yin and yang (Bright, 2002). **Yin** was viewed as the female element associated with negative energy, passiveness, destruction, the moon, darkness, and death. **Yang** was viewed as the male element associated with positive energy, action, generativity, the sun, light, and the creativity of life. Maintenance of this balance resulted in perfect health of the mind, body, and spirit. From the earliest records in 1400 BC, the ancient Chinese philosophy of yin and yang has lasted throughout the centuries and remains integral to concepts of health and health promotion practices not only for the Chinese but for people in many other cultures throughout the modern world.

The Middle Ages, Renaissance, and Early America

Religious beliefs formed the basis for health concepts and practices in early civilizations and continue to have great influence in the modern world. Over time, technology evolved within cultures and had great impact on the development and practice of health promotion. Coinciding with evolving technology was the development of the field of study known as **epidemiology**, which examines the relationships among disease, the environment, the individual, and the community. Epidemiology has been defined in many ways, but it is basically concerned with the time, place, and person components of disease, defect, disability, or death (Timmreck, 2002). Epidemiology specifically studies when disease occurs, how it is distributed in a population, the cause of the disease, the natural history or course of a disease, and factors influencing health promotion and protection. Table 1-1 shows how disease and life expectancy have changed over the last 600 years.

Health Promotion in the Middle Ages (AD 500–1500)

After the fall of Rome, during the period known as the Dark Ages, much of what was known about the health and medicine of ancient worlds was lost (Cockerham, 1978). The Roman Catholic Church claimed authority for

TABLE 1-1 Causes of Death, 1300 to Present

Epoch 1 1300–1800	Age of pestilence	Endemic diseases, chronic undernutrition and malnutrition, periodic epidemics of infectious diseases (bubonic plague, smallpox, measles, malaria, typhus, typhoid, etc.), and famine	Life expectancy of 20 years
Epoch 2 1800–1900	Age of declining pandemics	Declining epidemics, increase in endemic infectious diseases (tuberculosis, pneumonia, enteritis)	Life expectancy of 40–47.3 years
Epoch 3 1900–Present	Age of degeneration and manmade diseases	Shift from infectious to chronic diseases (heart disease, cancer, stroke, injuries)	Life expectancy in 1900 of 47.3 years and in 2002 of 79.9 years for women and 74.5 years for men

Sources: McLeroy, K. R., & Crump, C. E. (1994). Health promotion and disease prevention: A historical perspective. Generations, 18(1), 9–17; Kramarow, E., Lentzner, H., Rooks, R., Weeks, J., & Saydah, S. (1999). Health and aging chartbook (Library of Congress Catalog No. 76–641496, p. 30), Washington, DC: U.S. Government Printing Office; and Arias, E. (2004). United States life tables, 2002. National Vital Statistics Reports, 53(6), Hyattsville, MD: National Center for Health Statistics.

the welfare of society, and purity of the soul became the highest of priorities. Caring for the body, such as daily bathing and exercise, was viewed as a sinful indulgence resulting in neglect of the soul. Illness and death were associated with famine and infectious disease epidemics.

For nearly 1,000 years (AD 500–1500), after the Dark Ages shifted into the Middle Ages, very little was accomplished to promote health or to treat illnesses. It was not until the Crusades that a heightened sense of responsibility for health emerged when healthy warriors were needed to fight in religious wars (Clark, 2003). Although the emphasis on health by early Christians was on treating disease and illness, they did much to increase the public's awareness of health. This was mainly accomplished with the development of the concept of quarantine in response to repeated epidemics of the bubonic plague during the latter part of the Middle Ages.

The Renaissance and Early America (AD 1500–1800)

The European Renaissance (1500–1700) brought about the return to scientific thought with attempts to understand and control life. This changed the holistic view of health and illness held by followers of Hippocrates to a disintegrated view maintaining that the body was separate from the mind.

Interestingly, a return to social consciousness emerged during this time in which the responsibility of society for public health and welfare was at least recognized. Even so, most efforts related to health were directed to the improvement of medical technology. Other than that, little effort was made directly to the promotion of health in this relatively short span of time.

It was during the European Renaissance that colonies in America were being established. Compared to crowded European cities, the colonies were sparsely populated and remained isolated from one another for many years. Thus, early colonial health was good compared to that of the crowded Europeans, and the problems with communicable disease were minimal (Clark, 2003). In many respects health promotion in colonial days was like that in ancient times: it was based on successful survival against the elements of nature.

The Industrial Revolution in the United States marked the transition of the country's economic foundation from agriculture to industry. With this transition came the arrival of poor immigrants, shifting the population from rural to urban settings and resulting in inadequate living and working conditions. General public health declined and death from preventable diseases increased, especially among the children. In response to the health impact of low social and economic conditions, social policy on health began to take form.

The Social Mandate for Health Promotion

The social problems that began to flourish in the aftermath of the Industrial Revolution generated great interest in disease prevention, epidemiology, and community health. Three major movements in the late 1800s throughout Western Europe and America began to shape a social mandate for health promotion (Novak, 1988). These movements included the developing consciousness of the people, the changes occurring in medicine, and the development of nursing as a profession.

The social mandate for health promotion gained a strong foundation through these three major movements.

Ask Yourself

The Evolution of Health Technology

How has your own health been affected by discoveries made over 100 years ago? What recent discoveries do you know about that have advanced health care even farther? Compare the state of health technology of underdeveloped countries to that of the United States and other developed countries. How do they differ? What accounts for the differences?

Ask Yourself

The Wellness-Illness Continuum

Florence Nightingale believed that "the same laws of health" govern sickness and wellness. What does this mean to you? Do you feel this represents your belief about wellness and illness?

Not only was social consciousness raised for the prevention of disease and protection of health, but also the eyes of society were opened to the crucial role of nurses in what was the beginning of progressive health reform.

The First Movement

The first of the three major movements in the social mandate for promoting health was a greater sense of consciousness and reform from the wealthy of society. It was this segment of the population that aimed to ease problems associated with poverty, substandard housing, child labor, poor prison conditions, and undereducation of the general public.

A major contribution to this heightened consciousness in the United States can be attributed to the efforts of a man named Lemuel Shattuck. A former teacher and book salesman, Shattuck worked for the passage of a law in Massachusetts establishing statewide regulation of vital statistics (Novak, 1988). Shortly thereafter in 1845, he published a census report of the city of Boston containing surprisingly high infant and maternity mortality rates. Recommendations in the report were made for organizing local and state boards of health, conducting surveys on sanitation, and educating nurses. Nearly ignored, the report recommendations were not implemented for almost 20 years. Even so, the Shattuck Report is renowned as one of the first public health documents in the United States and earned Lemuel Shattuck the title of Father of Public Health.

The Second Movement

The attack on public health problems by the population prompted the second major movement for health promotion. The American Medical Association, founded in 1847, began responding to public pressure for disease prevention. As a result, medicine began shifting from an exclusive focus on disease cure to disease prevention. Consequently, changes in the structure and function of the medical community began to take form.

Also of major importance during this time was new knowledge of the nature of infection and major discoveries which changed medical practice and education for-

ever. For example, Louis Pasteur (1822–1895) discovered that heat killed bacteria; Joseph Lister (1827–1912) applied pasteurization and disinfection methodologies for surgical procedures; Robert Koch (1843–1910), a German physician, made the connection between specific organisms and specific infections; William Röentgen (1845–1923), also German, discovered x-rays; and Pierre Curie (1859–1906) and his wife Marie Curie (1867–1934) discovered radium in 1898 (Kelly & Joel, 2002; Stanhope & Lancaster, 2004).

The Third Movement

Although the practice of nursing has traditionally functioned in a framework of health promotion, the third movement, evolution of the practice of nursing into a profession, can be largely attributed to the accomplishments of Florence Nightingale. It was during the Crimean War in Europe in the late 1850s when Florence Nightingale implemented her philosophy of nursing that included care for the well and the sick and numerous improvements in health care of the military. She forged improvements in housing, sanitation, nutrition, physical fitness, and recreation for the military. As a result of these efforts, in only six months, the death rate in the military hospitals was reduced from 42 percent to 2.2 percent (Novak, 1988).

Nightingale's belief in health as a wellness-illness continuum is evident in her *Notes on Nursing*, originally published in 1859, in which she wrote that "the same laws of health or of nursing, for they are in reality the same, obtain among the well as among the sick" (Nightingale, 1859/1969, p. 10). She further wrote that the breaking of these laws "produces only a less violent consequence among the former than among the latter,—and this sometimes, not always" (Nightingale, 1859/1969, p. 10). She referred to disease as a "reparative process" of nature that resulted from lack of knowledge or attention (Nightingale, 1859/1969, p. 8). Education of clients and families, in her point of view, was a major responsibility of nurses and not limited to physicians only.

The works and deeds of Florence Nightingale spread to the United States in the early 1860s, greatly influencing nursing care during the Civil War years, and they continue to affect nursing education and practice in the modern world.

SOCIOPOLITICAL INFLUENCES FOR HEALTH PROMOTION IN THE TWENTIETH CENTURY

Scientific and sociopolitical events beginning in the twentieth century combined to become powerful determinants for reforming health care and stimulating political intervention. The epidemiology of disease shifted as hygienic and living conditions began to improve, antibiotics became routine for fighting infections, and scientific advancements were made in combating chronic illness. As a result, the morbidity from infectious diseases decreased and the life expectancy of those with chronic illnesses increased.

Also occurring at the turn of the century was the enormous national and personal economic growth resulting from industrialization. In turn, great population shifts took place with people leaving their rural lives for the promise of economic splendor in urban areas. This same hope for a better life attracted thousands of immigrants, especially from Europe.

The combined effects of rapid and uncontrolled industrialization, urbanization, and immigration resulted in congestion, poverty, malnutrition, and disease and set the stage for renewed interest in promoting health. With this heavy health care burden, innovations in health care and mechanisms for government intervention were set into motion to reform the way in which health care was provided, in order to improve the health of all Americans.

Health Reform

An early contribution to reforming health care was a nurse-inspired innovation that resulted in the establishment of public health nursing and the endorsement of health promotion by insurance companies. By the turn of the century, Lillian Wald had led the way for visiting nurses in New York City to incorporate health promotion in the form of education as they provided care at the Henry Street Settlement, treated children in public schools, visited sick workers in their homes, and treated the ill in rural areas. By enlisting the services of the nurses of the Henry Street Settlement, the Metropolitan Life Insurance Company was the first insurance company known to attempt to control costs by promoting the health of its policyholders (Novak, 1988).

The progressive movement of nursing and health reform toward health promotion in the United States was altered by involvement in World War I and again in World War II. The medical model of disease treatment gained re-emphasis during both wars with the finding that large percentages of military recruits were not fit for duty because of infectious diseases such as tuberculosis, typhoid fever, and gonorrhea. However, nurses during and after World War II made some progress toward health promotion when the role of the nurse was expanded to include caring for military families and veterans.

Federal Government Involvement in Health Care

The concept that healthy mothers produced healthy children who become healthy adults spawned maternal and infant care programs throughout the 1920s and 1930s. Additionally, the increasing shift in illness from infectious diseases to chronic diseases was also becoming apparent during this period. As a result, the involvement of the U.S. government in health issues increased with the enactment of legislation and establishment of agencies designed for improvement of the health of the nation's people. For example, Congress enacted the Sheppard-Towner Act of 1921 that funded maternal and child health services in 45 states (Novak, 1988). This legislation provided for access to entire families resulting in increased health education programs, management of individual cases, and decreased infant mortality rates.

The hardships imposed by the stock market crash of 1929 resulted in even more federal government intervention for the basic necessities of life for much of the population. As part of Roosevelt's New Deal, help was made available through federal relief programs and government legislation. The most significant legislation was the **Social Security Act** of 1935. This legislation provided an immediate boost to the American family with public aid, social services, and aid to the elderly. The Social Security Act is significant not only because it provided immediate help for the American people but also because it marked the emergence of the federal government as a dominant force in health care delivery and health care finance.

Following World War II, major advances in medical technology and disease control approached the miraculous. New drugs, diagnostic methods, and treatment regimes in the 1940s and 1950s heralded a new era in medical care, resulting in the saving of millions of lives, and forever altered the practice of medicine and nursing. Penicillin and other antibiotics, limited to the military during the war, became available to the public; sulfanilamide was proven effective for fighting infections; antihistamines were discovered; cortisone was synthesized; anticoagulants were developed; psychotherapy advances were made; polio vaccines were developed; the diagnosis and treatment of heart disease and heart failure were dramatically improved; and surgical techniques, including open heart surgery, were becoming more sophisticated (Kelly & Joel, 2002; Jonas & Kovner, 2002). The boundaries for life itself were literally expanded. It is no wonder that the American public became enamored with medicine, doctors, and hospitals.

It is no surprise that the wondrous advances in medicine and health care came with a higher price tag. Hospitals began charging higher rates for services, and health insurance companies charged higher premiums for their policies. These costs were compounded by the fact that physicians' office visits were sparsely reimbursed, if at all, which led to increased admissions to hospitals and increased orders for diagnostic testing by physicians.

Unfortunately, inherent in such a system is the potential for fraud with unnecessary admissions and diagnostic testing. It is easy to see how those who could afford insurance had access to care while the underinsured, poor, elderly, and chronically ill had great difficulties.

Medicaid and Medicare

Coming to the rescue of those having difficulties with access to health care were Medicare and Medicaid, 1965 amendments to the Social Security Act, and their subsequent amendments. Not only did these amendments facilitate access to health care for the disadvantaged, but they also attested to the increasing magnitude of the federal government's involvement in financing health care costs. Refer to Chapter 20 for more detailed information on health care costs.

The **Medicare program** was designed to provide hospital insurance and supplement medical insurance for people over age 65, people with disabilities who receive Social Security benefits, and clients in end-stage renal disease. The **Medicaid program** was designed to provide a share of payments made by state welfare to health care agencies caring for the poor, medically needy, aged, disabled, and their dependent children and families (Hoffman, Klees & Curtis, 2006). Once the federal government began paying for services, health care costs began to soar. Enrollments and usage by participants spiraled upward along with greed and fraud by providers. Additionally, the public began to consider health care as a basic right. Figure 1-1 shows the spiraling health care expenditures in the United States between the years 1960 and 2004. The table shows health care expenditures as an ever-increasing share of U.S. gross domestic product

(GDP), the government's primary measure of economic activity. Expenditures in the United States on health care were nearly $1.9 trillion in 2004, more than two and a half times the $717 billion spent in 1990, and more than seven times the $255 billion spent in 1980. The approximately $1.9 trillion in national healthcare expenditures in 2004 represents 16.0 percent of the gross domestic product, three times that in 1960 (CMS, 2006).

GOVERNMENT INITIATIVES FOR HEALTH PROMOTION IN THE TWENTIETH CENTURY

Beginning in the 1960s, as the United States was slowly awakening to the jolt of the economic crisis in health care, a movement toward the same concerns of the nineteenth century began to gain momentum. By the early 1970s, the public, who had become enraptured by the awesome advances in disease diagnosis and treatment, began to make the connections between health and lifestyles.

Facilitating these connections were major epidemiologic studies completed in the United States and Britain that provided valid evidence linking human behavior with chronic disease. Examples include the Framingham study, begun in Massachusetts in 1948, which linked cardiovascular disease with smoking, obesity, and hypertension (Gordis, 2004); the 1964 Doll and Hill study in Britain that associated smoking with disease (Chapman, 2005); and the 1964 U.S. Surgeon General's report *Smoking and Health,* which linked smoking with cancer (Parascandola, Weed, & Dasgupta, 2006).

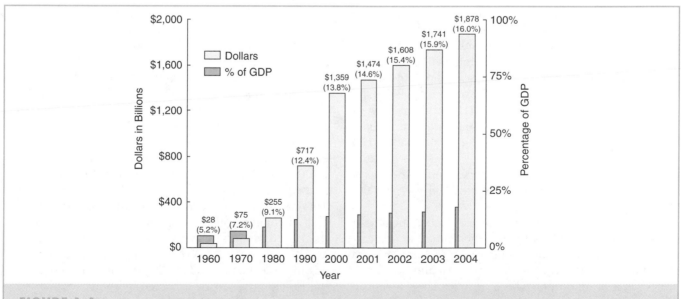

FIGURE 1-1 *Summary of National Health Care Expenditures and Share of the gross domestic product (GDP), 1960–2004. (Source: Centers for Medicare and Medicaid Services, Office of the Actuary, National Health Statistics Group.)*

In recognition of the effects of lifestyle and behavior on disease, the U.S. government established the Office of Disease Prevention and Health Promotion (ODPHP) in 1976 (Office of Disease Prevention and Health Promotion, n.d.). Today, the ODPHP continues to be a vital federal health agency devoted to promoting the health of Americans.

Canadian Influence on Health Promotion

The United States, however, is not known to have taken the lead in the health promotion movement. It is Canada that has been recognized as having launched health promotion to the world and presented theoretical frameworks from which other countries have modeled their health promotion programs. The government of Canada was the first to publicly acclaim health promotion as a major disease prevention strategy with the 1974 publication of *A New Perspective on the Health of Canadians,* known since as the **LaLonde Report.** In this classic document, LaLonde, then the Canadian Minister of National Health and Welfare, introduced the idea that human biology, social and physical environments, lifestyle behaviors, and health care organizations share equal importance and should receive equal consideration as determinants in chronic illness and/or a healthy life (Graff & Goldberg, 2000).

The report explicitly indicated that money spent on disease treatment could be saved if the disease could be prevented. This report gave rise to the concept of health care policy development and also to changing the way health care professionals practice.

International Goals for Health

By shifting the emphasis of health care away from the medical model of treatment to a more holistic one of prevention, the LaLonde Report linked the individual with society and the world. This insight stimulated a cascade of major global and national social initiatives. The first major action was taken in 1977 by the World Health Organization (WHO) at the World Health Assembly at Alma-Ata in the Soviet Union. Along with the United Nations International Children's Education Fund, WHO issued the Alma-Ata Declaration, which committed member countries to the goal of "an acceptable level of health for all the people of the world by the year 2000" (WHO, 1978).

At the time of the Declaration, the goal of "health for all" seemed achievable with strategies aimed at decreasing health disparities, increasing health technology, and providing primary health care for all. Health was envisioned as a human right. Three decades later, however, achievement of the goal remains elusive. The efforts of the WHO are compounded by existing, new, and emergent infectious diseases.

The United Nations has also continued the quest for international health. The 2005 World Summit of the United

Nations included international health among many global challenges. Two major areas of attention were identified: (1) heightened response to HIV/AIDS, TB, and malaria; and (2) support for international health regulations and the work of the World Health Organization (United Nations Department of Public Information, 2005).

The United States and National Goals for Health

Subsequently, the United States Public Health Service published *Healthy People: Surgeon General's Report on Health Promotion and Disease Prevention* (U.S. Public Health Service, 1979). This classic document outlined three major strategies for reaching national goals for health: preventive services for individuals provided by health professionals; individual protection measures to be taken by the government and industries; and health promotion actions to be taken by individuals and communities. Five priority areas for health promotion across the life span were identified: smoking, hypertension, alcohol and drug misuse, poor nutrition, and lack of exercise. The report identified the obligation that nurses have, along with other health care professionals, in providing health promotion and disease prevention services.

One year later, in 1980, in concert with the Surgeon General's report, 226 specific measurable objectives were identified to decrease mortality rates and disability from disease by the years 1990 and 2000 (U.S. Public Health Service, 1980). These objectives were developed even further with the publication of **Healthy People 2000:** *National Health Promotion and Disease Prevention Objectives, 1990* (U.S. Public Health Service, 1990). This document was developed by the U.S. Surgeon General, in conjunction with health care constituents across the nation, and it delineates 22 priority areas with 300 specific measurable objectives for health promotion, health protection, and surveillance and data systems for the United States to be achieved by the year 2000.

In the late 1990s, **Healthy People 2010** (U.S. Department of Health and Human Services, 2000) was similarly developed and organized into two major goals with 28 specific focus areas and 467 related objectives to improve health. Table 1-2 lists the 28 focus areas for collaboration

TABLE 1-2 *Healthy People 2010* Leading Health Indicators and Focus Areas for Collaboration

10 Leading Health Indicators

28 Focus Areas	Physical Activity	Overweight and Obesity	Tobacco Use	Substance Abuse	Responsible Sexual Behavior	Mental Health	Injury and Violence	Environmental Quality	Immunization	Access to Health Care
1. Access to Quality Health Services	•	•	•	•	•	•	•		•	•
2. Arthritis, Osteoporosis, and Chronic Back Conditions	•	•					•			
3. Cancer	•	•	•	•	•				•	•
4. Chronic Kidney Disease	•	•	•					•		
5. Diabetes	•	•	•							•
6. Disability and Secondary Conditions	•	•	•	•		•			•	•
7. Educational and Community-based Programs	•	•	•	•	•	•	•	•	•	•
8. Environmental Health								•		
9. Family Planning				•	•					•
10. Food Safety								•		•
11. Health Communication	•	•	•	•	•	•	•	•	•	•
12. Heart Disease and Stroke	•	•						•		
13. HIV				•	•	•				•
14. Immunization and Infectious Diseases									•	•
15. Injury and Violence Prevention			•	•		•	•			
16. Maternal, Infant, and Child Health	•	•	•	•	•	•	•		•	•
17. Medical Product Safety					•					
18. Mental Health and Mental Disorders			•	•	•	•				•
19. Nutrition and Overweight	•	•	•			•				
20. Occupational Safety and Health				•			•	•		
21. Oral Health		•	•	•					•	•
22. Physical Activity and Fitness	•	•	•		•	•		•		
23. Public Health Infrastructure	•	•	•	•	•	•	•	•	•	•
24. Respiratory Diseases	•		•					•		
25. Sexually Transmitted Diseases				•	•					
26. Substance Abuse			•	•	•		•			•
27. Tobacco Use			•					•		•
28. Vision and Hearing										•

Source: Healthy People 2010, *U.S. Department of Health and Human Services. Retrieved March 30, 2005, from* http://www
.healthypeople.gov/lhi/touch_fact.htm.

as they relate to 10 leading health indicators identified in *Healthy People 2010*. The purpose of *Healthy People 2010* is to build on initiatives set forth in and pursued by *Healthy People 2000* over the past two decades. It incorporates recent scientific advances in preventive medicine, disease surveillance, vaccine and therapy development, and information technology. It reflects the changes in the demographics of the country, the delivery of health care, and the effect of global influences on health by focusing on two major goals: (1) to increase the quality and years of healthy life and (2) to eliminate health disparities for those individuals who do not have access to quality health care.

HEALTH CARE COST CONTAINMENT

The mandate for cost containment beginning in the 1980s ushered in a new era of problems and challenges for both consumers and providers that continue today. Whether inspired by technology or deemed medically necessary, the ordering of expensive procedures and diagnostic tests prevails in spite of containment efforts. Gaining access to health care has become confusing and unattainable for some individuals and groups. Those gaining admission into hospitals are often sicker from delays in meeting criteria and are discharged earlier, and often more ill, than when they arrived. Reductions in hospital staff and early discharges have left many wondering about the quality of care provided. The issues of cost, access, and quality of health care have become the core elements affecting health care in America today.

Changes in Nursing Practice

A backlash from the effects of cost containment has actually resulted in many new and innovative actions with positive implications. Cost containment forced providers into increased competition, which, to some extent, has served to increase the quality of care provided. Also, more opportunities to provide for unmet health needs gave rise to an entirely new segment of health care in the form of home health agencies and rehabilitation centers. Of major importance is the development of increased empowerment and professional entrepreneurship within the profession of nursing. With teaching and advocacy always at the heart of nursing practice, empowerment of the nursing profession has served to rejuvenate and legitimize the incorporation of health promotion in nursing practice. In essence, cost containment and efforts directed at health care reform redesigned the way nurses practice. Community nurse-managed centers, models of nursing case management, and advanced practice models of nursing have replaced traditional modes of care (Tiedeman & Lookinland, 2004). For example, home health care agencies, many of which are owned and operated by nurses, seemed to literally spring forth overnight and practically on every

corner in the 1990s. All of these events, in combination with the changing paradigm for health care and nursing practice, have propelled the role of the nurse into one of high importance and extreme necessity in promoting the health of the American people.

As previously noted, the nursing profession has long maintained health promotion as integral to the practice of nursing. Client education and advocacy by nurses, unacceptable by many with a paternalistic and/or medical model orientation, was often accomplished in clandestine ways. Fortunately, the social initiatives set forth in 1980 for achieving national health goals by 1990 and 2000 called for the inclusion of health promotion, among which is client education and advocacy, in the practice of all health professionals. Such inclusion not only legitimized this facet of care for nurses but also helped to extend nursing practice into new realms.

Changes in Nursing Policy

By the end of the 1970s the profession of nursing had undergone dramatic changes, including diversified educational preparation, proliferation of specialty practice roles, practice control, and restructuring of the professional organization. Such diversity resulted in confusion among nurses and the public regarding the nature and scope of nursing. In response to this confusion and in an effort to unify the profession, the American Nurses Association (ANA), in 1980, prepared the classic publication entitled ***Nursing: A Social Policy Statement*** (American Nurses Association, 1980). This document, prepared by leaders in the profession, was the first of its kind to describe nursing and the profession's responsibility to society. The definition of health provided in this document related to biological, developmental, environmental, and behavioral components.

In 1995 the ANA published a revised policy statement titled *Nursing's Social Policy Statement* (American Nurses Association, 1995). The newer policy statement expands the definition of health and reflects an even greater commitment to the well-being of individuals in health and in illness. These documents are significant in that they embody health promotion and disease prevention as unifying concepts for the profession. The ANA's social policy statements are closely aligned with the ethical guidelines set forth in the ANA's *Code for Nurses* and the International Council of Nurses' (ICN) *Code for Nurses*.

Revised in 2005, the ANA's *Code for Nurses* reiterates the ethical commitment to health promotion that is inherent in the obligation of the nurse to the individual needs of the client and in the collaboration with other health professions and citizens. Through collaboration nurses can work to promote efforts in communities and the nation to meet the health needs of the public.

The creators of the ICN's *Code for Nurses* used foresight in explicitly identifying the ethical commitment of nurses to the promotion of health. The ICN's *Code for*

Nurses identifies the four major responsibilities of the nurse: promoting health, preventing illness, restoring health, and alleviating suffering (See Chapters 2 and 21 for related information). These responsibilities are further delineated in the nurse's responsibility to four entities: people, practice, co-workers, and the profession (International Council of Nurses, 2006.)

HEALTH PROMOTION: WHERE IS IT GOING?

After decades of disease-oriented care, health promotion, as a descendant of the World Health Organization's goal of health for all, is now recognized as a powerful health care strategy for the enhancement of the quality of life. *Healthy People 2000* set the stage for the future of health promotion in the United States. But promoting health for all is not without its problems. Health promotion can be seen as an idealistic concept and, when viewed realistically, raises many issues reflective of the diversity of populations involved. Cost, access, and quality of health care for all people are emerging as major issues as the government struggles with health care reform.

Because of the importance being placed on promoting health, and because it is understood that it is the nurse who is ever present in all phases and stages of health care, health promotion was identified as the emerging frontier in nursing. As a profession, nursing has been greatly involved in the many changes, challenges, and opportunities for health promotion. Where is health promotion going? Will nurses be prepared to meet new challenges? How can we manage the changes? These are just a few of the questions that nurses who are looking to the future might ask.

Forces Shaping the Future of Health Promotion

Today, it is clear that forces shaping changes in health care will directly affect health promotion needs and practices of the future. These forces are the changing dynamics of the demographics and behaviors of the people of the world. We know, for example, that people are becoming better informed and are living longer, chronic health problems are increasing, the numbers of disadvantaged young and old are increasing, and there are increasing cultural diversity and varying lifestyles among the population.

Futurists have envisioned both encouraging and discouraging prospects for health in the twenty-first century. Industrialized countries have seen increased quality of health, not because of medical care, but because of economic, social, and environmental improvements. This increase can be attributed to the adoption of healthier lifestyles. Environmental effects, however, such as global atmospheric changes, depletion of natural resources, and pollution, have been identified as major health threats to the people of the world in the future.

Sociopolitical unrest, manifested in terrorism, has presented even greater threats to health and well-being. **Terrorism** can be defined in many ways. Basically, it is the unlawful use of force and violence against persons or property to intimidate or coerce a government, the civilian population, or any segment thereof, in furtherance of political or social objectives (Grisit & Mahon, 2003, p. 117). On Tuesday, September 11, 2001 (9/11), the world changed forever when a series of coordinated attacks were inflicted upon the United States. Nineteen hijackers affiliated with al-Qaeda, an Islamic terrorist group led by Osama bin Laden, simultaneously took control of four U.S. domestic commercial airliners. The hijackers crashed two planes into the World Trade Center in Manhattan, New York City. A third hijacked plane crashed into the U.S. Department of Defense in the Pentagon, located in Arlington, Virginia. A fourth plane crashed into a rural field in Somerset County, Pennsylvania, following apparent passenger resistance. The official count records nearly 3,000 deaths in the attacks, including the 19 hijackers (September 11, 2001 attacks, n.d.).

The 9/11 attacks are among the most significant events to have occurred thus far in the twenty-first century, affecting millions of people in a multitude of ways: physically, politically, psychologically, spiritually, and economically. The attacks, and the subsequent U.S.-led wars in Afghanistan and Iraq, have made U.S. homeland security concerns much more prominent than they were in the previous decade. The effects of 9/11 in terms of health and health promotion are further addressed in Chapter 7.

A Framework for Thinking About the Future

Those who study health care offer frameworks that can be useful for envisioning the health promotion of the future and for planning its destiny. Using trends, scenarios, and

Ask Yourself

Consider the Future of Nursing

Using Norman Henchey's Four Ways of Thinking About the Future, what do you think about the future of nursing in health promotion in terms of what is possible, plausible, probable, and preferable?

vision as aspects of health futures is a proactive, rather than a reactive, approach to the future of health. Nearly three decades ago, Canadian futurist Norman Henchey suggested thinking about the future in four distinct ways:

1. Possible future—what *may* happen, including "wild-cards" and everything possibly imaginable no matter how unlikely.

2. Plausible future—what *could* happen, integrating possible future events with what is currently known, creating a range of alternatives.

3. Probable future—what *will likely* happen, one of the plausible futures based on the current situation and appraisal of likely trends.

4. Preferable future—what we *want* to have happen based on shared visions, empowering us to design the best future using our creative abilities.

Organizations, operating from a foresight perspective, can use this proactive approach in planning for the future (Vores, 2003). Using the metaphor of looking at the future from a narrow-angle or a wide-angle perspective helps in understanding two opposing views of making change happen. The narrow angle represents interventions through social control, implying forced change that is focused on statistical analysis of the population, identification of weaknesses, a health outcome, disease organization, and ways to motivate people. The wide angle encompasses a more comprehensive view of health and well-being with a focus on social-behavioral factors, identification of strengths, a health outcome that extends into the community, and ways to incorporate the motives of the people.

Facilitating Your Role in Health Promotion

The effect of nursing practice on promoting health for all people in the future can be profound. Whether you are working in a rural or urban setting, in a hospital, clinic, home health agency, workplace, school, or community agency, you can influence the health of each and every one of your clients.

Challenges facing nurses and health promotion practice today are numerous and varied. Among those challenges are: keeping current with new knowledge, technology, and information systems; understanding the changing demographics of society and the world; engaging in partnerships and collaborative relationships with individuals, families, and groups; becoming involved in health promotion policy development and implementation; participating in evidence-based practice; developing a worldview perspective; and embracing a proactive philosophy for professional practice.

The following can facilitate meeting the challenges of health promotion:

- Expand the frontiers of your own knowledge. By being knowledgeable about new research and technologies you will build a solid foundation to guide you in helping your clients. Keeping current with legislation affecting health care and your practice is also powerful knowledge.

- Make collaboration with other health providers a basic part of your practice. Nurses have historically maintained a "do all" attitude for client care. Most nurses have been educated to give total client care. Overlap of care already exists with physicians, nutritionists, physical therapists, and others. Working in a complementary manner with other providers can strengthen the health plan for your clients. Remember, too, that empowering the client is important to the effectiveness of the collaborative network.

- Place the emphasis of your care on outcomes, cost, and quality. Because health care will continue to be cost-driven, it is important that you exercise a cost-conscious model of care while maintaining a focus on quality in achieving goals.

- Enhance your sensitivities to biological factors, lifestyle choices, environmental factors, cultural diversities, and educational readiness of your clientele. Rather than diagnosis and treatment of disease, health promotion is particular to the individual.

- Adopt a wellness focus to guide your practice. Under the umbrella of wellness, health promotion activities, including health maintenance and disease prevention, must be granted the same esteem and professionalism as nursing activities involved in caring for clients with disease diagnoses.

SUMMARY

This chapter has presented an overview of the historical, social, economic, and political developments that have forged the foundation for health promotion and provided direction for the future. It is clear that health promotion is a dynamic process in constant change. The health promoting practices and policies of the past have gone through major alterations to adjust to the reality of the world today and to flow into the future.

Nursing practice has also undergone major changes but has continually maintained a commitment to promoting health. Today, the nursing profession, with its variation of roles and scope of practice, play has a vital part in the promotion of health that extends from individuals to families, groups, communities, and the world.

Key Concepts

The following summarizes the key concepts presented in this chapter:

1. Health promotion is a relatively recent term that has various meanings among individuals and societies reflective of values, beliefs, politics, and philosophies. Health education is a major component of health promotion.

2. The history of health promotion is a tapestry woven from ancient cultures, practices based on beliefs and values of the population, changing health behaviors, effects of technological and scientific advances, and powerful sociopolitical forces.

3. Heightened consciousness of society, the change of medical focus from disease treatment to illness prevention, and the development of nursing as a profession are the major movements behind health promotion in the nineteenth century.

4. The contributions of science and the effects of economic, environmental, and sociopolitical forces in the twentieth century profoundly affected health promotion in the United States. World War II was a major catalyst in technology advancement, immunization development, and disease treatment that changed medical practice forever. The United States prospered with industrial technology, resulting in national and individual economic gains, shifts from rural to urban populations, alterations in disease epidemiology, and changes in lifestyles. The Social Security Act provided the foundation for socialization of health care that was further developed by Medicare and Medicaid. Government spending for health care brought relief to many people as well as cost inflation and fraud. Cost, access, and quality have become major issues prompting support for health promotion.

5. Canada was an early leader of nations for health promotion with publication of the *LaLonde Report*. WHO enlisted the support of member nations in reaching the goals of *Health for All by the year 2000*. The United States has set new national goals for health as described in *Healthy People 2010*.

6. The profession of nursing, transformed by the social mandate for health promotion, continues to change in practice and policy to meet the dynamic needs of society. Consumer involvement, expanded roles for nurses, changing practice settings, and collaborative health care management highlight the importance of health promotion in professional practice. The *Code for Nurses, Nursing's Social Policy Statement,* and *Standards for Clinical Nursing*

Practice emphasize the commitment of the nursing profession to health promotion.

7. The future of health promotion and nursing practice will be affected by the manner in which nurses articulate their unique contributions. A personal commitment to increasing knowledge, collaboration, individualization of health care, and focus on wellness will expand from a narrow perspective to a wide perspective of health promotion.

Learning Activities

1. Identify five examples of efforts to promote the health of people in your community.

2. Match each example from above to a focus area of *Healthy People 2010*.

3. Explain how nurses and other health professionals could be involved in these efforts.

True/False Questions

1. T or F   Health promotion and health education are terms that have the same meaning.

2. T or F   Organized health promotion practices were not evident before 1935.

3. T or F   Politics and government have little influence on promoting health.

4. T or F   Health care providers, including nurses, physicians, and administrators of health care facilities, are responsible for creating *Healthy People 2000*.

5. T or F   The Social Security Act of 1935 provided the foundation for Medicare and Medicaid.

6. T or F   The Mosaic Code is a major part of the American Nurses Association's *Code for Nurses*.

7. T or F   The three major movements of the 1800s causing a social mandate for health promotion include the developing consciousness of the people, changes and advances in medicine, and the development of nursing as a profession.

8. T or F   Reforming health care throughout the twentieth century resulted from both scientific and sociopolitical events.

9. T or F   Diagnosis-related groups (DRGs) were designed by physicians to increase Medicare payments for health care services.

10. T or F   Canada is the nation known to have launched the concept of health promotion to the world.

Multiple Choice Questions

1. The Ottawa Charter was developed for which one of the following purposes?
   a. To guide Canada's health promotion initiatives
   b. To solidify the United States and Canada in coordinated health care services
   c. To expand health education for healthier lifestyles
   d. To achieve health for all by the year 2000 and beyond

2. Dualism in health care, rooted in the past and currently existing, refers to the
   a. Combination of values, attitudes, and beliefs with modern health care practices
   b. Conflicts that exist between two different cultures regarding health care
   c. Differences between society's needs and programs developed by health care administrators
   d. Recognition that individuals are often multicultural

3. Which one of the following is a long-term study known for linking cardiovascular disease with smoking, obesity, and hypertension?
   a. Doll and Hill study
   b. Framingham study
   c. *Healthy People 2000*
   d. *LaLonde Report*

Websites

http://www.healthpromotionjournal.com Contains contemporary articles and current information on conferences, resources, and careers related to health promotion.

http://odphp.osophs.dhhs.gov A U.S. government site for the Office of Disease Prevention and Health Promotion that provides information on a wide range of national disease prevention and health promotion strategies.

http://www.healthypeople.gov Provides information related to *Healthy People 2010* and other national health promotion and disease prevention initiatives involving a multitude of individuals and agencies to improve the health of all Americans.

http://www.ahrq.gov Site for the Agency for Health Research and Quality that offers practical health care information, research findings, and data helpful to clients, health care providers, and administrators.

Organizations/Agencies

The U.S. Department of Health and Human Services
200 Independence Avenue, S.W.
Washington, DC 20201

Tel: (202) 619-0257

Toll Free: (877) 696-6775

U.S. Department of Health and Human Services is the U.S. government's principal agency for protecting the health of all Americans and providing essential human services through more than 300 programs covering a wide spectrum of activities.

Office of Disease Prevention and Health Promotion

Office of Public Health and Science, Office of the Secretary

1101 Wootton Parkway, Suite LL100

Rockville, MD 20852

Tel: (240) 453-8280

Fax: (240) 453-8282

http://odphp.osophs.dhhs.gov

Office of Disease Prevention and Health Promotion works to strengthen disease prevention and health promotion priorities through a collaborative framework of Health and Human Services agencies.

The Centre for Health Promotion

100 College Street, Suite 207

The Banting Institute

Toronto, Ontario M5G 1L5 Canada

Tel: (416) 978-1809

Fax: (416) 971-1365

Email: centre.healthpromotion@utoronto.ca

http://www.utoronto.ca/chp/

The Centre for Health Promotion is an internationally recognized organization that is committed to excellence in education, evaluation, and research through multidisciplinary collaboration to activate, develop, and evaluate innovative health promotion approaches in Canada and abroad.

United States Army Center for Health Promotion & Preventive Medicine

5158 Blackhawk Road

Aberdeen Proving Ground, MD 21010-5403

Tel: (800) 222-9698

http://www.apgea.army

United States Army Center for Health Promotion & Preventive Medicine exists to provide worldwide technical support for implementing preventive medicine, public health, and health promotion/wellness services in all aspects of America's Army and the world community with a vision to be a world-class Center for Health Promotion and Preventive Medicine.

References

American Nurses Association. (1980). *Nursing: A social policy statement* (Publ. No. NP-63). Kansas City, MO: American Nurses Association.

American Nurses Association. (1995). *Nursing's Social Policy Statement* (Publ. No. NP-107). Washington, DC: American Nurses Publishing.

Anonymous. (1986). Ottawa charter for health promotion. *Canadian Journal of Public Health, 77*(6), 425–430.

Arias, E. (2004). United States life tables, 2002. *National Vital Statistics Reports, 53*(6). Hyattsville, MD: National Center for Health Statistics.

Babylonia, a history of ancient Babylon. (n.d.). Retrieved March 13, 2006, from http://history-world.org/babylonia.htm

Bright, M. A. (2002). *Holistic health and healing.* Philadelphia: F. A. Davis.

Chapman, S. (2005). The most important and influential papers in tobacco control: Results of an online poll. *Tobacco Control, 14.* Retrieved March 13, 2006, from http://tobacco.health.usyd.edu.au

Clark, M. J. (2003). *Community health nursing: Caring for populations* (4th ed.). Upper Saddle River, NJ: Prentice Hall.

Cockerham, W. C. (1978). *Medical Sociology.* Englewood Cliffs, NJ: Prentice-Hall, Inc.

Centers for Medicare and Medicare Services (CMS), Office of the Actuary, National Health Statistics Group. (2006, June 7). National Health Expenditure Overview. Retrieved November 27, 2006, from http://www.cms.hhs.gov/NationalHealthExpendData

Ellis, J. R., & Hartley, C. L. (2004) *Nursing in Today's World* (8th ed.). Philadelphia: Lippincott Williams & Wilkins.

Gordis, L. (2004). *Epidemiology.* Philadelphia: W. B. Saunders.

Graff, P., & Goldberg, S. (2000). *The health field concept then and now: Snapshots of Canada.* Ottawa, Ontario: Canadian Policy Research Network.

Griset, P. L., & Mahon, S. (2003). Terrorism in perspective. (p. 117). Thousand Oaks, CA: Sage Publications.

Guisepi, R. A. (2001). *A history of ancient Greece.* Retrieved March 13, 2006, from http://ancient_greecetwo.htm

Hoffman, E. D., Klees, B. S., & Curtis, C. A. (2006, November). *Brief summaries of medicare and Medicaid.* Retrieved November 27, 2006, from http://www.cmshhs.gov/MedicareProgramRatesStats/02_SummaryMedicareMedicaid.asp

International Council of Nurses. (2006) *The ICN Code of Ethics for Nurses.* Geneva, Switzerland: Author.

Jonas, S., & Kovner, A. R. (Eds.). (2002). *Health care delivery in the United States.* New York: Springer Publishing.

Kelly, L. Y., & Joel, L. A. (2002). *The nursing experience: Trends, challenges, and transitions* (4th ed.). New York: McGraw-Hill.

Kramarow, E., Lentzner, H., Rooks, R., Weeks, J., & Saydah, S. (1999). *Health and aging chartbook* (Library of Congress Catalog No. 76-641496, p. 30). Washington, DC: U.S. Government Printing Office.

MacDonald, G., & Bunton, R. (1992). Health promotion: Discipline or disciplines? In *Health promotion: Disciplines and diversity.* New York: Routledge.

McLeroy, K. R., & Crump: C. E. (1994). Health promotion and disease prevention: A historical perspective. *Generations, 18*(1), 9–17.

Moore, P. V., & Williamson, C. C. (1984). Health promotion: Evolution of a concept. *Nursing Clinics of North America, 19*(2), 195–207.

Nightingale, F. (1859/1969). *Notes on nursing: What it is and what it is not.* New York: Dover Publications.

Novak, J. C. (1988). The social mandate and historical basis for nursing's role in health promotion. *Journal of Professional Nursing, 4*(2), 80–87.

Nutbeam, D. (1996). Health promotion glossary. In *Health promotion: An anthology.* Washington, DC: Pan American Health Organization.

Office of Disease Prevention and Health Promotion. (n.d.). Fact Sheet. Retrieved March 13, 2006, from http://odphp.osophs.dhhs.gov

Parascandola, M., Weed, D. L., & Dasgupta, A. (2006, January 10). Two Surgeon General's reports on smoking and cancer: A historical investigation of the practice of causal inference. *Emerging Themes in Epidemiology* 2006, 3:1. Retrieved March 13, 2006, from http://www.ete-online.com/content/3/1/1

September 11, 2001 attacks. (n.d.). Retrieved March 9, 2006, from en.wikipedia.org/wiki/September_11,_2001_attacks

Stanhope, M., & Lancaster, J. (2004). *Community and public health nursing* (6th ed.). St. Louis: C. V. Mosby.

Tiedeman, M. E., & Lookinland, S. (2004). Traditional models of care delivery: What have we learned? *Journal of Nursing Administration, 34*(6), 291–297.

Timmreck, T. C. (2002). *An introduction to epidemiology.* Boston: Jones and Bartlett Publishers.

U.S. Department of Health and Human Services. (2000). *Healthy people 2010.* Washington, DC: U.S. Government Printing Office.

U.S. Public Health Service. (1979). *Healthy people: Surgeon General's report on health promotion and disease prevention* (DHHS Publication no. 79-55071). Washington, DC: U.S. Government Printing Office.

U.S. Public Health Service. (1980). *Promoting health/preventing disease: Objectives for the nation.* Washington, DC: U.S. Government Printing Office. HE 20.2:D63/4, 1980.

U.S. Public Health Service. (1990). *Healthy people 2000: National health promotion and disease prevention objectives, 1990.* Washington, DC: U.S. Government Printing Office.

United Nations Department of Public Information. (2005, September). *2005 World summit outcome.* Retrieved November 29, 2006, from http://www.un.org/summit2005/presskit/fact_sheet.pdf

Vores, J. (2003). A generic foresight process framework. *Foresight, 5*(3), 10–21.

Whitehead, D., Keast, J., Montgomery, V., & Hayman, S. (2004). A preventative health education programme for osteoporosis. *Journal of Advanced Nursing, 47*(1), 15–24.

World Health Organization (WHO). (1978). Declaration of Alma-Ata. International Conference on Primary Health Care, Alma-Ata, USSR, 6–12 September, 1978. Retrieved March 13, 2006, from http://www.who.int/hpr/NPH/docs/declaration_almaata

Bibliography

Allender, J. A., & Spradley, B. W. (2005). *Community health nursing: Promoting and protecting the public's health.* Philadelphia: Lippincott Williams & Wilkins.

Delaney, F. G. (1994). Nursing and health promotion: Conceptual concerns. *Journal of Advanced Nursing, 20,* 828–835.

Harris, J. (1994). The health benefits of health promotion. In M. P. O'Donnell and J. S. Harris (Eds.), *Health promotion in the workplace.* Clifton Park, NY: Thomson Delmar Learning.

Kalisch, P. A., & Kalisch, B. J. (2004). *American nursing: A history.* Philadelphia: Lippincott Williams & Wilkins.

Palmer, I. (1977). Nightingale: Reformer, reactionary, researcher. *Nursing Research, 22,* 101–110.

Spellbring, A. M. (1991). Nursing's role in health promotion: An overview. *Nursing Clinics of North America, 26*(4), 805–815.

Terris, M. (1996). Concepts of health promotion: Dualities in public health theory. In *Health promotion: An anthology.* Washington, DC: Pan American Health Organization.

Chapter 2

NURSING CONCEPTS AND HEALTH PROMOTION

Carolina G. Huerta, EdD, MSN, RN

KEY TERMS

adaptation
career ladder
concept
conceptual framework

cultural congruent care
general systems theory
holistic
homeostasis

metaparadigm
needs theory
paradigm

theory
transcultural nursing
theory

OBJECTIVES

Upon completion of this chapter, the reader should be able to:

- Identify concepts essential in defining professional nursing practice.

- Describe how the concept of health promotion provides a framework for professional nursing practice.

- Explain how a metaparadigm is useful in defining a profession.

- Describe the four concepts central to nursing's metaparadigm.

- Describe nursing educational levels and their relationship to health promotion.

- List assumptions basic to integrating health promotion into nursing practice.

- Identify selected nursing theoretical frameworks.

- List various definitions of nursing.

INTRODUCTION

The concept of health promotion is not a new one to the nursing profession. It should be noted that health promotion has evolved over the centuries and traces its roots to ancient times (see Chapter 1). In fact, Florence Nightingale's (1860) writings focused on health practices and health promotion within the context of the environmental impact on health. Nursing practice has long considered the concept of health promotion as integral to the prevention of disease, maintenance of health, identification of optimum health, and restoration of well-being.

A health promotion focus provides nursing and health care professionals with a heightened consciousness in assuming responsibility for personal health and welfare as well as the health and welfare of others in society at large. It is unfortunate that lifestyle or behavioral changes needed to achieve a state of health are not easy tasks.

It is extremely difficult to implement health promotion strategies if individuals lack motivation to do those things that will result in good health. In fact, many people, nurses included, are guilty of making lifestyle choices that seem to sabotage opportunities for achieving optimal health and living a long, prosperous life. Change, especially in relation to improving health, is difficult to achieve. Individuals need a lot of support and encouragement from knowledgeable health care professionals if they are to make lifestyle changes that will result in a state of optimal health.

The previous chapter introduced the concept of health promotion and provided a historical perspective on its evolution and impact on contemporary society. This chapter will focus on nursing's metaparadigm, professional nursing today, and its relationship to health promotion. Nursing theories, health promotion as a conceptual framework, and the four concepts that define nursing's metaparadigm are described. Professional nursing practice's influence on personal as well as community health care behavior changes will be emphasized.

PROFESSIONAL NURSING PRACTICE AND HEALTH PROMOTION

The concept of health promotion is found in much of the current nursing literature. The interest in health promotion has evolved because the idea of increasing levels of well-being, life expectancy, and health potential fits well with nursing as a caring discipline. Health promotion strategies also decrease health care costs and morbidity. Because the concept of health promotion is integral to everything that nurses do, it provides a framework useful in defining and describing nursing. The nursing profession has always included health promotion in one form or another in its attempt to define itself and identify the various nursing responsibilities.

The American Nurses Association's (ANA) *Code of Ethics for Nurses* (ANA, 2001), for example, which was originally adopted in 1950, clearly indicates the profession's responsibility to the public in promoting efforts to meet health needs (Box 2-1). This document highlights nursing's responsibility for protecting, promoting, and restoring the health of the community it serves.

The ANA's *Scope & Standards of Practice* (ANA, 2004), which addresses the profession's concern with quality of nursing service and accountability, also highlights health promotion in nursing. These standards describe nursing's concern for ensuring that nursing actions provide for client participation in health promotion, health protection, and optimization of health, and that they assist clients in maximizing their potential. The ANA's subsequent *Standards of Clinical Nursing Practice* (ANA, 1998) sets standards applicable to all nurses engaged in clinical practice and delineates nursing responsibilities in meeting client needs. According to these standards, nurses are required to educate their clients regarding the clients' health care and treatment, including health promotion and disease prevention (ANA, 2001). The concept of health promotion in these clinical practice standards is subsumed among all other standards.

The ANA documents are intended to reflect the scope of nursing practice and its theoretical or conceptual basis. Thus, it is evident that one of nursing's most highly prioritized responsibilities is to promote healthy behaviors among the constituents it serves. Table 2-1 identifies ANA documents important to professional nursing and their relationship to the concept of health promotion as a nursing goal. These documents are important to professional nurses in practice in that they identify nursing's role in the promotion of health.

NURSING'S METAPARADIGM

Health promotion is an integral part of nursing practice and is essential in defining nursing as a profession. Health promotion is always included in nursing's definition when viewing the nursing discipline on a broad basis. It is part of what nurses do in nursing practice and is reflected in what is called the paradigm or metaparadigm on nursing. A **paradigm** is an example that serves as a pattern or model for something (Tabers, 2005). A nursing paradigm provides a clear or typical example of nursing as a discipline. Paradigms have been used in recent years by theorists to illustrate how concepts and theories fit into the actual practice of a discipline.

BOX 2-1   American Nurses Association Code of Ethics for Nurses

1. The nurse, in all professional relationships, practices with compassion and respect for the inherent dignity, worth, and uniqueness of every individual, unrestricted by considerations of social or economic status, personal attributes, or the nature of the health problem.
2. The nurse's primary commitment is to the patient, whether an individual, family, group, or community.
3. The nurse promotes, advocates for, and strives to protect the health, safety, and rights of the patient.
4. The nurse is responsible and accountable for individual nursing practice and determines the appropriate delegation of tasks consistent with the nurse's obligation to provide optimum patient care.
5. The nurse owes the same duties to self as to others, including the responsibility to preserve integrity and safety, to maintain competence, and to continue personal and professional growth.
6. The nurse participates in establishing, maintaining, and improving health care environments and conditions of employment conducive to the provision of quality health care and consistent with the values of the profession through individual and collective action.
7. The nurse participates in the advancement of the profession through contributions to practice, education, administration, and knowledge development.
8. The nurse collaborates with other health professionals and the public in promoting community, national, and international efforts to meet health needs.
9. The profession of nursing, as represented by associations and their members, is responsible for articulating nursing values, for maintaining the integrity of the profession and its practice, and for shaping social policy.

Source: Printed with permission from American Nurses Association. (2001). Code of ethics for nurses with interpretive statements. *Washington, DC: American Nurses Publishing.*

TABLE 2-1 ANA Professional Nursing Practice Standards/Statements and Their Relationship to Health Promotion Concepts

Standards/Statements	Purpose of Document	Relationship to Health Promotion
Scope & Standards of Practice (2004)	Describes a means for determining the quality of nursing services received by client. The standards reflect the values and priorities of the nursing profession.	Concerned with the health status of the client, not just illness. Specifies that health status determines the nursing care needs and subsequent actions; highlights nursing's actions that promote, maintain, and restore well-being and health, and that optimize health.
Code of Ethics for Nurses (2001)	Establishes a code of ethics that provides guidance for professional nursing conduct and responsibilities.	Makes explicit nursing's responsibilities in relation to protecting, promoting, and restoring health in the care of individuals, families, groups, and communities. Delineates nursing's responsibility to assist clients in maximizing own potential and requires the client to participate in promoting own health.
Standards of Clinical Nursing Practice (1998)	Describes a competent level of professional nursing services and sets standards for professional nurse performance, regardless of practice setting.	Specifies that nurses are in a position to assist clients to make informed decisions regarding health care, treatment, health promotion, disease prevention, and attainment of a peaceful death. Utilizes nursing process to delegate nursing responsibilities such as culturally congruent care, safety, client teaching, and health promotion or self-care activities.
Nursing: A Social Policy Statement (2003)	Provides a framework for understanding professional nursing's relationship with society and its obligations for those receiving care. Expresses the social contract between society and the profession of nursing.	Focuses on nature of nursing and recognizes nursing practice as being restorative, supportive, and promotive. Emphasizes protection, promotion, and optimization of health. Nursing actions include promotion practices which mobilize health patterns of the body. Recognizes nurses' role of advocacy in the care of individuals, families, communities, and populations.

A **metaparadigm,** on the other hand, is usually used by an individual discipline to provide a global perspective of the field. The prefix *meta* refers to a more highly organized form at a later stage of development. A metaparadigm describes a later or more highly organized form of a paradigm. Nursing uses a metaparadigm as a unifying force to describe those common concepts specific to nursing. In fact, nursing theorists usually identify concepts that are congruent with their view of nursing and refer to these in their totality as nursing's metaparadigm. A metaparadigm is preferred to a paradigm because it is thought to represent a more organized framework than a paradigm. Nursing's metaparadigm helps to critically unify and evaluate concepts which are characteristic of nursing.

A description of nursing must include those concepts and theories that collectively or individually describe the profession. Definitions of nursing invariably include conceptual or theoretical frameworks that serve the purpose of explaining what nursing is and what actions are specific to nursing. For example, the concept of health promotion can be useful in defining or describing the nursing profession in relation to those actions that assist clients, their families, or both to prevent illness, maintain health, and promote optimum well-being. A nursing metaparadigm that uses health promotion will, then, make certain that this concept is integrated throughout the description of the four concepts commonly used to organize nursing's metaparadigm. The four concepts that are found in most theorists' descriptions of nursing's metaparadigm are *person, health, environment,* and *nursing* (Fawcett, 2005). These will be used in this chapter to define nursing and its relation to health promotion.

Prior to describing the profession in terms of nursing's metaparadigm, it is necessary to clarify the terms *concept, theory,* and *framework*. A **concept** is a generalized notion or idea useful in describing facts or occurrences. Person, environment, and health, for example, are major concepts used in defining nursing. Concepts provide a broad view or perspective of the nursing profession. **Theory,** on the other hand, is narrower and provides specificity in its description. Theory is defined as a set or group of interrelated concepts, facts, definitions, and propositions that specify relationships among variables and are useful in describing, explaining, predicting, and controlling phenomena (Kerlinger, 1973). Theory's primary purpose is to generate new knowledge and make scientific findings meaningful and generalizable. Theory takes into account observable or empirical facts in the environment, relates these facts to each other, and makes sense out of them. Generation of theory or theory building is important to the discipline of nursing which, for the most part, describes itself as an art and a science. As a science, nursing is expected to generate new knowledge and expand existing knowledge by building theory. The linking of concepts and propositions through theory building makes the accumulated body of knowledge easily accessible and organized. Nursing theory is useful in differentiating the various areas of practice (Hickman, 2002a).

A framework is a structure that provides support in organizing and shaping something. It is much like the frame of a house that lends support to its roof, walls, and existing structures. A **conceptual framework** as applied in a nursing theory context refers to those concepts, facts, and propositions that are useful for defining nursing (Polit & Hungler, 2004). This framework provides a way to shape nursing and nursing practice into a meaningful configuration. Frameworks used to define nursing may include theoretical frameworks that specify a certain theory or theorist or conceptual frameworks that identify the interrelated concepts important to nursing. A conceptual framework is less formal and less well developed than a theoretical framework. Because frameworks useful to describing nursing are not always based on a particular nursing theory, the terms *theoretical framework* and *conceptual framework* will be used interchangeably in this chapter.

DEFINING NURSING

Fawcett (2005) has attempted to conceptualize the essence of nursing in her description of nursing's metaparadigm. She has defined nursing in terms of the concepts that are central to nursing practice. Fawcett's metaparadigm provides organization in describing nursing as a practice discipline that has evolved from theory and nursing research. She uses the concept of person as the recipient of care (whether as an individual, a family, or a group). She also includes the concepts of environment as encompassing both animate and inanimate objects, health to include wellness and illness states of the client, and nurs-

ing actions to mean those actions taken by nurses in caring for a client. Fawcett's metaparadigm is frequently used to define and delineate the scope of nursing.

Nursing: A Social Policy Statement (ANA, 2003) illustrates how definitions of nursing include promotion of well-being in the recipient of care. These definitions are congruent with nursing's metaparadigm and also include human experiences, responses to health and illness, a knowledge base, and provisions for nurse-client relationships that foster health and healing. The scope of nursing practice is identified as one that includes practices that are restorative, supportive, and promotive. The definition and scope of nursing in this ANA document demonstrate the connection of the four concepts described by Fawcett's metaparadigm on nursing. Nursing's definition and scope include the concept of person in relation to human responses, the concept of health and nursing's role in relation to its promotion, the environment as reflected by a person's experiences and responses to health problems, and those nursing actions that involve restoration, support, and promotion of health.

PERSON, ENVIRONMENT, HEALTH, AND NURSING

Nursing's metaparadigm provides the substance and character of nursing as a profession. It is the strength upon which nursing practice is built. Figure 2-1 depicts nursing's metaparadigm and illustrates how the four concepts—person, environment, health, and nursing—interact dynamically in practice.

Person

A thorough description of the concept of person is essential to providing direction for nursing as a practice discipline. The person as the recipient of care is perceived to possess attributes that must be considered in the performance of nursing actions. These attributes are useful in the assessment, planning, implementation, and evaluation activities performed by a professional nurse. Nursing models using a health promotion approach describe recipients of care as holistic, biological, spiritual, psychological, social beings made up of more than a sum of their parts.

That is, person-centered nurses care for individuals in their totality as opposed to only those areas that are diseased. Because clients are also seen as capable of thinking critically, they are given the opportunity to have input into their own care. The client is seen as interacting with the environment, having energy, and being dynamic, and is also perceived as constantly changing and adapting. Clients are cultural beings whose uniqueness sets them apart from all others, although they may possess a shared culture. In the performance of nursing care, the nurse considers persons holistically and

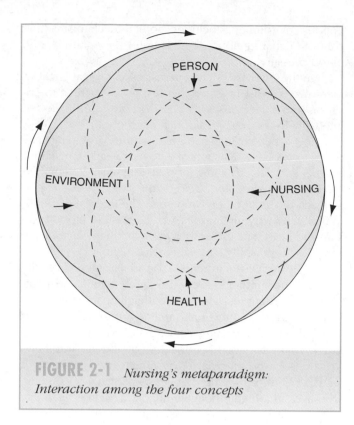

FIGURE 2-1 *Nursing's metaparadigm: Interaction among the four concepts*

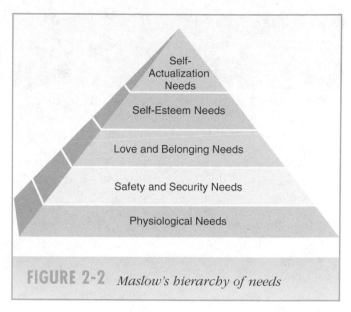

FIGURE 2-2 *Maslow's hierarchy of needs*

places great importance on their life experiences. People's experiences are a part of their very essence of being, and thus knowledge of their past, present, and possible future experiences must be considered when planning their care and health promotion activities.

Individual uniqueness in terms of total functioning must also be considered when planning and performing client care. As recipients of nursing care, clients are entitled to full disclosure and to active participation in the development of their health promotion or nursing care plans. A person is perceived as having many needs and as being capable of achieving and maintaining optimum health. For example, Maslow (1970, 1999), a social psychologist, describes the person as a social being having many common needs that motivate behavior. The meeting of these needs is important to the maintenance of health throughout the life span.

Maslow's Hierarchy of Needs

Maslow identifies what he calls the *hierarchy of needs* that encompass the physiological, safety and security, love and belonging, self-esteem, and self-actualization needs of all people. These needs are ranked in relation to their importance. Figure 2-2 illustrates a pyramid depicting the hierarchy of needs.

Imagine that the pyramid has a staircase that consists of five flights to get to the top floor. If the intent is to get to the top floor, then a person must climb each level of stairs first. Maslow's hierarchy of needs can be described in the same manner in that needs at one level must be met before a person can reach the next level.

The first flight of steps represents the physiologic needs. These physiologic needs form the base of the staircase and consist of basic life-sustaining needs such as food, water, air, rest, sleep, and activity. If basic needs are met, the individual is ready to climb the next flight. The needs at the next level are safety and security needs. Satisfaction of these needs allows the person to meet love and belonging needs found on the third level and the self-esteem needs found on the fourth level of the staircase. Ascending this fourth flight of stairs does not ensure that the person will make it to the top floor. Maslow describes this top floor as the highest level and as representative of a person's self-actualization needs. There may be many barriers that prevent most people from reaching this fifth level, but according to Maslow people continuously strive to achieve this level. The fifth level is represented as the top level because it is elusive and difficult to achieve. Box 2-2 depicts the specific needs that might surface within each category of needs.

There are many factors that can influence a client's pursuit of optimum health. It is nursing's responsibility to identify some of these factors. Self-prioritization of needs by clients, for instance, occurs all of the time and may impact their health-related outcomes. For example, a mother may choose to provide the only available water to her child so that the child's thirst may be satisfied. In doing this, she has chosen to satisfy her need for love and belonging instead of meeting her own physiological need for water. It is fortunate that people have the ability to communicate, think independently, and prioritize, because these characteristics are essential to meeting needs and promoting health. Knowledge of a human needs framework is useful in nursing practice because this framework provides a method for prioritizing client care activities and also provides a means for understanding the nurse's personal behavior as well as that of the client.

BOX 2-2   Maslow's Hierarchy of Needs
Subcategories

Self-Actualization
- Fulfillment
- Perception
- Peacefulness

Self-Esteem
- Approval
- Maturity
- Respect
- Self-worth

Love and Belonging
- Intimacy
- Comfort
- Closeness
- Family
- Self-acceptance

Safety and Security
- Protection
- Rules
- Laws
- Structure

Physiological
- Food
- Oxygen
- Water
- Rest
- Sex
- Warmth
- Elimination

Nursing attests to the importance of the concept of person by caring for, educating, directing, and assisting people in their attempt to achieve optimum health. The concept of person in nursing's metaparadigm focuses on a person's ability to direct his or her own health and determine the most favorable actions to acquire it.

Environment

The environment is a major influence on a person's overall functioning and health promotion activities. Because of this, it is critical for nurses to have an understanding of how the internal as well as external environments impact a client's everyday life. Nurse theorists throughout the history of modern nursing have identified the environment as an important concept in determining what nursing is and what nurses do. In fact, Florence Nightingale, who is recognized as the founder of contemporary nursing, described her whole philosophy of nursing in terms of environmental factors that influence health and disease. In her *Notes on Nursing* (1860/1969), which Nightingale wrote in 1859, she delineates symptoms of disease as environment related and expounds on environmental factors that cause or prevent disease. Pure water, fresh air, light, cleanliness, and efficient drainage are described as environmental factors essential to disease prevention.

The environment consists of both an internal and external environment that continuously interface with each other. People's internal environments include their ideas, biological makeup, emotions, and the psychosocial elements that influence them. Included in this psychosocial entity are a person's spiritual, cultural, and social needs and experiences. A person's internal bio-

logical environment includes bodily mechanisms that control such functions as heart rate, temperature, and blood pressure.

On the other hand, the internal psychosocial environment may consist of emotional responses such as to crisis or stress. Responses to crisis or stress are reflected internally in the biological functioning of our bodies. For instance, a person living in a stressful environment may worry excessively. This worry state may result in reactions by the internal environment that might lead to hypersecretion of hydrochloric acid by the stomach resulting in stomach ulcers or other symptoms. The internal response to this stress may also result in an increase in blood pressure and heart rate. Obviously, there are many factors that can upset a person's internal environment.

The external environment consists of more than the physical surroundings. It consists of all events and influences that occur externally and that impact a person's health status and functional abilities. Responses to our external environment are contextually based and reflect our own individual interpretation of the environment. Reactions to the external environment may or may not lead to health-promoting changes. A person, for example, who lives in a highly polluted area of a metropolitan city may decide to move to a less polluted area in order to improve his or her health. On the other hand, there are people who, because of their living conditions, believe that they can do little to effect healthy changes. These people, however, can be self-directed and do as much as possible to change their external environment. For example, people living in housing projects or tenements that are filthy and drug or cockroach infested will be impacted by these conditions. They may not have the choice to move elsewhere or change very much about their living conditions, but they can implement changes that impact their health, such as cleaning their homes. People can be catalysts in changing the external environment and thus promote changes in themselves and others.

Recognition of the interdependence and continuous interaction between the internal and external environments is important. This interdependence and subsequent interaction can lead to either health promotion or illness. Choices that people make impact them and their environment. These choices are reflected internally, such as might occur because of poor eating habits, or externally as might occur as a result of overexposure to the environment or our relationships with our family, peers, friends, and society. Figure 2-3 demonstrates how our external environment can affect our well-being.

Health

Although the concept of health is essential to defining nursing's metaparadigm, it is important to note that there is no current consensus on what actually constitutes good health. In fact, there is probably more agreement on what constitutes poor health. Within the last three

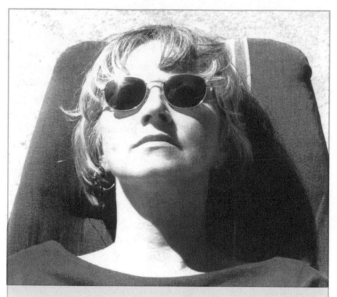

FIGURE 2-3 *Excessive exposure to the sun can be harmful to our health.*

Ask Yourself

The External Environment and Health

The sun is important in maintaining health. Studies have shown that lack of sunlight can cause depression in some people. The sun is also important for our nutritional health. Excessive exposure to the sun, however, can cause detrimental effects. What do you consider excessive exposure? What kind of damage can occur if a person is overexposed to the sun? How many hours do you expose yourself to the sun?

decades, the view of health has changed dramatically. In the late 1950s and the 1960s, for example, the health care field was influenced by Dunn's (1959) definition of health. This definition indicated that the concepts of health and illness were two diametrically opposed views; that is, a person who had experienced any symptoms of disease, whether in an acute or a remission state, could not be considered healthy. Since that time, the definition of health has evolved to include the view that health and illness exist on a continuum ranging from health and wellness on one end to illness and death on the other. Accordingly, then, there are degrees of health and illness. Most contemporary nursing leaders agree with this view.

The concept of health is central to nursing because all the actions and responsibilities integral to nursing involve aspects of health. Health is a central concept because nurses and clients interact when there is a health need. Today's nurse is taught to view health as an always changing, never static state that is determined by internal or external influences. These influences can be self-directed, as in the case of a young woman who decides to smoke although she is aware of the risks involved. Other influences are external, such as in the case of the youth who decides to drink or do drugs because of peer pressure. In any case, these internal and external influences can result in health or illness depending on the value placed on health by the individual involved.

Definitions of Health

There are several approaches to describing the health status of an individual. One approach is to describe health in terms of the role of the person in society. This approach views persons as being healthy if they are able to meet their role obligations; that is, if a person can still work or can assume the role of a parent, then that person is considered healthy. Other approaches to defining health include determining health status by finding out if a person is free from disease, can adapt to changes in the internal or external environment, or is in a state of self-identified complete well-being where the focus is self-actualization (Smith, 1983). Nursing, too, usually describes health in relation to a person's functioning in society. If a person is functioning at the best level possible, then that person is considered healthy.

Loveland-Cherry (2000) takes Smith's ideas farther and defines health in terms of the total functioning of the family. Family health is seen as the abilities and resources that are available to a family to accomplish its developmental tasks. If the family is able to perform effectively as a unit, then the family is healthy. There are other definitions of health that focus on the community. Community health is dependent on individual health as well as on the social, physical, and political arenas that are present to support a healthy life (Pender, Murdaugh, & Parsons, 2006).

Health is not only a state of physical functioning but is also a concept that encompasses the total functioning of a person. That is, health refers to the ability of persons to function effectively physically, socially, psychologically, and spiritually. In this context, effective physical functioning refers to the ability of the body structures to change and adapt, thus resulting in a positive health status. Effective social functioning relates to the ability of a person to interact in a meaningful fashion and to form relationships with others, recognizing that people are all different and come from diverse backgrounds.

Likewise, an individual who is in a positive state of psychological health has the ability to problem solve, manage stress and crisis, and respond in an appropriate emotional manner to the situations confronted. A positive health status also includes the spiritual domain of a person. The belief in a higher power, whether it is God or some other power source, is essential to maintaining overall health. Spirituality also includes other aspects of a person's total health such as ethical standards, moral character, and values. It is the total positive functioning of a person within the domains just described that constitutes a healthy state, leads to a fulfilling life, and results in **homeostasis,** or a state of equilibrium within the body.

Nursing

The last concept found in nursing's metaparadigm is probably the most important one to consider. Although it is difficult, if not impossible, to use a concept to describe itself, nurse theorists usually describe nursing in terms of what the nurse does for the client (Fawcett, 2005). Nursing is the reason nurses come together with the client and interact with him or her. While it is important to consider the concepts of person, environment, and health, it is the interaction among these three concepts that becomes the focus of nursing care.

Nurses work with culturally diverse people in a variety of settings and assist in meeting health care needs of individual clients, groups, society, and the world community. As such, nursing practice extends into all areas of the health care delivery system. Nursing provides a service which assists people to increase their knowledge, prevent illness, maintain or regain an optimum state of health, or cope with death and the dying process. It is obvious, then, that nurses have multiple responsibilities and assume the roles of care provider, teacher, counselor, helper, and health promotion resource in addition to those roles commonly associated with the profession. See Chapter 4 for the roles that nurses commonly assume when engaged in health promotion.

NURSING AS A PROFESSION

The characteristics of the discipline of nursing fit well with criteria commonly found in a profession. Nursing is considered to be a profession in that it is based on a body of knowledge, abides by its own ethical code, has established professional standards, and requires that nurses assume accountability for their own actions. In addition, professional nursing is taught in institutions of higher learning, usually a university or college, whose curriculum includes education in the research process and the science of inquiry. Nursing also has its own professional associations which espouse the principles of the profession and safeguard nursing's interest. The most recognized of these associations is the American Nurses Association. Other broad nursing associations include the National League for Nursing and the American Association of Colleges of Nursing, the primary voice for baccalaureate and graduate education.

NURSING EDUCATIONAL LEVELS AND HEALTH PROMOTION

Knowledge and competencies of registered nurses directly relate to educational preparation. Nurses function to meet the demands placed on them by society and the nursing profession according to their educational background. Education has a significant impact on the competencies and knowledge base of nurse clinicians (American Association of Colleges of Nursing, 2005a). Employers are urged to take note of and capitalize on the education and experiences provided by the various educational programs that lead to the registered nurse designation. Nurses should be used according to their educational capacities.

There are several routes to becoming a registered nurse. These educational pathways include diploma, associate degree in nursing, and baccalaureate degree programs. Graduates of all RN programs sit for the same National Council Licensure Exam-RN (NCLEX-RN). Education for these RN pathways can take place in a variety of settings.

The registered nurse with a diploma or associate degree can be further educated through a **career ladder** or a degree completion program. A career ladder approach focuses on transitioning from one educational level to the next. Registered nurses choosing a career ladder approach can expect to improve their nursing care and general nursing practice. A career ladder approach leads to a better educated nursing workforce. Clinical competencies and improved patient outcomes can be expected with additional nursing preparation.

All registered nurse preparation programs include a foundation of basic sciences and focus on critical thinking, problem solving skills, leadership skills, and health promotion. The amount of preparation on each concept depends on the type of program undertaken. The acquisition of knowledge on health promotion concepts, skills, and behaviors can be differentiated according to competencies of the program graduates.

Graduate nursing education programs also differ in terms of the expected competencies related to health promotion. Graduate nursing education programs include Master of Science in Nursing (MSN) and doctoral nursing preparation programs with a particular focus area. MSN programs may be clinical practice oriented or may be more theoretical or research directed. Nursing doctoral programs are more research oriented and prepare students to pursue intellectual inquiry (American Association of Colleges of Nursing, 2001). There are several pathways to receiving a doctorate in nursing. Doctoral programs are varied and may include a PhD in Nursing (PhD), a Doctor of Nursing Science degree (DNS, DSN, or DNSc), and a Nursing Doctorate degree (ND). AACN members endorsed a position statement on the Practice Doctorate (DNP), which will move the current level of preparation for advanced nursing practice from the master's degree to the doctorate level by 2015 (AACN, 2005b). Table 2-2 on page 28 demonstrates how health promotion competencies differ according to educational preparation.

INTEGRATING HEALTH PROMOTION CONCEPTS INTO NURSING PRACTICE

Any definition of nursing will include those activities that are specific to nursing. These definitions focus on what nurses do for clients, their families, and significant others and usually include such activities as caring for clients, assisting those that cannot do for themselves, and teaching clients how to care for themselves. All these activities involve the concept of health promotion and lead to formulation of several assumptions essential to integrating health promotion into nursing practice. These assumptions help blend health promotion with those concepts found in the metaparadigm on nursing and are an eclectic view of some of the assumptions described by several nursing theorists, including Imogene King, Dorothea Orem, Martha Rogers, and Sister Callista Roy (see Box 2-3).

Assumptions

The first assumption listed in Box 2-3 is critical to professional nurses engaging in health promoting activities. Nurses who are effective in implementing health promotion strategies realize that people are self-directing and make important decisions daily that have long-lasting consequences. These decisions can make the difference in terms of achieving optimum health. The fact that people can direct their own life means that, for the most part, they can promote or destroy their health. The ability to think abstractly and critically is only found in humans and is essential to making appropriate decisions. Choices affecting health can range from simple to very complex. For example, a client's health promotion decision can be as simple as deciding to exercise for 30 minutes a day. On the other hand, a client's decision to undergo coronary bypass surgery instead of conservative treatment with cardiotonic drugs is infinitely more complex. The nurse's knowledge of the consequences associated with any of the client's choices is essential. For a nurse who recognizes professional responsibilities in promoting health, it is important to provide clients with accurate information that may influence their decisions and, ultimately, their lives.

Professional nurses engaged in health promotion activities should also recognize the influences of the environment on client outcomes. As stated in assumption two, the effects of the environment can have long-standing consequences on a person's health. That is, if the environment is not a healthy one that is conducive to promoting quality of life, health promotion may no longer be possible unless certain changes occur in the environment. A positive environment increases quality of life and adds to inner and outer stability and wellness. A household environment, for example, where there is constant bickering or strife or one that has mentally ill members can be very stressful. Long-term stress can have deleterious effects on the body and mind (Selye, 1974; Frisch & Frisch, 2006). The nurse who recognizes the impact of environmental factors on clients understands the importance of treating people in a **holistic** manner—that is, in their unique totality.

The assumption that everyone is capable of learning and adapting is critical to promoting health in our society. However, although human beings are quite capable of learning, there are several factors that can limit learning. For example, if people are not motivated to learn those things that will lead to healthy and productive lives, their capacity to learn is irrelevant. People decide what they need to know and are willing to do or not do regardless of any disabilities (Craven & Hirnle, 2004). Additionally, the ability to adapt internally or externally can be either effective or ineffective. A reason for stressing people's capacity to learn and adapt in this assumption is that a major nursing focus is to improve the health behaviors of clients and to assist them to adjust to changes in their lives. Nurses impact health behaviors of clients through their roles as caregivers and client educators.

BOX 2-3 Assumptions Essential to Integrating Health Promotion into Nursing Practice

1. People have the capacity for self-direction, abstraction, and critical thinking.
2. The environment can affect a person's ability to live a long and prosperous life.
3. People are capable of learning and adapting and can be made aware of those things that promote well-being.
4. As open systems, people are capable of change.
5. People are biological, psychological, social, and cultural beings who form families and/or networks.
6. Communication, both verbal and nonverbal, is essential to the achievement of health throughout the life span.

TABLE 2-2 Nursing Educational Preparation and Health Promotion Competencies

Program Preparation	Typical Years of Study	Educational Setting	Select Health Promotion Competencies
Associate Degree	2	Community College	Provide nursing care for a limited number of individuals, families, or both. Collaborate with individuals to provide or coordinate health promotion. Develop and implement teaching plans for individuals, families, or both concerning health promotion and maintenance and restoration of health. Implement nursing care to promote health and manage acute and chronic health problems.
Diploma	3	Hospital	Provide nursing care for a limited number of individuals, families, or both. Collaborate with individuals to provide or coordinate health promotion. Develop/implement teaching plans concerning health promotion and maintenance and restoration of health. Implement nursing care to promote health and manage acute and chronic health problems.
Baccalaureate Degree	4	Senior College or University	Includes all of the above plus: Provide nursing care for individuals, families, and groups. In-depth knowledge of health promotion concepts. Implement comprehensive teaching plans to meet health promotion learning needs of patients, families, and groups. Perform comprehensive assessments relative to factors impacting health status and needs. Possess holistic understanding of health care and approaches to health care, including health promotion.
Master of Science in Nursing	2–3 years following BSN	Senior College or University	Includes all of the above plus: Use epidemiological, social, and environmental data in assessing the health status of populations (individuals, families, groups, and communities). Develop and monitor holistic plans of care addressing health promotion and disease prevention needs of populations (individuals, families, groups, communities). Incorporate theories and research in developing strategies to promote and preserve health. Empower populations (individuals, families, groups, communities) in attaining and maintaining functional wellness.
Nursing Doctorate	3–6 years following MSN	University	Includes all of the above competencies plus: Influence regulatory, legislative, and public policy to promote health and preserve healthy communities. Incorporate theories and research in developing strategies to promote and preserve health. Empower populations (individuals, families, groups, communities) in attaining and maintaining functional wellness.

Sources: *American Association of Colleges of Nursing, (2005a),* The Impact of Education on Nursing Practice; *American Association of Colleges of Nursing, (1995),* A Model for Differentiated Nursing Practice; *The Board of Nurse Examiners for the State of Texas & Texas Board of Vocational Nurse Examiners, (September 2002),* Differentiated Entry Level Competencies of Graduates of Texas Nursing Programs.

Everyone is capable of changing his or her behavior, whether in a positive or negative direction. Belief in this assumption is vital in order for nurses and their clients to effectively carry out health promotion activities. People never remain static, but are always interacting and communicating with their environment. The ultimate goal is the achievement of homeostasis or stability while continually adjusting and changing. Nurses promote positive changes in clients through client teaching, client advocacy, caregiving, and consulting and collaborating with other members of the health care team.

Assumption five recognizes that people have sociocultural characteristics and cannot be cared for in isolation. It is important to realize that the word "client" does not necessarily refer only to the person receiving the care, but may include the person, her or his family, significant others, social group, or community. For instance, dietary teaching for a diabetic client might be ineffective if the client is the only one to receive instruction. To increase the effectiveness of instruction and future compliance with the diet, the lesson on diabetic diet planning logically may include the client, spouse, family, significant other, or anyone else who cares and cooks for the client.

Communication ability is essential to promoting a healthy lifestyle. It is important to note that one of the unique characteristics of people is their ability to communicate both with words and with actions and expressions. This ability allows them to communicate their needs to others and proves to be quite useful in satisfying needs. Appropriate communication skills can assist people in achieving optimum well-being. This ability to communicate also provides a means to interact socially, an essential component of a full and productive life.

We primarily rely on our verbal communication skills as well as those of our clients in order to obtain an adequate interpretation of a situation. For a competent nurse, the ability to determine what a client has said or not said or to interpret other forms of nonverbal communication enhances caring skills and assists in achieving desired outcomes for client care. Astute observation of the client's verbal and nonverbal behaviors is essen-

tial to providing quality nursing care. Likewise, it is essential to remember that the nurse's own verbal and nonverbal behaviors can communicate many things to the client as well. The quality of the nurse-client relationship is related to the quality of communication between the nurse and the client (Craven & Hirnle, 2004). Chapter 5 provides further discussion on the impact of communication skills on educating others about health promotion.

Research Note

Use of the Health-Promoting Self-Care System Model to Predict Health Behaviors in Older Men

Study Problem/Purpose: To explore the relationships among health motivation, self-rated health, and health behaviors among community-dwelling older men. Elderly males are thought to value health less, participate in fewer health screenings, have shorter life expectancies, and allow illness to progress longer than their female counterparts. This study examined the motivational systems that lead older males to adopt health-promoting behaviors. The Health-Promoting Self-Care System Model was the conceptual framework which guided this study.

Methods: The sample consisted of 135 community-dwelling men 55 years old and older. A descriptive correlational design was used. The sample was given a questionnaire packet consisting of a demographic tool, the Older Men's Health Program and Screening Inventory, the Health Promotion Activities of Older Adults Measure, and the Health Self-Determinism Index.

Findings: Older men with more internal motivation rated their health as better and assessed their lifestyles as healthier. Anticipated benefits of health-promoting behaviors were significantly related to health-promoting behaviors, health program attendance, and health screening participation. There was no significant relationship between the Health Self-Determinism Index and any of the three variables.

Implications: Self-motivation may be the key to increasing perceptions of health and well-being in older men. A knowledge of the benefits of health promotion activities may increase older men's health screenings and program attendance.

Loeb, S. (2004). Older men's health: Motivation, self-ratings, and behaviors. *Nursing Research, 53*(3), 198–208.

THEORETICAL FOUNDATIONS

Theoretical or conceptual frameworks that encompass some of the assumptions discussed in the preceding section and that define nursing and its metaparadigm are useful in delineating health promotion activities. These theoretical/conceptual frameworks not only guide the nursing profession by addressing the four central concepts found in nursing's metaparadigm, but also serve as the bases for hypotheses testing that adds to nursing's body of knowledge. These frameworks, then, can serve as a springboard for nursing research through theory building and their application in problem solving. There are several theoretical frameworks and conceptual models that are commonly used in defining nursing. Although the following theoretical frameworks are found in most of the literature describing nursing, they are not totally inclusive. Among the most common frameworks used are systems theory, adaptation theory, needs theory, human becoming and human care theory, and transcultural theory. The accompanying research note demonstrates how a theoretical framework can be used in nursing research related to health promotion.

Systems Theory

General systems theory was described by Von Bertalanffy in 1968 and has been helpful to nursing theorists in describing the relationship between people, health, and their environment. This theory focuses on the exchange of energy between the individual and the environment and has as its central concept that a person is whole and more than a sum of parts. The person interacts with the environment continuously in a reciprocal and open manner; that is, people influence and change their environment, and the environment influences and changes people. Health promotion activities thus result from client self-direction. The environment has an impact on the health promotion activities and direction that an individual chooses to take. An overweight person, for example, can choose to diet and stock only healthy food in the refrigerator and pantry or

may choose to ignore obesity and keep fattening foods available for snacking. Regardless of the choice, the person's environment does include choices on the healthy or unhealthy foods that influence the individual's health. Systems theory proposes that change is self-directed, that the environment influences the course of this direction, and that change occurs continuously. Change creates energy fields and these energy fields include the client and his or her internal and external environments. The energy fields created by change are always evolving and never remain static (Fawcett, 2005). A client's choices on what foods to eat, such as in the above example, create these energy fields that eventually result in changes in health status.

Systems theory identifies systems and subsystems and proposes that these can interact and exchange energy with the environment. The individual, client, group, society, and community are considered to be systems. Other theorists have also incorporated aspects of this theory in their frameworks describing nursing.

Adaptation Theory

Adaptation theory has also been used by several nurse theorists to describe and define nursing. The major concepts in this theory include change, adaptation, and coping. **Adaptation,** in this context, refers to the process of changing behavior in response to external or internal stimuli or surroundings. That is, the client is seen as an adapting system capable of controlling individual responses. The environment, whether it is internal or external, stimulates the individual to respond or change accordingly (Carper, 2002). Everyone has adaptation levels that are unique and constantly changing. Not all of the adaptive responses, however, are considered appropriate or effective. Health and illness are responses to the adaptation process. Sister Callista Roy's *Adaptation Model* is based on adaptation theory and focuses on how this process affects nursing and health (Gallagher-Galbreath, 2002).

Adaptation theory is useful in describing why people behave in certain ways and in explaining why people choose or do not choose to participate in their own health promotion. The previous example of the overweight person is useful in demonstrating how this person might adapt and also illustrates the relationship between adaptation theory and health promotion. If an overweight male cannot climb a flight of stairs without experiencing difficulty catching his breath, he may respond or adapt by taking the elevator instead of the stairs next time. In much the same way, this person's internal environment makes several attempts to adapt. The increased effort required to climb those stairs forces the lungs to increase their respiratory efforts and thus provide needed oxygenation for the entire body. This obvious adaptive response will result in the overweight person's huffing and puffing and experiencing facial flushing while he climbs the stairs.

Needs Theory

Needs theory may be used interchangeably with goals theory or self-deficit theory. This theory describes all people as having common needs that must be met and that are essential for maintaining optimum health. People's needs may sometimes be confused with what they want, but these are two separate concepts. A need is usually defined as a requirement that has not been met. A want is something desirable, but not essential. **Needs theory** describes people as whole with many complex needs that motivate behavior. Everyone meets his or her needs in a unique way and may defer satisfying needs if they are not viewed as a priority at that time. Health promotion activities and needs are person-centered unless they cannot or will not be met by the person.

Needs theory may be used to explain health promotion activities because health promotion behaviors are motivated by need. For example, a student may stay up all night to cram for an exam on the following day. This student may respond to the need for sleep by going home to bed after the exam. This, however, may not happen because health behaviors are also influenced by individual values. If the student has another important exam the next day, the student may choose to forego sleep in favor of staying awake and studying. Dorothea Orem's *Self-Care Deficit Theory* (2001) is based on needs theory.

Human Becoming Theory and Human Care Theory

Human becoming and human care theories, developed in the late 1980s, have common philosophical roots. Both of these theories are useful in describing the nature of nursing and are based in humanistic and existential philosophy. These theories may also be useful in describing nursing's metaparadigm.

Rosemarie Parse's theory is based on human becoming and existence. Her book *Illuminations: The Human Becoming Theory in Practice and Research* (1995) was developed from her theory entitled *Man-Living-Health* (1981). This theory, in turn, evolved from some of Martha Rogers's principles and concepts, stated in her *Science of Unitary Human Beings Theory* (Hickman, 2002b). Parse's theory revolves around the concept of person and a person's interactions within the environment. Parse sees people as having choices in providing meaning to situations and as bearing responsibility for decisions. Parse maintains that people choose values, have their own way of living, and grow more diverse and complex in time (Fawcett, 2005).

Many caring conceptual frameworks are based on Jean Watson's original work. Watson is best known for her theory on caring, in which she sees the nursing role as a collective caring-healing role (1979). She is one of the first theorists to support the concept that people have souls and a spiritual dimension to their being. The

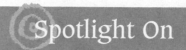
Spotlight On

Culture and Health

In certain cultures, the role of the woman is to take care of the children and the spouse. If this woman is unable to care for her children, her spouse, or her house, she is considered to be ill-equipped to be a parent or spouse. Consequently, she may be thought to exhibit symptoms commonly associated with poor health.

essence of her theory of human caring, also referred to as *Watson's Theory of Transpersonal Caring* (1996), is authentic caring that preserves dignity and the wholeness of humanity. The major conceptual elements of the theory are transpersonal caring, ten carative factors, and caring in general (Kelly & Johnson, 2002, p. 408).

In some respects, both the human becoming and caring theories are central to the discipline of nursing. Concepts in these theories can be easily incorporated into nursing practice. These theories provide a framework for working with human beings, taking into consideration the uniqueness of each.

Transcultural Theory

According to George (2002), Madeleine Leininger was the first nurse theorist to use the term "transcultural nursing" (p. 490). Since then, **transcultural nursing theory** has become quite popular and reflects nursing's and society's beliefs regarding the importance of culture and its effects on the total functioning of an individual. The major concepts found in this theory are human care, influence of culture, worldwide view of individuals, cultural congruence, commonality of needs, and diversity.

Transcultural theory focuses on the individual and describes how culture influences and provides meaning to everything that a person does, thinks, feels, or hears. A person is perceived to be a complex biological, psychological, social, spiritual, and caring being with meaningful patterns that vary among cultures. A person's culture provides meaning to health and illness and must be appreciated by the nurse in assisting clients with their health promotion activities and behaviors. If the person's culture is not considered in planning care, noncompliance with treatment will occur and will result in further delay in recovery.

According to this theory, health and illness cannot be defined because there are no universally accepted definitions for these concepts. Transcultural theory, however, proposes that health and illness are determined by the particular views of individual cultures.

Human behavior is influenced by the cultural context within which it occurs. It is the nurse's responsibility to bring cultural congruence and **cultural congruent care** to clients by utilizing the client's cultural lifeways and norms. Cultural congruent care is care that is provided to fit with an individual's, group's, or institution's values, beliefs, and lifeways. Cultural congruent care is necessary to provide meaningful and satisfying health care services to those in need of health care (Leininger, 2001). Transcultural theory maintains that nurses are responsible for linking the client's culture with the health care delivery system. Transcultural nursing theory can be used in planning client care and promoting, restoring, and maintaining health. The competent nurse uses a transcultural theory framework in all aspects of her or his professional role.

ORGANIZING NURSING THEORY

One of the goals of nursing theory is to describe nursing's metaparadigm in terms of those concepts essential to professional nursing practice. These same concepts are useful in organizing the theoretical frameworks previously described and may be useful in the development of a personal definition or philosophy of nursing.

Nursing's Metaparadigm and Nursing Theory

The various nursing theorists have used the concepts of person, environment, health, and nursing in their development of nursing theory. Virginia Henderson (1966), for example, in her development of a definition for nursing, viewed the human being as a biological, psychological, spiritual, and social being. She refers to people as having basic needs that can be categorized into 14 components of nursing functions. In much the same way, King (1971), in her Theory of Goal Attainment, describes the person as a social, sentient, rational, reacting, perceiving, time-oriented, cognitive human being. Pender (1996), the leading nurse proponent of a health promotion model, states that people are capable of determining their own health status and that they create conditions in order to express their uniqueness. Other theorists view the concept of person as just described but also include cultural characteristics as well as transcultural variances of human beings (Leininger, 1978). All of the major nursing theorists organize their theories by addressing nursing's metaparadigm concept of person.

Likewise, nursing theory addresses the concept of environment. King (1971), for example, sees people and their environment as being in continuous interaction. She identifies the environment as consisting of both a person's internal and external environments. Likewise, Sister Callista Roy (1974a, 1974b) in her adaptation model describes the interactions that occur between

Spotlight On

Providing Cultural Congruent Care

A Mexican-American mother brings her irritable baby to the clinic. In talking to the nurse, the mother states that her baby has been sick since she took him to a birthday party where he was admired by all of the guests but no one touched him. She fears that he has been given *mal de ojo*, or evil eye. The mother has attempted to cure him through prayer and rubbing his body with an egg. The nurse assesses the child and takes into consideration what the mother has told her and the mother's cultural beliefs. A nurse who accepts the client's own approach to health care is accepting of the client and family's cultural worldview and is providing cultural congruent care.

people and their environment. She, too, sees the environment as consisting of all that surrounds or influences a person. According to Callista Roy, the environment can be described as including both the internal and external environments. Martha Rogers, too, focused on the role of the environment and included this concept in her Science of Unitary Human Beings Theory (Roger, 1970; Garon, 2002). Rogers identified people and their environment as energy fields interacting as whole entities and having their own identity. People and their environmental fields are integral to one another.

The concept of health is also described by nursing theorists. King (1971) describes health as a dynamic state occurring in all life cycles. Roy (1974a, 1974b, 1999), too, describes health and illness as part of life's processes. She believes that if people adapt to their surroundings then health will be achieved. It is only when adaptation does not occur that a person becomes ill. Nursing theorists have also described health as being defined according to society's perception. For instance, in some societies, obesity is an acceptable norm. Leininger (1978, 2001) recognizes society's influence on health and notes that health is primarily culturally defined. She describes health as being influenced by the value that the culture places on a person's abilities to perform certain tasks. Pender, Murdaugh, and Parsons (2006), on the other hand, focus on the concept of health in relation to health promotion. They state that being free of symptoms of disease does not necessarily mean that a person is healthy. They describe health always in the context of illness and believe that optimum health as well as poor health can exist with or without illness (p. 19). Pender (1996) acknowledges that a healthy status provides a sense of empowerment. She believes that a person engaging in health promoting behavior can achieve health and, ultimately, can be quite powerful in achieving life's goals. Chapter 3 discusses Pender's and other nurse theorists' models of health and health promotion in more detail.

The concept of nursing, of course, is of major importance in developing and organizing nursing theory. It is a generally held belief that nursing is an art and a science. The art of nursing involves the actual skills that are used in administering care to clients. The science of nursing relates to the ability of the discipline to apply knowledge of scientific principles to caring for clients and to generate new knowledge through research. Orem's (2001) description of nursing seems to capture the essence of this concept. She defines nursing as a service that helps human beings who are unable to help themselves. Nursing is based on actions deliberately selected and performed by nurses to help individuals or groups to maintain or change their conditions (Renpenning & Taylor, 2003). King (1971), on the other hand, sees nursing as a process of action, reaction, interaction, and transaction used to meet basic needs of individuals (p. 25). The major nursing theorists describe nursing concerns, goals, and functions. Table 2-3 describes selected nurse theorist's views of nursing's metaparadigm and the relationship of health promotion to each.

SUMMARY

Health promotion is an essential concept within contemporary society. This concept is continuously highlighted by the various health professions and is a driving force in the establishment of initiatives useful to the achievement of optimum health. The importance of this concept to nursing is evident by the number of documents that cite promotion of health as a nursing goal. These documents clearly identify nursing's responsibility in promoting efforts to meet health needs in the community served.

Health promotion as a conceptual framework is useful to defining nursing practice and is reflected in nursing's metaparadigm. This metaparadigm uses concepts and theories that collectively or individually describe the profession and organizes nursing's metaparadigm around four central concepts: person, health, environment, and nursing. A nursing metaparadigm integrating health promotion concepts describes the profession in relation to activities that assist individuals and families, prevent illness, maintain health, and promote optimum well-being.

Several assumptions are critical to integrating health promotion concepts into nursing practice. These assumptions are primarily related to characteristics inherent in human beings. In order to successfully incorporate health promotion into practice, nurses must assume that a person is self-directing, is capable of learning, is capable of change, possesses a complex makeup, and is able to communicate her or his own needs. It is also important to assume that the environment can have a dramatic effect on a person's optimum health and life span.

Theoretical frameworks are useful in defining nursing and its metaparadigm and in delineating health promotion activities. These frameworks form the bases for hypotheses testing and for formal nursing research, and add to nursing's body of knowledge through research findings. Among the most common frameworks used are systems theory, adaptation theory, needs theory, human becoming and human care theory, and transcultural theory.

The concept of health is central to nursing because all actions integral to nursing involve aspects of health. Nursing is the reason we come together with the client. It is the interaction of the concepts of person, environment, and health that becomes the focus of our nursing care. Nursing provides a service that assists people to increase their awareness, prevent illness, maintain or regain health, or cope with death and the dying process.

Key Concepts

1. The concept of health promotion is essential to prevention of disease, maintenance of health, and defining of optimum health.

2. Health promotion provides an organizing framework useful in defining nursing.

3. Metaparadigms provide a global perspective of nursing and help to critically evaluate concepts characteristic of the nursing discipline.

4. Nursing theories utilize the four concepts described in nursing's metaparadigm: person, health, environment, and nursing.

5. People are holistic, biological, psychological, social, and spiritual beings with common needs.

6. The environment consists of internal and external influences that can affect personal functioning.

7. There is no consensus on what constitutes health; health may be viewed as a continuum or as the opposite of illness.

8. Knowledge on health promotion concepts, skills, and behavior can be differentiated according to graduate competencies.

9. Systems theory focuses on exchanges of energy between systems and subsystems and/or people and their environment; adaptation theory focuses on change and effective adaptive responses; needs theory can explain client and nurse behaviors; human becoming and human care theories focus on humanistic and existential philosophies; transcultural theory focuses on the cultural meaning of health and illness.

Nurse Theorist	Concept of Person	Concept of Environment
Florence Nightingale (1860) Environmental Theory of Nursing	Consists of physical, intellectual, spiritual, and social attributes. Concept of person defined only in terms of the individual's relationship with her or his environment.	Environment is major cause of disease.
Virginia Henderson (1966, 1991) Nature of Nursing	Biological, psychological, spiritual, social being; individual is a whole person with various fundamental needs. The person has 14 basic needs.	No major emphasis placed on environment; however, she does state that friends and family impact health status.
Martha Rogers (1970, 1990) Science of Unitary Human Beings Theory	Open systems, composed of more than the sum of their parts and characterized by their energy systems, and capacity for abstraction, imagery, language, and thought.	People and their environment are central to one another and are defined as energy fields; environmental fields are whole, irreducible, indivisible, and characterized by wave patterns that change continuously.
Imogene King (1971) Theory of Goal Attainment	Responsive, perceptive, goal-directed, time-oriented, cognitive, social being; utilizes mind, body, and energy in reacting to past and present experiences and events. A person functions in social systems through interpersonal relationships in terms of individual perceptions that influence his or her life and health.	Continual exchange between people and their environment; environment consists of both internal and external environments. All of society must be involved in achieving health.
Dorothea Orem (2001) Self-Care Theory	Persons who provide own self-care or care for others have specialized capabilities for action. All human beings have requisites for self-care, some of which are common to all human beings.	Total environment consists of psychosocial and physical environments.

Concept of Health	Definitions of Nursing	Relationship to Health Promotion
Emphasizes impact of environmental factors on health. Symptoms of disease are due to lack of fresh air, light, cleanliness, pure water, and efficient drainage.	The goal of nursing is to "put the client in the best condition for nature to act upon him" (p. 75). "Nursing ought to assist the reparative process" (p. 6).	Health promotion is primarily environment- and nurse-centered; disease occurs because of nature. "Real knowledge of the laws of health alone can check this" (p. 73). Health promotion focuses on eliminating environmental factors that cause disease.
Health is present if a person is not deprived of what he values or needs and is, then, able to maintain his own independence.	"The unique function of the nurse is to assist the individual sick or well, in the performance of those activities contributing to health or its recovery (or to peaceful death) that he would perform unaided if he had the necessary strength, will, or knowledge. And to do this in such as way as to help him gain independence as rapidly as possible" (1991, p. 21).	Health promotion is person-centered. Individuals are responsible for own health promotion. If individual is unable to perform duties that promote health, a nurse assists the client by providing what is lacking, carrying out prescribed treatment, and reducing discomfort if death is imminent.
Health is a value term and consists of those behaviors valued by individuals or cultures. Health and sickness are part of life processes.	Nursing science is the study of unitary, irreducible, indivisible human and environmental fields (1990).	In order to promote health, people must be considered in their totality, which must include the environment. Health promotion focuses on people and their environment. Health promotion activities are client-centered.
Health is a dynamic state that occurs as a result of continuous adaptation to stress; health is an ever-changing state of being; it cannot be completely achieved because it is not a static state.	"Nursing is a process of action, reaction, interaction, and transaction whereby nurses assist individuals of any age and socio-economic group to meet their basic needs in performing activities of daily living and to cope with health and illness at some particular point in the life cycle" (p. 25).	The importance of health promotion to a person is dependent on his or her perceptions of its value. Health promotion consists of utilization of resources to achieve maximum potential.
Self-care requirements that are not met constitute a health deviation. Health describes the state of wholeness or integrity of human beings. Temporary indispositions do not mean a person is not healthy.	"Nursing has as its special concern the individual's need for self-care action and the provision and management of it on a continuous basis in order to sustain life and health, and recover from disease or injury, and cope with their effects".	Person-centered health promotion consists of self-care activities that sustain life and regulate disease; health promotion activities consist of knowledge-seeking actions, assistance if necessary, control of external factors, resource-using actions, and self-control.

Nurse Theorist	Concept of Person	Concept of Environment
Sister Callista Roy (1974a, 1974b) Roy Adaptation Model	Open adaptive systems influenced by the world within and around; individual is a biopsychosocial being consisting of elements linked in such a way that force on the linkages can be increased or decreased.	People and their environment are in constant interaction with each other; the environment consists of all that surrounds or influences the development of a person.
Madeleine Leininger (1978) Culturel Care Diversity and Universality Theory	People are holistic and possess common cultural care values, beliefs, and practices. Human beings vary transculturally. Concept of person includes individuals, families, institutions, and cultures. Best source of information is the client.	Consists of totality of events, situations, or experiences; relates to physical, ecological, sociopolitical, and cultural settings.
Rosemarie Parse (1995) Theory of Human Becoming	Humans are open, unitary; they freely choose meaning in situations and bear responsibility. Humans are central to human becoming theory; they coexist while forming rhythmical patterns with the universe.	People and the universe are continuously interacting, co-constituting patterns of relating. Human beings and the universe are inseparable, complementary, and evolving together. The universe is made up of everything in a person's lived experience.
Jean Watson (1979, 1996) Theory of Transpersonal Caring	Human is a valued person greater than and different from the sum of his or her parts. A person can use the mind to attain higher levels of consciousness. People need each other in a caring way.	Environment is considered in the context of the human-environment field, perceived within a specific context, such as social or physical, or within the greater context of interacting within a phenomenological field.

10. The characteristics of the nursing discipline fit well with criteria commonly describing a profession.

11. Nursing theorists organize nursing theory by addressing nursing's metaparadigm concepts.

Learning Activities

1. Describe your nursing philosophy in writing. List at least 10 statements that reflect this philosophy.

2. Categorize the above statements in relation to the four concepts found in nursing's metaparadigm. (Some statements may fit in more than one category.)

   Person Health Environment Nursing

3. Describe why you selected the particular category(ies) for your belief statements. Be specific in your rationale by stating why the statement fits in a particular category.

True/False Questions

1. T or F The concept of health promotion is a new one to the nursing profession.

2. T or F Health promotion concepts are evident in the nursing profession standards.

3. T or F Nursing uses a metaparadigm to provide a global perspective of those concepts specific to nursing.

4. T or F Nursing theories reflect the concepts found in nursing's metaparadigm.

5. T or F The only nursing theoretical frameworks that are in current use are: adaptation theory, systems theory, transcultural theory, and needs theory.

6. T or F Maslow's hierarchy of needs describes the need for self-actualization as the highest level and most difficult to achieve.

Concept of Health	Definitions of Nursing	Relationship to Health Promotion
Health and illness are inevitable dimensions of life. Health is a state and process of being and becoming a whole person.	Goal of nursing is to promote adaptation and contribute to health by focusing on psychosocial needs, self-concept, roles, and interdependence relations.	Health promotion is goal of individuals and society. Health promotion activities focus on concept of adaptation.
Culturally defined state of well-being related to an individual's ability to perform daily role activities.	Conceptualized nursing as a transcultural human care discipline and profession. Goal of nursing is to provide cultural congruent care to individuals worldwide.	Society's cultural values influence health-promoting and care practices of individuals; health promotion activities occur only if cultural diversity is considered an important aspect.
Health is people's lived experience. It can be defined as a way of living, a personal commitment. It is a continuously changing process mutually cocreated through the human-universe experience.	Nursing is a basic science whose practice is a performing of art. Nursing involves innovation and creativity. Nursing's responsibility to society is to guide individuals in choosing possibilities in changing the health process.	Health promotion must consider the total lived experiences of an individual. Health promotion does not involve prescriptive approaches; rather, the client is the authority figure in the relationship and the prime decision maker in areas involving his health.
Health refers to unity and harmony within the mind, body, and soul; health is the degree of congruence between the perceived self and the self as experienced. Disease results from incongruences.	Nursing is carried out through human care and caring. Caring is the moral ideal of nursing, with the goal of helping another to gain self-knowledge, control, and healing.	The goal of health promotion is human care. Health promotion is directed toward care of the physical body within the context of the unity of mind, body, spirit, and nature.

Multiple Choice Questions

1. ANA's Standards of Nursing Practice:
   a. Describe a means of determining the quality of nursing services received.
   b. Establish a code of ethics that guides practice.
   c. Set competency levels for clinical only.
   d. Provide a framework for understanding nursing's relationship to society.

2. Of the following, which nurse would be most likely to incorporate theories and research in developing strategies to promote and preserve health?
   a. A nurse with an associate degree in nursing.
   b. A nurse with a Bachelor of Science in Nursing degree.
   c. A nurse with a doctorate in nursing.
   d. A nurse with a Master of Science in Nursing degree.

3. General systems theory focuses on:
   a. Goals and self-deficits identified by client.
   b. Changing behaviors through adaptation process.
   c. Complex needs that motivate behavior.
   d. The exchange of energy between an individual and the environment.

4. Transcultural nursing theory was originally described by which of the following nursing theorists?
   a. Sister Callista Roy
   b. Dorothea Orem
   c. Madeleine Leininger
   d. Martha Rogers

Websites

http://www.nche.edu Official website for the American Association of Colleges of Nursing (AACN); addresses education, research, advocacy, and data collection and provides a search site map for publications relevant to professional nursing.

http://www.nursingworld.org Official website for the American Nurses Association (ANA); provides information on ANA services, programs, and publications, and includes a search site map for items, articles, and issues of interest to professional nursing.

http://heapro.oxfordjournals.org Responds to the move for a new public health throughout the world and supports the development of action related to health promotion; contains refereed articles, reviews, and current debates related to health promotion.

http://www.enursescribe.com Provides a lifelong learning resource for nursing students, staff nurses, educators, and authors.

http://www.ncsbn.org For not-for-profit organizations whose members include the boards of nurse examiners for 50 states, the District of Columbia, and the five U.S. territories.

Organizations/Agencies

American Association of Colleges of Nursing (AACN)
One Dupont Circle, NW
Suite 530
Washington, DC 20036
Tel: (202) 463-6930
Fax: (202) 785-8320

This organization is the national voice for America's baccalaureate and higher-degree nursing education programs.

American Nurses Association (ANA)
8515 Georgia Avenue, Suite 400
Silver Spring, MD 20910
Tel: (800) 274-4ANA

This organization is the only full-service professional organization representing the nation's 2.7 million registered nurses through its 54 constituent member associations.

References

American Association of Colleges of Nursing. (1995). *A model for differentiated nursing practice.* http://www.aacn.nche.edu/Publications/DIFFMOD.PDF

American Association of Colleges of Nursing. (2001). Indicators of quality in research-focused doctoral programs in nursing. *AACN Position Statement.*

American Association of Colleges of Nursing. (2005a). The impact of education in nursing practice. *AACN Media Fact Sheets.*

American Association of Colleges of Nursing. (2005b). Frequently asked questions: Doctor of nursing practice (DNP) programs. *AACN Position Statement.*

American Nurses Association. (1998). *Standards of clinical nursing practice.* Washington, DC: American Nurses Publishing.

American Nurses Association. (2001). *Code of ethics for nurses with interpretive statements.* Washington, DC: American Nurses Publishing.

American Nurses Association. (2003). *Nursing: A social policy statement.* Washington, DC: American Nurses Publishing.

American Nurses Association. (2004). *Scope & standards of practice.* Washington, DC: The Publishing Program of ANA.

The Board of Nurse Examiners for the State of Texas & Texas Board of Vocational Nurse Examiners. (September 2002). *Differentiated entry level competencies of graduates of Texas nursing programs.* Austin, TX: Author. http://www.bne.state.tx.us

Carper, B. A. (2002). Fundamental patterns of knowing in nursing. In J. W. Kenney (Ed.), *Philosophical and theoretical perspectives for advanced nursing practice* (pp. 22–29). Sudbury, MA: Jones & Bartlett.

Craven, R. F., & Hirnle, C. J. (2004). *Fundamentals of nursing: Human health and function* (4th ed.). Philadelphia: Lippincott.

Dunn, H. (1959). High level wellness for man and society. *American Journal of Public Health, 49,* 786–792.

Fawcett, J. (2005). *Contemporary nursing knowledge: Analysis and evaluation of nursing models and theories.* Philadelphia: F. A. Davis.

Frisch, N. C., & Frisch, L. (2006). *Psychiatric mental health nursing* (3rd ed.). Clifton Park, NY: Thomson Delmar Learning.

Gallagher-Galbreath, J. (2002). Roy adaptation model: Sister Callista Roy. In J. B George (Ed.), *Nursing theories: The base for professional nursing practice* (pp. 295–338). Upper Saddle River, NJ: Prentice Hall.

Garon, M. (2002). Science of unitary human beings. In J. B. George (Ed.), *Nursing theories: The base for professional nursing practice* (5th ed.). Upper Saddle River, NJ: Prentice Hall.

George, J. B. (2002). Theory of culture care diversity and universality: Madeleine M. Leininger. In J. B George (Ed.), *Nursing theories: The base for professional nursing practice* (pp. 489–518). Upper Saddle River, NJ: Prentice Hall.

Henderson, V. (1966). *The nature of nursing: A definition and its implications for practice, research, and education.* New York: Macmillan.

Henderson, V. (1991). *The nature of nursing: Reflections after 25 years.* (Publ. No. 15-2346). New York: National League for Nursing.

Hickman, J. S. (2002a). An introduction to nursing theory. In J. B. George (Ed.), *Nursing theories: The base for professional nursing practice* (5th ed.). Upper Saddle River, NJ: Prentice Hall.

Hickman, J. S. (2002b). The theory of human becoming. In J. B. George (Ed.), *Nursing theories: The base for professional nursing practice* (5th ed.). Upper Saddle River, NJ: Prentice Hall.

Kelly, J. H., & Johnson, B. (2002). Theory of transpersonal caring: Jean Watson. In J. B. George (Ed.), *Nursing theories: The base for professional nursing practice* (5th ed.), pp. 405–425. Upper Saddle River, NJ: Prentice Hall.

Kerlinger, F. N. (1973). *Foundations of behavioral research* (2nd ed.), New York: Holt, Rinehart, & Winston.

King, I. (1971). *Toward a theory of nursing: General concepts of human behavior.* New York: John Wiley & Sons.

Leininger, M. M. (1978). *Transcultural nursing: Concepts, theories, and practice.* New York: John Wiley & Sons.

Leininger, M. (2001). *Culture care diversity and universality: A theory of nursing.* Boston: Jones & Bartlett.

Loeb, S. (2004). Older men's health: Motivation, self-ratings, and behaviors. *Nursing Research, 53*(3), 198–208.

Loveland-Cherry, C. J. (2000). Family health risks. In M. Stanhope & J. Lancaster (Eds.), *Community and public health nursing* (5th ed.). St. Louis: Mosby.

Maslow, A. (1970). *Motivation and personality.* New York: Harper & Row.

Maslow, A. (1999). *Toward a psychology of being.* New York: John Wiley & Sons.

Nightingale, F. (1860). *Notes on nursing: What it is and what it is not.* London: Gerald Duckworth.

Orem, D. E. (1980). *Nursing: Concepts of practice* (2nd ed). New York: McGraw-Hill.

Orem, D. (2001). *Nursing: Concepts of practice*. St. Louis: Mosby.

Parse, R. (1981). *Man-living-health: A theory of nursing*. New York: Wiley.

Parse, R. (1995). *Illuminations: The human becoming theory in practice and research*. New York: National League for Nursing Press.

Pender, N., Murdaugh, C. L., & Parsons, M. A. (2006). *Health promotion in nursing practice* (5th ed.). Upper Saddle River, NJ: Pearson Prentice Hall.

Pender, N. J. (1996). *Health promotion in nursing practice* (3rd ed.). Norwalk, CT: Appleton & Lange.

Polit, D. E., & Hungler, B. P. (2004). *Nursing research: Principles and methods* (7th ed.). Philadelphia: Lippincott Williams & Wilkins.

Renpenning, K. M., & Taylor, S. G. (2003). *Self-care theory in nursing: Selected papers of Dorothea Orem*. New York: Springer Publishing.

Rogers, M. (1970). *The theoretical basis of nursing*. Philadelphia: F. A. Davis.

Rogers, M. (1990). Nursing: Science of unitary, irreducible, human beings: Update 1990. In E. A. M. Barrett (Ed.), *Visions of Rogers' science-based nursing* (pp. 5–11). New York: National League for Nursing.

Roy, C. (1974a). *Introduction to nursing: An adaptation model*. Upper Saddle River, NJ: Prentice Hall.

Roy, C. (1974b). The Roy adaptation model. In J. P. Riehl & S. C. Roy (Eds.), *Conceptual models for nursing practice* (pp. 135–144). New York: Appleton & Lange.

Roy, C. (1999). *The Roy adaptation model*. Stamford, CT: Appleton & Lange.

Selye, H. (1974). *Stress without distress*. Philadelphia: Lippincott.

Smith, J. A. (1983). *The idea of health*. New York: Teachers College Press.

Taber. (2005). *Taber's cyclopedic medical dictionary* (20th ed.). Philadelphia: F. A. Davis.

Von Bertalanffy, L. (1968). *General systems theory: Foundations, development, and application*. New York: Braziller.

Watson, J. (1979). *Nursing: The philosophy and science of caring*. Boston: Little, Brown.

Watson, J. (1996). Watson's theory of transpersonal caring. In P. Hinton Walker & B. Neuman (Eds.), *Blueprint for use of nursing models* (pp. 141–184). New York: NLN Press.

Bibliography

Alligood, M. R., & Tomey-Mariner, A. (Eds.). (2002). *Nursing theory: Utilization and application*. St. Louis: Mosby.

Andrews, H. A., & Roy, C. (1986). *Essentials of the Roy adaptation model*. Norwalk, CT: Appleton-Century Crofts.

Boykin, A., & Schoenhofer, S. O. (2001). *Nursing as caring: A model for transforming practice*. Boston: Jones & Bartlett.

Catalano, J. (2006). *Nursing now! Today's issues, tomorrow's trends*. Philadelphia: F. A. Davis.

Chesnay, M. (Ed.). (2005). *Caring for the vulnerable: Perspectives in nursing theory, practice, and research*. Sudbury, MA: Jones & Bartlett.

Chin, P., & Kramer, M. K. (2004). *Integrated knowledge development in nursing*. St. Louis: Mosby.

Johnson-Lutjens, L. R. (1991). *Callista Roy: An adaptation model*. Newbury Park, CA: Sage.

Kenney, J. (2002). *Philosophical and theoretical perspectives for advanced nursing practice*. Sudbury, MA: Jones & Bartlett.

King, I. (1981). *A theory for nursing: Systems, concepts, process*. Clifton Park, NY: Thomson Delmar Learning.

King, I., & Fawcett, J. (1997). *The language of nursing theory and metatheory*. Indianapolis: Sigma Theta Tau International Nursing Press.

Leddy, S. K. (2003). *Integrative health promotion: Conceptual bases for nursing practice*. Thorofare, NJ: Slack.

Leininger, M., & McFarland, M. R. (2002). *Transcultural nursing: Concepts, theories, research, and practice* (3rd ed.). New York: McGraw-Hill.

Leininger, M., & Watson, J. (1990). *The caring imperative in education*. New York: NLN Press.

Leininger, M. M., & McFarland, M. (2005). *Culture care diversity & universality: A worldwide nursing theory* (2nd ed.). Boston: Jones & Bartlett.

Roy, C., & Andrews, H. A. (1999). *The Roy adaptation model: The definitive statement*. Norwalk, CT: Appleton & Lange.

Tomey-Marimer, A., & Alligood, M. R. (Eds.). (2006). *Nursing theorists and their work* (6th ed.). St. Louis: Mosby.

Young, I. F., & Hayes, V. (2002). *Transforming health promotion practice*. Philadephia: F. A. Davis.

Chapter 3

THEORETICAL FOUNDATIONS OF HEALTH PROMOTION

Janice A. Maville, EdD, MSN, RN
Carolina G. Huerta, EdD, MSN, RN

KEY TERMS

Consumer Information Processing Model
Diffusion of Innovations Model
disease prevention
health
Health Belief Model
health promotion plan

health protection
high-level wellness
model
O'Donnell Model of Health
   Promotion Behavior
Pender Health Promotion Model

Precede-Proceed Model
Protection Motivation Theory
self-efficacy
Theory of Planned Behavior
Theory of Social Behavior
Transtheoretical model

OBJECTIVES

Upon completion of this chapter, the reader should be able to:

- Explore the meaning of health.
- Examine definitions of health promotion.
- Differentiate health promotion from wellness, disease prevention, and health protection.
- Compare and contrast theories and models of human behavior, human behavior and health, and human behavior and health promotion.
- Relate theoretical concepts of human behavior to the promotion of health.
- Discuss the application of theories and models for health-promoting behavioral outcomes.
- Describe strategies for development of a health promotion plan.

INTRODUCTION

The promotion of health has assumed increasing importance in today's society. Health promotion is continuously highlighted by nurses and other health care professionals through the establishment of initiatives that are vital to the achievement of optimum health. Before health promotion can be applied to nursing practice, however, it is necessary to examine the various ways that health promotion has been defined and differentiated from other health-related concepts, and how theories and models have been developed in an attempt to explain this concept. In doing so, a firm foundation may be established on which practice can be implemented. This is the nature of a profession. This is the nature of nursing.

The concept of health promotion and those issues instrumental in its development were previously discussed in Chapter 1. Chapter 2 introduced the metaparadigm of nursing and emphasized assumptions basic to the integration of health promotion in nursing care. This chapter will focus and expand on the many definitions of health and differentiate health promotion from concepts of wellness and disease prevention. The various theories and models related to health promotion will also be described, and guidelines essential to developing a health promotion plan will be introduced.

CLARIFYING TERMS

Defining health and describing what constitutes a healthy status is quite complex because there are many varying perspectives. As previously discussed in Chapter 2, there is no consensus on what constitutes health. There is agreement, though, that **health** encompasses the total functioning of an individual. That is, in order for individuals to attain a state of health, they must effectively function in several areas: physical, psychological, social, cultural, environmental, and spiritual. When viewed in this manner, health reflects the holistic nature of individuals. Although there are several approaches to describing the health status of an individual, there is usually no one definition for the terms *health* and *health promotion*. In fact, there are several terms related to health and health promotion that are used frequently in nursing and health care and throughout this text that need clarification. For example, the concept of health promotion is different from the concept of wellness. Likewise, health promotion and disease prevention are not necessarily the same. *Health protection* and *health promotion* are also terms that do not necessarily mean the same thing, yet may be used to describe the same phenomenon. The following section will attempt to clarify some of the terms related to health promotion.

Wellness

The concept of wellness has existed for over four decades. This concept was heavily influenced by Dunn (1959), who recognized that health and illness were often described as being direct opposites of each other when, in fact, they could be viewed on a continuum that also includes high-level wellness. Dunn's theory of high-level wellness has served as a focal point for the discussion of health promotion and is frequently described to differentiate it from the concept of health.

If the concept of health refers to effective personal functioning, then wellness refers to this effective functioning and more. Wellness includes individual functioning at the highest potential and can be viewed as the actualization of the human potential (Pender, Murdaugh & Parsons, 2006). The concept of wellness is an expanded term that is not as restricting as the concept of health. Accordingly, **high-level wellness** describes the dynamic state of wellness that occurs at the individual, environmental, cultural, and social levels. Key to this state are the capability and potential of the individual.

Dunn (1973) perceived high-level wellness as a step above health. This concept of high-level wellness is congruent with systems theory in that individuals are seen as open systems interacting continuously with their environment (refer to Chapter 2 for a discussion on systems theory). This interaction involves energy. People are made up of various forms of dynamic energy, including expendable energy that is used to carry out daily activities of living. There is no one optimal level of wellness; however, all people are capable of moving toward a personal level of wellness. A wellness approach requires a holistic view of people and may include many degrees of wellness.

Disease Prevention and Health Protection

Like the term *wellness*, the terms *disease prevention* and *health protection* are frequently used when discussing health and the concept of health promotion. While the

concept of wellness has a positive connotation with a focus on the individual's expanded potential for health, **disease prevention** has a negative connotation as it focuses on reduction of disease and severity of disease. Disease prevention thus looks at actions that modify the environment, behaviors, or bodily defenses in eliminating, slowing, or changing a disease process. **Health protection,** which is frequently used interchangeably with disease prevention, also reflects a disease-related focus that is consistent with the medical model supported by the discipline of medicine.

Because both disease prevention and health protection activities are aimed at prevention of disease or disorder, their focus is on particular groups or individuals at risk for the development of that disease or disorder rather than on all people, whether individually or as a family, society, or community. As such, these terms do not imply a positive representation of health that moves forward, but are concerned with maintaining the status quo of certain individuals or groups by reducing risks for disease.

Describing health and health promotion by using such terms as disease prevention and health protection implies that there are others who are expert at knowing what is best for an individual. These experts use strategies such as health education to persuade individuals to assume responsibility for their own health. In turn, knowledge may be gained, skills may be learned, and behaviors may be changed to avoid disease, but health may not be enhanced as occurs when using a health promotion approach.

Human behavior incorporated into lifestyle is responsible for the status of health for most individuals. It has been reported that approximately 40 percent of all premature deaths are the result of unhealthy lifestyle choices related to tobacco use, misuse of drugs and alcohol, poor diet, sedentary lifestyles, and accidents (McGinnis, Williams-Russo, & Knickman, 2002). In fact, statistics reported by the National Center for Health Statistics show that in 2002 nearly 45 percent of deaths in the United

States resulted from six leading causes: heart disease (28.3 percent), cancer (22.8 percent;), stroke (6.7 percent), respiratory disease (5.1 percent), accidents (4.4 percent), and diabetes (3.0 percent) (Anderson & Smith, 2005).

Health Promotion

It is important to note that although *wellness, disease prevention*, and *health protection* are terms used individually in defining health, they are all also used in defining the term *health promotion* and those activities that promote health. That is, these terms are in concert with the concept of health promotion as defined in Chapter 1 because the definition includes any activity useful in enhancing the quality of health and well-being of individuals, families, groups, communities, and nations. Certainly the activities necessary to achieve the goal of high-level wellness enhance the quality of health. These activities can also include endeavors directed toward disease prevention and health protection. Thus, the concepts of wellness, disease prevention, and health protection are subsumed in the definition of health promotion.

The major themes of empowerment, lifestyle change, health enhancement, and well-being, as described in Chapter 1, are central to defining health promotion. Health promotion differs from wellness, disease prevention, and health protection in that it seeks to empower people to change through personal choices regarding their lifestyles and health enhancement and well-being activities. The major difference is in the underlying motivation for the behavior. Whereas terms such as *disease prevention* and *health protection* imply behavior that avoids disease or maintains the status quo, health promotion is motivated by the desire to increase wellness and actualize human health potential (Pender, Murdaugh, & Parsons, 2006). Health promotion thus includes any activity that helps people to adopt or maintain lifestyles that support a state of optimal health or balance of physical, emotional, social, spiritual, and intellectual health.

THEORETICAL FOUNDATIONS

Individuals have their own thoughts and perceptions. People use their impressions of what is going on within and around themselves to form ideas or concepts about a phenomenon or area of interest such as health. These concepts can become connected or related to form a theory that helps to explain a phenomenon or area of interest. (See Chapter 2 for further clarification on theory and theoretical frameworks.) **Models** are visual representations of the concepts that work together to become a theory.

Researchers who have studied human behavior have developed and tested theories that help to explain why people behave in a certain manner. Researchers who have analyzed human behavior and health have developed theories that seek to explain factors and interactions among factors that influence the health of individuals or a group of individuals. Building upon these factors, researchers interested in health promotion have developed theories and models to explain human behavior for the enhancement of health. Predominant theories and models relative to each of these areas are presented in the following sections.

THEORIES OF HUMAN BEHAVIOR

Promoting health has been part of national and international agendas particularly within the past 20 years. Governments can make laws that are designed to protect individuals from harm. But, at a more fundamental level, it is the individual who determines personal health status and what can be done to improve it. Planning strategies for health promotion depends upon having an understanding of human behavior.

With a focus on personal responsibility for promoting and protecting health, theories developed by social psychology scientists and researchers have gained much interest and attention. In developing theories, social psychologists have tried to explain why people act or behave in the manner that they do. Although these theories were not created with health-related behaviors directly in mind, they have been very useful in helping to develop an understanding of why people behave the way that they do in regard to their health. The theories of Planned Behavior and Social Behavior are particularly helpful in this respect.

Theory of Planned Behavior

The Theory of Planned Behavior was developed by social psychologist Icek Ajzen (Ajzen, 2002). Prior to this theory there were others that explained how attitudes and intentions influenced behavior. Building on this, the **Theory of Planned Behavior** took into account that control of behavior is not always voluntary, and that a type of behavior control continuum exists with lack of control at one end and extending to total control at the other end. If people have the resources, support, or skills needed for a certain behavior, they would be at the control end of the continuum. See Figure 3-1 for an illustration of the behavior control continuum.

Complete lack of control ⇒ ⇒ ⇒ ⇒ TOTAL CONTROL

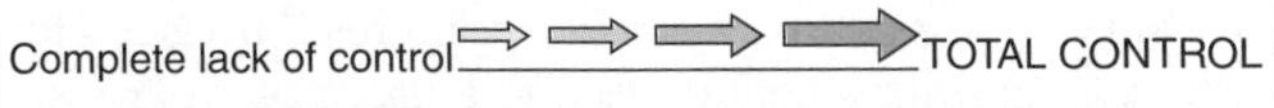

FIGURE 3-1 *Behavior control can be viewed as a continuum with lack of control at one end and total control at the other end.*

Perception of control of behavior was also an important element of the Theory of Planned Behavior. In later theories and models, this concept is expressed as **self-efficacy**, or self-conviction or belief that one can be successful in achieving the desired behavior. For example, Figure 3-2 shows how the Theory of Planned Behavior might be applied in a real-life situation. If a person knows that exercise as the outcome expectation (behavior) is necessary to promote health (subjective norm), the attitude toward exercise and the individual's self-efficacy (perceived control) influence the intention to carry out this behavior.

Ask Yourself

Theory of Planned Behavior and Monthly Breast Self-Exam Performance

Monthly breast self-exam is recommended for all women as a means of early detection of breast cancer. Is knowledge of how to do a breast self-exam all that is necessary for a woman to carry out this activity monthly? If not, what resources are necessary? Is a woman's perception of her ability to do an accurate self-exam important?

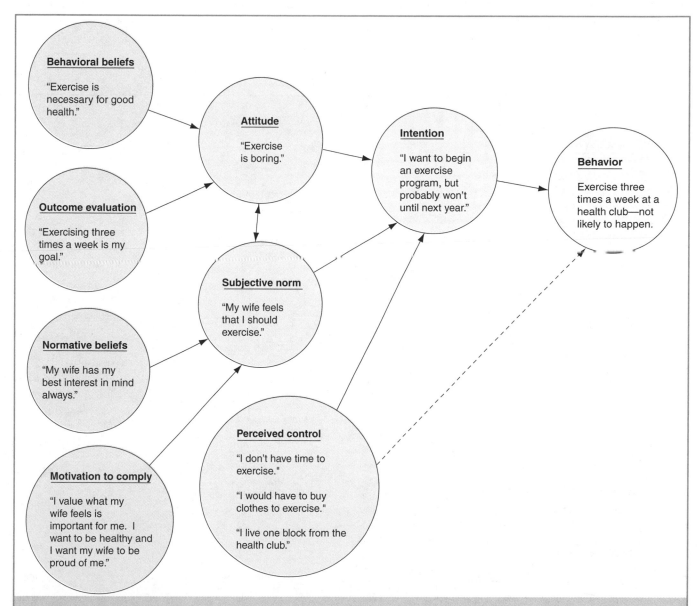

FIGURE 3-2 *The Theory of Planned Behavior helps to examine factors influencing a health-promoting activity such as exercise. (Adapted from* Theory of planned behavior, *by I. Ajzen, 2002, retrieved December 3, 2005, from www.people.umass.edu)*

Theory of Social Behavior

Similar to the Theory of Planned Behavior, the **Theory of Social Behavior** was not intended to explain health behavior. Developed by sociologist Henry Triandis, this theory introduces the concept of habit in that it distinguishes behavior under the individual's control from behavior that has become automatic or habit (O'Donnell, 2002). As depicted in Figure 3-3, the likelihood of an individual engaging in a behavior or action is equal to the sum of the person's habits and intentions which are affected by internal values, personal attitudes, and social factors. The likelihood of the health behavior action is further influenced by the connection between the physiologic effects (physical arousal) the habit has on the body and the supporting effects (facilitating conditions) that favor the change.

THEORIES OF HUMAN BEHAVIOR AND HEALTH

There are many theories and models developed by researchers interested in studying factors related to health behaviors in particular. Concepts from the psychosocial models previously described are reflected in these theories and models. Selected for discussion here are the Health Belief Model and the Protection Motivation Theory. Because of their emphasis on risks and threats of disease, these theories and models are strongly aligned with health protection rather than health promotion.

Health Belief Model

The **Health Belief Model** is a well-known model that became significant because of its emphasis on predicting

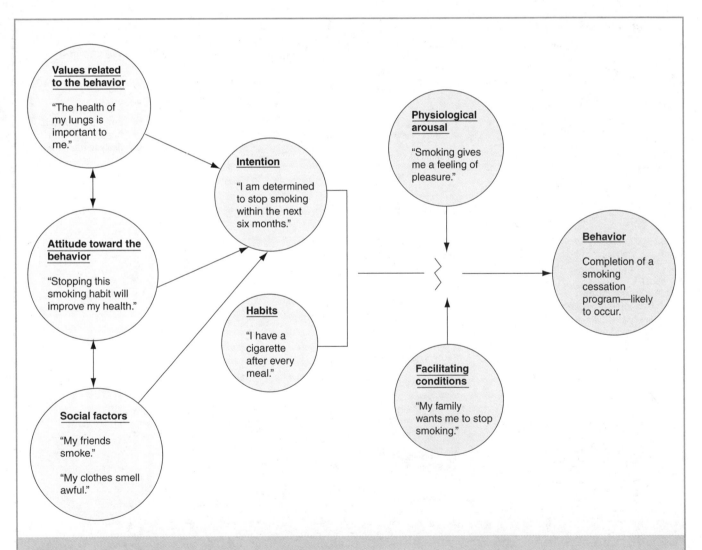

FIGURE 3-3 *This is an example of the Theory of Social Behavior reflecting how habit can affect the outcome behavior of smoking cessation. (Adapted from* Health promotion in the workplace, *by M. P. O'Donnell, 2002, Albany, NY: Delmar.)*

individual preventive health behavior. It was developed by four social psychologists—Hochbaum, Kegeles, Leventhal, and Rosenstock—for the U.S. Public Health Service, to offer an explanation for nonparticipation by people in disease prevention programs (O'Donnell, 2002). Consequently, this theory is based on an individual's ideas about and appraisal of perceived benefits compared to perceived barriers and costs of taking a health action. The Health Belief Model suggests that a person's susceptibility to a health threat and its seriousness influence the decision to engage in a preventive health behavior.

The model helps to identify the strengths as well as weaknesses of the individual that could affect the success of a plan of action for disease prevention. The model assumes that individuals value health. The original model, developed in the 1950s, was later revised to include nonhealth reasons, such as finances, knowledge about disease, or personality, that could modify perceptions about susceptibility to disease. Although intended as a disease-prevention model, the Health Belief Model could be applied when considering stress as a disease risk factor, as shown in Figure 3-4.

Protection Motivation Theory

The **Protection Motivation Theory,** developed in the mid-1970s, is a fear-driven model. It proposed that a perceived threat to health activates thought processes regarding the severity of the threatened event, the probability of its occurrence, and coping mechanisms (Rogers, 1975). The motivation to protect results from the perception of the threat and the ability of self-efficacy for coping. This theory is oriented more toward disease prevention than health promotion. The Protection Motivation Theory contains components from the Health Belief Model (vulnerability, severity, and response efficacy) and from social learning theory (self-efficacy).

The major areas where the Protection Motivation Theory has been applied include alcohol use, healthy lifestyle enhancement, promotion of diagnostic health behaviors, and disease prevention. The original theory and model have been revised many times. A schematic representation of this model for smoking cessation is shown in Figure 3-5.

Transtheoretical Model of Behavior Change

The **Transtheoretical Model (TTM)** was the result of smoking cessation research in adults by Prochaska and DiClemente (1984). These researchers concluded that changes in health behaviors progress through five distinct stages that contain elements of thought, action, and time. These components are depicted in Table 3-1 on page 48. Adjunct to this model are nine processes of change that affect the individual across all stages of change. These processes of change are categorized as experiential (what the individual is experiencing in relation to self, the environment, and others) and behavioral

Spotlight On

Motivation Theory and Change

Changing a client's behavior is very difficult. Sometimes it takes a life-threatening illness, such as a heart attack, to motivate individuals to change their lifestyles. In order to protect themselves and prevent further illness, clients may be willing to change their nutritional intake, increase their levels of exercise, and adopt healthier habits.

Research Note

Behavior Change and WIC Mothers

Study problem/purpose: To examine the relationship of the Transtheoretical Model (TTM) of behavior change to the physical activity behavior of mothers receiving assistance from the Women, Infants, and Children (WIC) program.

Methods: A descriptive correlational design was used. A sample of 30 mothers was selected with six women at each of the five stages of readiness as depicted in the TTM for behavior change. Scales used in this study included the Stage of Exercise Adoption tool, the Seven-Day Physical Activity Recall tool, the Exercise Benefits/Barriers Scale, the Self-efficacy for Exercise Scale, the Processes of Exercise Adoption tool, and the Social Support for Exercise Scale.

Findings: Analysis of the data showed statistically significant relationships between stage of behavior change, two physical activity energy expenditures, daily minutes spent in moderate to hard physical activity, pros, cons, decision balance, and self-efficacy. Self-efficacy was found to increase in all stages. It was also found that the use of the 10 processes of change differed according to the stage of change for the individual participant. The advantages, or pros, found for physical activity included a sense of accomplishment, increased strength, stress relief, and getting in shape after pregnancy. The disadvantages, or cons, included fatigue, childcare, and cold weather. The results of this study support the TTM as relevant to WIC mothers. The authors offered further suggestions for strategies to increase physical activity in this population that focus on increasing the pros and decreasing the cons.

Implications: The use of models, such as the TTM, can be valuable in providing structure, direction, and focus in examining areas of concern or interest in promoting health of individuals, groups, and communities.

Fahrenwald, N., and Walker, S. N. (2003). Application of the transtheoretical model of behavior change to the physical activity behavior of WIC mothers. *Public Health Nursing, 20*(4), 307-317.

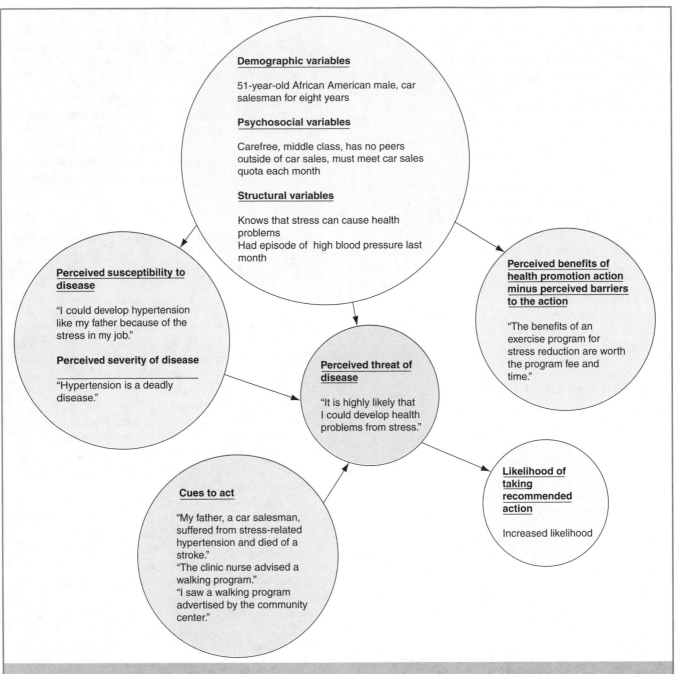

FIGURE 3-4 *The Health Belief Model could be applied when considering a health promotion intervention for a disease risk factor such as stress. (Adapted from* Health promotion in the workplace *(3rd ed.), by M. P. O'Donnell, 2002, Albany, NY: Delmar.)*

(the processes that enhance success for change). These two categories include the following factors (Fahrenwald & Walker, 2003):

1. Experiential
   a. Conciousness raising
   b. Dramatic relief
   c. Environmental reevaluation
   d. Social liberation

2. Behavioral
   a. Counterconditioning

b. Helping relationships
c. Reinforcement management
d. Self-liberation
e. Stimulus control

The Transtheoretical Model is valuable in helping to understand why individuals do or do not become involved in making a healthy behavior change, in evaluating their personal situations, and in tailoring efforts and strategies according to each individual's stage of change.

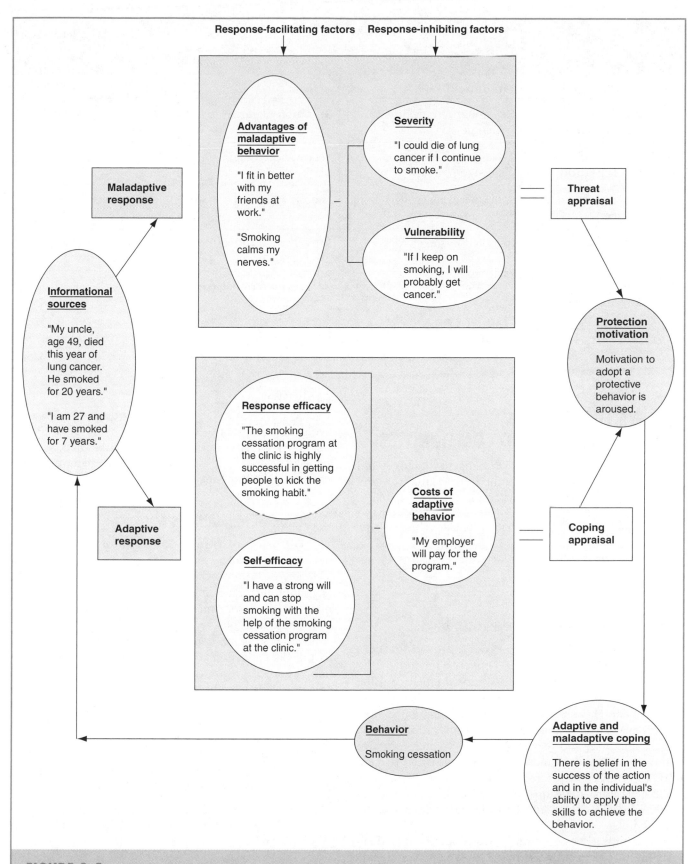

FIGURE 3-5 *This illustration of the Protection Motivation Theory shows how elements related to threat of disease and coping could affect a health promotion activity such as smoking cessation. (Adapted from* Health promotion in the workplace *(3rd ed.), by M. P. O'Donnell, 2002, Albany, NY: Delmar.)*

TABLE 3-1 Summary of Stages of the Transtheoretical Model of Behavior Change

Stage	Thought	Action	Time
Stage 1 Precontemplation	No thought to making a change	No action planned	Not within the next six months
Stage 2 Contemplation	Thoughts of making a change	Actions considered	Within the next six months
Stage 3 Preparation	Seriously thinking of making a change	Actions identified	Within the next month
Stage 4 Action	Involved in the change	Actively involved in the behavior change	Involved in the change for six months
Stage 5 Maintenance	Processing effects of change	Continuation of behavior change	Indefinite

Adapted from "The Transtheoretical Model and Stages of Change," by J. O. Prochaska, C. A. Redding, and K. E. Evers (pp.60–82), in K. Glanz, F. M. Lewis, and B. K. Rimer (Eds.), Health Education and Health Behavior: Theory, Research, and Practice, *1997, San Francisco: Jossey-Bass.*

MODELS FOR GROUPS, ORGANIZATIONS, AND COMMUNITIES

Most theories and models for behavior change and health have focused largely on the individual. There are, however, a few that offer structures to guide families, groups, communities, and even nations in making changes for healthier environments. Those selected for discussion here include the Consumer Information Processing Model, the Diffusion of Innovations Model, and the PRECEDE-PROCEED Model.

Consumer Information Processing Model

The **Consumer Information Processing Model (CIP)** (Bettman, 1979) incorporates concepts related to the use of information and the motivational effect of using this information in making choices (National Cancer Institute, 2003). Essentially, this model recognizes that individuals (1) have limits on the amount of information they obtain, use, and recall; (2) actively search for information based on their motivation, attention, and perception; (3) create rules for more rapid decision making; (4) base future decisions on the outcome of choices made; and (5) desire information that is relevant and convenient.

Although it may seem that this model is individual-specific, its application is most helpful to families and communities. A prime example is the information that is presented to consumers regarding food. Applying the concepts of the CIP model, the labels are concise and pertinent, for the most part. Information needed to make a selection, such as "low salt" or "sodium-free," is relatively easy to locate and compare with other items. Health promotion information, similarly, needs to be available, useful, and designed for convenient cognitive processing by the consumer.

Diffusion of Innovations Model

The **Diffusion of Innovations Model** addresses how new ideas, products, and social practices spread within a society or from one society to another (Rogers, 2003). Decisions by organizations and communities to adopt new programs or practices (innovations) depend on how successful they were in other areas.

Diffusion is the communication process that is vital to the dissemination of information about the innovation, whether it is an idea or a product or practice. The communication method is vital to the actual adoption. Involving community leaders, using mass media, and choosing interpersonal modes of communication enhance the likelihood of practice adoption.

The Diffusion of Innovations Model reflects characteristics of innovations that can impact their adoption. These characteristics include the following:

1. Relative advantage: The extent to which an innovation is seen as better than the idea or practice it is replacing

2. Compatibility: The extent to which the innovation fits with existing values, habits, experience, and needs

3. Complexity: The extent to which the innovation is understood

4. Trialability: The extent to which the innovation can be tried or practiced before it is adopted

5. Observability: The extent to which results of the innovation can be seen or observed (National Cancer Institute, 2003)

Time, communication systems, the social structure, and the innovation itself intertwine to create a complex model designed for long-range change on a broad-based level. The Diffusion of Innovations Model has been used successfully in communities the world over for smoking cessation campaigns. Most recently it has been found successful for use in designing effective technology implementation systems to promote client safety (Karsh, 2004), for a worksite sun protection program in the outdoor recreation industry (Buller, 2005), and as a framework for evaluating comprehensive community initiatives (Lafferty & Mahoney, 2003).

PRECEDE-PROCEED MODEL

The PRECEDE-PROCEED model evolved over the past 40 years from two separate frameworks created by Green, Kreuter, and colleagues (Green & Kreuter, 2005). These frameworks unite to form a model to guide the development of health promotion programs for groups, communities, states, and nations. Over time, the intent of this model has shifted from health education program planning to health promotion planning. The purpose is to focus on the outcomes of rather than the inputs for program planning. Simply, the outcome of quality of life forms the beginning of the model, which then works backward to determine components for success in the following order:

1. Assessment of health, behavior, lifestyle, and environment

2. Analysis of factors that predispose, reinforce, and enable the project or program

3. Implementation of educational or health-promoting program(s) with evaluation of influences by health policy organizations and regulations

The PRECEDE portion of the model was developed between 1968 and 1974. The model's title is an acronym for its components—*p*redisposing, *r*einforcing, and *e*nabling *c*onstructs in *e*ducational/ecological *d*iagnosis and *e*valuation. The focus of PRECEDE is to use a multidimensional approach in diagnosing a problem in a target population in order for appropriate health education to be implemented as an intervention. Because this model is founded in the social/behavioral sciences, epidemiology, administration, and education, it recognizes that health and health behaviors have multiple causations that must be evaluated in order to assure appropriate intervention. Table 3-2 lists the five phases of the PRECEDE portion of the model.

The PROCEED (*p*olicy, *r*egulatory, *o*rganizational constructs in *e*ducational and *e*nvironmental *d*evelopment) portion of the model was added in the 1980s to encompass the wider environmental, policy, and organizational factors that Green and Kreuter had recognized during their involvement with national programs of community health promotion. The intent of the model shifted from

TABLE 3-2 Phases of the PRECEDE-PROCEED Model

PRECEDE		PROCEED	
Phase 1	Social Diagnosis: evaluation of social problem(s)	Phase 6	Implementation: operationalization of program
Phase 2	Epidemiological Diagnosis: analysis of health problem(s)	Phase 7	Process Evaluation: evaluation of the process used to implement the program
Phase 3	Behavioral and Environmental Diagnosis: identification of health practices linked to problem(s)	Phase 8	Impact Evaluation: assessment of the achievement of objectives
Phase 4	Education and Organizational Diagnosis: identification of learning objectives	Phase 9	Outcome Evaluation: measurement of overall goal achievement and effect on quality of life
Phase 5	Administrative and Policy Diagnosis: analysis of policies, resources, and management components		

an educational program planning approach to one that is centered on population health promotion. At its core is the belief that behavior change will occur when the people involved have become empowered with understanding, motivation, and skills and active engagement in community affairs that improve their quality of life. Note that in Table 3-2 the administrative diagnosis is the final planning step to "precede" implementation. From there, "proceed" is activated to implement the plan or policy in phase six. Phases seven, eight, and nine evaluate the process for factors that enhance or impede it, organize the resources and services as required by the plan or policy, assess achievement of objectives that are established for each phase, and evaluate the overall objective relating to quality of life. The addition of PROCEED extends the model beyond educational interventions to the political, managerial, and economic areas for action that are necessary to create social environments that are more conducive to healthy lifestyles.

According to Green and Kreuter (2005), the PRECEDE-PROCEED Model has been applied, tested, studied, extended, and verified in over 960 published studies and thousands of unpublished projects in community, school, clinical, and workplace settings over the last 10 years. Its multidimensional, multilevel nature creates a complexity that is compounded by time and effort by those involved at every phase. Although it is more suitable for broad-based interventions with long-term goals, it has been successfully implemented in a variety of settings and target populations. Recent examples of implementation include health promotion programs for African Americans with diabetes (Gary, 2003), wellness of American Indian elders (Bumsted, 2003), nutrition of low-income mothers (Chang, 2004), and workplace interventions (Connon, 2004).

HEALTH PROMOTION MODELS

Chapter 1 described how health promotion evolved from global concerns of the World Health Organization nearly 30 years ago and how efforts have grown at the local, national, and international levels. Several models of health promotion have been developed as a result of this concern. In Europe, for example, the United Kingdom has made major contributions to the philosophy, policy, and practice of health promotion. One such contribution is the Tannahill Model of Health Promotion developed by Scottish scholar Andrew Tannahill in the early to mid-1980s. In the United States the leading health promotion model, and the one most often used in nursing, is the Health Promotion Model developed and later revised by nurse researcher Nola Pender. The O'Donnell Model of Health Promotion Behavior created by Michael O'Donnell, founder of the *American Journal of Health Promotion*, is one of the most recent of the health promotion models. The Pender and O'Donnell models will be described in the following sections.

Pender Model of Health Promotion

In spite of all the efforts to explain why people behave the way they do, internal and external variables included, no one theory has been developed to integrate or link all the diverse circumstances into one health promotion theory. Psychologist and nurse educator Dr. Nola Pender, however, has proposed a model that integrates perspectives from the areas of behavioral science and nursing.

The Pender Health Promotion Model has been used extensively to provide the framework and guidance for innumerable health promotion activities. These activities have included the preparation of individual client health promotion plans, health promotion programs for worksites, and community health promotion programs. Additionally, the Health Promotion Model has been used and studied in scores of health promotion research endeavors.

The **Pender Health Promotion Model** integrates concepts from the expectancy-value model of human motivation and social cognitive theory to form the theoretical basis (Pender, Murdaugh & Parsons, 2006). In other words, people will work toward what they feel is of value to them and are influenced by internal and external factors unique to the individual. Self-efficacy is predominant in the model. What makes this model unique, however, is its holistic perspective, which is integral to professional nursing care.

The Health Promotion Model variables are grouped into three major categories: individual characteristics and experiences, behavior-specific cognition and affect, and behavior outcome. As such, the Health Promotion Model shows how individual characteristics, including prior related behavior, personal factors, and biopsychosocial factors, have a direct effect on the desired health-promoting behavior. These same characteristics have an indirect effect on behavior-specific cognitions and affect, or the perceptions and feelings a person has regarding benefits and barriers of the action, self-efficacy, and sensitivity to the desires and demands of others. All of this combined directly affects the individual's commitment to a plan of action and ultimately the performance of the health-promoting behavior. Figure 3-6 shows the application of this model for an individual whose behavioral outcome is weight loss.

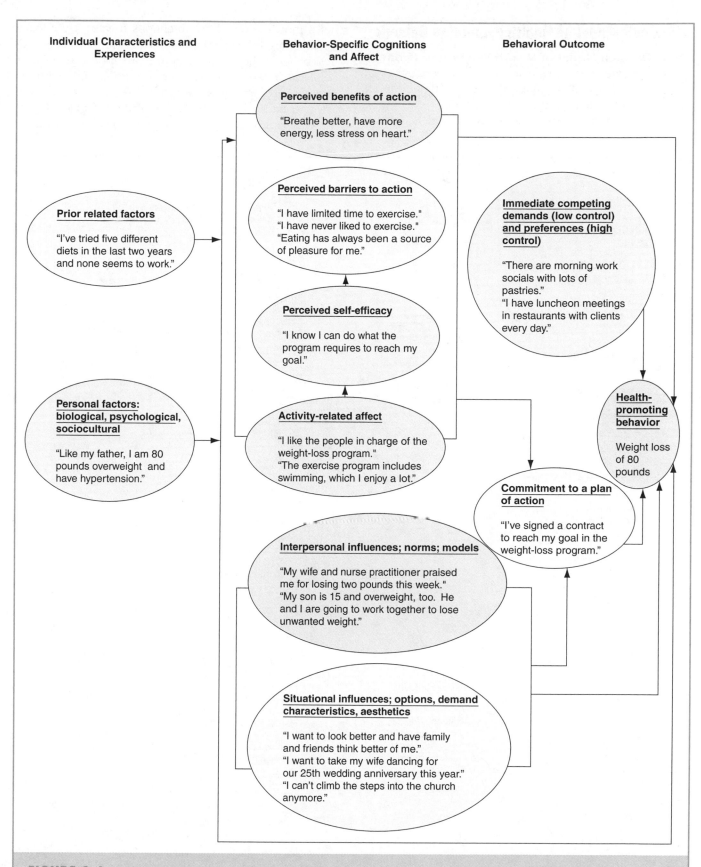

Individual Characteristics and Experiences

Prior related factors

"I've tried five different diets in the last two years and none seems to work."

Personal factors: biological, psychological, sociocultural

"Like my father, I am 80 pounds overweight and have hypertension."

Behavior-Specific Cognitions and Affect

Perceived benefits of action

"Breathe better, have more energy, less stress on heart."

Perceived barriers to action

"I have limited time to exercise."
"I have never liked to exercise."
"Eating has always been a source of pleasure for me."

Perceived self-efficacy

"I know I can do what the program requires to reach my goal."

Activity-related affect

"I like the people in charge of the weight-loss program."
"The exercise program includes swimming, which I enjoy a lot."

Interpersonal influences; norms; models

"My wife and nurse practitioner praised me for losing two pounds this week."
"My son is 15 and overweight, too. He and I are going to work together to lose unwanted weight."

Situational influences; options, demand characteristics, aesthetics

"I want to look better and have family and friends think better of me."
"I want to take my wife dancing for our 25th wedding anniversary this year."
"I can't climb the steps into the church anymore."

Behavioral Outcome

Immediate competing demands (low control) and preferences (high control)

"There are morning work socials with lots of pastries."
"I have luncheon meetings in restaurants with clients every day."

Commitment to a plan of action

"I've signed a contract to reach my goal in the weight-loss program."

Health-promoting behavior

Weight loss of 80 pounds

FIGURE 3-6 *The Pender Health Promotion Model can be applied to many health promotion activities, including weight loss. (Adapted from* Health Promotion in Nursing Practice *(5th ed., p. 50), by N. Pender, C. L. Murdaugh, and M. A. Parsons, 2006, Upper Saddle River, NJ: Pearson Prentice Hall.)*

O'Donnell Model of Health Promotion Behavior

The **O'Donnell Model of Health Promotion Behavior** is a composite of Ajzen's Theory of Planned Behavior, the Theory of Social Behavior, the Health Belief Model, and Pender's Health Promotion Model (O'Donnell, 2002). As in the two theory of behavior models, O'Don- nell's model shows how intentions toward a particular behavior are influenced by behavioral beliefs, health values, belief in those that prescribe or support the desired behavior (referents), and motivation to comply with the referents. The model also includes self-efficacy, cues to act, and barriers and facilitators of the behavior. Figure 3-7 depicts how the components of O'Donnell's model

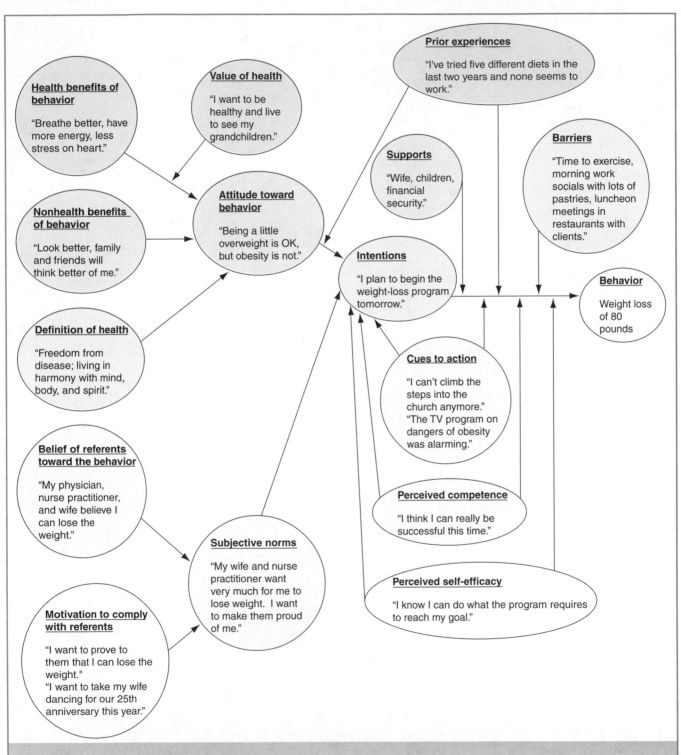

FIGURE 3-7 *The O'Donnell Model of Health Promotion Behavior is a combination of several previous models. (Adapted from* Health Promotion in the Workplace *(3rd ed.) by M. P. O'Donnell, 2002, Albany, NY: Delmar.)*

are essentially the same as in the Pender Health Promotion Model with a few adjustments in configuration.

DEVELOPING A HEALTH PROMOTION PLAN

The theories of health promotion and human behavior described in the previous sections provide nursing with the tools necessary to develop a comprehensive health promotion plan for clients, as individuals, families, communities, and groups. A **health promotion plan** looks beyond the client to the family and the community because the client does not exist in isolation.

The health promotion plan focuses on achieving wellness and, along with the client (identified as an individual, a family, or a community), determines the activities that are necessary to achieve optimum health. The plan examines the client's vulnerability to health imbalance, assesses client weaknesses and strengths, and determines potential for illness. Unlike the nursing process plan, which includes existing or potential health problems, the health promotion plan emphasizes the achievement of optimum health outcomes for clients.

Critical to the development of a health promotion plan is the nurse's recognition that the client is the expert regarding her or his own health needs. The client has the right to be an active participant in the determination of her or his own health. Consequently, client participation in the planning process is essential if the goals of the plan are to be attained. It is also important for the nurse to have an understanding of the motivation for human behavior and for changing health behaviors. The successful health promotion plan identifies the interactions among all of the factors that influence the health of the individual (Pender, Murdaugh, & Parsons, 2006). Development of a health promotion plan involves collection of assessment data, recognition of resources, supports, and constraints or barriers to the achievement of goals, identification of outcome measures, planning/implementation, and evaluation.

Assessment and Data Collection

The collection of data to be used in making a client assessment is a critical phase in the development of a health promotion plan. This phase involves looking at the client holistically. The client's health status is viewed not only in terms of physiological needs but also in terms of total biological, psychological, social, spiritual, cultural, intellectual, and environmental functioning. This assessment phase goes beyond the individual client to the family, community, and related influences. The family assessment is important in order to assess the client's ability to handle a health problem or an activity aimed at eliminating a risk factor such as smoking. The community assessment is essential because the community is where the client exists, and changes to the surrounding

community may be necessary (Pender, Murdaugh, & Parsons, 2006).

The assessment phase identifies resources and individual supporting systems available to the client. Barriers or constraints that may prevent the client from achieving health promotion goals are also identified. The identification of resources, supports, and constraints is critical in that these may enhance or limit the client's ability to accomplish activities in the health promotion plan. Incentives for client change are also identified. The client's health, health beliefs, and behaviors are also assessed because these provide the data for identification of outcome measures needed for achieving optimal health (Pender, Murdaugh, & Parsons, 2006). These outcome measures are determined by the client together with the nurse and must be measurable and realistic.

Planning and Implementation

The health promotion planning phase looks at possible problems and weaknesses of the client that increase health risks. This planning phase is based on the assessment data collected and the outcome measures determined. Again, the plan capitalizes on the resources and supports previously identified in order to enhance the client's ability to change health behaviors. Active participation by the client in planning the care is important. Both the client and the nurse identify health priorities and objectives and determine a time frame that is reasonable for achieving the previously identified outcome measures. Nursing facilitates learning, provides support, assists in identifying possible plan options, and decreases barriers to the achievement of goals (Pender, Murdaugh, & Parsons, 2006).

Evaluation

Determining whether the health promotion plan achieves the needed behavior changes—whether in client lifestyle, health beliefs, or practices—involves the process of evaluation. The nurse and client review and evaluate the client's progress. They then determine whether the identified outcomes were achieved and if they were achieved in a timely manner. If the goals or outcome measures were not achieved, the question of what needs to be included in the plan or eliminated must be asked. The last step in the evaluation phase is determination of whether any plan revisions are needed. According to Pender, Murdaugh, & Parsons, (2006), periodic revisions of the plan provide a systematic approach to move a client toward a higher level of health. Once the plan for health promotion is developed, the implementation of the nursing process can begin. For information on how the health promotion plan and nursing process can be used in planning client care, refer to Chapter 4. Table 3-3 provides an example of a health promotion plan for the community. This format may also be used in health planning for individuals and families.

TABLE 3-3 Sample Health Promotion Plan for the Community

Health Promotion Need: Need for community program to augment retirement life for older adults.
Assessment Data: Community of 35,000 with 30 percent over age 65 (United States has average of 12 percent over age 65). One community center but no programs for older adults. No senior citizen centers.
Outcome Measure(s): The community will establish a program to enhance retirement life for older adults.

Plan of Action: Objectives	Implementation	Resources	Supports/ Constraints	Evaluation
1. Identify retirement issues of older adults in the community	Form a task force Develop a needs assessment survey Recruit volunteers to conduct survey	Churches, garden club, and barber shop Community newspaper volunteered printing and copying	Several older adults among city leaders Lack of monetary resources	Task force of six members formed, including two city leaders 600 needs assessment surveys completed at seven churches, four supermarkets, and two hardware stores
2. Develop program to address retirement issues	Establish a community action committee Develop program Present program to City Council	Financial planner, community health nurse, recreation coordinator, and retirees willing to develop program	Community center has space and time for planning and conducting meetings and program No budget for program	Program developed addressing six major retirement issues Program presented to City Council and approved with allocation of budget
3. Implement program	Develop schedules, market program, and implement program	Part-time program coordinator hired with City Council funds to manage implementation	Community action committee to serve as advisory to coordinator	Use questionnaires to evaluate program effectiveness

This health promotion plan for a community reflects a general format that could be used in planning for individuals, families, and groups.

SUMMARY

The promotion of health is extremely important today. Nurses and other health care providers are involved in identifying needed changes in behavior, lifestyle, or both for the achievement of optimum health or wellness. Defining the different terms that are used in describing health is important in identifying health promotion outcomes. It is important for the terms used in defining health to reflect the holistic nature of individuals. High-level wellness, for example, involves a dynamic state of wellness that occurs at the individual, environmental, cultural, and social levels. Key to high-level wellness is an understanding of the capacity and potential of the biological, psychological, sociological, cultural, and spiritual human being. The concepts of wellness, disease prevention, and health protection are subsumed in the definition of health promotion.

Several theories have been developed to explain, describe, or predict human behavior and how this behavior is related to health outcomes and the promotion of health. Each one of us is an individual with unique characteristics, personalities, qualities, intentions, and motivations. There is no one exactly like us in the entire world. Because of this, there is no one theory or model that can be applied universally. Theories and models, however, are not only useful but necessary in providing a foundation for practice that is grounded in science. There are theories and models that attempt to explain

1. Human behavior (Theory of Planned Behavior, Theory of Social Behavior)

2. Human behavior and health (Health Belief Model, Protection Motivation Theory, Transtheoretical Model)

3. Organization and community health promotion (Consumer Information Processing Model, Diffusion of Innovations Theory, PRECEDE-PROCEED Model)

4. Individual health promotion (Pender Health Promotion Model, O'Donnell Model of Health Promotion Behavior)

The theories of health promotion and human behavior provide nursing with the tools necessary to develop comprehensive health promotion plans for clients, families, and communities. These health promotion plans are developed jointly with a client because the client is considered the expert regarding her or his own health. The client's plan focuses on wellness and determines the factors that act in concert to influence health. Development of the health promotion plan involves assessment, identification of outcomes, planning, and implementation and evaluation phases.

Key Concepts

1. Defining what constitutes health is quite complex. There is agreement that health encompasses the total functioning of an individual.

2. The concept of health refers to high-level personal functioning; the concept of wellness refers to high-level functioning and more.

3. Health promotion is any activity useful in enhancing the quality of health and well-being of individuals, families, groups, and communities.

4. The terms wellness, health protection, and disease prevention are all subsumed under the concept of health promotion.

5. Theories and models of human behavior originated in the field of behavioral psychology in an attempt to explain or predict why humans do what they do. Health care researchers added a disease prevention/health protection focus. The recent emphasis on the promotion of health has resulted in the generation of theoretical frameworks and models aimed at enhancing health and well-being. Biological, psychological, cultural, and social factors are predominant in these theories and models.

6. Personal responsibility and sense of control inherent in the client (individual or group) are key concepts for promotion of health. Belief in the ability to do what is required for the desired health-promoting behavior (self-efficacy) along with the necessary skills, resources, and support are major components influencing the behavioral outcome.

7. Theories and models can be used in planning for health-promoting behavioral outcomes of individuals, families, groups, communities, or nations. For nurses, using a systematic approach, or a combination of approaches from different theories or models, serves to empower the client through introspec-

tion, communication, and coordination of resources directed toward commitment to the achievement of a health promotion outcome.

8. Strategies for development of a health promotion plan include empowerment of the client through active involvement in development of the plan, collection of data for assessment, and a recognition of resources useful in supporting the plan.

9. A positive nurse-client relationship is important in the promotion of client health.

10. The nurse facilitates client learning, provides support for clients undergoing behavioral and lifestyle modifications, and identifies options in the achievement of client health promotion goals.

Learning Activities

1. Describe your personal definition of health. Remember at least three different situations or occasions when you felt extremely healthy. Include how you felt during those times in your personal definition of health.

2. Develop a health promotion plan for Mr. and Mrs. M, a young couple in their early 20s with a 1-month-old daughter. This couple wants to know how to keep themselves and their baby healthy. There is a history of cancer on the wife's side. They do not seek regular screenings in relation to their health risks.

True/False Questions

1. T or F Health promotion theories and models helped to form the basis for theories of human behavior.

2. T or F The PRECEDE-PROCEED Model is helpful in designing a health promotion plan for an individual.

3. T or F The Pender Health Promotion Model is unique to nursing because of its holistic perspective.

4. T or F A universal theory for health promotion is needed to guide all health promotion programs and activities.

Multiple Choice Questions

1. Which one of the following terms is defined as any activity useful in enhancing the quality of health and well-being of individuals, families, groups, and/or nations?
   a. Disease prevention
   b. Health protection
   c. Health promotion
   d. High-level wellness

2. Which one of the following models conceptualizes change in behavior through a five-stage progression with related elements of thought, action, and time?
   a. Consumer Information Processing Model
   b. Health Promotion Model
   c. PRECEDE-PROCEED Model
   d. Transtheoretical Model

3. Which of the following statements most accurately represents a health promotion plan as opposed to a nursing process plan?
   a. A health promotion plan includes existing or potential health problems.
   b. A health promotion plan emphasizes the achievement of optimal health outcomes.
   c. A health promotion plan recognizes the health care provider as the expert regarding the client's health needs.
   d. A health promotion plan focuses on process rather than outcomes.

Websites

http://www.cancer.gov Provides an overview of health promotion theories and describes their importance in planning, implementing, and evaluating health promotion programs.

http://lgreen.net Web page of the originator of the PRECEDE-PROCEED Model for planning health education and health promotion programs.

http://www.ihpr.ubc.ca Official website for the Institution of Health Promotion and Research, University of British Columbia, Canada, with the mission to provide a focus for interdisciplinary collaboration on research, education, and community partnerships in health promotion.

References

Ajzen, I. (2002). *Theory of planned behavior.* Retrieved December 3, 2005, from www.people.umass.edu

Anderson, R. N., & Smith, B. L. (2005, March 7). Deaths: Leading causes for 2002. *National Vital Statistics Reports, 53*(17). National Center for Health Statistics. Retrieved November 23, 2005, from http://www.cdc.gov/nchs/data/nvsr/nvsr53/nvsr53_17.pdf

Bettman, J. R. (1979). *An information processing theory of consumer choice.* Reading, MA: Addison-Wesley.

Buller, D. B. (2005). Randomized trial testing a worksite sun protection program in an outdoor recreation industry. *Health Education & Behavior, 32*(4), 514–535.

Bumsted, M. M., Smith, S. N., Cross, P. S., Cochran, T. M., Bromm, M. M., & Jensen, G. M. (2003). Using the PRECEDE-PROCEED model to improve health and wellness of American Indian elders. *Journal of Geriatric Physical Therapy, 26*(3), 41.

Chang, M. (2004). Development of an instrument to assess predisposing, enabling, and reinforcing constructs associated with fat intake behaviors of low-income mothers. *Journal of Nutrition Education & Behavior, 36*(1), 27–34.

Connon, C. L. (2004). Linking practice and research. Developing more effective workplace interventions: Use of the precede-proceed model. *American Association of Occupational Health Nursing (AAOHN) Journal, 52*(5): 188–190.

Dunn, H. L. (1959). High-level wellness for man and society. *American Journal of Public Health, 49,* 786–792.

Dunn, H. L. (1973). *High-level wellness.* Arlington, VA: Beatty.

Fahrenwald, N., & Walker, S. N. (2003). Application of the transtheoretical model of behavior change to the physical activity behavior of WIC mothers. *Public Health Nursing, 20*(4), 307–317.

Gary, T. L. (2003). Randomized controlled trial of the effects of nurse case manager and community health worker interventions on risk factors for diabetes-related complications in urban African Americans. *Preventive Medicine, 37*(1), 23–32.

Godin, G., & Kok, G. (1996). The theory of planned behavior: A review of its applications to health-related behaviors. *American Journal of Health Promotion, 11*(2), 87–95.

Green, L. W. (2005). *The Precede-Proceed Model of health program planning and evaluation.* Retrieved December 3, 2005, from http://lgreen.net

Green, L. W., & Kreuter, M. W. (2005). *Health program planning: An educational and ecological approach* (4th ed.). New York: McGraw-Hill Higher Education.

Karsh, B. (2004). Beyond usability: Designing effective technology implementation systems to promote patient safety. *Quality & Safety in Health Care, 13*(5): 388–394.

Lafferty, C. K., & Mahoney, C. A. (2003). A framework for evaluating comprehensive community initiatives. *Health Promotion Practice, 4*(1), 31–44.

McGinnis, J. M., Williams-Russo, P., & Knickman, J. R. (2002). The case for more active policy attention to health promotion. *Health Affairs, 21,* 78–93.

National Cancer Institute. (2003). *Theory at a glance: A guide for health promotion practice.* Retrieved November 26, 2005, from http://www.cancer.gov/aboutnci/oc/theory-at-a-glance

O'Donnell, M. P. (2002). *Health promotion in the workplace* (3rd ed.). Albany, NY: Delmar.

Pender, N., Murdaugh, C. L., & Parsons, M. A. (2006). *Health promotion in nursing practice* (5th ed.). Upper Saddle River, NJ: Pearson Prentice Hall.

Prochaska, J. O., & DiClemente, C. C. (1984). *The transtheoretical approach: Crossing traditional boundaries of change.* Homewood, NJ: Dow Jones-Irwin.

Prochaska, J. O., Redding, C. A., & Evers, K. E. (1997). The transtheoretical model and stages of change. In K. Glanz, F. M. Lewis, & B. K. Rimer (Eds.), *Health behavior and health education: Theory, research, and practice* (pp. 60–82). San Francisco: Jossey-Bass.

Rogers, E. M. (2003). *Diffusion of innovations* (5th ed.). New York: Free Press.

Rogers, R. W. (1975). A protection motivation theory of fear appeals and attitude change. *Journal of Psychology, 91,* 93–114.

Chapter 4

THE ROLE OF THE NURSE IN HEALTH PROMOTION

Carolina G. Huerta, EdD, MSN, RN
Janice Welborn, MSN, RN

KEY TERMS

advocate
community
coordinator of care
culture broker

domains
empowerment
expected outcomes
interventions

nursing diagnosis
nursing process
primary disease
   prevention

secondary prevention
spiritual health
taxonomy
tertiary prevention

OBJECTIVES

Upon completion of this chapter, the reader should be able to:

- Identify domains fundamental to nursing practice in health promotion.
- Describe how the technological domain impacts the domains fundamental to nursing practice in health promotion.
- Define holistic nursing practice in relation to health promotion.
- Describe the role of the professional nurse in health promotion for the individual, family, and community.
- Describe the steps of the nursing process in health promotion.
- Define specific nursing responsibilities for promoting health during each phase of the nursing process: assessment, diagnosis, planning, and evaluation.
- Utilize the nursing process in promoting health in individuals, families, and communities.
- Identify risk factors or potential problems influencing health.
- Identify current factors affecting nursing roles in health promotion.

INTRODUCTION

The role of the nurse in health promotion has expanded over time. Nursing's role in the care of patients has evolved from a physician-focused model of medical management to one that includes independent nursing function and practice, advocacy, and leadership with the goal of promoting individual, family, and community health. Health promotion in nursing is a continual, active process necessary to achieve and maintain the condition of wellness. Health promotion encompasses those activities that help people change their lifestyle in order to move toward a state of optimal health (O'Donnell, 1986).

Promoting health has been a fundamental goal of nursing for years, but only recently has it been emphasized in the public arena as a key to optimum wellness. The desired outcome has obvious benefits for individuals and society as a whole. Not only does the concept of health promotion decrease medical costs and morbidity, but its focus on health maintenance also increases the quality of life and life expectancy. By limiting the number of people requiring hospitalization, treatment, and continued care, health promotion and maintenance provide a solution to the health care dilemma. Nursing's role in health promotion, although expanded, has changed little over time. Technological developments have impacted the delivery of nursing care, yet nursing's focus continues to be alleviation of suffering and enhancement of health and wellness.

Previous chapters have defined health promotion, identified nursing concepts related to health promotion, and addressed health promotion models and theoretical foundations related to health promotion. This chapter will focus on domains fundamental to nursing practice and health promotion, concepts related to health and wellness, holism, nursing roles in health promotion, and the nursing process.

DOMAINS FUNDAMENTAL TO NURSING PRACTICE IN HEALTH PROMOTION

There are many factors which can influence whether an individual achieves a state of optimal health or wellness. These factors consist of internal and external influences that can be considered separately or combined. These internal and external factors can be classified in terms of domains and dimensions that provide the nurse with a holistic approach to nursing practice. These **domains,** or areas of concern affecting optimal health, are fundamental to health promotion and include biological or physiological, psychological, sociological, environmental, political, spiritual, intellectual, sexual, and technological factors. Figure 4-1 depicts domains and dimensions affecting optimal health. These domains are described in this chapter and referred to throughout this textbook.

Biological Domain

Physiological and genetic composition predispose individuals to disease or wellness. Biological factors can influence our susceptibility to disease and serve as predictors of potential health problems. No disease is entirely ethnicity-specific; however, many health problems are identified among specific ethnic groups. For instance, persons from African American and Native American populations are more likely to experience hypertension. A higher incidence of diabetes mellitus has been found among the African American, Native American, Mexican American, Filipino, and Jewish American populations. Stomach cancer is more prevalent among

the Japanese population (Giger & Davidhizar, 2004). Such a client's health, then, may be dependent on conditions beyond his or her control, but they may respond to health-promoting lifestyle changes. It is becoming apparent among health care workers that lifestyle education may promote health among all people.

Psychological Domain

The psychological or the mental health of an individual plays a significant role in promoting wellness and preventing disease. Feelings of depression can make the difference between whether a person gets up and goes to school or work or whether that person stays in bed and calls in sick. A person's perceptions of health and well-being are reflected in behavior and attitude. The relationship between psychological factors and physical illness is recognized when individuals respond to stress. Persons who are compulsive, obsessively clean, and prompt are more likely to develop ulcerative colitis than persons who are not perfectionists. Self-knowledge and desire are necessary to initiate healthy behaviors (Craven & Hirnle, 2006). For example, persons with hypertension and high cholesterol who exercise regularly and follow prescribed dietary instructions likely recognize

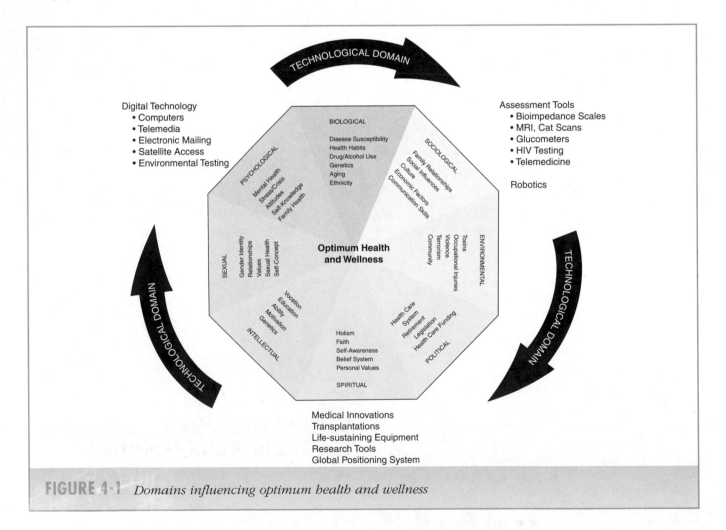

FIGURE 4-1 *Domains influencing optimum health and wellness*

the potential health problems that could develop without changes in lifestyle. A person's negative perceptions about his or her body limitations resulting from illness, such as heart failure or cancer, may hinder the ability to comprehend needed instruction and limit the benefit of health teaching.

Clients use their developmentally determined sense of self-esteem and identity to meet their basic needs. Obviously, individuals respond to crisis depending on their personal development and individual needs (Frisch & Frisch, 2006). Nurses are in a unique position to facilitate the processes of adapting and coping in their interactions with clients.

Sociological Domain

The way a person relates to others in the family, community, or society influences individual responsiveness to health promotion activities. Social mores often affect the health practices of an individual within a community. For instance, some African Americans or Mexican Americans may seek guidance from folk healers before seeking assistance from local health professionals (Giger

& Davidhizar, 2004). Trusting in the health care professional and valuing one's health are the foundation of health promotion practices.

Accessibility to health care is an additional sociological factor influencing positive or negative outcomes of health promotion. Economic factors must also be considered. In low-income families, transportation or money may not be available to seek medical attention or buy necessary food or medication. Lack of information is also a barrier to health care for persons living in rural, underdeveloped communities.

As mentioned in Chapter 2, there are many nursing theorists who consider sociological influences as integral parts of their theoretical frameworks. These theorists view people holistically and recognize that a person is a biological, psychological, social being. One theorist who focused extensively on the influence of sociological as well as cultural factors is Madeleine Leininger (1978), whose theory recognizes society's influence on health and its cultural definitions.

Environmental Domain

Primary environmental hazards are found in the home, workplace, and community. Obviously, safety is a chief concern in all these areas but especially in the home. Potential hazards are often overlooked until an accidental drowning, fall, or burn occurs. Most individuals think their home is poison proof or that firearms are stored properly. We seldom think of garbage, radon, lead, formaldehyde, carbon monoxide, and tobacco as home hazards. Yet statistics show that the home is often the most dangerous place encountered. It is far from unusual to read about child poisonings or accidental shootings in our daily newspapers. For example, accidents were the fifth leading cause of mortality reported in our country in 2001 (U.S. Department of Health and Human Services, Centers for Disease Control and Prevention, 2003). Educational programs and community assessments by health care professionals on the hazards found in our own backyard could prevent the thousands of accidents that occur yearly and take people's lives. An example is the deaths of 14 children whose school bus was sideswiped by another car and went over a ravine into a creek. Obviously, a protective fence around the creek or the use of seat belts could have saved some of these lives. Perhaps if the school district or the community health care workers had conducted an assessment of the potential hazards, such a senseless tragedy could have been avoided.

In addition to the obvious hazards (such as sanitation and chemicals), noise, temperature, infectious agents, physical agents (such as motor vehicles), radiation, and psychological stress pose threats at work. Environmental toxins and pollutants found in water, air, and food cause a large percentage of all cancers (Murray & Zentner, 2001). The community may provide public information describing environmental hazards and safety precautions. As a nurse with a holistic approach, you will be in a unique position to raise awareness of the importance of environmental factors in promoting health. For further description on how the environment relates to health promotion, refer to Chapter 7.

Political Domain

Bureaucratic policies influence and fund health care programs. Government policy directly affects community health goals. In the past three decades, policies influencing health care changed drastically. Decentralization of health care has led to the duplication of services and excessive health care costs. Today, health care programs are often limited or eliminated. Limited funding is a major concern to the public as well as to health care professionals. Federal, state, and local fund reductions may limit or totally eliminate specific health care programs.

Health care professionals provide necessary health promotion activities needed in the community and require political support for them. Professional nurses may be involved in health promotion at the national and local government levels through lobbying and actively participating in national nursing organizations and in community or regional health task forces. Disease prevention is the primary focus of the health care system today. The government is focusing on health promotion and prevention to encourage a healthy society and reduce health care costs. *Healthy People 2010*, a U.S.-government publication, describes health problems and objectives for health promotion for the United States. This document has proven beneficial in providing a political impetus for the creation, expansion, and funding of health care legislation and programs in the United States.

Spiritual Domain

Individual beliefs and value systems are inherent within everyone and may affect decisions regarding health and life. Spiritual values and beliefs may be barriers to health care among certain population groups. For example, Jehovah's Witnesses do not believe in blood transfusions

Research Note

Effects of Social Support in Motivating Cardiac Risk Factor Modification

Study Problem/Purpose: To examine risk factors that contribute to coronary artery disease and that are useful when health behaviors must be modified. The purpose of the study was to identify categories of instrumental social supports that clients with coronary artery disease find most helpful in health behavior modification and lifestyle changes.

Methods: A purposive sample of 63 adults agreed to participate in this study. All were admitted to a telemetry unit. Eligibility criteria included a documented history of cardiac disease and at least one behavior-related cardiac risk factor. A qualitative design was used. The participants were interviewed using a semi-structured questionnaire that inquired about demographic characteristics, health habits, and duration of coronary artery disease. Participants were also asked questions to determine the types of instrumental supports that were perceived as most useful.

Findings: The most frequently cited lifestyle changes reported included making dietary changes, reducing responsibilities, keeping doctor's appointments, taking medications, and exercising. Instrumental supports perceived as being most helpful in making changes were those that made it easy to engage in healthy behaviors, alleviated stressful situations, and facilitated receiving medical care.

Implications: The study supported the concept that social supports can promote risk factor modification and contribute to improving the risks for future coronary incident.

Boutin-Foster, C. (2005). Getting to the heart of social support: A qualitative analysis of the types of instrumental support that are most helpful in motivating cardiac risk factor modification. *Heart and Lung: The Journal of Acute and Critical Care, 34*(1), 22-29.

or the injection of blood products. Caring for clients of faiths different from ours may necessitate a personal spiritual assessment and perhaps the development of alternate approaches to nursing problems. All nurses should identify individual beliefs to ensure that any barriers to health are identified and preventive measures are implemented.

Spiritual health may be identified as a balance between self and others. Spiritual distress may occur when there is an imbalance. Individual faith and hope promote health and foster coping ability in times of stress. The spiritual dimension is essential for accepting life's demands, and it allows people to confront, deal with, and reconcile crisis (Cavendish et al., 2003). The nurse should recognize a person's need for rituals and respect family roles.

The health-promoting nurse recognizes that all people have diverse spiritual and family role needs. Professional nurses may care for clients whose beliefs are much different than their own; consequently, it is essential that nurses perform a spiritual self-assessment that will reveal biases as well as spiritual strengths. It is only through an honest recognition of personal spiritual beliefs that nurses are able to assist others in their health-promoting decision making.

Intellectual Domain

In considering the domains that influence nursing practice and health promotion, it is important to recognize the influence of the intellectual domain. A person's intellect may determine his or her understanding of illness, needed lifestyle changes, and hospitalization.

People are born with certain intellectual abilities that are primarily defined genetically. However, the intellectual domain is also influenced by environmental, psychological, and biological factors. Individuals are born with some degree of intellectual ability, yet a person's desire or motivation to achieve or not achieve may determine the level to which the ability is developed. Environmental influences within the home, school, and community contribute to an individual's perception of success or failure. Although nurses do not perform IQ tests on their clients, it is important that the nurse recognize the impact of the intellect on all health promotion and health-promoting activities.

Sexual Domain

The sexual domain is private to the individual and is a subject that may or may not be openly discussed. Values based on upbringing and social influences, perhaps, may underlie sexual identity. Sexual expression, attitudes, and orientation may change or become more evident as one matures from adolescence to young adult-

hood (Murray & Zentner, 2001). A nonjudgmental attitude toward the client's sexuality is demonstrated by the health professional in order to promote trust and confidence. However, sexual identity and sexual history should be determined in order to recognize potential health problems not only for the individual but for others as well. For example, a nurse working with a population at risk for human immunodeficiency virus (HIV) would be remiss if the nursing approach did not also include an assessment of the clients' sexual practices that may, in turn, affect health practices and lifestyle behaviors.

Technological Domain

Although considered as a separate domain in this text, the technological domain affects all the other domains. As depicted in Figure 4-1, technology can affect biological, psychological, sociological, environmental, political, intellectual, spiritual, and sexual functioning. For example, technology affects the biological domain by influencing outcomes that are brought about by life-threatening situations. Technology is largely responsible for organ transplantation, a fairly common procedure that can lead to a longer and fuller life for those afflicted with a debilitating organ injury or failure. The psychological domain, too, is influenced by technology that allows viewing of the structures of the entire brain, thus assisting in the diagnosis of causes for defects in psychological functioning. In the sociological and intellectual domains, technology has made it possible for individuals to research symptoms and conditions on the Internet, communicate with health care specialists, and socialize via email with their peers and family members who may not be with them during their illness.

Innovations such as computers, digital technology, telemedia, electronic mailing, satellite access, various assessment tools, robotics, and other medical discoveries have influenced the achievement of health promotion and wellness. Technological advances increase learning and the speed of processing information. Globalization and knowledge sharing are expending through technology. Shared practices assist researchers in evaluating outcomes.

HOLISTIC PHILOSOPHY

The holistic philosophy views the total individual in all domains in an accepting, caring manner to promote optimum health and wellness. Health promotion from a holistic perspective involves the total person, biological and psychological, affected by numerous external and internal influences. An individual may have multiple nursing diagnoses that represent separate systems or domains, yet holistic practice continues to look at the person as a whole being.

HOLISTIC NURSING PRACTICE

As described in Chapter 2, the holistic approach to nursing refers to a view of people in their entirety or totality. Holistic nursing practice, then, involves caring for an individual in his or her entirety, including all the aforementioned domains. **Nursing process,** on the other hand, refers to a problem-solving method for developing an appropriate plan of care and wellness outcomes for clients. Nursing care is delivered through this process, and the given subject matter (individual, family, and community) is viewed in a systematic manner with the ultimate goal being individualized care (Craven & Hirnle, 2006). Holistic nursing centers on the individual and family, and on an individual's rights and ability to cope. All domains are considered in order to provide holistic care.

Cultural, spiritual, psychosocial, intellectual, and biological domains contain differences that must be addressed to selectively and purposefully meet individual needs. Each domain possesses a dichotomy in that health promotion can be helped or hindered, depending upon the characteristic found or adhered to by the individual client or aggregate. Because cultural influences may block positive actions toward healthy lifestyle changes, the nurse must be knowledgeable regarding cultural variables and individual beliefs. This knowledge is vital to formulate positive health action plans.

In a holistic approach, the nurse recognizes how spiritual beliefs may influence health-promoting actions by individuals and will act accordingly. Understanding spiritual beliefs enables the nurse educator to collaboratively select appropriate approaches to promoting care with individuals. Although some spiritual beliefs may limit health promotion choices (no exercise from sundown Friday to sunup Sunday for Seventh Day Adventists), other beliefs expand options.

A holistic approach also recognizes psychosocial influences. An astute nurse is well aware that an individual's psychosocial status may affect the way health and wellness are viewed. For example, financial strain limits the frequency of physician visits for routine health evaluations for some individuals; however, persons with insurance or financial resources may visit health care settings more frequently than necessary. Some individuals may not visit health care settings because they do not understand the need even though the financial means are present. Differences may create interest in one area of health promotion and less in another.

Probably one of the most important domains to consider when the nurse cares for a client holistically, and one that may be ignored, is the psychological domain. This domain includes mental as well as intellectual variables that also affect individual perception of health and health-promoting activities. For example, special populations such as the mentally challenged may require that client education by nurses be addressed according to the individual levels of understanding of the client. This client population may also require special learning activities and more frequent assessments.

Biological differences may predispose persons to a weak or strong constitution. Susceptibility to specific disease may be prevalent among particular ethnic groups. The African American population is more likely to suffer from sickle cell anemia than are European Americans (Giger and Davidhizar, 2004). A holistic nurse practitioner is aware of individual biological differences and incorporates these differences into the client's plan of care.

An effective nurse will focus on interest areas first to encourage compliance and trust. As a result, the client will be ready to receive additional information regarding the disease processes and potential health hazards. Looking at individuals holistically provides a nonbiased, personal approach to health and disease prevention.

ROLES OF THE NURSE IN HEALTH PROMOTION

The role of the nurse in health promotion is complex, enveloping several roles into one (see Box 4-1). The nurse involved in health promotion assumes the usual roles commonly identified with the nursing profession. These include the roles of advocate, educator, coordinator of care, leader or member of the profession, provider of care, research user, and role model. In a health promotion approach, the nurse empowers clients to care for and maintain their own health. There is a need for nurses to shift from simply fulfilling their traditional functional roles to assuming greater responsibility in a much wider arena of action focusing on healthy people, on healthy environments, and on the challenges that occur in trying to transform nursing (Kearney, 2005). Consequently, the roles of the nurse involved in health promotion include those of empowering agent, proactive change agent, consultant, and, for those nurses with doctoral degrees, researcher testing health promotion models.

Activist/Proactive Change Agent

Inherent in the role of the nurse in health promotion is functioning as an activist and proactive change agent. Nurses should view themselves as clinical practitioners as well as social activists who can bring about social change (Green & Daniel, 2002). Change is essential in transforming the future. Nurses can make a difference beyond the clinical level by challenging institutional and political barriers that impede the progress toward wellness and health promotion goals. The nurse who embraces a health promotion approach to nursing care recognizes that the client is capable of initiating change and is competent in knowing self-needs. In the role of proactive change agent, the nurse performs a thorough assessment of the client, family, and community. Once strengths and weaknesses are identified, the proactive change agent nurse builds on those strengths, enhances existing resources, and fosters support systems that will enhance the client's ability to change (Pender, 1996).

Advocate

The nurse represents the client and the client's needs at all times. An **advocate** is one who takes the client's side and provides complete information to allow him or her to make decisions concerning individual health care (Craven & Hirnle, 2006). When a client's condition warrants an immediate appointment, the nurse may act as a referral agent and assist the client in obtaining the care deserved. As such, the nurse is the client's representative. The nurse is responsible for facilitating the client's well-being and for maintaining the client's best interest.

Educator

The nurse-educator role does not require a specific setting. Education may occur in formal or informal places, in the hospital, home, or community. The role of the nurse as educator is one of the most important. Education to remedy health promotion deficits is essential for solving problems. Post-hospital telephone contact, for example, may lead to clarification and information pertaining to medication or diet regimen. Questions asked in the physician's office or clinic also afford the nurse the opportunity to instruct and explain health-promoting activities. Formal education programs may be offered to the public regularly so that public awareness of potential and actual health risks is heightened.

Empowering Agent

In contrast to other approaches to health care that focus on fear or threats to motivate behavior changes, the health promotion model considers personal values and a person's feelings about his or her ability to achieve goals as the primary motivation for health behavior changes (Pender, 1996). Clients receiving health care are

thus empowered through their ability to self-direct and self-regulate. Nurses who recognize their responsibilities in health promotion also assume the role of empowering agents. As an empowering agent, the nurse emphasizes the active role of the client by including the client in every aspect of care. The nurse empowers the client, the family, community, and other groups that may relate to the client's situation. This empowering process can be the impetus for improving the health of communities and the quality of life for individuals, families, and communities (Pender, Murdaugh, & Parsons, 2006).

Communicator

The role of the nurse as a communicator is especially important and is closely linked to the role of the nurse as empowering agent. **Empowerment,** in relation to health promotion, is the process of helping others to help themselves. For the nurse this involves persuasion, support, and encouragement, all of which are conveyed through various modes of communication. Empowerment can best be accomplished through education. This education is communicated in many ways to a client. The role of the nurse as a communicator also involves communication with all who are involved in the care of the client. This collaborative, multidisciplinary approach to client empowerment requires that the nurse be skillful in communicating. In fact, health promotion and health education cannot be achieved without the power of the nurse as a communicator. See Chapter 5 for further information on concepts related to communication in teaching/learning.

Consultant

In the management of client care, the nurse may be frequently called upon to act as a consultant if a client is unable to solve a personal health problem. The role of the nurse can include being a consultant on a formal or informal basis. In the role of consultant, the nurse assesses the problem situation, collects information, identifies the actual problem, and, in conjunction with the client, determines appropriate solutions.

Coordinator of Care

The nurse acts as a **coordinator of care** to assure the appropriate sequence of events in the client's plan of care. Leadership skills are required to coordinate the plan of care and refer clients to appropriate sources when indicated. In the role of coordinator of care, the nurse also functions as a facilitator. As a facilitator, the nurse directs client care within the health care system to meet client needs and prevent duplication of services. The nurse is knowledgeable regarding nursing issues and trends, societal changes, and community resources. A working relationship between the nurse and the individual, family, and community may determine the achievement of health care goals.

Leader/Member of the Profession

Nurses are responsible for their own actions, being health care advocates, and serving as leaders of the nursing profession (Board of Nurse Examiners for the State of Texas & Texas Board of Vocational Nurse Examiners, 2002). To ensure accountability, the nurse must maintain current education in the field of practice and implement research findings in day-to-day nursing. Leaders maintain the standards of care and edify the professional practice of nursing. Nurses apply the historical development of the profession to current trends in order to direct the profession to meet societal changes. As a leader, the nurse promotes ethical and legal standards, innovative practices, and service to the public to maintain a positive image for nurses.

Graduates of registered nursing programs are prepared to function in three major roles, including provider of care, coordinator of care, and member of the profession. Registered nurses are skilled in using a systematic approach in providing or coordinating health promotion, maintenance, and restoration. Nursing management and nursing care supervision are two responsibilities of the nurse. The nurse is to act as a leader in promoting nursing as a profession (Board of Nurse Examiners for the State of Texas & Texas Board of Vocational Nurse Examiners, 2002).

Provider of Care/Caregiver

As a caregiver for health restoration, the nurse is actively involved in the nursing process, a problem-solving method for developing an appropriate plan of care and wellness outcomes for a client, while continually assessing the client's responses to nursing interventions. Direct client care may be delivered in the home, hospital, or community setting. The nurse assesses all domains of the individual, family, or aggregate and, along with the client, develops a plan of care. Through inclusion of the client in the planning process, the caregiver has a better understanding of the community composition and resources available that may influence the outcomes of care. The plan of care is implemented after the nurse and client establish appropriate, realistic goals. Through direct care, the nurse can evaluate the client and determine if client needs are being met. After analysis and evaluation, the plan of care may be restructured at any time to further promote client comfort and well-being.

Research User and Health Promotion Models Researcher

As a research user, the nurse can play a significant role in advancing a theoretical knowledge base for health promotion and in facilitating client outcomes utilizing contemporary, current knowledge and practice. Statistical evidence of nursing theory supports nursing actions and expands nursing science. The conscientious nurse will continue using research findings, increase personal knowledge, and thereby improve client care. The graduate educated nurse, usually one prepared at the doctoral level, can assume the role of a researcher who empirically tests health promotion models, thus increasing the predictive value of health promotion in health care.

Role Model

Nurses represent standards and quality of care defined within the limits of education, experience, and state licensing bodies. The general public has the right to expect safe, conscientious practice from nurses. Professionally, optimal standards of practice must be maintained for the achievement of the desired health care outcomes. As role models, experienced nurses exemplify the highest ideals of nursing practice, and they command admiration, trust, and respect from all health care professionals and persons receiving care.

Although nurses rarely view themselves as role models for future nurses, it is important to recognize that nurses will be seen by others as just that. As students and later on as professionals, these individuals will be expected to abide by the highest standards of care and to show through their actions that they are truly worthy of the professional title "registered nurse."

OVERVIEW OF THE NURSING PROCESS

The nursing process is a problem-solving method that involves gathering and interpreting data to formulate a plan of care. The nurse is significant in determining the needs of the client and acting as a representative of the individual. The nurse and client jointly must identify nursing needs before the health promotion nursing process plan can be formulated.

Nursing theories may be used in clinical practice within the nursing process and guide and structure each phase of that process (Reeves & Paul, 2002). Nursing theorists describe the various steps of problem-solving as the nursing process. The method is ongoing and continually involves the following steps: (1) assessment of the client, (2) identification of a need or potential need, (3) development and implementation of a health care plan, and (4) evaluation of all areas (Duldt, 1995).

The nursing process is a continual, ongoing process used to determine if a health problem or potential health problem exists. The steps of the nursing process supported by the majority of nursing theorists and subsumed by the preceding four steps are the following:

1. Assessment

2. Nursing diagnosis

3. Outcome identification

Role Modeling

Do you know any ideal nurse role models? As a nurse, would you want to model their behaviors? What professional behaviors are exhibited which you find appealing? What about the nurses' personal behaviors related to health promotion and lifestyle choices? What if a nurse smokes or drinks in public? Do you think that the nurse should always comport herself or himself in a professional manner even when enjoying activities in the nurse's personal life?

4. Planning

5. Implementation

6. Evaluation (Reeves & Paul, 2002)

Client responses are continually monitored to determine effectiveness of care. Using the data collected, the nurse and client determine what action is necessary to provide correction or prevention of the client's condition (Fawcett, 2005).

The nursing process in health promotion utilizes the original steps of assessing, diagnosing, planning, implementing, and evaluating. The primary foci in the nursing process when utilized for health promotion appear to be its emphasis on wellness without a primary physical or mental condition, empowerment of the client, promotion of lifestyle changes, and health enforcement. Health promotion seeks to expand positive potential for health with emphasis on strength, resiliencies, capability, and resources rather than on existing pathology (Pender, Murdaugh, & Parsons, 2006). The nurse looks at potential illnesses or problems and then seeks to provide preventive measures. For the nurse to be instrumental in health promotion, it is imperative to consider potential risk factors within the individual, family, or community. Among teenage girls, for example, the nurse would consider potential risk factors such as smoking, sexually transmitted diseases (STDs), and pregnancy and their potential effects on the individual, family, community, and society. Use of the nursing process in health promotion is congruent with the Pender Health Promotion Model (1996) in that it seeks to increase wellness and actualize human potential.

Assessment (Acquiring Information)

The first step occurs with the assessment of an individual, family, or community. The term **community** when used in a health promotion context refers to a collection of people who interact with each other and who have common interests that form a sense of unity or belonging (Allender & Spradley, 2001). Members of a community identify themselves as such. They participate in activities to improve their community through planned change (Pender, Murdaugh, & Parsons, 2006). Assessment includes collection of data, asking questions to learn as much information as possible about the client, identification of resources, and recognition of barriers to goal achievement. Past medical history is important to assist the nurse in formulating a diagnosis and developing a plan of action. Environment, culture, family background, work ethic, educational level, social standing, and gender may contribute to the individual's perception of health or illness (Fawcett, 2005). Assessment involves observing, questioning, inferring, and clarifying information to determine appropriate nursing action.

Observation begins when the nurse first sees the client. Skin color, gait, poise, demeanor, facial expression, and speech are among characteristics to be noticed. Psychiatric or neurologic impairment may be suggested on first encounter with the client.

Interviewing the client gives inside information into the client's personal habits, perceptions, current state of mind, medical history, and spirituality. The nurse should ask open-ended questions and give the client time to speak. The nurse needs to be an active listener. A trusting, friendly rapport with the client will encourage a relaxed atmosphere.

Questions (who, what, where, when, why) are helpful in assessing the client. Who is the client? Who else lives in the home? Who is the caretaker? What does the client do? What symptoms are present? What has the client done to relieve the problem? Where does the client work? Where was the client when symptoms began? When did symptoms begin? When did the client first seek treatment? Why is the client here? Why has previous treatment not been successful? There are numerous assessment forms that can be used. Institutions may choose to develop forms specific to their client population. Refer to Chapter 15 for an example of an assessment form.

Nursing Diagnosis

The **nursing diagnosis** consists of the actual identification of a client's need and is formulated after "the nurse establishes a database that includes the simultaneous consideration of the dynamic interactions of physiologic, psychological, sociocultural, developmental, and spiritual variables" (Fawcett, 2005, p. 178). Based on nursing knowledge and the client history, the professional nurse establishes one or more nursing diagnoses specific for the client.

The nurse does not confuse the nursing diagnosis with the client medical diagnosis. The nursing diagnosis is specifically developed from the nursing perspective and is separate from the physician treatment plan. The diagnosis leads to the plan of care that the nurse will implement. The nursing diagnosis identifies a client need and forms the basis for adopting a plan for nursing action.

Several recognized languages have been developed to document nursing care using the nursing process. These languages are used to track the clinical care process for an entire episode of care for clients in various care settings (American Nurses Association, 2005). Developing a standardized language that reflects the complexity and diversity of nursing practice is an extremely challenging task (NANDA, 2001).

Organizations such as the North American Nursing Diagnosis Association (NANDA) develop terminology to describe important clinical decisions made by nurses for individuals, families, and communities (NANDA, 2007). The nursing diagnosis may be an actual need identified or a potential need that could develop in the future. NANDA has developed one of the most recognized classification systems that have a listing of approved diagnoses. These nursing diagnoses are crucial to the selection of interventions and outcomes. Because of this, NANDA (2007) provides a **taxonomy,** or common classification structure that links nursing diagnoses, interventions, and outcomes. *The NNN Taxonomy of Nursing Practice* has been created and refined within the last several years to link nursing diagnoses, interventions, and outcomes. It was developed through the NNN Alliance of NANDA International, the Nursing Interventions Classification (NIC) and the Nursing Outcomes Classification (NOC). Box 4-2 lists several classification systems, including NANDA, used to support clinical decision making and organize and categorize nursing phenomena.

Not all institutions have adopted the NANDA-approved diagnoses, but many have. The three parts of the nursing diagnosis for actual problems are (1) diagnosis, (2) cause, and (3) sign/symptom. Previous work by the NANDA focuses primarily on describing illness problems. For example, the actual nursing diagnosis for the client with a decubitus ulcer should state: "Impaired skin integrity (diagnosis) related to decreased circulation (cause) as evidenced by an open sore on sacral area (sign/symptom)." For potential problems, only the first two parts of the nursing diagnosis are necessary. The potential nursing diagnosis for a client with a family history of breast cancer should state, "Ineffective health maintenance (diagnosis) related to knowledge deficit regarding self-breast examinations (cause)."

Nursing theorists view health promotion and health maintenance as two distinct concepts. The NANDA developed two diagnoses for applying health maintenance and health promotion in clinical practice: ineffective health maintenance and health-seeking behaviors. Essentially, health maintenance behaviors are those that seek to maintain health—avoid illness, disability, and so forth. Health-seeking behaviors, by contrast, are those that seek to promote or improve health. Assessment is

BOX 4-2	Select Classification Systems

North American Nursing Diagnosis Association (NANDA)
North American Nursing Diagnosis Association International (NANDA International)
Nursing Interventions Classification (NIC)
Clinical Care Classification (CCC)
Omaha System
Nursing Outcomes Classification (NOC)
Nursing Management Minimum Data Set (NMMDS)
Patient Care Data System (PCDS)
International Classification for Nursing Practice (ICNP®)

the key determining factor. Is the client able to identify health-promoting activities? Does he or she recognize negative health behaviors?

Examples of health maintenance interventions include a balanced diet, use of seat belts, and quitting smoking. Health interventions related to health-seeking behaviors are more aggressive: vigorous aerobic exercise three times a week, avoidance of food additives, and stress management.

Planning

From the nursing diagnosis a plan of care is formulated and implemented. Outcome identification, or goal setting, is an important part of the planning stage. Once a nursing diagnosis is established, the nurse determines what outcomes are important to resolving the patient's problems. **Expected outcomes** are measurable goals set by the nurse and the client for the client and derived from the nursing diagnosis (Sparks-Ralph & Taylor, 2005). Outcomes or goals are either short or long term. Short-term outcomes are those directed toward problems that require immediacy. "Long-term goals take more time to achieve and usually involve prevention, patient teaching, and rehabilitation" (Sparks-Ralph & Taylor, 2005, p. 13). The patient's setting may also dictate the type of outcome expected. A goal for a patient in the emergency room, for example, might differ from one for the same patient receiving home health care.

The nursing care plan represents the goal or outcome the client should reach. Realistic goals are stated specifically and within a designated time frame. A correctly stated goal reads: "Client will turn, cough, and deep breathe every two hours during the immediate eight hours post-op" or "client will reduce the number of cigarettes smoked from two packs to one pack per day within two weeks' time." The goal should be stated in measurable terms for evaluation purposes.

The nursing care plan is developed with potential problems or needs in mind. Who is the client? With whom does the client live? To what sociocultural group does the client belong? What may occur if teaching or knowledge is not given? Where can the client go to receive information? When can the client go? Does the client have transportation? Why does the client need information?

Implementation

Nursing interventions are determined based on the nursing diagnoses. **Interventions** are nursing actions that enable the client to achieve the desired goal. Interventions for health promotion are determined by primary, secondary, or tertiary prevention. In **primary disease prevention,** high-level wellness is the goal. Primary disease prevention includes activities and lifestyle factors that can be changed or maximized. Behaviors that include adequate nutrition, exercise, immunizations, and stress prevention are good examples of primary disease prevention. **Secondary prevention** focuses on screenings that identify abnormalities within a population. Secondary prevention includes all health screenings and assessments. **Tertiary prevention** seeks to address the situation once symptoms have occurred. It is directed toward minimizing disease or disability and optimizing health (Craven & Hirnle, 2006).

Educating individuals about primary prevention may involve addressing unhealthy behaviors and mutually determining a plan to achieve wellness or optimum health. Secondary prevention involves assessing individual awareness of the importance of health screenings such as lab tests for assessment of diabetes or cholesterol. Tertiary prevention focuses on helping the ill person get well or live within certain limitations. Individual variables affect the lines of defense present among physiological, psychological, sociological, developmental, or spiritual domains.

Critical to using the nursing process in health promotion is consideration of the interactions among all of the factors influencing the health of the client, whether the client be a family, a community, or society at large (Pender, 1996). In health promotion, interventions may occur less frequently or over a longer period of time. Immunizations may be given to adults and children once a month in a community clinic. Nutrition classes for heart-healthy living or diabetes education may be conducted weekly or monthly. Interventions for health promotion may occur in the clinical setting or in the community. Tables 4-1 and 4-2 describe nursing diagnoses and interventions across the life span.

Evaluation

The plan of action and the results of implementation should be evaluated regularly to determine if the desired goals have been achieved. Accurate record keeping is essential to establish reference logs. Evaluation occurs after action has been implemented. Did the action do what was intended? Does the action need to change? Is the client worse? The evaluation process is ongoing.

Any change in the client's condition will warrant a look at the current implementation of care and its merit. Has the goal been achieved? What has been accomplished? In all settings for health promotion, the nursing care plan is used for evaluation. The care plan may change hourly, daily, weekly, or monthly, depending on the client's progress toward goal achievement.

NURSING PROCESS AND HEALTH PROMOTION FOR THE INDIVIDUAL, FAMILIES, AND COMMUNITIES

The nursing process involves looking at all domains affecting an individual, families, and communities. Motivation to seek action is determined by a desire to protect health, avoid illness, or enhance one's level of health regardless of illness (Pender, Murdaugh, & Parsons, 2006). The culture and social environment of the community influence health promotion for individuals, families, and communities. The models of health promotion described in Chapter 3 focus on preventive measures, educational efforts, policy making, and client empowerment. All of these measures and concepts should be included in the nursing process health promotion plan.

Individual

The individual may be viewed separately from the family and community as a sole being with unique physiological and psychological complexity. The individual's perception of health and health risks determines specific health-seeking behaviors. In assessing an individual, careful attention must be focused on the health history regarding previous diseases or disabilities, lifestyle patterns, and knowledge of health condition/status. The individual may live alone or be a member of a family unit.

Family

The family may be considered a separate open population system composed of a varying number of individuals. Families may be defined as couples, nuclear, blended, or extended. Relationships within the family among one or more individuals form subsystems within the family as a whole. Interpersonal relationships affect the family dynamics and create an atmosphere of stress or tranquility. Crises occur at differing frequencies and intensities among families. Coping abilities are represented in families with strong organization, positive personal values, and purposeful lifestyles. Dysfunctional families may promote disorganization within the family unit and create disharmony among family members. The nursing process, applied to the family unit, assesses the family structure, relationships, risk factors, and health education.

Age Level	Nursing Diagnosis Examples	Interventions
Infant (Birth–1)	Ineffective breast-feeding pattern related to mother's deficient knowledge	Assess the mother's knowledge regarding breast-feeding. Identify barriers that may impact successful breast-feeding. Demonstrate appropriate breast-feeding technique. Assess mother's level of anxiety. Educate on anxiety-reducing techniques. Provide written information regarding successful breast-feeding practices. Evaluate baby's sucking ability. Keep baby awake and alert during feedings.
Children (1–14)	Risk for injury related to delayed developmental skills	Identify motor, mental, sensory, or musculoskeletal deficits. Include parents in educational session describing risks in the child's environment. Orient child to home environment. Instruct child and family on how to avoid accidents. Caution parents regarding dangers of playground and home, including information on use of electrical equipment, water from bathtub, placing toxic chemicals out of child's reach. Promote early childhood development programs. Begin educating children on lifelong health promotion habits and health protection.
Adolescent and young adult (15–24)	Risk for poisoning related to lack of knowledge on risks associated with substance abuse	Provide information to adolescent and parents on the harmful and potentially lethal effects of abusing drugs and alcohol. Discuss consequences of peer pressure. Provide appropriate written materials related to abuse of drugs. Help identify potential stressors, depression, and related family issues. Provide available community resources to prevent or treat substance abuse. Discuss differences between medications that are prescribed and those available without a prescription. Listen nonjudgmentally.
Adult (25–64)	Risk for ineffective health maintenance related to chronic disease, stress, cardiovascular disease, and smoking	Discuss need for health maintenance routine. Encourage regular exercise, fitness, and sound nutritional practices. Provide information on appropriate health screenings for age. Teach effective stress reduction and coping skills. Involve person in decision making by providing choices. Identify barriers to performing activities unassisted. Review dietary habits. Educate on risk factors associated with a sedentary lifestyle.
Older adult (65 and older)	Activity intolerance related to the aging process	Mutually establish realistic goals for activity levels. Identify assistive devices helpful in increasing activity (e.g., cane, walker, shopping cart on wheels, or trapeze). Encourage rest period in between exercise activity. Determine realistic activity goals. Encourage person to take part in exercise and social activities. Monitor for signs of weakness or fatigue. Educate on home safety to prevent accidents and reduce risk of falls.

TABLE 4-2   Nursing Diagnoses for the Individual, Family, and Community

Individual

DIAGNOSIS: Decreased Cardiac Output

INTERVENTIONS:	• Educate client re: diet, exercise, medical screenings • Provide activity information re: type of exercise, time required for effective prevention	• Counsel client re: diet and cholesterol • Monitor client vital signs, blood cholesterol at regular intervals
EVALUATION:	• What lifestyle changes are observed? • Does client exercise regularly? • Are nutritional goals met? Is weight desirable?	• Does client seek regular physical exams and attend wellness/illness clinics?

DIAGNOSIS: Ineffective Health Maintenance Related to Uncontrolled Diabetes

INTERVENTIONS:	• Educate client re: disease, medication, diet, exercise • Provide information re: community resources	• Advise client re: necessity for regularly scheduled appointments with health personnel • Counsel client
EVALUATION:	• Does client follow medication regimen? • Can client describe correctly the diet, exercise, and health regimen to follow and parameters for blood glucose?	• Does client seek resources for assistance?

Family

DIAGNOSIS: Ineffective Health Maintenance Related to Safety Hazards in the Home

INTERVENTIONS:	• Determine age of family members • Stress health promotion activities	• Educate family re: risk factors (wet floors, toys, visual disturbances, fire hazards, motor vehicle safety, etc.)
EVALUATION:	• Lifestyle changes? • Is family demonstrating health-seeking behaviors?	• Does family attend safety seminars in the community or call for assistance?

DIAGNOSIS: Impaired Parenting Related to Loss of Spouse

INTERVENTIONS:	• Counsel client re: primary role of lost partner • Determine roles within family	• Refer to counseling center
EVALUATION:	• Do child and parent communicate daily? • Does child behave appropriately?	• Does parent discipline and seek assistance in caring for child?

Community

DIAGNOSIS: Ineffective Health Maintenance Related to Sexually Transmitted Disease

INTERVENTIONS:	• Counsel community regarding safe sex practices • Determine knowledge base of community	• Monitor regular physical exams to ensure infection is eradicated
EVALUATION:	• Is community demonstrating health-seeking behaviors?	• Is community demonstrating understanding of prevention?

DIAGNOSIS: Ineffective Health Maintenance Related to Deficient Knowledge Regarding Smoking Risk Factors

INTERVENTIONS:	• Provide information re: risk factors related to smoking • Educate community re: ways to reduce risk factors	• Provide health screenings (chest x-rays) • Monitor individuals' and community's willingness to reduce smoking hazard
EVALUATION:	• Is community demonstrating health-seeking behaviors?	• Do community members seek regular physical exams and attend wellness/illness checks?

Community

A community is a particular population of people with common interests and common values. A community may be determined by geographical proximity or by a common social structure (Pender, Murdaugh, & Parsons, 2006). Examples of a community include teenage pregnant girls, persons who smoke cigarettes, and persons with tuberculosis. Assessment of communities includes careful history, demographic information, lifestyle, and knowledge of health risks. The nursing process can be applied to individuals, families, and communities to (1) systematically assess health needs and concerns that could lead to a change in health status; (2) formulate a plan of prevention or care that will reduce identified problems; and (3) evaluate prevention plans and goal attainment and modify the plan to achieve the best results in promoting health, preventing disease, and creating a well society (Allender & Spradley, 2001).

RISK FACTORS AND HEALTH PROMOTION

A risk factor includes anything that can increase the vulnerability of an individual, family, or community to an unhealthy event (Craven & Hirnle, 2006). Risk factors may or may not be controllable. For example, cigarette smoking, blood pressure, weight, exercise, cholesterol, and stress may be controllable while factors such as age, heredity, and sex cannot be. Health Risk Appraisal tools assist the nurse in the assessment of potential health problems of an individual throughout the lifespan (Stanhope & Knollmueller, 2001). An example of a health risk appraisal tool utilizing Domains is demonstrated in Figure 4-2.

Some risk factors to be considered in the area of health promotion include environment, work, socioeconomic level, education, gender, cultural influences, and spiritual beliefs. The role of the nurse as educator is essential to resolving client problems and providing direction on how to decrease risk factors.

Environment

The environment often predisposes a person to disease processes. Living conditions may promote illness. For instance, tuberculosis, among the bacterial and viral infections, is more prevalent in crowded living conditions. Persons in areas of contaminated water are at an increased risk for intestinal infections if sanitation measures are neglected. The role of the nurse as advocate requires that nurses be cognizant of the environmental risk factors that exist and speak up in order to alleviate them.

Work

Work influences health and wellness. Many employers today provide health screenings and health prevention programs for employees. Such employers often include

hospitals, factories, and large institutions. Work safety is imperative for optimum health and wellness. The number of dependents living in the home and the head of the household play a large part in the status of the family and individuals within the household.

The nurse may take an active role in developing community programs for individuals and their families. Often the small business owner is not able to provide health education programs routinely. The nurse may collaborate with small business owners to provide needed information to employees.

Socioeconomic Level

The socioeconomic level of an individual influences the affordability of health care and health promotion activities. Often, funds are limited and the resources are unavailable to access the care required for optimum health. Persons may delay seeking treatment or information due to lack of money. Nutrition and living conditions may affect the health risk of the individual as well.

Education

Education may influence the level of understanding among the public. Laypersons often do not have the knowledge base to know what causes a disease, much less how to prevent the development of the disease. Public education announcements and offerings of health information provide a beginning knowledge level and will promote further learning. Education must be simple, clear, and understandable. Intellectual differences may influence the type and length of educational offerings. Nurses will want to speak at the educational level of their clients, communicating the message in simple terms. The caregiver may also require explicit information regarding client needs. This information should be given at the educational level of the caregiver.

Health-seeking behavior is critical to implementing health promotion. For instance, if a person does not believe immunizations are necessary, immunizations will probably be rejected. Health-seeking behavior is more readily taught through education. The level of education and ability to learn may influence the success or failure of health promotion. A nurse must first know the audience and recognize its needs. Information should be presented in simple terms, using appropriate pictures, vocabulary, and literature for the education level being taught. Often health promotion is not achieved because the general public does not know the requirements for good health.

Providing information through community, private, and corporate educational facilities will generate public knowledge. Media presentation is an excellent means of disseminating information. Types of media useful for health education include radio, television, and the Internet. Persons may be contacted via media at the rural, urban, district, regional, state, national, and international levels. In order to achieve the maximum outcome of health promotion and wellness in the world, individuals

Health Risk Appraisal According to Domains

Please complete the following:

Client Profile

Name _____	Age _____
Gender _____	Ethnicity _____
Occupation _____	Marital Status _____
Height _____	Weight _____
HDL _____	LDL _____
Total cholesterol _____	B/P _____

Biological Domain
Usual source of health care _____
Present health problem _____
Current perception of health (poor, fair, good, excellent) _____
List home treatment/complementary therapies _____
Current medications _____
Immunization status   DPT _____   Influenza _____   MMR _____
                      Varicella _____   Hepatitis _____   Polio _____
                      Pneumonia _____   Others _____
Screening tests   HIV_____   TB _____   PSA_____
                  Mammogram _____   Cervical Pap Smear _____
                  Other _____
Date of last health exam _____
Date of last dental exam _____
Date of last vision exam _____
Exercise routine_____
Numer of times exercise per week _____
Intensity of exercise (mild, moderate, intense) _____
Diagnosed   Diabetes _____   Heart disease _____   Other _____
Smoker (Yes/No) _____   No. of cigarettes per day _____

page 1 of 3

Psychological Domain
Engage in therapy (Yes/No)_____   Meditation _____   Yoga_____
Sleep patterns _____
Description of activities of daily living _____
Patterns of coping (poor, good, excellent) _____
Coping activities _____

Social Domain
Annual income_____
Living arrangements _____
Alcohol use (Yes/No) _____
Drug/substance use (Yes/No) _____
Coffee drinker/Cola drinker (Yes/No)_____   Amount _____
Recreational activities _____
Frequency of travel _____
Meal patterns_____
Person who cooks (self, mother, spouse, other) _____

Environmental Domain
Allergies (Yes/No) _____   To what _____
Home environmental concerns _____
Neighborhood concerns _____
Work-related risks _____
Sun exposure (never, occasionally, often)_____
History of violence (domestic, self-inflicted, other) _____
Number of accidents/speeding tickets in last year_____

Political Domain
Use of seatbelts (Yes/No) _____
Use of child safety seats _____
Use of helmet when on ATV, motorcycle, etc. _____
Insurance (Yes/No) _____
Medicare/Medicaid (Yes/No) _____

page 2 of 3

Spiritual Domain
Religion _____
Religious restrictions (describe) _____
Religious beliefs/practices _____

Intellectual Domain
Educational background _____
Reading proficiency_____
Language(s) spoken _____
Preferred language _____

Sexual Domain
Monogamous (Yes/No) _____
Number of sexual partners in previous year _____
Last Pap smear _____
Last mammogram _____
Last testicular exam_____

Technological Domain
Use of assistive devices (wheelchair, walker, cane, prosthesis, etc.) _____
_____
Any hearing aids, glasses, LASIK surgery _____
Computer literate (Yes/No) _____
Email, Internet accessibility_____

page 3 of 3

FIGURE 4-2 *Health Risk Appraisal According to Domains*

must be educated. Nurses are influential in their individual communities and should network with other health professionals to enhance the public knowledge of health and wellness.

Gender

Individuals are susceptible to gender-specific health alterations. Males develop testicular cancer and females uterine/ovarian cancer due to genetic composition. Women have a higher incidence of breast cancer. Men develop cancer of the head and neck more often than women. Men experience high blood pressure and are diagnosed with diabetes more often than women. Women encounter the health care system more frequently than men because of issues centered on their social definition as women, such as reproduction, child rearing, and caring for the elderly (Black & Hawks, 2005).

Cultural and Spiritual Influences

As discussed previously, many cultures own preset beliefs regarding health, religion, and wellness. Knowledge of various cultural beliefs will enable the nurse to prepare an appropriate teaching tool relevant to specific cultures and religions. Cultural and spiritual differences must be recognized to enhance learning and allow for the development of appropriate health prevention measures for a client. Christian Scientists rely on prayer to heal while some cultures observe rituals to rid the body of "evil spirits" (See Chapter 6). Cultural "brokering" may be required. A **culture broker** is a go-between, one who advocates on behalf of another individual, family, or community. Cultural brokering is an effective approach to community engagement (National Center for Cultural Competence, 2004). "The culture broker is one who bridges the gap in cultural meanings or gaps in understanding between health professionals, the client, his community and the broader social system" (Jezewski, 1994, p. 167). Most clients will respond to a nurse's suggestion if the nurse first listens carefully. The nurse must first understand cultural beliefs before stating reasons for intervention. Listening sessions can present opportunities to educate the client and adapt the program accordingly. Nurses seeking to reach compromises with the client will build trust and ultimately community support for educational programs. Community support of educational programs may be difficult for some persons to follow if cultural differences abound.

CURRENT FACTORS AFFECTING NURSING ROLES IN HEALTH PROMOTION

Health promotion is the key word in the health care workplace today. Nurses are essential for promoting public health. Factors influencing health promotion today are (1) the health care system, (2) nursing roles, (3) increasing technology, (4) the economic environment, and (5) individual behavior.

Health Care System

Change is absolute in nursing. The health care system is changing rapidly due to rising costs of medical care and treatment. Different approaches to health care concerns have resulted in managed care of clients. Insurance parameters, hospital regulations, and physician diagnosis regulate client health care. To reduce the costs of medical care, hospitals are encouraged to provide optimum care to expedite discharge from the unit as soon as possible. The hospital is reimbursed a set dollar amount for each client admission. Extended stays in the hospital result in less monies for care. The current trend is to keep clients away from the hospital unless absolutely necessary.

Nursing Roles

New nursing roles are developing as the profession expands with the changing health care environment. Until recently, nurses carried out physicians' orders and worked predominantly in hospitals at the client's bedside. The role of the nurse today has expanded with specialization and increasing health information. Nurses may become certified in their areas of expertise, such as cardiology, medical-surgical, critical care, pediatrics, or neonatology. Increased knowledge enhances the nursing role. Some nurses today are educated to be nurse practitioners to work in underserved areas of the country. Nurse practitioners work in rural settings, hospitals, or clinics and provide services parallel to the physician specialist: family practice physician, pediatrician, cardiologist, or gynecologist.

Nurses are available to assess additional clients for the physician. Thus, health care is easier for persons to access. The nurse works in collaboration with the physician and provides similar services. Nurse practitioners work in family planning clinics, neonatal units, and physicians' offices. In many areas, the nurse has prescriptive authority to dispense medications when indicated. Increased knowledge leads to increased responsibility and community esteem. Nurses are the leaders in health promotion activities.

Leadership will be vital to the success of health promotion involving the appropriate integration with health care systems. The nurse collaborates with other disciplines to achieve the desired results for the client. Networking will be a selected tool to design and distribute information throughout the country to determine if outcome criteria have been established.

Increasing Technology

Technological advances have greatly impacted the role of the nurse in health promotion. Technology has advanced so much that sometimes it is difficult to keep up with the latest developments. For example, using digital technology, clients now have a wealth of information literally at their fingertips. Some medical practices are now offering results of physicals, electrocardiograms, and other diagnostic tests that can be loaded on a thumb or jump drive. Records can then be updated on visits to specialists and beamed to other health caregivers. Websites such as WebMD and HealthRecord.com let individuals manage their own and their family's health history. Data can be gathered and stored and then shared with physicians, nurses, and other members of the health care team (Saporito, 2005). Computer technology also helps clients research their health concerns and email their providers questions related to their health care.

High-tech equipment is also available for specific diagnostic testing and treatment. Mammography, magnetic resonance imaging, and computerized axial tomography will visualize specific tumors and their size and depth, if present within an individual. Radiation and nuclear medicine are two modes of treatment for persons with diagnosed disease.

Equipment is available to monitor diseases such as diabetes. One example is the One-Touch Glucometer that reads the blood sugar level and may be carried in a small, transportable case for home or hospital use. The test results are immediately displayed.

Health promotion may be achieved more rapidly through technology. Media channels and interactive computer networks are tools to reach a greater number of persons in areas where accessibility to health care is limited or there is a lack of information. Schools, libraries, and many homes have televisions and computers which can be used for the transfer of information.

Economic Environment

Rising medical expenses, health maintenance organizations, and managed care reflect the increasing cost of maintaining health. Public awareness of the state of health care in this country is high today. The federal government is attempting to develop a national health plan. The aging population is increasing. There are dwindling funds to support the aged population when health needs are the greatest. See Chapter 19 for further information on health care cost and quality issues.

Individual Behavior

Each individual must assume responsibility for his or her own health. Genetic predisposition to specific diseases may influence health. Nurses educate individuals about health maintenance and disease when a genetic predisposition exists. For example, the African American population has a predisposition to develop sickle cell anemia, and hereditary factors predispose Hispanics to diabetes. Predisposition is beyond a person's control; however, knowing that a predisposition exists is imper-

ative in preventing serious medical consequences. Perceived benefit of behavior is valued for promoting health (Pender, Murdaugh, & Parsons, 2006).

SUMMARY

Many factors can influence achievement of optimal health or wellness. These factors can be classified according to domains that allow the nurse to view the client in a holistic manner. These domains affecting optimal health are fundamental to health promotion and include biological or physiological, psychological, sociological, environmental, political, spiritual, intellectual, sexual, and technological domains.

Health maintenance and promotion may occur in a variety of settings such as the hospital, home, and community. Types of health-promoting activities include counseling, screening, and education. These activities may occur in any area of health promotion. In the hospital, the nurse addresses the client, family, or caregiver. Factors regarding precipitating symptoms, health history, and support system are obtained at this time. At home, the client, family, and nurse may interact to determine various age spans within the family unit. A primary goal of the nurse in the home, hospital, or community is to develop rapport and trust with the individual, family, or community.

An accepting, trusting relationship between the nurse and client will further lead to compliance and respect for the health care profession, while creating a sense of empowerment for the individual. If nurses can give clients empowerment for the direction of health and wellness in their lives, this empowerment will be passed to the next generation. When the individual assumes personal responsibility for health, the value of health and well-being is also recognized.

Nurses are the persons in the forefront today to encourage health values and responsibility. As a result, disease can be detected earlier with less treatment cost. Health and wellness will increase among general populations. Health services are becoming increasingly accessible in urban and rural areas. Health promotion may occur in any setting at any time when instigated by a qualified health care professional. Resources, public awareness, and public interest for improving quality of life create a positive health perspective for the twenty-first century. Nurses lead the parade in promoting wellness of future generations.

Key Concepts

1. Domains fundamental to effective nursing practice include biological, psychological, sociological, environmental, political, spiritual, intellectual, and technological.

2. Health promotion is a continual, active process designed to achieve and maintain wellness.

3. Holistic nursing practice views health care in terms of the whole individual.

4. The role of the nurse is complex and includes activist/advocate, educator, coordinator of care, leader/member of the profession, provider of care, research user, role model, empowering agent, and change agent.

5. The nursing process is the accepted guide for developing appropriate nursing care and wellness outcomes for clients. The four phases of the nursing process are (1) assessing and establishing a nursing diagnosis, (2) planning, (3) implementing, and (4) evaluating.

6. Health promotion is designed to prevent illness before it begins and to maintain current health status.

7. Promoting individual responsibility for health is significant for long-term health outcomes and compliance.

8. Nursing responsibilities for promoting health care should include understanding of the (1) political and social changes in the government process, (2) risk factors for potential health problems and their respective preventive measures, and (3) health education resources.

9. Risk factors to be considered in developing a health promotion plan include environment, work, socioeconomic level, education, gender, culture, and spiritual beliefs.

10. Current factors influencing health promotion are (1) the rapidly changing health care system, (2) expanded role of the nurse, (3) technology, (4) the economic environment, and (5) individual behavior.

Learning Activities

1. Describe five situations that you have experienced that influenced your achievement of an optimal state of health.

2. Categorize the above in terms of the domains described in the chapter.

3. Take one of the following situations and utilize the nursing process in:

   Listing two factors to be assessed.

   Identifying one nursing diagnosis for each.

   Describing three actions to alleviate the nursing diagnosis.

   Evaluating each action and its efficacy in solving the nursing problem.

Situation A

Mr. Jones, a 55-year-old male, borderline diabetic, is five-feet, 11 inches tall and weighs 200 pounds. His physician reported elevated cholesterol levels and recommended a fitness and weight reduction program. Mr. Jones states he works at a "high pressure" job and eats snacks a lot.

Situation B

Mrs. Smith, an 80-year-old female, lives alone since the death of her spouse two months ago. The family is not able to persuade Mrs. Smith to participate in her usual activities such as grocery shopping and needlework. Her daughter Sue also states Mrs. Smith skips meals, is anemic, and cries a lot.

4. Using the following case study, categorize the data according to identified domain. Describe how each of these domains influences health promotion.

Laura is a 35-year-old single mother of three who has recently been diagnosed with type 2 diabetes. She is a college-educated finance broker for a large company, and she works 50 hours per week. She has few hobbies but does like to read and spend time outdoors with her children. She and her children live in a large apartment complex, and she knows very few of her neighbors. She has low self-esteem and does not like to go out, not even to church, because she has gained 30 pounds over the years. She is computer literate, and she does email old friends occasionally. She knows how to use the Internet to research her newly diagnosed condition.

True/False

1. **T or F**   Health promotion is a continual, active process necessary to achieve wellness.

2. **T or F**   Physiological and genetic composition have no relationship to individual wellness.

3. **T or F**   Another name for the nursing process is problem-solving method.

Multiple Choice Questions

1. Of the following, which role of the nurse is essential when using a health promotion approach to client care?
   a. Coordinator of care
   b. Empowering agent
   c. Member of a profession
   d. Provider of care

2. Immunizations to prevent diphtheria, polio, and tetanus are considered which of the following?
   a. Initial intervention
   b. Primary prevention
   c. Secondary intervention
   d. Tertiary prevention

3. When the nurse initially treats a known problem, the nurse is working at which of the following levels of prevention?

a. Intermediate prevention
b. Primary prevention
c. Secondary prevention
d. Tertiary prevention

Websites

http://galenet.galegroup.com Health and Wellness Resource Center. An online "go to medical reference" center that provides access to references in libraries everywhere.

http://nmfn.com Longevity Game (2005). Includes a game developed by Northwestern Mutual that gives tips on daily lifestyle changes and identifies factors that can lead to a healthier, more productive life.

http://www.ana.org Online Journal of Issues in Nursing. (2005) Provides access to online articles related to professional nursing.

http://pegasus.cc.ucf.edu Resources for Nurses and Families. Nursing Informatics and Technology. Online site provided by the University of California–San Francisco that provides nursing references, Nursing Center, teaching, writing, and search engine resources.

Organizations

ILSI Center for Health Promotion (CHP)
2220 Parklane Drive, Suite 528
Atlanta, GA 30345
Phone: (770) 456-0778
Fax: (202) 659-3617
Nonprofit research and education organization dedicated to the promotion of health in individuals and populations on a global basis.

NANDA International
1211 Locust Street
Philadelphia, PA 19107
Phone: (800) 647-9002
Fax: (215) 564-2175
NANDA International develops terminology to describe the important judgments nurses make in providing nursing care.

Stanford Prevention Research Center
Stanford University School of Medicine
Hoover Pavilion, Mail Code 5705
211 Quarry Road, Room N229
Stanford, California 94305-5705
Phone: (650) 723-6254
Fax: (650) 725-6906
Disseminates information on disease prevention and control. Research conducted through the Center seeks methods to improve the overall level of community health by favorable modifying the social and personal factors known to influence chronic disease incidence: nutrition, physical activity, tobacco use, social and economic factors, and stress.

References

Allender, J. A., & Spradley, B. W. (2001). *Community health nursing: Concepts and practice* (5th ed.). Philadelphia: Lippincott.

American Nurses Association. (2005). Nursing information and data set evaluation center. http://nursingworld.org/nidsec/CLASSLST.HTM

Black, J. M., & Hawks, J. H. (2005). *Medical surgical nursing: Clinical management for positive outcomes.* St. Louis: Elsevier Saunders.

Board of Nurse Examiners for the State of Texas & Texas Board of Vocational Nurse Examiners. (2002). *Differentiated entry level competencies of graduates of Texas nursing programs.* Austin: Board of Nurse Examiners for the State of Texas.

Boutin-Foster, C. (2005). Getting to the heart of social support: A qualitative analysis of the types of instrumental support that are most helpful in motivating cardiac risk factor modification. *Heart and Lung: The Journal of Acute and Critical Care, 34*(1), 22–29.

Cavendish, R., Konecny, L., Mitzelliotis, C., Russo, D., Kraymyak, B., Lanza, L. M., Medefindt, J., & Bajo-MacPartlan, M. A. (2003). Spiritual care activities of nurses using nursing interventions classification (NIC) labels. *International Journal of Nursing Terminologies and Classifications, 14*(4), 113–124.

Craven, R., & Hirnle, C. (2006). *Fundamentals of nursing: Human health and function* (5th ed.). Philadelphia: Lippincott Williams & Wilkins.

Duldt, B. W. (1995). Nursing process: The science of nursing in the curriculum. *Nurse Educator, 20*(1), 24–29.

Fawcett, J. (2005). *Contemporary nursing knowledge: Analysis and evaluation of nursing models and theories.* Philadelphia: F. A. Davis.

Frisch, N. C., & Frisch, L. (2006). *Psychiatric mental health nursing.* Australia: Thomson Delmar Learning.

Giger, J. N., & Davidhizar, R. E. (2004). *Transcultural nursing: Assessment and intervention.* (4th ed.). St. Louis: Mosby.

Green, L. W., & Daniel, M. (2002). Transforming practice, dodging false dichotomies, and avoiding ideological quicksand. In L. E. Young & V. Hayes (Eds.), *Transforming health promotion practice: Concepts, issues, and applications.* Philadelphia: F. A. Davis.

Jezewski, M. A. (1994). Cultural brokering as a model for advocacy. In E. Hein & M. Nicholson (Eds.) *Contemporary leadership behavior: Selected readings* (4th ed., pp. 165–73). Philadephia: Lippincott.

Kearney, R. (2005). *Advancing your career: Concepts of professional nursing.* Philadelphia: F. A. Davis.

Leininger, M. M. (1978). *Transcultural nursing: Concepts, theories, and practice.* New York: National League for Nursing.

Murray, R., & Zentner, J. (2001). *Health promotion strategies through the life span* (7th ed.). Upper Saddle River, NJ: Prentice Hall.

NANDA. (2001). *NANDA Nursing Diagnoses: Definitions and Classification 2001–2002.* Philadelphia: North American Nursing Diagnosis Association.

NANDA. (2007). *NANDA Nursing Diagnoses: Definitions and Classification 2007–2008.* Philadelphia: North American Nursing Diagnosis Association.

National Center for Cultural Competence. (2004). *Community engagement: Culturally and linguistically competent approaches.* Georgetown University. http://nnlm.gov/projects/2004ncc

O'Donnell, M. (1986). Definition of health promotion. *American Journal of Health Promotion, 1,* 4–5.

Pender, N. J. (1996). *Health promotion in nursing practice* (3rd ed.). Norwalk, CT: Appleton & Lange.

Pender, N., Murdaugh, C. L., & Parsons, M. A. (2006). *Health promotion in nursing practice* (5th ed.). Upper Saddle River, NJ: Pearson Prentice Hall.

Reeves, J. S., & Paul, C. (2002). Nursing theory in clinical practice. In J. B. George (Ed.), *Nursing theories: The base for professional nursing practice* (5th ed.). Upper Saddle River, NJ: Prentice Hall.

Saporito, B. (2005, June 27). The e-health revolution. *Time* magazine, Special Report, 55–57.

Sparks-Ralph, S., & Taylor, C. (2005). *Sparks and Taylor's nursing diagnosis reference manual* (6th ed.). Philadelphia: Lippincott Williams & Wilkins.

Stanhope, M., & Knollmueller, R. (2001). *Handbook of public and community health nursing practice: A health promotion guide.* St. Louis: Mosby.

U.S. Department of Health and Human Services. (2000). *Healthy people 2010.* Washington, DC: U.S. Government Printing Office.

U.S. Department of Health and Human Services, Centers for Disease Control and Prevention. (2003). Deaths: Leading causes for 2001. *National Vital Statistics Report.* http://www.cdc.gov/nchs/data/nvsr/nvsr52/nvsr52_09.pd

Bibliography

Barnes, D. M., & Almasy, N. (2005). Refugees' perceptions of healthy behaviors. *Journal of Immigrant Health, 7*(3), 185–193.

Health Source. (2005). Prevention to-do list. *Prevention, 57*(7), 42.

Hellman, E. A. (2005). Health promotion. In J. M. Black & J. H. Hawks (Eds.), *Medical-surgical nursing: Clinical management for positive outcomes* (7th ed.). St. Louis: Elsevier Saunders.

Institute of Medicine. (2002). *Health and behavior: The interplay of biological, behavioral, and societal influences.* Washington, DC: National Academy Press.

Janz, N., Champion, V., & Stretcher, V. (2002). The Health Belief Model. In K. Glanz, B. Rimer, & F. Lewis (Eds.), *Health behavior and health education: Theory, research and practice* (3rd ed.). San Francisco: Jossey-Bass.

Reedy, J., Haines, P. S., & Campbell, M. K. (2005). The influence of health behavior clusters on dietary change. *Preventive Medicine, 41*(1), 268–275.

SECTION II

FACTORS INFLUENCING HEALTH PROMOTION

CHAPTER 5
Communication

CHAPTER 6
Cultural Considerations

CHAPTER 7
Environmental Factors

CHAPTER 8
The Mind-Body Connection

Chapter 5

COMMUNICATION

Verolyn Barnes Bolander, MS, RN, C
Janice A. Maville, EdD, MSN, RN

KEY TERMS

active listening	caring	kinesics	sensory channel
agraphia	communication	message	therapeutic
alogia	context	motor aphasia	communication
andragogy	decoder	nonverbal	touch
aphemesthesia	empathy	communication	unconditional positive
ataxic aphasia	empowerment	nonverbal vocalizations	regard
auditory amnesia	encoder	paralanguage	verbal communication
auditory aphasia	expressive aphasia	pedagogy	visual aphasia
authenticity	feedback	personal presentation	word blindness
body language	global aphasia	proxemics	word deafness

OBJECTIVES

Upon completion of this chapter, the reader should be able to:

- Define communication.
- Discuss the six elements of communication.
- Contrast the two types of communication.
- Relate human behavior to communication.
- Explain the importance of communication in therapeutic relationships as found in selected nursing theories.
- Describe four nurse characteristics that promote effective communication.
- Identify therapeutic techniques for effective communication.
- Discuss the role of the nurse in the use of communication for health promotion.

INTRODUCTION

Marianne Forester is teaching the dangers of steroid use to a group of exceptionally healthy athletes at the prime of their lives. Latonya Washington holds out her arms to a 4-year-old boy as he practices walking with crutches for the first time since his amputation. Carlos Rodriguez works in a hospice where he is stroking the hands of a man dying of AIDS. These are common actions of nurses doing what all nurses must do well. They are teaching, they are encouraging, and they are caring as they seek to promote higher levels of health in their clients. But, they are all doing something even more basic. These nurses are communicating. And, in communicating, they are engaging in one of the cornerstones of health promotion, one of the basic activities upon which all other health-promoting activities are built.

COMMUNICATION AND NURSING

Communication is the process of conveying ideas, thoughts, opinions, or facts from one person to another. In the work setting, nurses communicate most with clients, with their clients' families, and with others on the health care team. When considering nursing care and the human interactions involved, it is difficult to think of anything a nurse does that does not involve communication.

Effective communication is important at all times because breakdowns may cause ill feelings and may result in other negative consequences. Poor communication might even have a devastating effect on a client's health. It is not surprising that health promotion depends to a great extent on communication between nurse and client.

To improve communication skills, nurses must be aware of the messages they are sending at all times. This is not an easy task. Some basic theories, models, and concepts have been created or adapted by nurses to help improve communication. These theories, models, and concepts were generated by a number of individuals from disciplines inside and outside nursing. Nurses

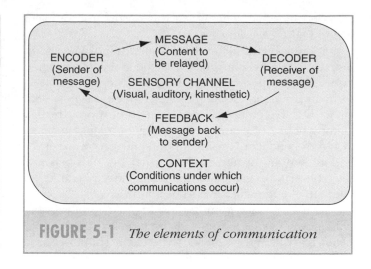

FIGURE 5-1 *The elements of communication*

should be able to use these in a very practical way to promote the health of others.

One widely accepted model suggests communication consists of six elements. These six elements are generally accepted as the basis for communication.

- **message**—the content (idea, thought, opinion, or fact) one person wishes another person to receive. Unfortunately, this content cannot be relayed directly from brain to brain. It must be put in a form that is transmissible and receivable.

- **encoder** (sender)—the person who initiates communication by placing a message in a form that is understandable to the intended recipient.

- **sensory channel**—the means by which a message is sent. There are three primary routes. They are the visual (sight), auditory (hearing), and kinesthetic (touch) channels. Sometimes all three channels are used together, such as when a nurse leans toward an accident victim, looks her in the eye while squeezing her hand, and says, "I can help you."

- **decoder** (receiver)—the intended recipient of the original message. This person must decode the encoded message to understand the sender's intended thought, opinion, or fact.

- **feedback**—the process whereby the overall communication is evaluated for effectiveness. This is the encoding and sending of a message from the receiver back to the original sender in order to let the sender know the message was received. Feedback says, in effect, "I read you loud and clear" or "I'm afraid I didn't quite get your message. Can you repeat it for me?" Without feedback, the sender can never really be certain the intended communication occurred.

- **context**—the conditions under which communication occurs.

Figure 5-1 is a graphic representation of the elements of communication. Awareness of these elements, and how they work, helps nurses and other health care profes-

sionals avoid misunderstandings and can strengthen the communication process. A closer look at the six elements provides a glimpse of how awareness may help a nurse in daily communication.

The Message

Communication will break down when the content (idea, thought, opinion, or fact) of a message is incomplete. The person who starts to talk without knowing (or before thinking through completely) what she or he wants to say often sends a garbled message. Consider, for example, the client with Alzheimer's disease who clutches at a nurse's arm to convey a feeling of discomfort. This client may be incapable of understanding the source of distress—disorientation, loneliness, or something else altogether. The message is vague because the client's thoughts and ideas are confused.

Vague messages are extremely frustrating to the receiver. A nurse who is unable to understand the message is likely unable to help. Health care providers must understand that clients may be communicating without completely understanding their own thoughts. Understanding that communication is breaking down at the point of message formation helps nurses consider ways to help clients focus or relax in order to clarify their thoughts. Where this is not possible, it is necessary to try to think for a client. What has happened that affected the client's ability to communicate clearly?

Encoding

For a variety of reasons, communication can break down with encoding. Much depends on the skill of the encoder. For example, the nurse may intend to ask about a client's stress management and asks, "How have you been?" The client may interpret this as a social greeting and respond with "Fine, How are you?" rather than responding about management of stress. The message the nurse wished to send differed from the actual encoded message sent. When this occurs, the problem lies in faulty encoding.

It is important for nurses to understand when communication is breaking down at the point of encoding rather than at message formation. If a client is unable to form a coherent thought, a nurse's approach to that client will be quite different from the approach to a client who is, for example, speaking a foreign language. When the encoder is using an unfamiliar term (or entire coding system), a nurse needs to let the person know that she or he is using a code that is indecipherable. An alternative code will have to be found.

As the encoder, a nurse must know that the receiver will understand the message. A common language, vocabulary, or code must be used. The client should also be able to understand any abstractions used and be able to concentrate. For example, it is usually helpful for health care professionals to avoid the use of medical terminology or jargon in speech and to use lay terms when communicating with clients.

The Channel

Communication will also break down if inappropriate sensory channels are used. For example, clients may try to tell you that they feel pain. They may have the ability to think clearly but lack the ability to speak (expressive aphasia), as, for example, if they are recovering from a stroke. Such clients may try to form the word for "pain," and it comes out "plant" or "fly." Because they lack the ability to form words appropriately, they are incapable of vocally expressing that they have pain. Worse still, they cannot express where that pain is being experienced. For one lacking verbal encoding ability (the ability to form words), the auditory channel is obviously not the best option.

In such cases, a nurse should understand that communication is breaking down at the auditory channel. Other channels should be explored. Is body language reflective of additional communication? Can the client write out the message? In worst case scenarios, it is also possible to have clients nod or blink in response to "yes" or "no" questions. In other situations a nurse might try the kinesthetic channel and touch a client, feeling for areas of increased warmth where inflammation might be present.

Any communicator should consider all possible channels and the receiver's ability to use them. If the auditory channel is used to convey a message, the receiver's sense of hearing must be unimpaired. It may be necessary move closer to the client or to augment auditory deficits by verifying that a client's hearing aid is in place, is turned on, and contains a working battery.

If the visual channel is used, the receiver must have the eyesight to see the message at the distance it is displayed. The lighting must also be adequate. An astute nurse will assure that needed eyeglasses or contact lenses are clean and in place as well.

If the kinesthetic channel is used, the receiver's reactions to touch should be assessed. This may be an ideal channel for certain messages, but for some individuals, touch may be intrusive. Violating a client's sensibilities may result in a complete rejection of intended communications. Nurses must always seek permission to touch a client.

In summary, it may be necessary to use more than one channel to communicate clearly. When teaching, for example, even clear verbal messages may be enhanced with charts, graphs, outlines, and other visual aids. The nurse in Figure 5-2, for example, is using the auditory channel and the visual channel. When teaching, the nurse might also use the kinesthetic channel when appropriate and desirable.

Decoding

Breakdowns in communication also occur if the receiver is unable to correctly decode the message. Most often, the inability to comprehend a message is the result of a breakdown in an earlier step in the communication process (i.e., an inappropriately encoded message, or an ill-suited channel); however, breakdown may occur even if all else goes well in the communication process. The recipient may not pay attention. This is very frequent in health care. The client may be worried about a family problem, may be depressed or in pain, or may be otherwise distracted. Additionally, the decoder may be so anxious about the expected message that she or he jumps to unwarranted conclusions. Nurses need to note communication blocks and work to overcome them.

Feedback

Communication will also break down without appropriate feedback. Frequently, this stems from a desire to avoid

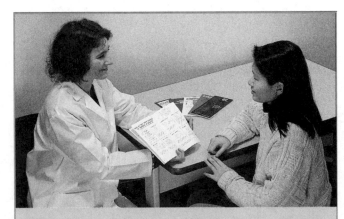

FIGURE 5-2 *Using visual materials enhances the messages the nurse wants to convey and increases the client's understanding.*

Enhancing Message Decoding

When receiving messages, do you ask for clarification whenever necessary? Do you pay close attention to the sender or do you fail to hear what is being said because you are thinking about what you will say next? Always focus on what is being said and really listen to the entire message before you start to formulate a response.

Validating Understanding of Messages

As a nurse who suspects a block in communication at the point of feedback, you should be able to assess the client's understanding by asking specific questions to verify understanding. Do not simply ask whether or not the client understands. A good idea is to ask a question that cannot be answered with a simple yes or no. A good example of this type of question is, "Tell me how you can alter your diet to reduce your cholesterol level."

embarrassment. Consider, for example, a client who may nod in apparent understanding when the physician explains measures to lower cholesterol. As soon as the physician leaves the room, the client turns to the nurse and asks, "What did the doctor mean by "lower my lipid level?"

Context

Finally, communication may break down because of conditions in which it occurs. Context affects all other elements of communication. Think about what a blizzard would do to the communication between a couple in a stranded car. They might be too distracted by the cold to think or speak clearly. Words sent over the auditory channel might be drowned out by the roar of the wind outside. Environmental context also applies in the health care arena. Role relationships and emotional factors frequently come into play in emotionally charged situations. For example, a parent may be so anxious about her child that she never even hears a nurse's attempts at communication.

Contextual variables affecting communication include:

- surrounding environment, including the geography, climate, weather, and ambient temperature

- social, cultural, and ethnic expectations for individuals as they communicate

- social, work, and educational positions and roles of the participants in the interaction

- history and experiences of the participants

- physical, mental, and emotional states of the participants

- goals and expectations of the participants

- effects of current events on the situation

- time constraints imposed on the participants

Each of these factors may have positive or negative effects on a given communication. Most allow for inter-

vention by the alert nurse who is aware of ways to enhance communication by taking the context into consideration.

TYPES OF COMMUNICATION

Communication theorists generally accept that there are two types of communication: verbal and nonverbal. **Verbal communication** is the use of words to convey messages. Most often these words are written or spoken, but they may be formed in other ways, such as by the use of the telegraph key, sign language, or braille. **Nonverbal communication** is the conveyance of messages without the use of words. Nurses can be more effective communicators if they are consciously aware of both the nonverbal and the verbal communication occurring between themselves and others.

Verbal Communication

It would seem that verbal communication should be very clear because of the use of a common language made up of defined words. Unfortunately, like all communication, the verbal arena is subject to faulty message formation, encoding, channel selection, reception, decoding, and feedback.

Speakers vary in their ability to use language to convey precise content. Additionally, dictionaries differ in their definitions of words. Worse yet, many words have more than one meaning, and those meanings often change over time and geography. For example, in 1958, a teenager might have asked for a "pop" in Toledo, Ohio; a "soda" in Beacon, New York; or a "phosphate" in Boston, Massachusetts. All three references indicate a carbonated beverage in a generic sense. Similarly, a teenage girl in the 1950s would likely refer to her steady date as her "boyfriend," but her grandmother would refer to him as her granddaughter's "beau." Some words last beyond their time. Some generalize and some become more specific over time. In some respects it is a wonder that verbal communication does not break down far more frequently than it does.

It is interesting to note that the ability to use verbal communication is so important that an inability to verbally communicate is considered a disease. Look at Table 5-1 for some terms related to the inability to communicate via various channels.

Teaching is a very large part of nursing. When teaching, verbal communication can be vital (but not essential). Think of how difficult it likely was for the teacher of Helen Keller. It was necessary to first teach her student to communicate verbally by touch before she could really begin her much wider education. When teaching, it is often helpful to send verbal messages over more than one channel at the same time. Educators, for example, make wide use of computers, movies, videos, television, slide-tape presentations, and lectures with the use of an overhead projector.

In addition to augmenting the spoken word with pictures, diagrams, music, and other nonverbal messages, audiovisual technologies are frequently used to present words in both speech and print. This uses both visual and auditory channels for the same verbal content. This reinforcement is helpful in communication and in learning retention. For example, a video might feature a speaker who is introduced only by the title "Dr." and a last name, which might be spelled "Wallick," "Walluch," "Walluck," "Wallach," or "Wallack." Presenting the speaker's name

visually in a subtitle makes it much less frustrating for the viewer to later find books or articles written by that particular speaker.

When teaching one-to-one, the nurse should reinforce the spoken word with the written word whenever possible. A printed handout or booklet allows the client to review key points in the message whenever necessary, and it allows the client to take the message home upon discharge from the health care facility, if needed. A handwritten message can do the same.

TABLE 5-1 Communication Channels, Deficits, and Descriptive Terms

Channel	Deficit	Descriptive Term
Auditory, expressive	Ability to think without the ability to speak Types include: • a general inability to speak • an inability to coordinate the muscles responsible for speech	Expressive aphasia Alogia Motor aphasia, ataxic aphasia
Auditory, receptive	Ability to think and hear without the ability to understand the spoken word heard	Auditory aphasia (auditory amnesia, word deafness)
Visual, expressive	In a literate person, the inability to coordinate hand muscles sufficiently to produce handwriting	Motor aphasia (agraphia)
Visual, receptive	In a literate person, the inability to decode the written word	Visual aphasia (word blindness)
Mixed auditory and visual, receptive	In a literate person with the ability to think, an inability to understand the spoken or the written word	Aphemesthesia
All channels	In a literate person, an inability to express or receive verbal messages in any form	Global aphasia

Working with an Interpreter

Interpreting for people with hearing impairments is very physical. It involves almost constant movement of the arms, hands, and fingers of the interpreter, resulting in expenditure of a great deal of energy. Allowing for intervals of rest is important, especially when interpretation is needed for extended periods of time.

Personal Presentation

Think about a female acquaintance you know fairly well. With this person in mind, think about your reaction if she shaved her head. What would this behavior communicate to you? For this individual, would this behavior have a specific meaning?

Is she the type who is merely looking for attention? Does she have a health problem, such as a skin condition, that requires shaving for treatment? Is she joining a religious cult? Is she protesting something? Did she lose a bet? Is she self-mutilating because of a mental illness? Does she have a role in a play or movie? Taking into consideration all that you know about her, you might make a correct guess. But it would only be a guess until confirmed.

Special attention needs to be paid to clients with impaired receptive channels. The visually impaired have much less trouble with verbal communication than do the hearing impaired. Communication with a receiver who is hearing impaired is often time-consuming, as is feedback. To avoid confusion, it is sometimes necessary to communicate through a third person, or interpreter, whose hearing is intact and who has the ability to use sign language (sign). The interpreter listens to a hearing speaker, interprets the words into sign language for the client with impaired hearing, and reverses the process for feedback to the sender. If no interpreter is available, the client with impaired hearing will usually be able to either read lips to some degree or read written language.

Clients who are hearing impaired and who use a sign language/system make up a very diverse population. Their diversity is reflected not only by their hearing impairment but also by individual differences in age, gender, race, ethnicity, national origin, religion, sexual orientation, and socioeconomic status as well as the sign language/system that they use. A client who identifies as a member of the deaf community/culture in the United States usually uses American Sign Language. Others who are hearing impaired or hard of hearing and who use a hearing aid will most likely use an invented sign system (Scott & Lee, 2003). In some situations it may be necessary to use the services of a sign language interpreter to facilitate communication and better serve the health needs of clients who are hearing impaired.

Those who sign use their hands to spell out letters of the alphabet or to indicate entire words. Signing letters one at a time is termed fingerspelling and can be laborious. Even so, to learn to sign entire words, learning to fingerspell is a first step—much like learning the alphabet to read words. See Additional Resources at the end of this chapter for resources helpful in learning to fingerspell and sign.

Writing is also an option when lip reading and signing are not. It is slow but it is a definite alternative. Paper and pencil should always be readily available for nurses to use with clients who are hearing impaired.

Nonverbal Communication

It is well known that over 90 percent of communication is nonverbal. No matter how hard we try, we cannot avoid communicating in a nonverbal manner. Our appearance, facial expressions, body language, and other behaviors all relay a message. How that message is interpreted by receivers can vary. Theorists agree that most communication takes place without the use of words. A large number of variables may alter messages, so they must be interpreted with caution.

Nonverbal communication consists of body language and paralanguage. **Body language** is the use of nonverbal communication behaviors that include personal presentation, proxemics, kinesics, and touch. **Paralanguage** is the use of nonverbal components of spoken language. These components consist of nonverbal vocalizations and vocalizations that alter the quality of verbal messages.

Personal Presentation

Personal presentation is how individuals show themselves to the world. It includes dress, grooming, and the use of cosmetics, perfumes, and deodorants. Personal presentation creates an identity that an individual wishes to portray to the outside world. Details may vary depending on where an individual will be going and whom he or she might see. For example, a person may choose to present herself or himself differently when going to school than when going out for a formal dinner.

The person who fails to meet societal expectations or who alters her or his normal pattern of personal presentation is communicating something to others. It may be a health care need that is communicated. For example, someone who has not attended to personal appearance may indicate a lack of needed resources (time, money, or energy). This behavior may also be communicating a change in level of health. Failure to attend to normal grooming frequently signals a lack of energy that may indicate a depression. Bear in mind, however, that changes in grooming may result from a number of factors, as may any change in behavior. The meaning of nonverbal behavior, including presentation of self, cannot be interpreted with certainty without verification by the sender of the message.

Proxemics

Proxemics is how we use the personal space around us, the distances we maintain from others. The scientific study of proxemics in humans began with Hall (1966), who theorized that people are surrounded, at all times, by a space considered to be an extension of that person. This is "personal" space. Most individuals allow only a select few—such as children or a spouse—to enter this space. They become very uncomfortable if others intrude into it. Most people tend to behave in ways designed to protect their space from accidental intrusion. The size of this personal space is culturally determined and varies considerably. In the United States, for example, most of us maintain personal distances of approximately 18 inches. Of course, there are also individual variations.

Most activities and relationships are governed by concepts of space. People tend to place themselves at socially and culturally determined distances from each other according to their relationships and according to their activities at the time. These distances have been determined to be approximately as follows (see Figure 5-3):

- intimate distance (0 to 1.5 feet)—the distance allowing touch and very close communications, usually only with a select few persons.

- personal distance (1.5 to 4.0 feet)—the distance allowing personal communications with persons known fairly well.

- social distance (4 to 12 feet)—the distance allowing casual, social-level communications with acquaintances.

- public distance (12 to over 25 feet)—the distance allowing formal communication among one person and a larger number of persons, as might occur with public speaking in an auditorium.

A person who fails to adhere to unwritten rules concerning appropriate distances for communication may be demonstrating a lack of socialization to cultural norms. Alternatively, a person who feels her or his personal space is being violated will often feel threatened. The normal response is to back away and thus increase personal space. Most people can read this subtle body language and back away from someone's personal zone after an accidental intrusion. Failure to back away, it is important to note, frequently causes extreme discomfort, especially if the person is, for example, confined to a hospital bed and cannot back away. Intrusions into personal space can result in unexpected behavior. In extreme cases, persons may even become violent as they seek to protect themselves.

Nurses need to be aware of space. They work closely with clients at intimate distances, meeting personal needs in a matter-of-fact manner. It is important

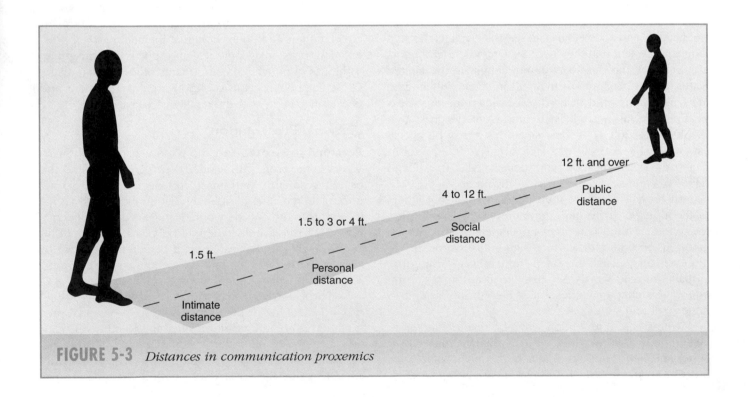

FIGURE 5-3 *Distances in communication proxemics*

to understand that individual clients have varying levels of tolerance for such closeness and intrusion into their space. Nurses must, therefore, be ever aware of, and respectful of, the personal space needs of clients. This requires being alert to slight body movements. It requires explaining to a client what will be done before making an intrusive action. It often requires asking permission.

Kinesics

Kinesics is the conscious or unconscious movement of the body. It includes changes in body posture, facial expressions, and gestures. As with other types of body language, kinesics may be conscious or unconscious, voluntary or involuntary. Kinesics are, therefore, not easy to interpret with precision. Is a person with a "ramrod" spine sitting up so straight because she is alert and on the defensive or has she merely spent a lifetime learning to maintain excellent posture?

People communicate a variety of emotions with their bodies, eye contact, and facial expressions. These communications are often culturally determined. For example, a young Asian woman who lowers her eyes when talking to an adult is showing respect. On the other hand, a young American woman who lowers her eyes when talking to an adult is often thought to be indicating dishonesty, guilt, or shame.

Touch

Touch is the manner in which people come into bodily contact with one another. It can be seen as a special way of moving your body or gesturing, or it may be seen as the most intimate distance in the study of proxemics. Touch is a very important part of human communication and, indeed, of human health and even human life. Touch can be comforting and pleasurable when it communicates caring, as seen in Figure 5-4, or it may cause physical and emotional pain. A firm handshake may communicate trust and the offer of friendship while a limp handshake, on the other hand, may flag boredom or distaste.

Paralanguage

Paralanguage is the use of sounds with and without words (verbal language). It is an intermediate area between nonverbal and verbal communication; it consists of **nonverbal vocalizations** (such as grunts, groans, sighs, and sobs) that alter the quality of verbal messages.

Vocalizations That Alter the Quality of Verbal Messages

Vocalizations that accompany verbal messages (such as accent, intensity, intonation, nasality, pause, pitch, range, rate, rhythm, stress, and volume) are closely associated

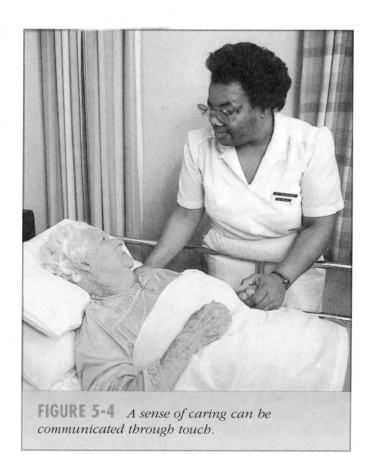

FIGURE 5-4 *A sense of caring can be communicated through touch.*

with, and often support and strengthen, the accompanying verbal message. It is best when this is so. This does not always occur, however, and the verbal message and its accompanying paralanguage message may disagree. Consider the person who rapidly snaps, "Oh, I just don't care. Do what you want to do!" Obviously she *does* care and cares enough to be angry about it.

COMMUNICATION AND THE THERAPEUTIC RELATIONSHIP

Nurses are expected to use communications with clients in a manner designed to promote health. The interactions with clients should be therapeutic relationships. Because the profession of nursing is a science as well as an art, it is important to recognize how nursing theories incorporate communication and what characteristics of nurses enhance the communication process.

Communication in Selected Nursing Theories

Throughout the years, nursing theorists have provided some guidelines to help professional nurses engage in therapeutic relationships. Some theorists have been explicit in explaining the role of communication in the therapeutic nature of nursing while others imply its importance. The following theories are presented as examples.

Peplau

Hildegard Peplau (1952), an early nurse theorist, believed that nurses promote trust by relating to their clients in an authentic manner, sharing feelings and thoughts appropriately. She supported closeness in a therapeutic relationship as a means to build trust, increase the client's self-esteem, and lead to the growth of the client.

Peplau identified six roles nurses use within the nurse-client relationship (see Table 5-2). Through the

use of appropriate communication strategies within each role, nurses may become excellent at meeting needs of the client.

Travelbee

Joyce Travelbee (1966), another respected nurse theorist, also discussed the interpersonal relationship between nurse and client. For Travelbee, the focus of the relationship was the client's needs. She believed that for the relationship to proceed therapeutically, it was vital that the nurse have an understanding of the client's experience. She felt that such understanding was impossible without appreciating the client's uniqueness without labeling or stereotyping. Travelbee characterized therapeutic communication as human-to-human communication and believed it to be reciprocal and dynamic.

King

Imogene King developed a conceptual framework for nursing in the 1960s that she further clarified throughout the 1970s and 1980s (Alligood & Marriner-Tomey, 2002). It initially consisted of four systems universal to nursing: social systems, perceptions, interpersonal relationships, and health. Communication was inherent within each of these systems and a major concept in the interpersonal systems.

In 1981 King expanded her framework to include goal attainment, which addressed how nurses interact with clients for health goal achievement (Alligood & Marriner-Tomey, 2002). She added concepts of personal space, learning, and coping. With emphasis on human characteristics and interaction, communication becomes vitally important.

Orem

Nurse theorist Dorothy Orem developed her self-care deficit nursing theory based on her dedication to the concept that humans have an innate need for self-care to manage life and health. Nursing strives to assist in overcoming limitations that humans may have in achieving self-care. Her theory places emphasis on nursing interventions for the purposes of maintaining health, preventing illness, or restoring health whether the actions are for or with the client (Hood & Leddy, 2003). When put into practice, Orem's theory intended for collaboration to occur between the nurse and the individ-

TABLE 5-2 Peplau's Nursing Roles in the Nurse-Client Relationship

Nursing Role	Nurse-Client Relationship
Stranger	At first both nurse and client are strangers. The client may view the nurse as fitting into some preconceived notion of what a nurse should be, which may or may not be factual. Mutual interest and respect will allow the nurse and client to inform each other simply and clearly about their mutual expectations for their interaction.
Resource person	As a resource person, the nurse provides the client with specific answers to any number of questions relative to health care. The nurse interprets technical information to the client in a straightforward manner that can be understood but also realizes when the client's questions involve problems that may require the use of counseling.
Teacher	As a teacher, the nurse does not merely hand down knowledge based on what some authority figure has declared to be true. Rather, the nurse develops novel learning experiences that can lead the client to fruitful outcomes. Peplau noted that this role is really a combination of all other roles and can lead the client to a habit of grappling with all of life's difficulties rather than responding to them as an automaton might.
Leader	In addition to the fact that leadership is demanded of nurses on the local, national, and international levels, client groups often expect nurses to be their leaders. For these client groups, the best type of leadership is a democratic style in which all group members make decisions together.
Surrogate	The client sometimes casts the nurse in the role of surrogate parent, sibling, teacher, or other significant person from the client's past. The nurse is not seen as an individual in his or her own right. This perception is not easily altered, but the nurse can help the client to recognize similarities and differences between the nurse and the person with whom the client has identified him or her. The nurse can best do this by being authentic and by being accepting of the client.
Counselor	In the counselor role, the nurse does not tell the client what to do. Rather, the nurse helps to facilitate the client's self-directed actions and promotes experiences leading to health.

ual or the person responsible for the individual if he or she were dependent.

Although mainly focused on the individual and his or her needs, most nursing interventions could not be accomplished without the use of good communication. Orem's self-care theory has been widely used in nursing education, practice, and research.

Nurse Characteristics That Promote Communication

Certain characteristics of nurses tend to promote communication. An astute nurse will cultivate these characteristics as personal attitudes to strengthen communication with clients.

Unconditional Positive Regard

Unconditional positive regard is an attitude that Carl Rogers (1942), the renowned psychotherapist, believed to be necessary for any therapist to have if positive results were to be attained from therapy. Nursing adopted this value. Showing **unconditional positive regard** for your client means accepting and respecting the client as a fellow human being, without imposing any conditions for that acceptance.

Nurses display this characteristic in verbal and nonverbal ways. By saying "I'm so glad to see you today" the nurse accepts the client and encourages the client to be herself. Using touch, such as a pat on the hand or back, offers further encouragement.

Unconditional positive regard is a characteristic that promotes trust between the client and nurse. When the nurse has this attitude, clients will feel more freedom to express themselves without anticipation of rejection.

Empathy

Empathy, or empathetic understanding, means identifying closely with a client because a nurse can imagine herself in the client's situation. Offering comments such as "I think I understand how you feel" or mirroring the client's facial expressions are examples of verbal and nonverbal ways of displaying empathy. When there is empathy, there is harmony between the nurse and client.

Authenticity and Genuineness

Authenticity means being real or genuine, as opposed to hiding behind a mask of professionalism. Being authentic helps to further establish trust with the client. Authenticity requires openness and sharing of true feelings. For instance, if an obese teenager on a weight management program sets a goal of losing 10 pounds in 10 days, it is honest to say "I think it would be better if we looked at a more realistic time frame" instead of "I just know you can do it!"

Caring

Caring is more than just the respect and valuing that occurs with unconditional positive regard. **Caring** is having a personal interest in the client; it is *feeling* for the client; it involves an investment of the self. Caring is exhausting, however. It entails a substantial drain of emotional energy. Many nurses become disappointed or hurt because a client's health care outcomes were not attained.

But there are rewards for caring. Nurses experience much relief or happiness as they see a client progress a great deal. Caring involves a risk but it can be one of the most beneficial aspects of nursing.

Caring can be shown in many ways both verbally and nonverbally. Just saying "I care about you" establishes a climate of acceptance and encouragement. Merely paying attention shows a sense of caring for a client.

Active Listening

Active listening is the act of perceiving what is communicated verbally as well as nonverbally. Active listening is critical to true communication between the client and nurse. Listening becomes active when it moves beyond mere hearing of the words being spoken and into an involvement with the client whereby feelings, meanings, or intentions behind spoken words are reflected by the nurse. In this sense, active listening helps the client to clarify and further articulate inner thoughts. For example, a client may say, "I can't follow this diet." A typical response could be "Don't worry; many people are successful with this diet." An active listening response could be "I understand that you feel you can't follow this diet. Could you tell me what makes you feel this way?" Active listening relays to the speaker not only that what she or he said was understood but also that the speaker's underlying feelings were comprehended.

There are many advantages to active listening. First, it enhances the relationship between the nurse and the client by creating a sense of mutual trust. Second, it minimizes the chances for misinterpretation. Third, it creates an atmosphere of acceptance that encourages clients to verbalize more than they might otherwise do.

In using active listening, nurses must be cognizant of verbal and nonverbal messages being conveyed by

Nursing Alert

Communicating Therapeutically

Never assume that because you are using one example of a therapeutic technique you are communicating therapeutically. Peplau (Parker, 2006) noted that it is important that nurses be able to use a wide range of therapeutic techniques and even more important that they are able to identify which technique they are using at a given time. Conscious awareness of interactions remains vital to therapeutic communication.

clients in order to respond appropriately. It is important also that nurses understand that their personal characteristics, their choice of communication techniques, and the manner and timing of their use of communication techniques can all affect communication (Estes, 2006).

Specific Techniques That Promote Communication

Therapeutic communication requires the use of verbal and nonverbal techniques that are focused on client needs. It also requires the avoidance of unhelpful or nontherapeutic techniques. The ability to use these techniques may only be developed if practiced. Table 5-3 provides a list of therapeutic communication techniques, their definitions, and examples of how they can be used in various age groups. Table 5-4 identifies some of the nonverbal and verbal barriers to communication that can interfere with the therapeutic relationship between the client and nurse.

USING COMMUNICATION FOR HEALTH PROMOTION

The organizing framework that nurses use to achieve the goals for health promotion is the nursing process, which was discussed in Chapter 4. For health promotion this involves collaboration with the client to identify needs, determine desired outcomes, plan actions, implement the plan, and evaluate the actual outcomes. Obviously, effective communication is vital in this collaborative process between the nurse and the individual, family, group, or community.

Communication and *Healthy People 2010*

As discussed in Chapter 1, *Healthy People 2010* is a national health initiative for Americans that has two major goals: (1) to increase the quality of life, and the number of years of healthy life, and (2) to eliminate health disparities (U.S. Dept. of Health and Human

TABLE 5-3 Therapeutic Communication Techniques

Technique	Description/Definition	Example
Provide broad opening	The nurse invites the client to select a topic.	Nurse with child: "What would you like to tell me about yourself?" Nurse with adolescent: "Tell me what's been on your mind." Nurse with adult: "I'm interested in hearing about issues of concern to you."
Provide silence	The nurse allows the verbal conversation to stop to provide a time for quiet contemplation of what has been discussed, for formulation of thoughts about how to proceed, or for tension reduction.	(Silence) Nurse observes client's behavior for what is not being expressed verbally. Child: Looks down at floor. Adolescent: Eyes well with tears. Adult: Fidgets with hands, adjusts in chair, and eyes dart around the room.
Select focus	The nurse selects one topic for exploration from among several possible topics presented by the client.	Nurse with child: "You said you hate all of your brothers. Tell me about Melvin first." Nurse with adolescent: "You've briefly mentioned three different suicide attempts. For now, I'd like to focus on just what was going on with you at the time of the first attempt." Nurse with adult: "Let's return to the last point you made and talk more about that."
Clarify	The nurse lets the client know that what was said was unclear. If necessary, the nurse asks for clarification or provides input regarding how to make the message clearer.	Nurse with child: "You say you fell in a hole. Tell me what you mean by this." Nurse with adolescent: "I didn't understand what you meant then. Can you say that in different words?" Nurse with adult: "Let me repeat back to you what I think I heard you say."
Interpret	The nurse pulls facts together to come to a conclusion and then verifies that with the client.	Nurse with child: "OK, your two friends pushed you into the slide and that's how you got the scar on your head." Nurse with adolescent: "Your stomach pains seem to happen whenever you have to give a report in class." Nurse with adult: "Your food and sleep diary shows that you sleep better when you have a light snack around 9 PM."
Restate	The nurse rephrases what the client has said. The rephrased message lets the client know the nurse is attentive and allows for further dialogue.	Child: "Ugh! That's yucky!" Nurse: "You don't like how the medicine tastes, right?" Adolescent: "I upchucked and it grossed me out." Nurse: "You vomited and it upset you." Adult: "I'm up and down all night." Nurse: "You are having difficulty sleeping."
Validate	The nurse attempts to verify with the client that a certain term means the same thing to both parties.	Nurse with child: "You want 'moo moo'? Does 'moo moo' mean milk?" Nurse with adolescent: "When you say your brother is crazy, does the word 'crazy' mean 'kind of wild'?" Nurse with adult: "Tell me if we both understand the term 'nap' the same way."

Adapted from Health Assessment & Physical Examination *(3rd ed.), by, M.E. Z. Estes, 2006, Clifton Park, NY: Thomson Delmar Learning.*

TABLE 5-4 Barriers to Effective Communication

Nonverbal Barriers of Client or Nurse		Verbal Barriers
Physical	**Psychological**	**Errors in message conveyed by nurse**
1. Speech impairment 2. Hearing impairment 3. Vision impairment 4. Cognitive impairment 5. Environmental distractions or disruptions	1. Personal perceptions 2. Personal prejudices 3. Fear of person, environment, subject 4. Lack of interest	1. Giving orders, advice 2. Threatening client 3. Lecturing 4. Criticizing, blaming, shaming 5. Overly praising 6. Too much or too little information

Services, 2000). *Healthy People 2010* has identified 10 leading health indicators and 467 related objectives. As such, *Healthy People 2010* provides for a framework for prevention of threats to health for individuals, groups, communities, and the nation.

Programs to meet the goals of *Healthy People 2010* are directed at preventing disease and promoting health. Prevention involves nurses working with clients individually or in groups to prevent disease by providing counseling and education on many health issues. It may also include expertise in performing and interpreting results of screening tests, administering immunizations, and giving medications aimed at preventing disease. Promoting health becomes both challenging and rewarding when nurses endeavor to encourage and empower people to adopt or adhere to healthy lifestyles.

Communication is not only a necessity but also a vital key in meeting the goals of *Healthy People 2010* whether the nurse is actively participating in a formal health program for many clients or caring for an individual client in a clinic, an institution, or the client's own home.

Nurses most often communicate with clients as they serve in five of the six roles identified by Peplau. Recall that, at first, clients and nurses are strangers and nurses and clients must communicate about their shared expectations for their interaction. Nurses then fulfill the roles of resource persons (answering questions and interpreting technical information), teachers (developing novel learning experiences for clients), leaders (encouraging the democratic process in client groups), and counselors (facilitating the clients' self-directed actions and promoting experience, leading to health).

It is important to remember that within each of these roles nurses may communicate with clients who are individuals, couples, families, small groups, or larger groups in communities or societies. Often it is a nursing goal to change the behavior of these clients. Changes may include:

- encouraging clients to behave in a manner more consistent with attaining higher levels of wellness, or

- discouraging them from behaving in a manner that could cause them to become ill.

The Health Promotion Model and Communication

Pender's Health Promotion Model and Revised Health Promotion Model (Pender, Murdaugh, & Parsons, 2006), as described in Chapter 3, is often used by nurses to assist clients in altering their behaviors relative to health. It is helpful in facilitating a change in behavior and in making decisions about health. This model proposes that individual characteristics (biological, psychological, and sociocultural) and experiences (past health behavior) have both a direct and an indirect effect on the likelihood of an individual engaging in behaviors to promote health. What the individual perceives about the health-promoting behavior (benefits of and barriers to action, perceived control of health, and perceived self-efficacy) and what influences exist (family, peers, societal norms and models, and personal and work environment) have a direct effect on the commitment to a plan of action and on the health-promoting behavior. Table 5-5 identifies some specific communication-related interventions according to domains which could be helpful.

Refer to the therapeutic communication techniques in Table 5-3. When using Pender's Health Promotion Model and Revised Health Promotion Model, nurses use a variety of these therapeutic techniques of communication to draw information from clients. In doing so, they discover their clients' definition of health, the importance of health, the perception of control of health, the ability to control personal health, and interpersonal as well as situational influences and support. A great deal of this information may be new even to the client.

TABLE 5-5 Communication-Related Nursing Interventions Categorized by Domain

Domain	Interventions
Biological	Assess clients for intact sensory perception abilities (vision, hearing, touch). Make sure clients use hearing aids or eyeglasses if available. Assess clients for physical conditions that may cause communication difficulties or limitations, including loss of sensory perception, stroke, injuries, disease, or birth defects. Monitor energy levels and expenditure during communication. Allow for rest periods as needed. Arrange for an interpreter if needed. Modify visual materials as necessary.
Psychological	Assess each client's readiness to communicate. Assess each client's understanding of messages sent or information provided. Provide clarification as necessary.
Sociocultural	Recognize the customs, beliefs, and values of each individual client. Modify communication to accommodate cultural beliefs and customs.
Spiritual/Religious	Recognize that spiritual and religious beliefs have varying influences on the client's perceptions of health and control of health.
Environmental	Ensure an environment conducive to good communication, including adequate lighting, comfortable temperature, and freedom from distracting noise.
Technological	Choose the appropriate technology for communicating: video, audiotape, computer-interactive, teleconference, email.

Empowering Through Communication

Empowerment, in relation to health promotion, is the process of helping others help themselves. For the nurse, this involves much persuasion, support, and encouragement. But empowerment can best be accomplished through education. In fact, health promotion and health education are seen as synonymous by many.

The rising cost of health care and the abundance of information on health care issues, made available to individuals from a variety of sources, are two major forces driving the increased demand by clients for knowledge and skills about self-care and prevention of disease (Bastable, 2003). The Internet has become a medium for both information and misinformation. Nurses can help to empower clients through introducing new information, clarifying misinformation, and validating clients' interpretations of information.

Healthy People 2010 (2000) delineates 28 focus areas (see Table 1-2, Chapter 1) related to two overarching goals: (1) to increase quality and years of healthy life, and (2) to eliminate health disparities. Teaching as related to these goals requires effective communication by all health professionals with all categories of clientele, whether they be children, adults, families, or groups in the community. Understanding what to teach, how learners learn,

the learning environment, and technological aspects of communication is important for nurses as they communicate with education as the focus. In order for the teaching to be effective, it must be tailored to the client.

What to Teach

In some work settings, nurses teach content or programs integral to the health agency or facility. For example, a clinic nurse teaches about the immunizations and chemoprophylaxis (drug therapy) that the clinic provides. The specific content taught to each individual or group depends on the clients' needs for specific information. Clients want to know about those things that have relevance or personal meaning for them, such as information that will help them avoid trouble, solve their problems, or live a better life.

How Learners Learn

Adults learn differently than children. Malcolm Knowles, renowned adult learning theorist, in his classic text, *The Modern Practice of Adult Education: Andragogy versus Pedagogy* (1970), described the difference between **andragogy,** the education of adults, and **pedagogy,** the education of children. Knowles's concepts are timeless and form the foundation for educating adults even today. His four andragogical assumptions are that adults

1. move from dependency to self-directedness;

2. draw upon their reservoir of experience for learning;

3. are ready to learn when they assume new roles; and

4. want to solve problems and apply new knowledge immediately.

Keeping these assumptions in mind is helpful when planning any educational intervention for promoting health of the adult, whether as an individual, a spouse/partner, or the parent of a child. Accordingly, nurses teaching adults should follow these guidelines:

- Include the client in the learning plan.

- Arrange for a diagnosis of learner needs and interests.

- Identify learning objectives based on the diagnosed needs.

- Build on learning from simple to complex components.

- Evaluate the quality of the learning as it is occurring.

- Re-diagnose needs for further learning.

Table 5-6 includes these assumptions and teaching design considerations in a comparison of pedagogy to andragogy. This comparison provides valuable information to be considered when developing the health promotion plan as described in Chapter 3.

The Learning Environment

Creating a supportive, nonthreatening environment for learning can greatly enhance the communication process in teaching. First, the nurse needs to recognize that learning can take place at any time or any place as long as the client feels comfortable. Sometimes learning is best done

TABLE 5-6 Pedagogy and Andragogy: A Comparison

	Assumptions			Design for Teaching	
	Pedagogy	**Andragogy**		**Pedagogy**	**Andragogy**
Self-concept	Dependent	Self-directed	**Climate for Learning**	Authority oriented, formal, competitive	Mutuality, respectful, collaborative, informal
Experience	Builds with age	A resource for learning	**Planning**	Nurse	Mutual between client and nurse
Readiness	Depends on biological development and social pressures	Depends on developmental task of social roles (parent, spouse, employee, etc.)	**Diagnosis of Needs**	Nurse	Mutual between client and nurse
Time Perspective	Postponed application	Immediate application	**Formulation of Objectives**	Nurse	Negotiated by client and nurse
Orientation to Learning	Subject-centered	Problem-centered	**Design**	Focus on subject and content	Developed in terms of client preference and need to problem-solve
			Evaluation	Nurse	Mutual evaluation by nurse and client with re-diagnosis of needs

Adapted from "Andragogy," by M. K. Smith, 1996, 1999, The encyclopaedia of informal education, *http://www.infed.org/lifelonglearning/b-andra.htm, last updated January 28, 2005.*

Research Note

Identification of Learning Needs of Professionals Who Teach Health Promotion

Study Problem/Purpose: To assess the self-perceived skills and preferred learning formats of maternal and child health educators who teach health promotion content in their professional practice areas.

Method: The study used a survey design whereby a self-administered instrument was developed and distributed via email to maternal and child health educators from medicine, nursing, dentistry, social work, and public health who were members of *Bright Futures,* a national health promotion workgroup. In addition to questions about background, experience, and continuing education for teaching, the survey asked respondents to rate their confidence and desire for improvement in teaching health promotion concepts related to the following six core areas: partnership, communication, health promotion/illness prevention, time management, education, and advocacy.

Findings: Of the 180 respondents, 41 percent had backgrounds in nursing, 27 percent in public health, 27 percent in medicine, 14 percent in dentistry, 8 percent in social work, and 6 percent in "other" areas. Forty-six percent of the respondents reported having attended seminars or lectures for continuing education on teaching. The majority agreed or strongly agreed that they were confident in their ability to teach the six health promotion concepts. Eighty-two percent of respondents indicated that time constraints were a barrier to integrating health promotion information into teaching settings, 58 percent indicated lack of funds, and 30 percent indicated lack of resources. Most were comfortable in using electronic technology (email, Internet, CD-ROM).

Implications: Health professionals, like their clients, learn in a variety of ways and have varied preferences for learning. Assessing the learning needs, skills, and preferences of educators, such as maternal and child health educators in this study, is important in developing supporting programs that will, in turn, affect the quality of care for their clientele. Electronic technology can be used as a communication tool for assessing the learning needs of health care professionals and for delivering content to enhance practice.

Bernstein, H. H., Rieber, S., Stoltz, R. A., Shapiro, D. E., and Connors, K. M. (2004). Assessing the learning needs of maternal and child health professionals to teach health promotion. *Maternal and Child Health Journal, 8*(2), 87-93.

informally on a one-to-one basis or perhaps in a group setting in the home where those with shared interests can gather. Proper lighting, room temperature, and seating should be considered whether in a clinic, hospital setting, or community gathering.

The attributes of the nurse as educator influence the learning environment. The nurse must be knowledgeable about the subject being communicated. Being open to listening to what the client wants to say creates an atmosphere of acceptance and encouragement.

Technology and Communication

The major influence of technology on communication in contemporary health care cannot be disputed or overemphasized. Technology has become an integral part of how nurses function. For example, the use of computerized charting and medication administration is becoming routine in a majority of health care institutions.

Client information such as health histories, signs and symptoms, laboratory tests, medications, and treatment plans can be obtained and shared among health care professionals via email and the Internet (Estes, 2006). The Institute of Medicine of the National Academies has advocated a national network of health information that is accessible by all health care organizations. Electronic records of clients' care, based on data standards that make health information uniform and understandable to all, will facilitate the exchange of information among providers and clients (National Academies, 2003). Although there is great benefit in using technology to facilitate communication for clients and health care providers, nurses need to be aware of associated legal issues.

Technological advances in communication, including the Internet, computer programs, videos, teleconference capabilities, email, and even cellular phones with picture and text messaging, have changed the way people interact, store and retrieve information, and learn. Nurses work to promote the health of clients of all ages and backgrounds and who have a wide range of technological abilities and capabilities. Therefore, choosing the appropriate technology to achieve the purpose intended, whether the client is an individual, a group, or a community, is important for the success of any health promotion endeavor.

SUMMARY

Nurses have a responsibility to promote the health of clients whether they are individuals, families, groups, or communities. This responsibility requires therapeutic communication with clients, verbally and nonverbally. It requires much skill to do this on different levels with children, adolescents, and adults, and with consideration of the various domains (biological, psychological, sociocultural, spiritual, and environmental). To be effective in promoting the health of clients, nurses must develop and exercise effective communication skills.

This chapter presented elements involved in communication, types of communication, and the use of therapeutic communication skills for health promotion. It is impossible to promote health without communication. Communication is a cornerstone for health promotion.

Key Concepts

1. Communication is the process of conveying ideas, thoughts, opinions, or facts from one person to another.

2. The six elements of communication include: message, encoder, channel, decoder, feedback, and context.

3. The two types of communication are verbal (the use of words to convey messages) and nonverbal (the conveyance of messages without the use of words).

4. Communication is inevitable because, as Paul Watzlawick suggested, we cannot *not* communicate.

5. Hildegard Peplau identified six nursing roles that involve communication between client and nurse. Joyce Travelbee characterized therapeutic communication as human-to-human communication and believed it to be reciprocal and dynamic. Communication was inherent within each system of Imogene King's systems framework for nursing (social, interpersonal, and personal) and a major concept in the interpersonal systems. Dorothea Orem's Self-Care Deficit Theory also involves use of therapeutic communication in the various roles.

6. Nurse characteristics that promote effective communication include unconditional positive regard, empathy, authenticity, caring, and active listening.

7. Nurses use therapeutic techniques of communication to gain information about clients and their perceptions, and nurses provide information to clients in order to assist clients to change health-related behaviors and to foster behaviors that promote health.

8. Teaching is a major role of the nurse in health promotion. Whether teaching occurs informally when a need arises or more formally in a care plan, the nurse must understand the differences in teaching adults and children. Knowledge of the teaching environment, what to teach, when to teach, and how to teach are vital to effective teaching.

9. Technology is an important adjunct to teaching clients and promoting health. Nurses can be facilitators in using and teaching the use of the appropriate technology for information exchange and for educating clients.

Learning Activities

1. With the assistance of your instructor, arrange to observe a health care professional in communication with a client. Identify the various types of therapeutic techniques you observe, nurse characteristics that promote communication, and how personal space is used.

2. Under the direction of your nursing instructor, select an actual client and interview this person about what she or he does to stay healthy. Include attention to the biological, psychological, sociocultural, spiritual, and environmental domains.

3. Explain the difference between the encoder and the decoder of a message.

4. What part does context play in communicating a message?

True/False Questions

1. T or F Therapeutic communication involves verbal techniques focused on client needs and with the avoidance of nonverbal communication.

2. T or F Proxemics is important to nurses in regard to awareness of and respect for personal space needs of clients.

3. T or F Active listening requires that the nurse allow the client to speak without interrupting or adding comments or questions.

Multiple Choice Questions

1. Mr. George is looking out the window, with his back to the door. A nurse opens the door and says, "You will not be able to eat or drink after supper because of tests tomorrow." Then the nurse leaves. Did communication take place?
   a. No; there was no feedback.
   b. No; there was no eye contact.
   c. Yes; Mr. George had to hear the message.
   d. Yes; there was a sender, receiver, and message.

2. What is the best way to communicate?
   a. It depends on what the message is.
   b. Nonverbally.
   c. Verbally.
   d. Verbally and nonverbally together.

3. When performing a nursing procedure on a client the nurse should:
   a. always have someone witness the procedure.
   b. avoid eye contact to reduce embarrassment.
   c. be aware of his or her own nonverbal messages.
   d. only listen to what the client says.

4. The nurse is aware that most nursing procedures are performed in which spatial comfort zone?
   a. Intimate
   b. Personal
   c. Public
   d. Social

5. Adult clients would most typically want to learn about health promotion when they:
   a. admit that they do not know enough.
   b. are told by the nurse that they need to know more.
   c. feel a social pressure to learn.
   d. feel the information relates directly to them.

Websites

http://www.handspeak.com Handspeak™
A subscription-based website consisting of the American Sign Language (ASL) online dictionary, lessons, and resources, including Baby Sign, International Sign Language, Emoticon + Bodicon (facial expression + body language), gestures, manual alphabet (fingerspelling) and numerals, sign stories, and arts.

http://www.ed.gov U.S. Department of Education
Provides an exploration of information literacy as it relates to schools, workplaces, individuals, and society.

Organizations

ASHA
10801 Rockville Pike
Rockville, MD 20852
Tel: (800) 638-8255
www.asha.org

The American Speech-Language-Hearing Association (ASHA) is the professional, scientific, and credentialing association for speech-language pathologists, audiologists, and speech, language, and hearing scientists in the United States and internationally.

Videos

A World of Differences

One of a series from the University of California, this video examines verbal and nonverbal ways that people from two different cultures can experience communication failures and conflict. Examples show mistranslation, the difficulty of understanding idioms from another culture, cultural differences in personal space, patterns of touch, etiquette and ritual, the expression of emotions, ideas about food, gestures, courtship differences, and parent-child interactions.

The following videos are also in the series.

The Human Voice: about both language and vocal paralanguage, i.e., what can be inferred about a speaker from spoken language

The Human Face: about emotions, identity, attractiveness, and other facial cues

A World of Gestures: about cultural and national differences in gestures, cross-cultural misunderstandings, etc.

IPT and **IPT-15:** two video self-tests that enable viewers to see how accurately they can decode nonverbal cues and interpersonal behavior

Videos are available from:
University of California Extension Center for Media
2000 Center Street, Fourth Floor
Berkeley, CA 94704
Tel: (510) 642-0460
Fax: (510) 643-9271
cmil@uclink.berkeley.edu

References

Alligood, M. R., & Marriner-Tomey, A. (2002). *Nursing theory: Utilization and application*. St. Louis: Mosby.

Bastable, S. (2003). *Nurse as educator: Principles of teaching and learning for nursing practice*. Sudbury, MA: Jones & Bartlett.

Bernstein, H. H., Rieber, S., Stoltz, R. A., Shapiro, D. E., & Connors, K. M. (2004). Assessing the learning needs of maternal and child health professionals to teach health promotion. *Maternal and Child Health Journal, 8*(2), 87–93.

Estes, M. E. Z. (2006). *Health assessment & physical examination* (3rd ed.). Clifton Park, NY: Thomson Delmar Learning.

Healthy People 2010: Leading Health Indicators: Priorities for Action. (2000). Washington, D.C.: U.S. Department of Health and Human Services.

Hood, L. J., & Leddy, S. K. (2003). *Conceptual bases of professional nursing* (5th ed.). Philadelphia: Lippincott Williams & Wilkins.

Knowles. M. (1970). *The modern practice of adult education: Andragogy versus pedagogy*. Chicago: Follet Publishing Company.

National Academies: Advisors to the Nation on Science, Engineering and Medicine. (2003, November 20). *Reducing medical errors requires national computerized information systems; Data standards are crucial to improving patient safety*. Retrieved May 20, 2006, from http://www4.nas.edu/news

Parker, M. E. (2006). *Nursing theories and nursing practice* (2nd ed.). Philadelphia: F. A. Davis.

Pender, N. J., Murdaugh, C. L., & Parsons, M. A. (2006). *Health promotion in nursing practice*. Upper Saddle River, NJ: Pearson Education.

Peplau, H. E. (1952). *Interpersonal relations in nursing*. New York: G. P. Putnam's Sons.

Rogers, C. R. (1942). *Counseling and psychotherapy: Newer concepts in practice*. Boston: Houghton Mifflin.

Scott, S., & Lee, J. H. (2003). *Serving clients who use sign language*. Retrieved May 21, 2006, from http://www.asha.org/about/publications/leader-online/archives/2003/q2/030401fa.htm

Smith, M. K. (1996, 1999). Andragogy. *The Encyclopedia of Informal Education*. Retrieved January 28, 2005, from http://www.infed.org/lifelonglearning/b-andra.htm

Travelbee, J. (1966). *Interpersonal aspects of nursing*. Philadelphia: F. A. Davis.

U.S. Department of Health and Human Services. (2000). *Healthy people 2010*. Washington, DC: U.S. Government Printing Office.

Chapter 6

CULTURAL CONSIDERATIONS

M. Sandra [Sandy] Sánchez, PhD, RN

KEY TERMS

acculturation
cultural competence
cultural tapestry
culture
emic knowledge

ethnicity
ethnocentrism
etic knowledge
folk health sector

lay/popular health
  sector
medicocentrism
nationality

professional health
  sector
race
worldview

OBJECTIVES

Upon completion of this chapter, the reader should be able to:

- Discuss the concept of culture, including its components.

- Differentiate among the concepts of culture, race, ethnicity, and nationality.

- Explain how culture is holistic.

- Describe how culture impacts each metaparadigm concept.

- Identify examples of bigotry, discrimination, prejudice, racism, and ethnocentrism.

- Describe how cultural assessment relates to the nursing process.

- Complete a cultural assessment of yourself and others.

- Become aware of your own culture and how it permeates your life.

- Describe how culture is interwoven with wellness and illness.

- Differentiate among cultural competence, cultural awareness, and cultural sensitivity.

- Specify ways of culturally advocating for clients.

INTRODUCTION

This chapter is not intended to serve as a comprehensive survey of culture. Rather, it is intended to provide a very basic introduction to concepts of culture. The more people understand about themselves and others, the better people may understand one another. That is how bridges are built instead of walls, and health promotion is all about building bridges. Understanding your own culture and those of others creates an awareness that is fundamental to providing competent nursing care.

THE CONCEPT OF CULTURE

Culture is holistic. It is more than the sum of its parts. It affects everything, including thoughts and behaviors. But what is culture? It is sometimes hard to talk about culture because it is all-encompassing. Entire books and journals are written about it. Undergraduate and graduate courses are devoted to it. Students major in it. Research focuses on it. Theories are developed about it. Yet a concrete definition remains elusive to many people, probably because much of culture is intangible. Culture is probably something most people do not think about until they are confronted with something or someone from a different culture. The natural reaction then is to say, "He's different."

What Is Culture?

Culture is a buzzword that is commonly thrown around today, and yet most people, even anthropologists, have slightly different ideas about it. So, what is culture? It is certainly more than ethnicity or religion, although those affect culture. It is much more than race, itself a superfluous label.

Culture is defined in various ways. Leininger, a recognized nurse leader and theorist on transcultural nursing, defined culture as the "learned, shared, and transmitted knowledge of values, beliefs, and lifeways of a particular group that are transmitted intergenerationally and influence thinking, decisions, and actions in patterns or certain ways" (Leininger & McFarland, 2002, p. 47).

Here are some interesting and thought-provoking definitions.

As a noun, culture is defined as:
- cultivation, tillage
- the act of developing the intellectual and moral faculties, esp. by education
- expert care and training
- enlightenment and excellence of taste acquired by intellectual and aesthetic training
- acquaintance with and taste in fine arts, humanities, and broad aspects of science as distinguished from vocational and technical skills
- the integrated pattern of human knowledge, belief, and behavior that depends upon man's capacity for learning and transmitting knowledge to succeeding generations
- the customary beliefs, social forms, and material traits of a racial, religious, or social group
- the set of shared attitudes, values, goals, and practices that characterizes a company or corporation
- cultivation of living material in prepared nutrient media; also, a product of such cultivation [in other words, culture is what you are prepared in *and* what you are!]

As a verb, to culture means to:
- cultivate (i.e., to foster the growth of)
- to grow in a prepared medium
- to start a culture from

As an adjective, cultured means:
- cultivated

Source: Merriam-Webster's Collegiate Dictionary *(Mish, 2004, p. 304)*

Each definition, including those listed in Box 6-1, offers something to the concept of human culture. Aspects of each definition are relevant. They may be incorporated into a meaningful understanding of human culture when viewed simply as "cultivation of living material in prepared nutrient media" (Mish, 2004, p. 304). In other words, culture is the expert cultivation of a human being in a nurturing milieu. As such, human growth and development begin in a rich womb and continue throughout life to foster an ingrained pattern of attitudes, beliefs, values, morals, knowledge, and behaviors. Of course, the reverse may be true as well.

In this chapter, **culture** is defined as dynamic adaptation, a learned way of life that includes interrelated attitudes, morals, beliefs, values, ideals, knowledge, symbols, artifacts, customs, traditions, and norms of a particular group that guide behavior, make life meaningful, and

are transmitted intergenerationally. An individual lives in the larger society and absorbs "culture" through his or her daily activities. Culture represents a particular group's overarching lifeways as well as a an individual's worldview and way of life. Culture affects what is seen and thought. It is the lens for each person's view of the world. And what is seen, consciously or not, often determines behavior. Box 6-2 lists attributes of culture.

Worldviews

There are many worldviews. **Worldview** refers to the way individuals perceive the world, including the inherent nature of its inhabitants. No two people, regardless of culture, are exactly alike or share the same worldview, not even people within the same family. Why? Recall that each person has his or her own unique culture derived from the overarching culture. Certainly, siblings may possess many cultural similarities that were transmitted from their parents and families, but they also have unique differences. Some of those differences might be attributed to age differences, personal preferences, and history. That is why it is critical to realize that although culture is pervasive, it is difficult to discern a person's culture without knowing or talking to that person.

Particular Group

Cultural traditions are passed down from generation to generation within a particular group. The group might be a tiny clan living in an isolated part of the world or a large collection of people in the United States. It could be the Catholic church or the Hindu religion. It could be Northern or Southern. The group could be Californian or Texan, Irish American or Mexican American. It could be Black or White, and so forth.

The number of potential groups is virtually limitless. Some of the more common particular groups include those bound by race, ethnicity, religion, and nationality, with each of those having its own subgroupings. Box 6-3 lists other particular groups.

Race

Race is a misunderstood term. It is not uncommon to hear people referring to the British race, the Jewish race, or the white race. This may result from the various definitions of **race** as "a family, tribe, people, or nation belonging to the same stock," or "a category of humankind that shares certain distinctive by physical traits" (Mish, 2004, p. 1024). Although these definitions offer value, the last

---

BOX 6-3   Examples of Particular Groups

In addition to race, ethnicity, religion, and nationality, other particular groups that share traditions include those groups delineated by:

- region of the country (East Coast, West Coast, North, South, Southwest)
- states (Alabama, Delaware, Florida, Maine, Oregon, Texas, etc.)
- agencies (IBM, 3M)
- professions (nursing, medicine, pharmacy, teaching)
- clubs (sororities, fraternities, Girl Scouts, Boy Scouts, 4-H)
- gangs
- prisons
- gender (female, male)
- socioeconomic status (upper, middle, lower; rich, poor)
- universities (students, alumni, faculty)
- athletics (basketball, tennis, cycling)
- acting (film, stage)
- degree major (art, business, engineering, journalism, math, nursing)
- homelessness
- sexual orientation (heterosexual, homosexual, bisexual)
- physical ability (able-bodied, disabled)

Spotlight On

Forgetful Foreigners

With few exceptions, the United States is made up of foreigners of one sort or another. Some came willingly, such as the Pilgrims or Ellis Island immigrants. Others such as Africans were not so willing. Their struggle to become full citizens of the United States has been difficult. Some foreigners mistreated the residents, such as Native Americans, Eskimos, Mexicans, and so forth, by taking their land and resources.

---

definition will be used in this chapter. Ideally, there would be one simple overarching term—*human* race.

For the most part, however, when people use the term *race*, they are referring to the anthropological usage. Anthropologically, race refers to physical characteristics that a particular group of people share. These shared characteristics, initially due to a common geography, include head shape, facial features, bone structure, hair texture, and skin color. Interestingly, the least important characteristic is skin color, as it is the one with the most variation within racial classifications. Yet, ironically, it is the one characteristic to which most people steadfastly cling. Additionally, many anthropologists point out that categorizing people according to race is "virtually meaningless" (Wali, 1992, p. 7), as there is at least as much variation within racial groups as among them. Nonetheless, throughout history, certain physical characteristics attributed to racial differences have been used as a basis for social discrimination and oppression.

Currently, according to the 2000 United States Census form, designations of race include:

- White
- Black, African American, or Negro
- American Indian or Alaska Native (with space for the name of the principal tribe)
- Asian or Pacific Islander (API)
- Other (with a space for the name of the race)

Even with these categories, race is an extremely broad category, providing only general information at best. This is especially true when a person may easily be a product of a biracial or multiracial union. For example, one's mother might be White and her or his father Asian. Interestingly, the U.S. Office of Management and Budget now allows people to check more than one race on census and other federal forms, a move that, ideally, will provide more precise statistics. See Table 6-1 for the most current profile of the U.S. population according to race.

TABLE 6-1 Demographic Profile of the U.S. Population by Race

Race	Percentage of Population
1. White	75.1%
2. Black or African American	12.3
3. American Indian and Alaska Native	0.9
4. Asian	3.6
5. Native Hawaiian and Other Pacific Islander	0.1
6. Some other race	5.5
7. Two or more races	2.4

From: United States Census 2000, *U.S. Census Bureau, 2000,* retrieved March 17, 2006, from www.census.gov/main/www/cen2000.html

Spotlight On

A World Without Race

"Within 200 years, the very concept of race will be meaningless. There will be more and more mixing of races, until the time comes when people stop defining themselves and other people on the basis of race."

"But if that really does happen—if race ceases to mean anything—then who will people hate?"

"Hopefully, no one," Maharidge said. (Greene, 1996)

Nursing Alert

Understanding Hispanic Ethnicities

Hispanic ethnicities include Argentinean, Colombian, Costa Rican, Cuban, Dominican, Ecuadoran, Guatemalan, Honduran, Mexican, Nicaraguan, Peruvian, Puerto Rican, Salvadoran, and Spanish. Knowing that your client is Hispanic is only part of his or her uniqueness.

It is important to note that Hispanic is not a race. Hispanic is an ethnicity. Hispanics may belong to any of the designated races. (See the Ethnicity section in this chapter.) Nonetheless, numerous people in government, education, industry, politics, and the press continue to refer to Hispanic as a race. This is erroneous. If, however, it is important to specify whether someone is Hispanic, the proper reference is Hispanic White, Hispanic Black, non-Hispanic White, non-Hispanic Black, and so on.

A similar note should be made about the term African American. Although it is common to use this term when referring to members of the Black race, the term itself literally refers to an ethnicity. That common usage resulted in its incorrect listing as a race on the 2000 census form.

Ethnicity

Ethnicity comes from the word *ethnos,* meaning nation and people, or "a shared sense of peoplehood" (Clinton, 1986, p. 571). In general, **ethnicity** refers to a large group of people classified according to common national, tribal, linguistic, or cultural origin or background *and* who feel a sense of shared identity. Examples of ethnicity include African, Cuban, English (usually termed Anglo), French, German, Haitian, Irish, Italian, Jamaican, Mexican, Nigerian, Polish, Scottish, Spanish, Turkish, and so on. It is important not to presume to know what a person's ethnicity is based on physical appearance or what that person wishes to be called. Ask, as that person may offer some other ethnic designation or multiple ethnicities.

Although Hispanic is a popular ethnic designation, it is probably too broad to be useful. It refers to people who "trace their family background to one of the Spanish-speaking . . . nations" (Marín & Marín, 1991, p. 18). Because there are a multitude of ethnicities subsumed under that heading, it is preferable to use a specific ethnicity, such as Cuban, instead of the overarching term Hispanic. It is also important to note that not all Hispanics appreciate the term, because many believe it to blur cultural identity and others consider it to be a label of convenience. Although there are ongoing movements to change the term, it is probably here to stay, unfortunately, because the government has latched onto it. Nonetheless, as with any label, it is vital that the health professional go beyond terminology and interact with each unique person.

African American is an ethnic designation as well; however, do not automatically assign that term to Black people because some may prefer another qualifier that best addresses their own cultural ancestry.

Race and ethnicity are not mutually exclusive terms. For example, a person may be of the Black race and of Haitian ethnicity. Or a person may be White and of Mexican ancestry. Although ethnicity is not as broad a term as race, it is still somewhat of an umbrella term. It is, thus, essential to recall that although there may be many similarities among people who share the same ethnic origin, there are wide intraethnic variations. No two people within the same ethnic group behave exactly the same—nor should they be expected to do so. It is incumbent upon health care professionals to recognize each person's uniqueness in order to avoid falling into

Don't Call Me That

The gifted actor Morgan Freeman says, "If you want to give me an adjective, call me black. . . . But don't call me African. I'm an American. Long, long bloody history, . . . just like every other American. When I was a kid, we were colored. . . . Then we became Negro. . . . Then we became Afro, in the '60s, Afro-American. . . . So this quest for identity—it's like, number 1, misguided. . . . This latest one, it just sets my teeth on edge. I think it's another one of those attempts to separate yourself. . . . I'm walking around with this one-man crusade saying, 'DON'T CALL ME THAT [African-American]!' " (Rowe, 1997).

- How can you use this information to provide culturally competent care?
- What do you want to be called?

Effect of Socioeconomic Status

People who share the same socioeconomic status (i.e., income, education) probably have more in common than those who do not, regardless of ethnicity.

past and it is time to build a better future. Their attitude is one of "How long do we have to be here in order to just be called American?" Because such varying attitudes exist, it is imperative that individual people be asked what they want to be called.

Labels

The bottom line is that these various terms are all just labels. The problem with labels is that they rarely serve any useful purpose other than convenience. Additionally, the use of labels when referring to people tends to depersonalize and/or dehumanize them. In many respects,

the trap of stereotyping. Consider the child pictured in Figure 6-1 who could be erroneously stereotyped as one race or ethnicity although she is uniquely multiracial.

Religion

Religion can be interpreted as belief in a higher power. However, it often refers to being affiliated with an organized religion, of which there are many.

Sometimes people may list a religion on health forms, but not practice that religion. Conversely, some people might be quite spiritual but have no specific religious affiliation. That is why a nurse should find out what religious or spiritual practices might be relevant for each of his or her clients.

Nationality

Although there are various connotations for the word **nationality,** in general, it refers to country of origin such as Canada, France, Mexico, or the United States of America. For example, if a child is born in Canada and has not changed citizenship, then his or her nationality is Canadian.

In the United States, it has become popular for people to identify with a larger ethnic group. Some examples are Chinese American, Irish American, Italian American, Mexican American, Polish American, and so forth. (See the section on Ethnicity.) When identifying self, those qualifiers can signify cultural pride. When identifying others, those same qualifiers can signify cultural discrimination. It depends on the tone.

It is equally important to note that some U.S. citizens only want to be identified as nonhyphenated Americans. Supporters of this stance indicate that the past is in the

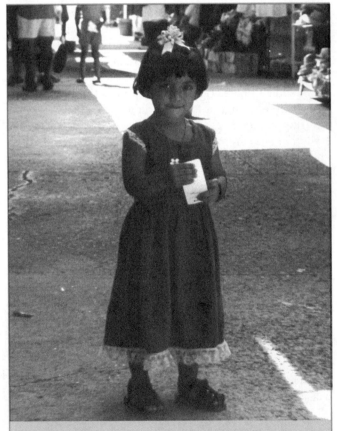

FIGURE 6-1 *This child represents the unique multicultural, multiracial tapestry of which we are all a part.*

Getting away from the use of labels is an uphill battle. Using precise labels is an even steeper climb (even among people who should know better). For example, White is not an ethnicity. It is a race. Hispanic is not a race. It is an ethnicity, albeit a broad term. So, if you must use a label for whatever reason, make sure you use a correct one.

Spotlight On

Build a Bridge

An old saying goes, "Build bridges instead of walls, and you will find a friend." When people focus only on differences, they build walls of fear and resentment instead of bridges of appreciation and joy. Don't waste energy building impenetrable walls. Walk across that bridge. Enjoy what you find there.

labels reflect a caste-system mentality that effectively categorizes and rank orders people. As such, the use of labels sometimes serves to create artificial boundaries, reinforce territoriality, and aggravate social discrimination.

Nonetheless, if labels are to be used for whatever reason, it is imperative that they be used precisely. For example, if a nurse is talking about race, he or she should use one of the accepted racial classifications. Often, people use incorrect terms due to ignorance and not malicious intent; however, it is puzzling that some people continue to use incorrect terms even when the distinctions among the various terms are known by the users. Is it habit or bigotry? Is it an easy way for an insecure ego to feel superior? In any case, the motivation for continued use of incorrect terms should be suspect.

Cultural Pride

For a long time, the United States was referred to as a melting pot where all cultural groups were supposed to be melted, blended, or homogenized into one culture. Instead of being proud of family legacies, people were made to feel ashamed if they were different in appearance, speech, dress, faith, or custom. Names were Americanized, native languages were banned, accents were silenced, family traditions were abandoned, and ethnic jokes were encouraged. Although the melting pot mentality seemingly prevailed, there were those who proudly held on to their cultural gifts. Slowly but surely the word got out that cultural differences should be sources of pride and not embarrassment and that having differences does not preclude having similarities as well. It is incumbent on health care workers to learn about similarities so that they may be used to build bridges that will help provide care.

Cultural Competence

Everyone, and just about every life event, is influenced by culture, and its impact extends into the health arena. A person's culture serves to assign meaning to various

Ask Yourself

What Does Your Cultural Heritage Look Like?

Does a **cultural tapestry,** woven with intricate yet distinctive strands that form a beautiful textured pattern, represent your unique cultural heritage? How about a meticulously pieced-together patchwork quilt? Or is a bland piece of assembly-line fabric more representative? Which symbol would you choose if you could?

Ask Yourself

Hospitalization and Culture Shock

People suddenly thrown into a strange environment can experience culture shock, causing them to feel lost and helpless. Sometimes people who are hospitalized can also experience culture shock. Can you imagine how they may feel? Can you think of ways to alleviate their disorientation?

health experiences. If nurses are to provide competent care, they should be culturally competent. They must realize that culture affects themselves as well as their clients.

To become culturally competent, a health care provider must first become culturally aware and learn what is culturally relevant for those people in his or her care. Essentially, **cultural competence** is being able to incorporate *emic* and *etic* cultural knowledge into holistic and cultural congruent client care. ***Emic* knowledge** refers to an insider's viewpoint, while ***etic* knowledge** is an outsider's viewpoint of a specific culture. Cultural competence also includes appreciating, respecting, and accepting people's cultural influences as well as incorporating them into appropriate wellness and illness client care. By enhancing communication, cultural competence facilitates positive health outcomes. Cultural competence is, indeed, a worthwhile goal. Box 6-4 offers some tips for enhancing communication for cultural competence.

CULTURAL ASSESSMENT

Because it is impossible to know everything there is to know about all cultures, a nurse's mission is to ask clients what is culturally relevant for them. Many caregivers conduct cultural assessments on their clients so that they may plan culturally appropriate care.

Cultural Assessment Tools

There are many cultural assessment tools, frameworks, and models (Andrews & Boyle, 2002; Giger & Davidhizar, 2004; Leininger, 1978; Leininger & McFarland, 2002). Most involve systematically collecting information about a person's particular group(s), spiritual beliefs, communication styles, interpersonal relationships, diet, wellness-illness practices, and lifestyles, in the hope of deriving that person's cultural attitudes, values, beliefs, knowledge, norms, customs, and so on. Because these assessment tools are designed to elicit so much cultural information via interviewing and observing, they will take a considerable amount of time to complete and are best done in the client's home and community. Even so, the cultural assessment is simply one source of client data, which should be placed in perspective and updated as needed. A sample framework for cultural assessment is provided, based on Leininger's (1978) Cultural Domains, in Box 6-5.

Cultural assessment, as any other assessment, is the first step of the nursing process. What is done with the

cultural information will determine how culturally competent a nurse is—that is, how well he or she incorporates culturally relevant information into cultural congruent client care. If the cultural assessment is done well, it is holistic insofar as the domains are interrelated, with each affecting the other; the product will be more than the mere sum of its domains.

Demographics/Individual Profile/Identifying Information

Demographic data must not be taken for granted. When viewed as a whole, an individual's demographic data provide essential information to derive a cultural profile that may effectively be incorporated into relevant wellness-illness care. For example, learning a woman's birthplace, age, marital status, years in the United States, and educational level will tell you much more about her than simply knowing her generation in the United States.

For the most part, demographic information indicates each client's preferred designation(s) regarding self-identity. Sometimes nurses may need to provide examples or probe to uncover relevant information, but they should not impose answers. For example, if a person's mother is French and his father is Irish, then that person should be allowed to claim both ethnicities. To claim only one is to disclaim the other. To claim only one is to conform to external expectations and is not an accurate representation of that person's identity.

BOX 6-5   Sample Cultural Assessment Framework

Demographics

Name _____ Gender _____ Religion _____

Race(s) _____ Ethnicity(ies) _____

Date of Birth _____ Birthplace _____ Where Raised _____

Marital Status _____ Generation in U.S.A. _____ Years in U.S.A. _____

Language(s) Spoken _____ Primary Language _____

Preferred Language _____ Education _____ Occupation _____

Cultural Domains (as identified by M. Leininger, 1978)

- General cultural life patterns or lifestyle
- Cultural values, norms, and expressions of an individual or a cultural group
- Cultural taboos and myths
- Worldview and ethnocentric tendencies
- Life-caring rituals and rites of passage

- Lay, folk, and professional wellness-illness cultural systems
- Specific caring behaviors and health care values, beliefs, and practices
- Cultural diversities, similarities, and variations
- Cultural changes and acculturation aspects

Adapted from M. Leininger's Cultural Domains *(1978).*

Name

An individual's name is part of a person's identity, and, as such, it is part of who that person is and should be treated with respect. Often a name is part of a family's culture as well. For example, it is not uncommon for a child to be named after a favored aunt or grandfather. Or clients may have hyphenated surnames passed on by their fathers. Hyphenated names also occur when individuals add a spouse's surname onto their own. Hyphenated names are fitting tributes to the families they proclaim. Whether or not a name reflects family traditions, it is still a big part of each individual.

Gender

Gender is part of a person's identity as well. Many cultural components are related to gender. These include norms, roles, self-worth, and body image. It is therefore important to note an individual's gender and then follow up with what cultural matters are gender-based. For example, are there different roles for the father and mother? Are there different chores assigned to sons and daughters? Are there different rites of passage? Household rules? Behaviors? Expectations? Are sons and daughters treated equally regarding dating practices, curfews, use of the family car, outside jobs, and so on? Are family attitudes about premarital sex the same for both the sons and the daughters? Are communication styles different for each gender? Are there rules about interacting with members of the opposite gender? Are male infants more prestigious than female infants?

Nursing Alert

Respecting People's Names

People should be called by their preferred name, and with correct pronunciation. If the nurse does not know how to do so, he or she should ask.

It is disrespectful to use only people's surnames, to call them by their first name without permission, to mispronounce their name, or to call them (familiar) names such as Grandma, Sweetie, Honey, Pop, Tía (aunt), or Bro. Such presumptions could very well be considered rude or impolite, as could referring to clients by their diagnoses, surgical procedures, or room numbers.

Religion/Spiritual Faith

Religious beliefs are integral to culture. Religious values extend into all aspects of life, such as attitudes about a higher authority, birth, death, good, evil, food, drink, sex, marriage, wellness, illness, health practices, choice, destiny, fate, afterlife, and so on. A nurse should be very careful when discussing religious or spiritual beliefs with clients so as not to inadvertently denigrate their views.

When asking about a client's religious or spiritual beliefs, it is not enough to merely list a person's religion on a form. Not all people from a given religion have the same spiritual beliefs or needs. Some people may list a given religion on their health records even though they have not practiced that religion in a long time. Others may not list a religion at all or even believe in a supreme being, but they may be quite spiritual. For that reason a health care provider should ask what religious or spiritual factors are important to each individual client. A nurse should not presume to know what the client believes or needs. For example, it could be rather unnerving to some people to see a religious leader walking into their hospital room.

Race(s)

Refer to the discussion on race earlier in this chapter. When nurses talk to clients, they should use only those races as outlined by the United States Census—that is, White, Black, American Indian, Alaska Native (include the principal tribe or nation), and Asian or Pacific Islander. Hispanic or African American should not be listed as race.

Ethnicity

Refer to the earlier discussion on ethnicity in this chapter. Bear in mind that people may be multiethnic, so a nurse should not force them to list only one ethnicity. Remember, too, that race should not be confused with ethnicity. For example, White or Black is not an ethnicity. Also, when people answer that they are Hispanic, it might be preferable to specify which particular ethnicity (e.g., Cuban, Mexican, Puerto Rican), because Hispanic is a very broad term.

Date of Birth/Age

Age has a bearing on culture in several ways, mainly the personal history lived by each individual. For example, a 5-year-old may have never experienced anything beyond her or his family's culture, whereas a 50-year-old might have been exposed to a variety of cultures, picking and choosing what is best for him. A teenager might feel quite differently about death than a centenarian. A school-age child might be much more in tune with the culture of computers than a 60-year-old, and so on.

Birthplace/Where Raised

As culture tends to vary with geography, finding out a person's birthplace is helpful. More important, however, is learning where the person grew up and the length of time in that location. A nurse should elicit the names of the city, state, and country.

Marital Status

In conducting a cultural assessment, a nurse should indicate whether the person is single (never married), separated, married, divorced, or widowed. It may also be helpful to know how long that person has been in the marital category. That information may provide added

insight into the client's present situation and, hence, in planning culturally competent care.

Generation in the United States

To a large extent, generational status affects cultural identity, affiliation, beliefs, attitudes, practices, and so on, because more recent immigrants generally cling to the culture of their homeland; however, much depends on the person's reason for immigrating as well as length of time in the United States.

Determining generational status may be complex. Strictly speaking, an immigrant is considered to be a first-generation resident. An immigrant's child who is born in the United States is considered second-generation. An immigrant's grandchild is considered third-generation, and so forth. The complexity occurs when there is a difference between the immigration status of a child's parents or grandparents.

Years in the United States

The length of time a person has lived in the United States affects that person's culture. For example, a person who has lived in New York for 40 years is more likely to have acculturated to the U.S. culture than someone who has lived there six months. That is not always the case, however, as much depends on the circumstances of each person's life.

All things being equal, how long a person has lived in the United States is probably more culturally influential than generational status. Consider the following examples of two 30-year-old people. The first person was born here, but has lived the bulk of her life elsewhere. The second person has lived here since being brought over by his parents when he was 6 months old. Who is more likely to be "American"?

Language(s) Spoken, Primary Language, and Preferred Language

Language and culture are intertwined. Language is one of the main means by which culture is transmitted. Language is also integral to intercultural communication. A shared language is a godsend, a welcomed familiarity, especially when two seeming strangers meet.

Primary language refers to the first language a person learned. It is sometimes also called native language. Occasionally, people may not have *one* primary language because they were taught two or more simultaneously. Preferred language is simply the language preferred by an individual. It may or may not be the same as the primary language. Where possible, a nurse should use a client's preferred language to enhance interpersonal communication, especially during times of stress. A multilingual person may not have a preference.

Practically all languages change after intermingling with other cultures. Dialects (regional language variations) may emerge. These frequently possess subtle yet significant differences from the main language. Cajun is an excellent example. Sometimes dialects reflect a combination of two or more languages (code switching, word borrowing, or word coining).

In the United States, speaking a language other than English has elicited both positive and negative responses. Throughout the twentieth century, some immigrants made a concerted effort to learn English and even encouraged their children to speak only English. Some did so in an attempt to adapt to the homogeneous melting pot mind-set. Others did so out of shame due to the stigma of being different. They wanted to blend in with the rest, so diversity was not valued in either case. Consequently, entire generations of people grew up without learning their culture's native tongue (e.g., German, Hebrew, Italian, Polish, Spanish, etc.). Recently people have realized that being multilingual is a gift because the world is not monolingual. As a result, there has been renewed interest—and pride—in learning and being able to speak more than one language.

Education

When conducting a cultural assessment, a nurse should specify the number of years of formal education. It is important to note, however, that the nurse should never confuse the lack of formal education with ignorance or diminished mental ability. Just because a client may have limited formal education does not mean that he or she is incapable of comprehending directions.

Occupation

A nurse conducting an assessment needs to determine the client's job. As with education, the health care provider should not presume that a blue-collar worker or unemployed person lacks intelligence.

Cultural Domains

In addition to factors such as marital status, birthplace, and years in the United States, there are several other considerations a nurse must be aware of while performing a cultural assessment. These include values, taboos, rituals, and more.

General Cultural Life Patterns or Lifestyle

Describe your life, focusing on what you do during a typical day. If your days vary due to work or school, then describe each day. It is also a good idea to compare weekdays to weekends.

Cultural Values, Norms, and Expressions of an Individual or Cultural Group

Value refers to the relative worth of a person, idea, thing, and so on. A value may be good or bad, desirable or not. For example, life might be valued above all costs, or it might be considered worthless unless a person is productive. A male child might be valued over a female and so on. While some values may easily be determined by watching or listening, others might be revealed only after questioning or inferred from behavior.

A norm is a cultural standard or rule that guides behavior. Norms are related to cultural values, because norms usually stem from whatever is valued. For instance, if a culture values virginity, then the norm might be to remain a virgin until marriage. If a culture values the

Personal space is the distance people maintain from others during interpersonal communication. Personal space, as an extension of the person, represents a sort of comfort zone that varies not only among cultures but also among people within the same broad cultural group. Personal space can be categorized (Hall, 1969) as intimate (physical contact up to 18 inches), personal (12–48 inches), social (4–12 feet), and public (12 + feet). What is a comfortable distance for your personal space? Does it vary depending on the other person?

Consider how these various worldviews might affect behavior.
- People are good.
- The world is magical.
- Trust no one.
- If you do not take care of yourself, no one else will.
- The human body is a machine.
- Humans have souls. There is life after death.
- Human beings are physical creatures. Once you die, there is nothing more.
- God looks after you.
- Health care professionals are cold and impersonal.

elderly, then old people will be treated with respect and dignity. Families might have their own norms, such as what university to attend, major to select, or club to join. Norms may also have ages associated with them, such as getting married by age 21 or having children by age 25.

Reflecting both cultural values and norms, expressions may be verbal or nonverbal, tangible or not. Expressions may include prayer, songs, music, art, food, dance, gifts, eye contact, language, voice tone or pitch, personal space, celebrations, smiles, laughter, crying, visits with loved ones, hugs, kisses, and other symbols.

Cultural Taboos and Myths

Taboos and myths are intertwined and related to values, norms, and expressions. A taboo is something that is forbidden, such as a dangerous thought or behavior. For example, divorce might be taboo in some cultures. It is interesting to note that many taboos pertain to life or sex, such as abortion, adultery, incest, or murder. A client's taboos may have profound implications in nursing care. For example, Jehovah's Witnesses consider it taboo to accept blood—even in cases of life and death.

A myth is a popular historical belief, tradition, or story that is unverifiable or unfounded, but may be hard to disprove. As a myth makes sense to particular groups, it often serves to reveal a person's cultural worldview as well as explain beliefs and behavior. Myths may also highlight taboos and their consequences. For instance, if a taboo forbids a pregnant woman from viewing an eclipse, the corresponding myth might reveal that if she does view it her child will be born with a cleft lip. Numerous myths about health exist, while others revolve around sexual situations.

A superstition is a belief or practice resulting from ignorance, fear of the unknown, trust in magic or chance, or a false conception of causation. A superstition may also be defined as an irrational idea or as a notion maintained despite evidence to the contrary. It is important to find out about people's superstitions, because they may have evolved from cultural taboos, myths, or even rituals. Although taboos and myths might be considered mere superstition by those who do not share similar cultural worldviews, it is important to recall that people's beliefs usually guide their actions. In other words, it does not matter whether anyone else considers those beliefs to be myths, superstitions, or fact.

Worldview and Ethnocentric Tendencies

A person's worldview reflects values, norms, expressions, taboos, myths, rituals, rites, and so forth. It refers to the way a person perceives the world, including issues of health, wellness, illness, sickness, death, human nature, and so on. Because culture affects worldview, and worldview usually affects actions, it is essential to understand how people see the world and what they think about it.

Ethnocentrism is the belief that one's cultural beliefs, worldview, and way of life are better than another's. It is rare to find a person who is not ethnocentric to at least a small degree. The important thing is to recognize internalized ethnocentrism so that it may be kept in rein.

Medicocentrism is the belief that professional health care practices are superior to any others, such as lay/popular or folk. It is not uncommon for some clients to be reluctant to reveal their health care practices to health professionals for fear of being ridiculed. A nurse's success as a health care professional will be enhanced if she or he truly appreciates, respects, and remains open to learning about other people's cultures.

Life-Caring Rituals and Rites of Passage

Rituals and rites of passage are intimately related to values, norms, expressions, worldview, taboos, health systems, and caring behaviors. Rituals and rites of passage are themselves intricately interwoven. A ritual is defined as a repeated act or series of acts. A rite of passage, on the other hand, is a ritual associated with a crisis or a person's change of status. Not all rituals signify rites of passage, but rites of passage are usually rituals of sorts.

Although some religious practices are considered rituals, some are also rites of passage (e.g., receiving the sacraments). Additionally, practices that deal with dying and death can be both rituals and rites of passage. For example, some people commemorate the dead by honoring them on special days (birthdays, Memorial Day, All Souls' Day/*Día de los Muertos*), placing flowers or food at their graves, homes, or death sites, or dedicating memorials (altars, statues, plaques, pictures, plants, trees, etc.) to them. (See Figure 6-2, which shows an altar commemorating *Día de los Muertos*/All Souls' Day.)

Lay, Folk, and Professional Wellness-Illness Cultural Systems

Cultural health systems are related to values, norms, caring behaviors, rituals, and taboos. According to Kleinman (1980), the overarching health care system in most societies is made up of three overlapping cultural health care arenas or sectors: lay/popular, folk, and professional. As health care professionals, it is important for nurses to recognize that these three health care arenas exist. To ignore even one of these arenas is to miss out on the holistic nature of an individual's health care experience.

Both the lay/popular and folk health care arenas are nonprofessional in nature. The **lay/popular health sector** is made up of the individual along with family and friends. An example of lay health care is a mother feeding her child hot oatmeal on a cold morning to keep him well. The **folk health sector** consists of unlicensed, nonprofessional specialists who are usually members of the local community. A *curandero* (Mexican healer) is an excellent example of a folk specialist who uses mental, spiritual, and physical levels in health care provisions. The **professional health sector,** by contrast, represents the formally organized, modern, scientific health community of licensed providers. Professional health care encompasses much more than medical care, because that is, for the most part, limited to care from physicians. A registered nurse is an example of a professional health care provider. See Table 6-2 for some other examples of health care providers within the various sectors.

No health care sector is necessarily better than another, although some are used more frequently. It has been estimated that most health care takes place in the nonprofessional sectors, with the bulk of that being wellness care within the lay/popular arena. Furthermore, both formal and informal research have documented that people tend to use the health care sectors simultaneously rather than unilaterally, picking and choosing what they want or need to stay well or get well again.

Although there are numerous terms in the literature to convey the notion that nonprofessional aspects of

health care are needed, "complementary" and "integrative" are perhaps the best. Complementary or integrative health care suggests that people enhance, complete, or complement their health by simultaneously engaging in multiple health care approaches from various nonprofessional and professional health providers within the three overlapping sectors, which blend into a unified whole. Think "holism." "Complementary" is also the most realistic term because health care rarely exists in isolation, that is, in only one sector. It is thus incumbent

TABLE 6-2 Health Care Arenas and Examples of Providers

Arena	Providers
Lay/Popular	Yourself
	Parents, grandparents
	Siblings, children
	Spouse
	Friends, roommates
Folk	Health food store employee
	Spiritual healer
	"Barefoot" doctor
	Intuitive nutritionist
	"Granny" midwife
	Spa worker
Professional	Registered nurse
	Registered pharmacist
	Registered massage therapist
	Licensed dentist
	Licensed physician

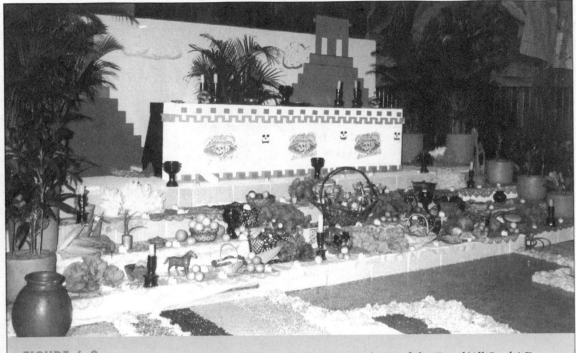

FIGURE 6-2 *An altar in celebration of Día de los Muertos/Day of the Dead/All Souls' Day.*

upon health care professionals to recognize that reality and ask about nonprofessional care in a nonthreatening way so that holistic and cultural congruent care may be provided. For example, in a Navajo reservation hospital, there is a special room for conducting traditional healing ceremonies by the shaman or various other healers. Thus, both nonprofessional and professional health care are provided, and cultural congruent care is facilitated.

It is important to note that certain approaches are not limited to one health care arena. Instead, a particular approach may be used by health providers from each arena. For example, an individual may choose to use ylang-ylang in a bath for its calming effect, an herbalist may recommend arnica for a sore ankle, and nurses may incorporate the scent of lavender to create a healing environment. These essential oils are used throughout the various health care arenas (lay/popular, folk, and professional).

Specific Caring Behaviors and Health Care Values, Beliefs, and Practices

Caring behaviors are intimately tied to values, norms, expressions, worldview, ethnocentrism, rituals, lay/popular, folk, and professional health cultural systems. Knowing how people view other people, wellness, illness, and healing can often help a nurse understand which health care values, beliefs, practices, and providers will be accepted by a client. Examples of these views about health include various health definitions, philosophies, meanings, expectations, or explanatory models. For instance, a person might define health as wellness, with wellness being the harmonious balance of mind, body, and spirit. Another person may believe that you are well as long as

you can get your work done. To yet another, health may mean being disease-free.

It is important for nurses to understand their own and their client's cultural health views, because caring behaviors usually stem from health beliefs and reflect cultural expectations or norms. For instance, cultural traditions may designate the recipient of care, the health care provider(s) (e.g., women, men, nonprofessionals, professionals), and the type of care. Cultural health practices may include getting acupressure, preparing special food, administering medications, laying on of hands, lighting candles, making *promesas* (promises), caring for the body after death, and so forth. There may also be forbidden health practices, such as blood transfusions, surgery, or being cared for by the opposite gender.

Cultural Diversities, Similarities, and Variations (Nonfamily)

Consider how you compare to those around you—your classmates, coworkers, friends, neighbors, etc.—regarding each of the other domains, such as values, norms, taboos, expressions, rites of passage, and so forth. What is the same, and what is different? Think about your religion, language(s), diet, clothes, physical appearance, recreation, music, parenting practices, job, income, degree major, lifestyle, worldview, health, and so on.

Cultural Changes and Acculturation (Family)

Acculturation refers to the process of adapting to or adopting aspects of another culture. Although something may be gained, something is also usually lost in the process. It is quite beneficial to reflect on your acculturation in comparison to your close family members, especially your parents, grandparents (both sets), brothers, sisters, and so forth. This comparison is especially striking when it involves the various generations. It is also interesting to compare yourself to your siblings who are either much older or younger than you. In essence, this domain integrates all the others—values, norms, expressions, taboos, worldviews, rituals, rites of passage, celebrations, etc.—as you compare yourself to your other family members regarding each domain.

Consider the ways you and your family members have acculturated, including similarities and differences. Think about your religion, language(s), diet, physical appearance, clothes, recreation, music, job, income, lifestyle, worldview, health conditions, and so on. Remember, you already compared yourself to your friends, classmates, neighbors, coworkers, and so forth in the section entitled Cultural Diversities, Similarities, and Variations (Nonfamily).

CULTURAL COMPETENCE IN A MULTICULTURAL SOCIETY

Culture permeates life. For that reason, it is essential that nurses become culturally conscious so that they may acknowledge when their attitudes, values, norms, taboos, and so forth may affect those around them, including clients. Although it is unrealistic to expect nurses or health care providers to always reconcile cultural differences, it is critical that they recognize and respect those differences in order to incorporate them into culturally realistic care.

There is no way to reduce cultural considerations to a simple cultural formula that may be memorized and used as needed. There are no key words providing ready-made answers to real-life situations. There are also

no *Culture for Dummies, Ten Steps to Cultural Competence,* or *All You Ever Wanted to Know About Culture but Were Afraid to Ask* books. Efforts to do so have failed abysmally, resulting in mere cultural cataloging, misguided messages, and inevitable stereotyping.

But all is not lost. A nurse may provide culturally competent care by realizing that although everybody has a culture, what is culturally relevant will vary from person to person. Where possible, a health care provider should willingly seek that which is culturally relevant for each individual.

Cultural Cataloging

There is no way a nurse may possibly know everything about everyone else's culture. Not all Catholics want to see a priest. Not all Californians surf. The best way a nurse can find out what is culturally relevant to any one person is to ask that person. A nurse should not make decisions impacting health care based on some cultural cataloging read in a handbook that highlighted points about various cultural groups. Stereotyping and negative prejudices may be inadvertently reinforced, resulting in cultural incongruence and distancing between the nurse and client. Information from a cultural catalog should be validated with a client before implementing it.

SUMMARY

Nurses are the logical mediators, teachers, enablers, and client advocates. They ensure that a client's cultural health rights are understood and respected in the professional health care arena as well as their fundamental human rights. Accordingly, it is vital for nurses to recognize both their own beliefs and those of their clients. By building cultural competence they may promote positive health behaviors outside the professional health care arena as well as deliver culturally competent care within it.

Key Concepts

1. The concept of culture is composed of an interrelated set of attitudes, morals, beliefs, values, ideals, knowledge, symbols, artifacts, customs, traditions, and norms of a particular group that are transmitted intergenerationally and reflected in the perceptions, cognitions, and behaviors that are unique to every individual, group, organization, and community.

2. Culture is holistic in that it is all-encompassing: It is pervasive in the life of every individual; integral to groups, organizations, and communities; reflected in thoughts, feelings, behaviors, and lifestyles; and, thus, greater than the sum of its parts.

3. Because they are not mutually exclusive, care must be taken to avoid confusion concerning the interrelated concepts of culture, race, ethnicity, and nationality.

4. Although often equated only with environment, in truth, culture impacts each of the four concepts of nursing's metaparadigm: person, health, nursing, environment.

5. Bigotry, discrimination, prejudice, racism, and ethnocentrism take many forms, including labeling others, being judgmental, and even committing hate crimes.

6. Cultural assessment, as any other assessment, is the first step of the nursing process; as such, it is vital to the analysis, planning, implementation, and evaluation phases of the nursing process.

7. Culturally competent care begins with completing a cultural self-assessment.

8. Performing a cultural self-assessment creates a keen sense of awareness of your cultural heritage and its evidence throughout all aspects of your life. Knowing how your culture influences the way you think, feel, and act will increase your appreciation of the influence that culture has in the lives of your clients.

9. Values, beliefs, customs, norms, and rituals are parts of culture that manifest themselves in how we strive to attain, maintain, enhance, or regain our wellness.

10. Cultural competence incorporates *emic* and *etic* cultural knowledge into holistic and cultural congruent client care; it involves cultural awareness, appreciation, and sensitivity.

11. Being a cultural advocate for your clients involves promoting positive health behaviors outside the professional health care arena as well as delivering culturally competent care within it to ensure that your client's culture is recognized, understood, and respected as a human right.

Learning Activities

1. Complete a cultural self-assessment.

2. How did you feel when you first enrolled in nursing school? Was your reaction in any way akin to culture shock? Were any of your beliefs, attitudes, values, etc., in conflict with those held by members of the professional health care system? Did you share those with your teachers and classmates? If not, why not? If so, what was their reaction?

3. Arrange a cultural celebration with your classmates. Bring in favorite foods, music, knickknacks, pictures, videos, clothing, etc., that reflect your culture. After each of you has discussed the cultural significance of your items, you can feast on the foods and browse through the various wares. You can learn a lot and have fun in the process.

4. What is meant by the culture of professional nursing? What components are involved? Language? Values? Norms? Expressions? Myths? Taboos? Superstitions? Rituals? Rites of passage? Foods? Caring behaviors? Celebrations? Ethnocentrism/medicocentrism? Acculturation?

5. At the end of each clinical day, do you reflect on the cultural congruent care you provided—or should have provided—to your client(s)?

6. If you still think you do not have a culture, read Miner's (1956) article on the Nacirema.

True/False Questions

1. T or F Ethnicity is synonymous with culture.

2. T or F Race is an extremely broad category, providing only general information at best.

3. T or F *Emic* knowledge refers to an outsider's veiwpoint of a specific culture.

4. T or F Complementary and integrative health care are terms that refer to multiple health care approaches from various professional and nonprofessional health care practitioners.

Multiple Choice Questions

1. A mother is observed breast-feeding her 4-year-old son, who is a client in the pediatrics wing of the hospital. A nurse is overheard talking in the nursing station about the "weird" way the mother has contin-

ued to breast-feed a 4-year-old. She comments that the American way is the best. The nurse is guilty of:
a. ethnocentrism.
b. stereotyping.
c. unusual break behavior.
d. not insisting that the mother stop breast-feeding.

2. Which of these clients would most likely refuse a blood transfusion, even if his or her life were in jeopardy?
a. Hindu
b. Jehovah's Witness
c. Jew
d. Mormon

3. It is important for the nurse to know the client's religion in order to:
a. chart it on his record.
b. give holistic care.
c. meet his physical needs.
d. know how to pray for him.

4. Which of the following is a characteristic of culture?
a. Culture is learned.
b. Culture stays the same.
c. Culture is biologically inherited.
d. Culture is individually determined.

5. "Hispanic" refers to:
a. a homogeneous culture.
b. a race.
c. an ethnicity.
d. Spanish speakers.

6. When a client says to the nurse, "I need to pray with my pastor in order to get well," the most appropriate response from the nurse is:
a. "The medicine you take will make you well."
b. "When you are released from the hospital, you can go to church and pray."
c. "May I call your pastor for you and ask him to visit you?"
d. "Why do you think prayer will make you well?"

7. It is important to be aware of cultural aspects of health because:
a. some cultural groups are represented in greater numbers than others.
b. cultural groups assign various meanings to health.
c. differences in care should not be based on culture.
d. reimbursement is related to ethnicity.

Organizations

Center for Cross-Cultural Health
P.O. Box 8184
St. Paul, MN 55108
International Institute of Minnesota
1694 Como Ave.
St. Paul, MN 55108
Tel: (651) 209-8999
Fax: (651) 209-8998
ccch@crosshealth.com
Center for Cross-Cultural Health is a research and information resource using information sharing, training, organizational assessments, and research to develop culturally competent individuals, organizations, systems, and societies.

National Center for Cultural Healing
2331 Archdale Road
Reston, VA 20191
Tel: (703) 626-1619
information@culturalhealing.com
www.culturalhealing.com
National Center for Cultural Healing provides training and education in cultural diversity.

Resources for Cross Cultural Health Care
8915 Sudbury Road
Silver Spring, MD 20901
Tel: (301) 588-6051
www.DiversityRX.org
Resources for Cross Cultural Health Care is a national network of individuals and organizations in ethnic communities and health care organized to offer technical assistance and information on linguistic and cultural competence in health care.

References

Andrews, M. M., & Boyle, J. S. (2002). *Transcultural concepts in nursing care* (4th ed.).

Clinton, J. (1986). Sociocultural issues relevant to health. In C. Edelman & C. L. Mandle (Eds.), *Health promotion throughout the life span* (pp. 570–583). St. Louis: Mosby.

Hall, E. T. (1969). *The hidden dimension*. Garden City, NY: Doubleday.

Giger, J. N., & Davidhizar, R. E. (2004). *Transcultural nursing: Assessment and intervention* (2nd ed.). St. Louis: Mosby.

Greene, B. (1996, November 10). United States with a white minority will be a significant change for the country. *The Monitor*, p. 7F.

Kleinman, A. (1980). *Patients and healers in the context of culture: An exploration of the borderland between anthropology, medicine, and psychiatry*. Berkeley: University of California Press.

Leininger, M. M. (Ed.). (1978). *Transcultural nursing: Concepts, theories, and practices*. New York: John Wiley & Sons.

Leininger, M. M., & McFarland, M. (2002). *Transcultural nursing: Concepts, theories, research, and practice* (3rd ed.). New York: McGraw-Hill.

Marín, G., & Marín, B. V. O. (1991). *Research with Hispanic populations*. Newbury Park, CA: Sage.

Miner, H. (1956). Body ritual among the Nacirema. *American Anthropologist, 58*(3), 503–507.

Mish, F. C. (Ed.). (2004). *Merriam-Webster's collegiate dictionary* (11th ed.). Springfield, MA: Merriam-Webster.

Rowe, D. J. (1997, October 28). Morgan Freeman: The hardest part of acting is "getting jobs." *The Monitor*, p. 7B.

U.S. Census Bureau. (2000). *United States census*. Retrieved March 17, 2006, from www.census.gov/main/www/cen2000.html

Wali, A. (1992). Multiculturalism: An anthropological perspective. *Report from the Institute for Philosophy and Public Policy* [University of Maryland at College Park], *12*(1), 6–8.

Chapter 7

ENVIRONMENTAL FACTORS

Janice A. Maville, EdD, MSN, RN
Ruth Tucker Marcott, PhD, RNC

KEY TERMS

anosmia
building-related
   illness
carcinogen
chemical sensitivity
chi
chromotherapy
disease cluster
ergonomics

environmental health
   hazard
environmental health
   risk
feng shui
mutagen
noise
outgassing
particulate matter

posttraumatic stress
   disorder (PTSD)
SAD syndrome
sha
sick building syndrome
simultaneous
   perception
tao
teratogen

terrorism
utter watchfulness
volatile organic
   compounds (VOCs)
weapons of mass
   destruction (WMDs)
weapons of mass effect
   (WMEs)

OBJECTIVES

Upon completion of this chapter, the reader should be able to:

- Identify factors influencing environmental health.
- Distinguish between the attributes of a supportive versus a threatening environment.
- Recognize common symptoms resulting from occupational and environmental pollutants.
- Describe the process of chemical sensitization.
- Discuss the nurse's role in promoting environmental health.
- Assess a variety of environments for sources of toxins.
- Select interventions to improve environmental health.
- Explain the relationship between natural, technological, or terror-related disasters and posttraumatic stress disorder.
- Discuss ways to empower citizens to protect a community's environmental health.

INTRODUCTION

Promoting a healthy environment is essential for people all over the world. No matter where nurses practice, they are involved with all that affects individuals—the air they breathe, the water they drink, the food they eat, the homes they inhabit, and the political and economic factors that influence their quality of life.

Creating an entirely pollution-free environment is virtually impossible. It is therefore critical to understand the way human bodies respond to the environment. A nurse's attention must focus on total health, including environmental surroundings, if health is to prevail or healing is to occur. It is possible to take steps to minimize the effects of environmental toxins, and all health professionals share the responsibility of promoting a healthy, supportive environment.

Interventions for air, water, and land pollution are well known. On a macro level, many of the changes needed to improve air, water, and land quality are expensive and complex, and require the involvement of many people. At the same time, interventions for promoting a healthy *personal* environment are often overlooked. These approaches are generally easy, inexpensive, and under individual control.

This chapter is a guide through the maze of environmental hazards. It provides an integrated view of the body and how it interacts with the environment. Identification of pollutants, environmental assessment, and methods to prevent or minimize the effects of toxins will be discussed. Other environmental factors (e.g., noise and color) will also be included. Suggested interventions are critical both as preventative and curative measures. Environmental disasters and terrorism are given special attention.

PROBLEM IDENTIFICATION

The environment encompasses all conditions, circumstances, and influences that may affect individuals and populations. The immediate environment includes home, school, or workplace. These are surroundings that an individual may encounter moving through normal daily activities. Factors affecting the local community, the global community, and its atmosphere are a larger part of everyone's environment.

Health is affected by complex and interrelated factors in the environment. It is impossible to view environmental health and threats in isolation. If an ecosystem is healthy, then individuals in that ecosystem will be healthier. As an ecosystem deteriorates, so does human health. Deterioration may be immediate (e.g., toxic chemicals, contaminated groundwater) or may accumulate over time (e.g., destruction of the ozone layer).

It has been estimated that there are some 3,000 chemicals produced in the United States and available in the marketplace that have not undergone any testing for toxicity, yet they are in materials used to furnish, clean, build, and insulate our homes, schools, public buildings, and workplaces. Although the Centers for Disease Control and Prevention (CDC) increased the tracking of hazardous agents from just 27 to 150 between 2001 and 2005, the agency is only monitoring exposure, not health effects ("10 ways to reduce your exposure to chemicals," 2005).

The CDC is one of many federal agencies that exist for the health of the people of the United States. Another major agency is the Environmental Protection Agency (EPA), created in 1970, the mission of which is to protect human health and the environment (EPA, 2006e). The EPA leads the nation's environmental science, research, education, and assessment efforts. These efforts are accomplished through enforcing regulations, providing grant funding for research and environmental education projects, and promoting education to enhance the public's consciousness in caring for the environment. Conserving water and energy, minimizing outdoor air pollution, controlling indoor air pollution, and eliminating pesticide risks are a few of the focus areas for education and research by the EPA.

Such agencies are instrumental in identifying environmental problems or diseases or both. Epidemiology is the study of the distribution and determinants of disease in a population as well as the occurrence and causes of health effects in humans (Gordis, 2005). Using the epidemiological approach, environmental health hazards and risks may be linked to the problem.

A substance or agent that has the ability to cause any type of adverse health effect is an **environmental health hazard.** The effect can range from a minor illness, to a serious illness, to death. An **environmental health risk** is defined as the probability that there will be actual consequences from the potential danger of the hazard. For example, asbestos-containing materials (such as ceiling tile) are usually considered relatively harmless (a *risk*). Ceiling tile, however, may release asbestos fibers if disturbed. These asbestos fibers, once airborne, can be inhaled and become a *hazard*. Environmental hazards are toxins, carcinogens, mutagens, or teratogens with specific consequences. Toxins cause harm or may be fatal to humans in low doses. **Carcinogens** promote the growth of or cause cancer. **Mutagens** change genetic material found in chromosomes. **Teratogens** cause birth defects.

A **disease cluster** is defined as a group of individuals experiencing the same disease in greater numbers than would otherwise be expected. An abnormally high level of colon cancer in a community is an example of a disease cluster. When a disease cluster is identified, biological and environmental factors are generally suspected (e.g., microorganisms or pollutants). Epidemiologists study disease clusters, identifying and studying patterns of health and illness in populations.

The EPA Model of Risk Assessment

The model used by the Environmental Protection Agency (EPA) involves four major steps to assess risk when a disease cluster is identified (Gordis, 2005). First, the potential environmental hazards are delineated. This includes identifying the type of agent, the way it works in the human body, and the seriousness of the damage done.

Second, the dose response process is delineated. The amount that is toxic and the human response must be determined. The model of response may be linear or threshold. Harmful effects coincide in proportion to the dose in the linear model. In the threshold model, certain levels of the substance may not be harmful; however, once a threshold is reached, harm occurs.

Estimation of the exposure is the third step. This includes determining the amount of the pollutant in the environment and the amount likely to reach a target site in the body. The fourth and final step is to characterize the risk in terms of seriousness of the harm and susceptibility of the population. When this process is completed, appropriate steps are taken to reduce risk to the public. Nurses are frequently among the first to recognize disease clusters and bring them to the attention of other individuals or agencies.

THE BODY'S RESPONSE TO ENVIRONMENTAL INFLUENCES

Nurses play a critical role in supporting individual health within a threatening environment. "Knowledge deficit related to risk of environmental hazards" and "potential for injury related to toxic exposure" are examples of nursing diagnoses related to environmental health. As disease entities are identified, the nursing plan of care can be expanded to include nursing diagnoses related to specific symptoms or illness.

The body produces internal toxins when under mental and emotional stresses. These toxins plus external pollutants significantly diminish the body's capacity to resist disease. Poor environmental conditions contribute either directly or indirectly to virtually all major chronic illnesses shown in a selected listing of adverse responses linked to known pollutants (see Table 7-1).

TABLE 7-1 Potential Adverse Responses Linked to Pollutants

Physiological	Adverse Responses
Gastrointestinal	Nausea, vomiting, diarrhea, cancer
Central nervous system	Headaches, sinus pain, sensory disturbances (auditory, visual, olfactory), dizziness and vertigo, blackouts, impaired mental functioning
Musculoskeletal	Weakness, muscle cramps, tremors
Respiratory	Nasal congestion, coughing, wheezing, asthma, emphysema, cancer
Genitourinary	Infertility, urine color changes, pain on urination, difficulty urinating or decreased urination
Integumentary	Rash, itching, hair loss
Immune responses	Irritated eyes, fever, chills, fatigue, chemical sensitivity
Psychological	Irritability, depression, loss of concentration, nervous breakdowns, short-term memory loss, mental confusion, personality changes, hyperactivity, learning disabilities, belligerence, temper outbursts, social withdrawal, criminal behavior, attention deficit disorder
Syndromes	Chronic Fatigue Syndrome, Epstein-Barr Syndrome, Gulf War Syndrome, Severe Acute Respiratory Syndrome (SARS)

Adapted from "Indoor Air Quality: Part II—What It Does," by A. Pike-Paris, 2005, Pediatric Nursing, 31(1), 39–49; "SARS: Key Factors in Crisis Management," by H. Tseng, T. Chen, and S. Chou, 2005, Journal of Nursing Research, 13(1), 58–62; Medical Toxicology, by E. M. Caravati and M. A. McCuigan, 2004, Philadelphia: Lippincott Williams & Wilkins; and Air Pollution, by J. F. Colls, 2002, London: Spon Press.

No body system is safe from environmental harm. Fortunately many of the physical illnesses and mental disturbances caused by environmental health hazards are reversible with removal of the pollutant.

Acute and Chronic Exposure

Illness may result from acute or chronic exposure to pollutants. Acute exposure is described as exposure to high concentrations of a pollutant for a short period of time. Examples of acute exposure include smog or chemical emissions. Consequences from acute exposure range from mild symptoms (e.g., headaches and itchy eyes) to death from high concentrations of a particular substance (e.g., carbon monoxide).

Exposure to low levels of a pollutant over an extended time is classified as chronic exposure. In the past this low-level but prolonged exposure was believed to be harmless. Definitive links have now been made between chronic exposure and the development of disease (Evans & Kantrowitz, 2003). Examples of chronic exposure include lead paint ingestion and inhalation of asbestos fibers. Pregnant women need to be especially alert as chronic exposure is more likely to be embryotoxic (toxic to a developing fetus) than is acute exposure.

Often it is the accumulation and combination of environmental threats that cause disease. One or two environmental stressors may be tolerated well. However, when another stressor is added, the biological system fails.

Pollutant sensitivity varies with the individual. Adverse reactions may be suffered by one individual while another remains symptom free. A formerly symptom-free individual may develop **chemical sensitivity** as a result of chronic exposure. Chemical sensitivity is the physiological response to a toxic substance following long-term exposure to low-level chemicals that were not recognized as harmful in the past. Following chemical sensitization, an individual develops a severe response with minimal exposure to the pollutant. Box 7-1 lists sample questions to ask when pollutants are suspected in causing physical symptoms.

SOURCES OF POLLUTION EXPOSURE

Common sources of widespread pollution exposure include the air, water, and soil. Other sources that are more localized are sound, light, and place. Disasters, not usually considered sources of pollution, cause both

Following is a selected sample of questions that may be used when pollutants are suspect.

- Do you think your symptoms can be associated with exposure to pollutants?
- When and where do your symptoms occur or worsen?
- Do others in the same setting experience the same symptoms and pattern of occurrence?
- Do symptoms diminish when you are away from the suspected setting for any length of time?
- Have you traveled or vacationed recently? Where?
- Have you flown on an airplane lately?
- Have you been swimming in rivers or lakes that might be contaminated?
- What cleaning supplies, fertilizers, herbicides, etc., are being used near you?
- Do you use any substances at work or in hobbies that may contain harmful chemicals?
- Have there been alterations in the growth patterns of your indoor plants? Signs that the inside air is heavy with unhealthy chemicals include: stems growing in strange, unnatural directions; abnormal growth rates; leaf tips that are curled or discolored.

Nursing Alert

Sensing Pollutants

The sense of smell can perceive between 2,000 and 4,000 different odors and is 10,000 times more sensitive than the sense of taste. Nonetheless, it is not an accurate tool for detecting pollutants because it begins to dull and adapt to odors during exposure. Also, even though an odor may be pleasing to an individual (e.g., perfumes, scented candles), it may not be harmless.

immediate and long-term devastating effects on the environment and its inhabitants.

Air Pollution

Contaminated atmosphere contributes to the full spectrum of physical ills. Fortunately, the environment has a very efficient cleaning system (e.g., wind, rain, temperature change) that purges the outside atmosphere periodically. Nevertheless, the body wages a constant battle for survival against inhaled pollutants from the atmosphere. Nasal hairs called cilia in the upper airway passages serve as filters. Coughs or sneezes are reflexes that expel many substances that get past the filtering system. Residual particles remain in the body to be fought by the immune system.

Indoor Air

The Environmental Protection Agency (2005b) estimates that indoor levels of many pollutants may be 25 to 100 times higher than outdoor levels, making indoor air pollution among the top five environmental risks to public

health. Indoor air quality has become a distinct field of study for environmental health.

The current air quality issue began in the early 1980s with building designs to conserve energy. Consequently, many buildings were constructed or remodeled to be airtight, with fresh air vents either plugged or omitted in the planning for air handling systems. As a result, rather than fresh air being circulated, stale air was recycled. One report suggested that up to 30 percent of new and remodeled buildings worldwide were responsible for excessive complaints related to indoor air quality (EPA, 2006c).

The term **sick building syndrome** was coined to describe situations in which building occupants experienced acute health and comfort effects that appeared to be linked to time spent in a building, regardless of location in the building, without having a specific illness or cause identified (EPA, 2006c). In contrast, the term **building-related illness** is used to describe a diagnosable illness that can be directly linked to airborne building contaminants (EPA, 2006c). An example is hypersensitivity pneumonitis, a nonallergic, immunologic pulmonary disease caused by inhalation of dusts from contaminated humidifiers, moldy organic debris, animal proteins, and certain chemicals (Ledford, 2002). Table 7-2 compares indicators for each of these terms. As seen in Table 7-3, the symptoms from various sources of indoor air pollutants vary. Therefore, determining whether the individual is suffering from sick building syndrome, building-related illness, or another cause can be difficult. For example, psychological factors (job or school stress, coworker conflict, work dissatisfaction, etc.) or health conditions (asthma, eczema, etc.) may be *caused* by or *exacerbated* by indoor air quality problems. Figure 7-1 depicts an example of internal and external sources of air pollution that may be found in schools.

Common sources for indoor pollutants include: tobacco smoke, unvented gas appliances, chemically treated building materials, foam insulation, synthetic

TABLE 7-2 Sick Building Syndrome versus Building-Related Illness: A Comparison of Indicators

Indicator	Sick Building Syndrome	Building-Related Illness
Building occupant complaints	Headache; eye, nose, or throat irritation; dry cough; dry or itchy skin; dizziness and nausea; difficulty in concentrating; fatigue; and/or sensitivity to odors	Cough; chest tightness; fever; chills; muscle aches
Cause of the symptoms	Unknown	Clinically defined and clearly identifiable
Relief from symptoms	Soon after leaving the building	Prolonged recovery times after leaving the building

From Indoor Air Facts No. 4 (revised): Sick Building Syndrome (SBS) *by Environmental Protection Agency (EPA), 2006a; Retrieved May 22, 2006, from http://www.epa.gov/iaq/pubs/sbs.html.*

TABLE 7-3 Checklist for Possible Symptoms and Related Indoor Air Pollutants

Symptoms	Environmental Tobacco Smoke	Other Combustion Products	Biological Pollutants	Volatile Organics	Heavy Metals	Sick Building Syndrome
Respiratory						
Rhinitis, nasal congestion	√	√	√	√		√
Epistaxis				√[1]		
Pharyngitis, cough	√	√	√	√		√
Wheezing, worsening asthma	√	√		√		√
Dyspnea	√[2]		√			√
Severe lung disease						√[3]
Other						
Conjunctival irritation	√	√	√	√		√
Headache or dizziness	√	√	√	√	√	√
Lethargy, fatigue, malaise		√[4]	√[5]	√	√	√
Nausea, vomiting, anorexia		√[4]	√	√	√	
Cognitive impairment, personality change		√[4]		√	√	√
Rashes			√	√	√	
Fever, chills			√[6]		√	
Tachycardia		√[4]			√	
Retinal hemorrhage		√[4]				
Myalgia (muscle aches)				√[5]		√
Hearing loss				√		

1. Associated especially with formaldehyde.
2. In asthma.
3. Hypersensitivity pneumonitis, Legionnaires' Disease.
4. Particularly associated with high CO levels.
5. Hypersensitivity pneumonitis, humidifier fever.
6. With marked hypersensitivity reactions and Legionnaires' Disease.

From Indoor Air Pollution: An Introduction for Health Professionals, *by Environmental Protection Agency (EPA), 2006b; www.epa.gov/iaq/pubs/hpguide*

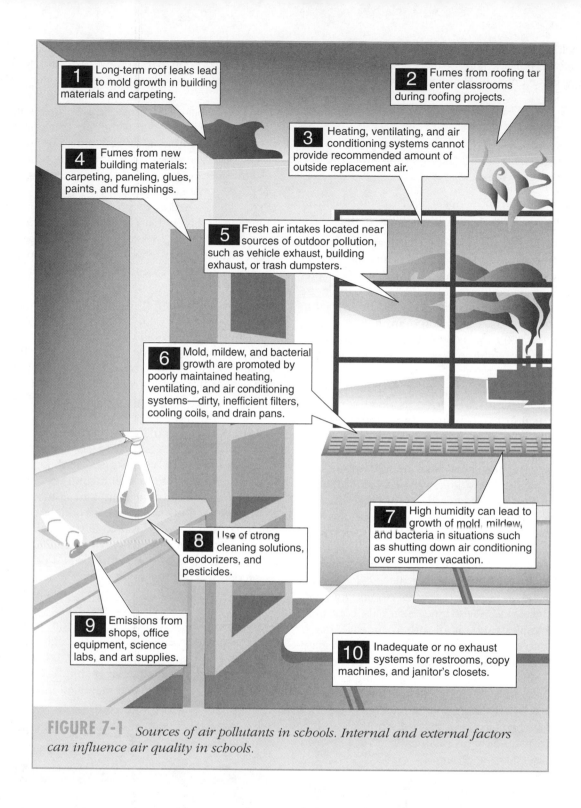

FIGURE 7-1 *Sources of air pollutants in schools. Internal and external factors can influence air quality in schools.*

carpeting, particle-board furniture, aerosol products, cleaning products, cooking fumes, and naturally emitted radon gas. These examples along with other indoor air pollutants can be categorized into three major areas:

- Particulate matter (e.g., environmental tobacco smoke, asbestos, dust)
- Biological contaminants (e.g., animal dander, fungal spores, bacteria, pollens, viruses)

- Gases and vapors (e.g., carbon monoxide, formaldehyde, radon, pesticides)
(Wigle, 2003, p. 270; EPA, 2006c)

Particulate Matter. **Particulate matter** refers to small particles or liquid droplets that can be suspended in the air. The amounts and sources of particulate matter in the air vary. The biggest sources of indoor particulates are windblown dust, house dust, and tobacco smoke. Other sources include woodstoves and appliances like furnaces and nonelectric heaters. The health effects of particulate matter vary in severity and may include the following:

- Coughing, wheezing, shortness of breath

- Aggravated asthma

- Lung damage (including decreased lung function and lifelong respiratory disease)

- Premature death in individuals with existing heart or lung diseases ("What is particulate matter?" n.d.)

Environmental tobacco smoke (ETS), also known as secondhand tobacco smoke, contains a mixture of over 4,700 chemical compounds and is the single most preventable indoor air pollutant (EPA, 2006d). Children are especially affected by ETS. It is estimated that 8,000 to 26,000 new asthma cases in children are linked to ETS, with another 150,000 to 300,000 new cases of bronchitis and pneumonia in children less than 18 months old (EPA, 2004, 2005a).

Asbestos is a source of particulate matter that is known to cause cancer. Asbestos was once commonly used in construction for insulation, fireproofing, soundproofing, and roofing and in other industrial work. It was even used in household products such as ironing board covers, hot pads, and oven mitts. Workers and their clothes would become covered with the white powder of asbestos. Years later, many of those exposed to the powder and fibers of asbestos were found to have developed gastrointestinal and lung cancers. A certain type of deadly cancer called mesothelioma is a direct result of asbestos exposure (American Lung Association, 2005, Mesolink.org, 2005). Because the substance was not known to be hazardous, asbestos-containing products were not labeled. Over time, materials containing asbestos disintegrate and, if disturbed, release microscopic fibers into the air to be inhaled. Removal of materials known to contain asbestos is recommended only as a last resort as this increases exposure; sealing or encapsulating the asbestos is recommended (EPA, 2006b; Mesolink.org, 2005). Buildings constructed before 1978 are considered suspicious for asbestos and should be inspected by construction professionals or local environmental agencies.

Biological Contaminants. Biological contaminants include bacteria, viruses, molds, mildew, animal dander and cat saliva, house dust, mites, cockroaches, and pollen (EPA, 2005d). Even protein in urine from rats and mice is a potent allergen when it dries and becomes airborne. Biological contaminants are found everywhere—in schools, offices, workplaces, stores, and homes. Contaminated central air handling systems can become breeding grounds for mold, mildew, and other sources of biological contaminants that can be spread throughout a building (EPA, 2005d). For example, Legionnaires'

disease, a potentially fatal bacterial pneumonia, and its lesser form, Pontiac Fever, were found to be spread indoors via moisture from contaminated air conditioning systems.

Three types of human disease can be attributed to biological contaminants in the air. These include infections, where pathogens invade human tissues; hypersensitivity diseases, where specific activation of the immune system causes disease; and toxicosis, where biologically produced chemical toxins cause direct toxic effects (EPA, 2006b). Action to protect against biological contaminants is directed at eliminating the sources as much as possible. Efforts should be taken to: repair leaks; dry areas where moisture has collected; keep the relative humidity between 30 and 50 percent; vent areas where moisture can collect such as bathrooms and kitchens; maintain clean filters in air conditioning systems; wash bedding and soft toys frequently in water at a temperature above 130°F to kill dust mites; and vacuum carpets and upholstered furniture regularly (EPA, 2006b). Sensitive individuals should avoid contact with pets and dust and use a commercially available HEPA (High Efficiency Particulate Air) filtered vacuum.

Gases. Gaseous pollutants can be emitted from a variety of indoor sources, including gas appliances, fireplaces, furnaces, wood or coal stoves, and kerosene stoves, heaters, or lights due to malfunction or improper use. In addition to natural gas emission, combustion sources can cause serious atmospheric pollution by releasing such gases as carbon monoxide (CO), nitrogen dioxide (NO_2), and sulfur dioxide (SO_2) (EPA, 2006b).

Radon is a tasteless, colorless, and odorless gas that is second to cigarette smoking as the leading source of lung cancer, accounting for approximately 20,000 deaths each year in the United States (EPA, 2006b). Radon is a decay product of uranium and occurs naturally in soil and rock. Radon enters a home through cracks in walls, basement floors, foundations, and other openings. It may also contaminate the water supply, especially in private wells. Radon has been identified in every state. It is

---

BOX 7-2   Testing for Radon

Low-cost radon test kits are available by mail order, in hardware stores, and through other retail outlets. Depending on whether a short-term or long-term test is used, it takes anywhere from 2 to 90 days for results. Long-term tests give a more accurate annual average radon level than do short-term tests because radon levels vary from day to day and season to season. Only home test kits labeled "meets EPA requirements" should be used.

estimated that 6 percent of U.S. homes, or one in 15, have elevated levels of radon. Box 7-2 highlights information on testing for radon.

Volatile organic compounds (VOCs) are gases released from certain solids or liquids and are found in thousands of products. Box 7-3 lists examples of VOC sources. Concentrations of many VOCs are up to 10 times higher than outdoors (EPA, 2005c). The effects from exposure to these VOCs can be short or long term; nonetheless, they can contribute to the creation of an indoor chemical crisis for some individuals.

Formaldehyde is the most well-known of volatile organic compound (VOC) pollutants. It is a common ingredient in plywood, particle board, laminated lumber, vinyl panels, wallpaper, glue adhesives, and insulating materials. In high temperatures and humidity, formaldehyde breaks down into a toxic gas. This process is called **outgassing.** The strength of the odor is usually directly proportional to the degree of outgassing. That "new carpet smell" or "new car smell" and the haze on a car's windows result from formaldehyde outgassing. The outgassing process from plastics and upholstery in a new car may last a couple of years. Formaldehyde is also found in permanent press fabrics, rubber, and consumer products ranging from cosmetics to medicines. Certain occupations (such as morticians and pathologists) are exposed to high levels of formaldehyde. Formaldehyde monitors are available. Monitors may be hung in a room and then submitted to a laboratory for analysis. Symptoms of exposure include eye irritation, heart palpitation, coughing, chest tightness, and headache.

It is important to note that some common household cleaners may be extremely toxic when combined. For example, when chlorine-based cleaners are mixed with ammonia, a deadly gas called chloramine is formed. Read-

ing and following instructions and warning labels on all products is essential for safe use and for avoiding exposure to harmful pollutants. See Table 7-4 for typical warning label terminology. Box 7-4 lists questions that could be used in assessing for risks from indoor air pollutants.

Worksite Air Quality Management

Occupational health nurses are concerned with indoor air quality management at the worksite. They work as facilitators or team leaders to improve environmental conditions, including air quality, at the worksite.

Indoor air quality problems at the worksite arise from various sources, as shown in Box 7-5. A multidisciplinary group of professionals may be required to assess the situation and to develop a plan to minimize or eliminate the problem. The team may be composed of an occupational health nurse, a physician, an industrial hygienist (environmental hygienist), a microbiologist, an epidemiologist, a toxicologist, and/or a professional engineer. The complexity and seriousness of the identified problem determine size and membership of the team.

A team should investigate a situation if at least 20 percent of the employees report a similar problem. Individual, nonrecurring problems can be addressed by the occupational health nurse. Once the problem is identified and resolved, employees will enjoy better health, which can lead to improved efficiency, decreased absenteeism, and increased worker satisfaction.

Sick Building Syndrome

- Are problems temporally related to time spent in a particular building or part of a building?
- Do symptoms resolve when the individual is not in the building?
- Do symptoms correspond to the need for heat or air conditioning?
- Have coworkers, peers had similar complaints?

Biological Contaminants

- Are symptoms related to the workplace, home, or other location?
- What are possible sources of contaminants in the suspected location?
- Is the relative humidity in the home or workplace consistently above 50 percent?
- Are humidifiers or other water-spray systems in use? How often are they cleaned?
- Are they cleaned appropriately?
- Has there been flooding or leaks?
- Is there evidence of mold growth (visible growth or odors)?
- Are organic materials handled in the workplace?
- Is carpet installed on unventilated concrete (e.g., slab on grade) floors?
- Are there pets in the home?
- Are there problems with cockroaches or rodents?
- Is adequate outdoor air being provided?
- Are bacterial odors present (fishy or locker-room smells)?

Sources of Combustion (Stoves, Heaters, Fireplaces, etc.)

- What types of combustion equipment are present, including gas furnaces or water heaters, stoves, unvented gas or kerosene space heaters, clothes dryers, fireplaces? Are vented appliances properly vented to the outside?
- Are household members exhibiting influenza-like symptoms during the heating season?
- Are they complaining of nausea, watery eyes, coughing, headaches?
- Is a gas oven or range used as a home heating source?

- Is the individual aware of odor when a heat source is in use?
- Is heating equipment in disrepair or misused? When was it last professionally inspected?
- Does structure have an attached or underground garage where motor vehicles may idle?
- Is charcoal being burned indoors in a hibachi, grill, or fireplace?

Heavy Metals (Airborne Lead and Mercury)

- Does the family reside in old or restored housing?
- Has renovation work been conducted in the home, workplace, school, or day care facility?
- Is the home located near a busy highway or industrial area?
- Does the individual work with lead materials such as solder or automobile radiators?
- Does the child have a sibling, friend, or classmate recently diagnosed with lead poisoning?
- Has the individual engaged in art, craft, or workshop projects?
- Does the individual regularly handle firearms?
- Has the home interior recently been painted with latex paint that may contain mercury?
- Does the individual use mercury in religious or cultural activities?

Volatile Organic Compounds (Formaldehyde, Pesticides, Solvents, Cleaning Agents)

- Does the individual reside in a mobile home or new conventional home containing large amounts of pressed wood products?
- Has the individual recently acquired new pressed wood furniture?
- Does the individual's job or a vocational pursuit include clerical, craft, graphics, or photographic materials?
- Are chemical cleaners used extensively in the home, school, or workplace?
- Has remodeling recently been done in the home, school, or workplace?
- Has the individual recently used pesticides, paints, or solvents?

Adapted from Indoor Air Pollution: An Introduction for Health Professionals, *by Environmental Protection Agency (EPA), (2006, March 6), www.epa.gov/iaq/pubs/hpguide.*

Outdoor Air

One of the most pressing worldwide problems in the new century is outdoor, or ambient, air pollution. Contributors to ambient air pollution include: factories releasing particulate matter, nitrogen, and sulfur oxides; vehicles emitting carbon monoxide; and natural phenomena diffusing particulate matter (i.e., volcanic eruptions and geysers). Diesel exhaust contains 20 to 100

BOX 7-5   Sources of Worksite Air Pollution

Indoor Sources

Housekeeping and Maintenance
Some cleansers, dusting, vacuuming, disinfectants, pesticides, and adhesives

Occupant
Tobacco products, office equipment (printers, copiers), microwaves, cooking appliances, art supplies, marking pens, personal products, tracked-in dirt/pollens

Shared Space
Dry cleaners, pet stores, laboratories (chemicals, moisture), print shops, art stores, beauty salons, restaurants, cafeterias, medical offices

Building
Construction materials and adhesives, asbestos, insulation, wall/floor coverings, wet building products, upholstered furniture, renovation materials, and transformers

HVAC System (Heating, Ventilation, and Air Conditioning)
Filters, ducts, humidifiers, drain pans, mechanical rooms, lubricants, combustion appliances, refrigerants

Vehicles
Underground/attached garage

Outdoor Sources

Vehicles
Traffic, loading docks

Commercial/Manufacturing
Dry cleaners, restaurants, automotive shops, gas stations, paint shops, electronics manufacturers

Utilities/Public Works
Utilities/power plants, incinerators, water treatment plants

Agriculture
Pesticide use, processing plants, ponds

Birds/Rodents
Droppings, nests

Building Maintenance
Painting, roofing, sanding, pesticides, trash, refuse

Water
Pools of water on roofs, cooling tower mist

Ground/Underground
Soil, water, sewer gas, underground storage tanks

From An Office Building Occupant's Guide to Indoor Air Quality, *by Environmental Protection Agency (EPA), 2006, Retrieved May 29, 2006, from www.epa.gov/iaq/pubs/occupgd; "Indoor environments and health: Moving into the 21st Century," by J. M. Samet and J. D. Spengler, September 2003,* American Journal of Public Health, *93(9), 1489–1493.*

times more particles than gasoline exhaust along with dangerous gases, including nitrous oxide, nitrogen dioxide, formaldehyde, benzene, sulfur dioxide, hydrogen sulfide, and carbon dioxide, carbon monoxide (AFSCME, n.d.). Not surprisingly, diesel exhaust from common sources, such as trucks, buses, and trains, is linked to increases in asthma, bronchitis, emphysema, and cancer. Landfills can also be a source of outdoor air pollution as they contribute to outgassing of methane and buried toxic chemical fumes.

Under normal conditions, warm air rises, dispersing pollutants and carrying them away from earth. Wind also dilutes pollutants. When a temperature inversion occurs, pollutants are trapped as the warm air settles to earth.

Atmospheric airflows, however, contribute to global transportation of pollutants. For example, the continental airflow across the United States distributes air pollution from the Midwest throughout the Northeast contributing to high levels of air pollution in the New England states (Kleim & Rock, n.d.). In fact, the New England states have been referred to as the "tailpipe" of

the United States as the airflow moves polluted air eastward across the Atlantic Ocean and on into Europe. Scientists have found that, in contrast to eastbound Pacific air that flows into North America, eastbound transatlantic air pollution from North America to Europe hangs closer to the surface of the earth, causing a greater effect on humans (Spotts, 2004).

In the past, the term *smog* was used to describe smoke, ashes, soot, and other particulate matter and substances in the air. Today the term also includes photochemical smog resulting from the sun's reaction with chemicals in the air. Ozone is one of the largest components of photochemical smog. Ozone in the upper atmosphere acts as a protective shield to earth's inhabitants while ozone in the lower layer of the atmosphere is associated with adverse health effects.

Another form of outdoor pollution is acid rain that forms when emissions of sulfur dioxide and nitrogen dioxide combine with other chemicals high in the atmosphere. As a result, droplets are carried by winds, perhaps far from the pollutant-producing area, and fall to earth as either dry or wet (rain, snow, fog) acid-contaminated droplets. Acid rain threatens ecology and defaces monuments and buildings.

Conflicting research reports create confusion about the effects of electromagnetic radiation (Zeman, 2004). Radio, television, wiring in the house, and household appliances, including electric blankets, have low levels of electromagnetic transmission. Higher levels (e.g., coming from high voltage power lines, heavy usage of computers, and microwave ovens) have been implicated in neurological damage and cataracts. As a precaution, recommendations are that exposure to electromagnetic radiation be kept to a minimum and that homes be at least 500 feet from high-voltage power lines (Peterson, 2004).

Health Promotion and Nursing Interventions for Air Quality

Strides have been made in developed countries to address the issues of indoor air quality. New issues, however, continue to emerge. Issues of concern relate to synthetic organic compounds, intentionally introduced viruses and other infectious organisms (addressed later in this chapter), and engineering and design factors in the workplace (Samet & Spengler, 2003). The role of the nurse will continue to be of great importance in current and emerging issues related to indoor air quality. The first step in this role is to identify problems and then determine the need for professional assistance. Improving out-

TABLE 7-5 Health Promotion Guide to Indoor Air Quality Management

Pollutant	Source		Possible Adverse Health Effects	
Environmental Tobacco Smoke (ETS)	Cigarettes Cigars	Pipes	Respiratory irritation Bronchitis SIDS in infants Pneumonia in children	Emphysema Cancers (lung, brain, leukemia, lymphoma) Heart disease
Carbon Monoxide	Unvented or malfunctioning gas appliances	Woodstoves Indoor vehicle work Tobacco smoke	Headache Nausea Angina Impaired vision	Impaired mental functioning Death at high concentrations
Nitrogen Oxide	Unvented or malfunctioning gas or kerosene appliances	Ice resurfacing equipment	Eye, nose, and throat irritation	Respiratory infections
VOCs (Formaldehyde, Chemical Solvents, Pesticides)	Aerosol sprays Solvents Glues, hobby products Cleaning agents Pesticides, paints Moth repellents Air fresheners Dry-cleaned clothes ETS	Cosmetics Pressed wood (plywood, particleboard) Furnishings (carpet, draperies, furniture) Wallpaper Durable press fabrics	Eye, nose, and throat irritation Allergic reaction Headaches	Loss of coordination Liver, brain, and kidney damage Cancer, leukemia
Respirable Particles	Cigarettes Woodstoves Fireplaces	Aerosol sprays House dust	Eye, nose, and throat irritation	Respiratory infections and bronchitis Lung cancer

door air quality is more difficult and requires cooperation among individuals, communities, and industries.

Prevention is the key to air quality problems. Not all air pollutants, however, can be prevented. Table 7-5 summarizes the major threats to indoor air quality and presents a health promotion guide to be used by the nurse with clients to prevent adverse effects.

Individuals with respiratory sensitivity can minimize their responses to outdoor air pollutants by remaining indoors when pollen and mold counts are high and during smog and ozone alerts. Print and electronic media provide information regarding smog and ozone alerts as well as pollen counts. Sun-sensitive individuals should pay particular attention to ultraviolet light level reports as well.

Individuals who have developed chemical sensitivity may be diagnosed as having environmental illness or multiple chemical sensitivity. Although such diagnoses are controversial among medical professionals, individuals who suffer health consequences from chemicals in their environment also suffer from the accompanying stresses, including strained or lost relationships with family and friends and reduced access to public places. A safe environment is imperative for the well-being of chemically sensitive individuals.

A safe environment is one that is, as nearly as possible, void of chemical pollutants. Protective steps must be taken for the individual to survive. These individuals spend a great deal of time in a chemically free

Health Promotion Guide

Do not smoke. Do not smoke in your home or permit others to do so. Seek nonsmoking restaurants and other public social venues.	Do not smoke if children are present, particularly infants and toddlers. If smoking indoors cannot be avoided, increase ventilation in the area where smoking takes place. Open windows or use exhaust fans.
Keep gas appliances properly adjusted. Consider purchasing a vented space heater when replacing an unvented one. Use proper fuel in kerosene space heaters. Install and use an exhaust fan vented to outdoors over gas stoves. Open flues when fireplaces are in use.	Choose properly sized woodstoves that are certified to meet EPA emission standards. Make certain that doors on all woodstoves fit tightly. Have a trained professional inspect, clean, and tune up the central heating system (furnaces, flues, and chimneys) annually. Repair any leaks promptly. Do not idle vehicles inside garage.
Refer to steps for Carbon Monoxide	
Use household products according to manufacturer's directions. Make sure you provide plenty of fresh air when using these products. Throw away unused or little-used containers safely; buy in quantities that you will use soon. Keep out of reach of children and pets. Never mix household care products unless directed on the label.	Use "exterior-grade" pressed wood products (lower-emitting because they contain phenol resins, not urea resins). Use air conditioners and dehumidifiers to maintain moderate temperature and reduce humidity levels. Increase ventilation, particularly after bringing new sources of formaldehyde into the home.
Vent all furnaces to outdoors; keep doors to rest of house open when using unvented space heaters. Choose properly sized woodstoves, certified to meet EPA emission standards; make certain that doors on all woodstoves fit tightly.	Have a trained professional inspect, clean, and tune up central heating system (furnace, flues, and chimneys) annually. Repair any leaks promptly. Change filters on central heating and cooling systems and air cleaners according to manufacturer's directions.

Pollutant	Source		Possible Adverse Health Effects	
Bioaerosols (Bacteria, Viruses, Fungi, Animal Dander, Mites)	House dust Pets Bedding Poorly maintained air conditioners,	humidifiers, and dehumidifiers Wet or moist structures Furnishings	Allergic reaction Asthma Eye, nose, and throat irritation Fever	Influenza and other infectious diseases (i.e., Legionnaires' Disease, Bird Flu)
Asbestos	Damaged or deteriorating insulation	Fireproofing and acoustical materials	Asbestosis	Mesothelioma, lung cancer and other cancers
Lead	Sanding or open-flame burning of lead paint	House dust	Nerve and brain damage, particularly in children	Anemia Kidney damage Growth retardation
Radon	Soil under buildings Some earth-derived construction materials	Well water	Lung cancer	

Adapted from California Air Resources Board (2001), "Indoor Air pollution: A Serious Public Health Problem," Sacramento, CA: Research Division; A. Pike-Paris, 2005, January–February, "Indoor Air Quality: Part II—What It Does," Pediatric Nursing, 31(5), 39–49; U.S. Environmental Protection Agency and the United States Consumer Product Safety Commission, 2005, "The Inside Story: A Guide to Indoor Air Quality," Office of Radiation and Indoor Air (EPA Document # 402-K-93-007), Retrieved January 10, 2005, from http://www.epa.gov/iaq/pubs/insidest.html.

environment and lead an isolated existence. Care must be taken so that pollutants are not reintroduced into the controlled environment. Creating a chemical-free living space has been rated the highest of all treatment methods for chemically sensitive individuals (Gibson, Elms, & Ruding, 2003). Box 7-6 provides a nursing checklist for creating a safe haven for the chemically sensitized individual.

Water and Soil Pollution

Pure water is essential to life. Surface water is the water source for most large metropolitan areas and comes from lakes, rivers, reservoirs, and streams. Organic contaminants from naturally decaying animal and vegetable materials pose a threat to surface water. Other sources of contamination include acid rain, urban storm water runoff, pesticide runoff, industrial waste, and synthetic chemicals.

Groundwater comes from underground aquifers. Underground aquifers are long stretches of underground rock formations filled with water. Wells, which are more commonly found in rural areas, tap into these aquifers. Sources of groundwater pollution include pesticides, herbicides, and fertilizers; hazardous industrial wastes; leaking underground gasoline storage tanks; discarded household chemicals; and other synthetic chemicals. Industries can work to prevent groundwater pollution and provide safe water recreation areas.

Contaminated soil affects people's surroundings and food and water supplies. Some workers, such as those working in landfills or at chemical dumps, may have exposure to high levels of soil-carried toxins. Most individuals are affected to a lesser extent. Gardeners and constructions workers may be exposed by digging in it. Children may be exposed by playing in it. Anyone may inhale dust from it or eat food grown in it.

Soil pollution may result from fertilizers and pesticides that leach into the ground, and from gas tanks or chemical barrels that leak. Soil may be contaminated from refuse brought to the surface with mining. Other sources include chemicals from chemical spills, disposal ponds, and landfills, and even leaks that wash off parking lots and highways.

Health Promotion Guide

Install and use fans vented to outdoors in kitchens and bathrooms. Vent clothes dryers to outdoors. Clean cool mist and ultrasonic humidifiers in accordance with manufacturer's instructions and refill with clean water daily.	Empty water trays in air conditioners, dehumidifiers, and refrigerators frequently. Clean and dry or remove water-damaged carpets. Use basements as living areas only if they are leak-proof and have adequate ventilation. Use dehumidifiers, if necessary, to maintain humidity between 30 and 50 percent.
Do not disturb. Use trained and qualified contractors for control measures that may disturb asbestos and for clean-up.	Follow proper procedures in replacing woodstove door gaskets that may contain asbestos.
Keep areas where children play as clean and dust-free as possible. Leave lead-based paint undisturbed if it is in good condition; do not sand or burn off paint that may contain lead.	Do not remove lead paint yourself. Do not bring lead dust into the home. If your work or hobby involves lead, change clothes and use doormats before entering your home. Eat a balanced diet, rich in calcium and iron.
Test the home for radon. Fix the home if radon level is 4 picocuries per liter (pCi/L) or higher.	Radon levels less than 4 pCi/L still pose a risk, and in many cases may be reduced. For more information on radon, contact the state radon office, or call 800-SOS-RADON.

BOX 7-6   Nursing Checklist for Creating a Safe Haven for the Chemically Sensitized Individual

1. Remove fabrics and synthetic items such as stuffed toy animals, curtains, tablecloths, upholstered furniture, etc.
2. Clean air conditioning vents and ducts and replace filters often.
3. Wash walls, windows, blinds, and other objects with water and unscented cleaner such as baking soda, vinegar, or hydrogen peroxide.
4. Replace carpet with untreated hardwood or terrazzo tile.
5. Encase pillows and mattresses in hypoallergenic material.
6. Use natural-fiber fabrics such as cotton.
7. Keep paper products at a minimum (chemicals, inks, and dyes may produce a reaction).
8. Do not use scented candles or air fresheners.
9. Use a room-size air purifier and replace filter frequently.
10. Assess grooming items for toxins.
11. Replace furniture made of particleboard.
12. Use electric appliances.
13. Do not use pesticides, exterminators, or lawn care companies.
14. Introduce new items individually to test tolerability and add other items after a four-day wait.

Each year at least 250 million tons of waste are labeled as hazardous. Oil refineries and chemical manufacturers generate at least half of this total toxic waste. Materials must be biologically or chemically treated to remove toxins prior to disposal. Guidelines for toxic waste disposal have increased in stringency over the years. Special sites are designated as toxic waste dumps. Soil structure or special linings prevent leakage of toxins into the ground and into underground water sources.

Health Promotion and Nursing Interventions for Water and Soil Quality

Individuals contribute significantly to the reduction of health risks caused by water and soil contamination. Nurses may assist in reducing risks for individuals by encouraging them to use nontoxic cleaning materials, such as vinegar and baking soda; substitute organic insecticides and compost for toxic chemicals and fertilizers; and select consumer products with minimal packaging to reduce waste. Home gardeners and do-it-yourself pest controllers must be made aware of the long-lasting dangers of pesticides and herbicides.

On a larger scale, nurses and nursing organizations may work to influence the agricultural industry's development of more insect-resistant crops and use of fewer pesticides. Many nurses have become involved with environmental groups and have paired with communities to sponsor massive clean-up campaigns and organize beach, waterway, and roadside pickups of litter. Long-term recycling programs, including organic and nonorganic materials, should be encouraged. Many communities sponsor composting classes and furnish compost bins to participants to encourage recycling of organic materials. Newspapers, glass, plastic, and aluminum are commonly recycled household wastes. Automotive repair shops recycle tires, batteries, and oil. Artificial reefs for water wildlife have been created from old tires and metal wastes.

Even though water looks, tastes, and smells fine it may still be hazardous. In fact, waterborne microorganisms can be lethal. Coliform, a harmless microbe, serves as an indicator organism in the coliform test. It usually coexists with disease-causing organisms such as *Escherichia coli* and *Klebsiella*. Water in public systems goes through a series of treatments, including filtering, treating, and aerating. This provides consumers a high level of protection. Those using private wells must test their water annually for contaminants to ensure the same protection. Adequate water testing and treatment must be enforced.

Improved landfill technology confines current hazardous wastes more effectively than in years past. Waste sites and dumps that have been filled or covered prior to use of improved technology must be identified and tested for toxicity. Consumer education regarding identification and proper disposal of toxic materials (e.g., leftover insecticides, paint, and batteries) will reduce improper disposal practices. Development of alternative waste technology and stricter guidelines for industrial and commercial emissions will reduce future risks.

Sound Pollution

Silence, the absence of sound, is something most people today experience all too infrequently. The ears remain open and working whether people are awake or asleep. Silence can be deafening if stimulation is needed, or

Research Note

Study Problem/Purpose: To examine the association between pesticide use and breast cancer incidence among farmers' wives in a large prospective cohort study in Iowa and North Carolina.

Methods: Participants included 30,454 women who had history of breast cancer prior to enrollment during 1993–1997. Demographic information and data on pesticide use were obtained by a self-administered questionnaire. A prospective design was used to determine incidence of cancer among the participants from a regional cancer registry.

Findings: There were 309 incident breast cancer cases identified between enrollment in the project and the year 2000. Some evidence of increased risk was associated with use of a particular pesticide chemical (2,4,5-trichloro-phexypropionic acid), but firm conclusions could not be drawn. There was clear association of breast cancer risk with the size of the farm or with the washing of clothes worn during pesticide application. Cancer risk, however, was modestly elevated among women whose homes were closest to areas of pesticide application. Continued research was recommended.

Implication: Knowledge from this study can be integrated into care by nurses in agricultural areas in expanding their assessment of clients who live on farms or in farming communities. Teaching about hazards should be incorporated into the plan of care.

Engel, L. S., Hill, D. A., Hoppin, J. A., Lubin, J. H., Lynch, C. F., Pierce, J., et al. (2005, January). Pesticide use and breast cancer risk among farmers' wives in the agricultural health study. *American Journal of Epidemiology, 161*(2), 121-135.

restorative if a period of relaxation is needed. Silence provides a shift or break from usual sounds.

Conversely, sound or noise can become an environmental pollutant when it is extremely annoying and potentially harmful to hearing when individuals are exposed to noise at high levels. Sound pollution has a long history. Indeed, the Romans went so far as to ban chariots on cobblestone streets at night. Today, sound pollution is growing to epidemic proportions. This type of pollution is invisible, odorless, and tasteless. People are almost constantly barraged with sounds, such as: office noises; voices in a crowded room; urban noise from vehicles and church bells; airport noise; recreational noise, including rock music and sports; and heating and air-conditioning gusts. Hearing becomes diminished as a result of prolonged exposure to loud sounds.

Nearly 31 million people in the United States have impaired hearing (Kochkin, 2005a). Whether it is

TABLE 7-6 Common Sound Measurements

Average dBa	Sound
0–1	Normal hearing possible
20	Whisper
60	Normal conversation
75	Washing machine
85	Busy city traffic
90	Lawn mower, motorcycle, hair blower
110	Snowmobile
115	Live rock music concert, chain saw
118	Health clubs and aerobic studios
125	Ambulance siren, jackhammer
125–155	Firecracker at 10 feet
135	Jet plane takeoff at 100 feet
140	"Boom" cars
165	12-gauge shotgun blast
180	Rocket engine

Adapted from Information Center: Hearing Loss, *by Dangerous Decibels, 2005, http://www.dangerousdecibels.org/hearingloss.cfm; and* Hearing Loss Prevention, *by R.W. Danielson, 2005, retrieved June 3, 2006, from www.betterhearing.org.*

referred to as a disability, a disorder, or an impairment, hearing loss is one of the most common chronic health conditions affecting all age groups, ethnicities, and genders. Box 7-7 provides some general demographic facts about hearing loss in the U.S. population.

All cells within the body act as sound receptors, eliciting physiological and psychological responses. Some individuals are particularly sound sensitive. The body reacts adversely to strong sounds. Behaviors are amplified. Tension develops. Energy is depleted. In contrast, welcome sounds trigger a relaxation response and create energy.

Noise is any loud, discordant, or disagreeable sound or sounds that may decrease body energy or cause auditory damage. Potential harm from a sound is determined by several characteristics: sound pressure level (loudness, intensity), frequency (pitch), rhythm, and duration. Even good music becomes noise if played so loudly that distortion occurs. Certain repetitive rhythms may be depressing. The damaging effects of noise are cumulative.

Exposure to noise is responsible for over 77 percent of all hearing loss (Better Hearing Institute, 2005). After exposure to loud noises, a person's hearing grows dull, causing a temporary hearing threshold shift. Hearing returns to its normal sharpness with cessation of the noise. A sudden, extremely loud noise, such as an explosion, creates pressure waves with enough intensity to cause actual physical trauma to the inner ear.

Sound loudness is measured in decibels (dBa) with 0 dBa being the lowest possible audible sound by a person with normal hearing. Standards set by the Occupational Safety and Health Administration (OSHA) indicate that hearing impairment can occur with continued exposure to noise over 85 decibels averaged over an eight-hour day (OSHA, 2002). See Table 7-6 for examples of common sounds and their decibel measurements.

Noise is probably the most common occupational hazard facing people today. It is estimated that as many as 30 million Americans are exposed to potentially harmful sounds at work. Even outside work, many people participate in recreational activities that can produce harmful noise (musical concerts, use of power tools, etc.). Sixty million Americans own firearms, and many people do not use appropriate hearing protection devices.

Noise-induced hearing loss is permanent. Other effects of long-term, low-intensity noise include tension headaches, lack of concentration, anxiety, hypertension, and insomnia. Warning signs of dangerous noise levels demand immediate action to preserve hearing.

Throughout life, from birth to death, individuals are able to adapt to noise. Adaptation occurs as the body diminishes its awareness of continuous or repetitive sounds. However, the body continues to respond to the noise even though awareness has decreased. Therefore, adaptation places us at risk for the continuing physiological and psychological effects of sounds as well as auditory damage. Recovery rates and quality of life can be improved through control of a client's auditory environment. Sensory messages are transmitted during sleep, even during deep anesthesia-induced sleep. The unconscious client may be able to hear, though other sensory stimuli are blocked. Hearing is believed to be the last sense lost during the dying process.

Health Promotion and Nursing Interventions Related to Sound

The body can discriminate between beneficial and detrimental sounds, responding physiologically and psychologically. Good music and most natural sounds have a therapeutic effect, strengthening the body.

Music is an integral part of behavioral kinesiology. Behavioral kinesiology suggests that each gesture or movement made is the body's response to a need to tonify or to correct an imbalance in a certain body system. Muscle tension and relaxation in response to sounds can be measured. Music elicits body movement (e.g., swaying or dancing to music). Orchestra conductors move with the music, experiencing the healing qualities of music while vigorously tonifying the body. Observe music conductors. Most are trim, healthy, and relaxed, and they live for many years.

Rhythm in music can stimulate or depress. Individuals tend to breathe with the rhythm of music. A 4/4 tempo corresponds to the normal heart rate, eliciting a relaxation response. Rapid, even drumbeats are highly stimulating while progressively slower rhythms lead to relaxation and sleep. Commercially produced intrauterine sounds quiet newborns within 30 seconds.

In the presence of biological symptoms, nurses must consider not only physiological causes but environmental causes as well. The nurse must work to achieve a balance between sensory deprivation and sensory overload. Taking research into the practice arena, nurses should minimize sources of loud sounds (e.g., conversations, radios, telephones, incubators, respirators, cardiac monitors, and other equipment). Routine nursing interventions must be evaluated for frequency and necessity. These include suctioning, inserting various tubes, and personal care (e.g., changing diapers on the preterm infant).

Nurses in many ways have used music as an environmental intervention. Music can help clients increase movement, mobility, and positive self-expression. Music can significantly decrease a client's awareness of pain.

Ask Yourself

Sound Awareness

Sit quietly for at least five minutes. Really listen. Jot down the sounds in your environment.
- Which sounds were already in your awareness?
- Which sounds came into awareness only with real concentration?
- What subtle changes occur in your body in response to these sounds?
- Are there sounds that irritate you, make you tense, and drain your energy?
- Which sounds are soothing and help to energize?
- How can you diminish the unwelcome sounds? Increase the welcome ones?

For agitated clients or hyperactive children, music can reduce activity level. For the developmentally disabled child, the rhythmic drive of music can aid in mental, emotional, and social maturation. It can help bring a sense of wholeness to scattered individuals and bring about positive interactions (Guzzetta, 2005).

What are the sounds that make us whole? Sounds of nature bring pleasure to the listener. Remember some of your favorite natural sounds. Maybe it was the rustle of fall leaves beneath your feet, the crunch of fresh snow, or rain splashing against the window. In some countries, nature's sounds are built into homes and temples. Bamboo steps in homes in West Java and Thailand produce sounds similar to those made by a bamboo musical instrument named the anklung. Before being installed as steps, the bamboo is carefully tuned (Papanek, 1995). Wind chimes are used in the garden to add music outside and to extend the defensive sound zone beyond the confines of the home. A trickling waterfall and the rustling sounds created by breezes blowing through trees and other garden greenery help to create an environment of renewal (Beattie, 2003). Fountains and waterfalls are becoming more popular as a part of interior decoration. The soothing and invigorating sounds of running water and birds are incorporated into many relaxation audiotapes.

Upholstered furniture, curtains, and carpet soften sounds. Acoustical consultants have identified approaches to reduce noise in the workplace, including substituting quieter processes or equipment, separating employees from noisy equipment, altering the direction of the noise, and absorbing the noise with specially designed noise dampeners (Mayo Clinic, 2005). Noise from building construction (e.g., jackhammers, riveting) can be baffled by hanging steel-mesh blankets.

Ear protection should be worn to prevent hearing loss. An informal test of noise level can be done. If you have to shout above noise to be heard an arm's length away from another person, the noise level is approximately 90 dBA, a level that can cause permanent hearing loss. Protective equipment is needed. Earplugs or over-the-ear muffs offer protection. Attention should be paid to the noise-reduction rating of these protective devices. Using both plugs and muffs simultaneously may be needed in extremely noisy environments.

Hearing screenings can be highly important in identifying individuals with hearing loss at any age. Most hospitals test the hearing of newborns, and schools have ongoing hearing testing for children. Adults, however, may not have their hearing disorder identified until it is well advanced. Only 13 percent of physicians include a hearing screen as part of a routine physical exam (Kochkin, 2005b). Health care providers need to include this screening as part of a comprehensive assessment.

Light and Health

The human response to light lies on a continuum. One individual may be more sensitive to a particular level and length of exposure to light than another person. Disturbances caused by lighting level may occur because of inadequate exposure, overexposure, or adequate amounts at the wrong time of day (e.g., jet lag). Exposure or lack of exposure to both natural sunlight and artificial light have an effect on our health.

As winter days get shorter and darker, humans tend to feel apathetic and depressed. Decreased daylight in the middle of winter can cause seasonal affective disorder, or **SAD syndrome,** believed to be related to increased melatonin levels. Symptoms associated with SAD syndrome include fatigue, increased craving for carbohydrates in the diet, weight gain, lethargy, and severe clinical depression. Physiological problems such as infertility, alterations in menstrual cycles, and premenstrual syndrome may also occur. Suicides occur most frequently during the late winter months. People with depression feel worse, and alcohol-related problems increase. Interestingly, those born in areas of prolonged darkness do not suffer from SAD to the extent of those transplanted from other parts of the country (Miller, 2005).

High levels of light from sunlight or prolonged exposure to fluorescent lighting may cause eyestrain, headaches, increased stress, and hyperactivity. Retinal damage may occur from fluorescent lighting in neonatal intensive care units. Biochemical and physiological changes in the retina may lead to later problems with visual acuity and color vision for those infants.

Adequate lighting in nurseries plays a significant role in early detection of skin color changes indicative of complications such as jaundice or lack of oxygen. Signs of seizures might be overlooked in lowered lighting.

Health Promotion and Nursing Interventions Related to Light

It is advisable to provide as much natural lighting in a space as possible. Flooding rooms with daylight and the longer and brighter days of spring and summer increase serotonin production, resulting in more positive attitudes and higher energy levels. SAD sufferers sit in bright-light boxes for about two hours a day. The light in these boxes is 5 to 10 times brighter than a normal room's lighting. Phototherapy (light therapy) has been successful in treating severe cases of SAD (Miller, 2005).

When adding light, a word of caution is necessary. Light from both natural and artificial sources can create a glare. In offices, a computer monitor acts like a mirror. To identify the source of glare or reflections, turn off the screen and use it as a mirror to locate the source. Antiglare screens are recommended. Dust accumulated on computer screens adds to glare (Mayo Clinic, 2006). Screens should be cleaned each day using treated screen wipes. This dust is electromagnetically charged and may cause skin problems if hands are used to clean the screens and then touched to the face.

The interplay of shafts of bright daylight, darkness, and shadows is called "visual acoustics" by some architects. Designers plan lighting to influence mood. Dim lighting (i.e., candlelight, fireplace fire) is romantic and relaxing. Brighter lighting and spotlights focus attention. Adequate lighting is a safety consideration in the home and in the workplace.

Nurses need to bear these suggestions in mind in order to promote health in their personal and work environments. When working with clients through infancy and old age, lighting practices that protect health and promote well-being should be integrated into care.

Space and Health

Generally speaking, an individual's living space is harmonized with his or her lifestyle. Individuals interact with the environment through all their senses. People are significantly influenced by these sensory interactions with the environment. The musculature of the body adjusts as a person experiences the surrounding space, whether it is expansive or cramped. The balancing mechanisms of the inner ear also become involved as one moves through the space, climbing stairs and turning corners. The body's reaction to space is referred to as the body "reading" a building. Architects use knowledge about these kinesthetic responses when planning and designing space in building.

Dwellings reflect social and societal needs. Consider the cultural and environmental influences of homes around the world. Construction reflects materials readily available in the environment: log cabins, grass/reed or mud huts, caves, adobe pueblos, igloos, brick or stone houses. Culture and class determine the home's size. Organization and meaning of spaces and rooms within a home evolve from social patterns of a culture. It is important that interior spaces be in harmony with the environment, ecology, and the people who live and work there.

Culture and building site determine not only the orientation of the house to the land but also the level of security. Security needs are less for primitive tribes who have few possessions and whose goods are freely shared with others in the group. Huts are built close together. There are no doors or locks or fences. As societies grow larger, possessions multiply. The potential for trouble escalates. The need for security increases.

A place must feel safe in order for simultaneous perception to occur. **Simultaneous perception** allows responses from each of our senses to be combined. In this secure setting one may also pay equal attention to everything at once, a characteristic called **utter watchfulness.** No incoming stimuli are eliminated or emphasized. A sudden change in stimuli, such as a loud noise or a sudden movement, diminishes or eliminates utter watchfulness. Incoming stimuli are no longer experienced as equal. That specific sensory stimulus takes precedence over all others. A potential threat has been identified. Utter watchfulness returns as the threat is dismissed or diminished (Hiss, 1990).

The site or setting of a home or workplace influences the sense of well-being. If settings and personal preferences are in synchrony, a sense of ease is experienced. For example, in a rural environment, change is gradual and periodic. Space is open and expansive. The pace is slow and relaxed. The urban environment is characterized by quick and continuous change with multiple and intense stimuli. Space is crowded. The pace is rapid, often frantic. A country dweller may become tense, stressed, and ill at ease in the city. A city dweller may experience similar feelings when placed in the country.

Crowding has been blamed for crime and violence. Crowding is neither good nor bad. An individual's typical negative or positive reactions to a given situation do intensify in crowding. Exposure to high-density situations is usually brief (e.g., heavy traffic, crowded subway or elevator). Generally, crowding is tolerated well.

Close physical proximity to other people almost forces some kind of interaction. Factors influencing the response to close proximity include individual personal characteristics, the relationship between those involved, the formality of the situation, and ethnicity. For example, close proximity is better tolerated with friends than with strangers. Social withdrawal is a coping strategy used to handle unwanted social demands that typically accompany prolonged crowding.

Dealing with others becomes increasingly difficult and stressful when there are insufficient resources and crowding. Competition for resources intensifies and produces negative effects such as increased tension and aggressiveness. High crime rates and poverty often coexist. In contrast, crime rates may be low in highly populated parts of the world if food, transportation, housing, energy, and other resources are adequate.

Architects work with design elements to reduce the sense of environmental crowding. Rooms with more light are perceived as less crowded than rooms with less natural light. Spaces that are subdivided decrease the perception of crowding and improve socialization and decrease social withdrawal. The layout of a home's floor plan influences interaction patterns within the home.

At the work site, the overall office design (e.g., how enclosed, how noisy) has an effect on job performance, job satisfaction, interoffice communication, and satisfaction with the surroundings. Personal health, safety, and productivity depend on how furniture and workstations are laid out. Reportedly, people generate most of their ideas from face-to-face contact but are reluctant to move from their work area to exchange thoughts/ideas with other.

Clutter has a potential physiological and psychological effect on health and safety. Clutter and disorganization in a room encourage frenetic and chaotic lives (Moran, 2002). Clutter junks up the environment, harboring dust and other unmentionables that degrade our environment. A disorganized desk may indicate a disorganized life. Cluttered spaces suggest confused or nonspecific goals, inefficient work methods, and an inability to complete projects.

Clutter interferes with the most important resource we have, which is time. Shuffling through clutter makes every job harder and takes more time. De-junking is a cheap, fast, and effective way to improve the quality of your life by altering your environment. Ability to focus improves. Productivity increases. Time management improves.

Health Promotion and Nursing Interventions Related to Space

Changing the usual indoor or outdoor environment may have restorative benefits. When one moves from the high-tech, high-stress level of a crowded work setting and takes a short walk in a nearby park, the internal gears shift. The body responds by relaxing and a sense of balance is restored. A mix of short- and long-term restorative experiences maintains inner balance. The following sections describe how manipulating the senses through color and smell and developing a sense of safety within our environmental space have health-promoting effects. The Asian philosophy of feng shui is also introduced as an integrative approach for a healthy environment.

Color and Health

People respond to colors. Color expresses personality. The same color may have a different influence on different people. If an individual sees a color and likes it, the whole body system relaxes. Outlook becomes more optimistic. Therefore, a color that brings about a favorable response should be incorporated into that individual's surroundings. Since biological and psychological changes can be attributed to color, it is important to be attentive to individual color preferences and their effects.

The goal is to achieve balance while avoiding monotony of color and overstimulation by color. Visualize a color. Place it along a continuum ranging from the lightest to the darkest shade. Limit use of the color on either extreme of the continuum or combine the extremes to achieve balance. Staying in the color midrange on the continuum also provides balance. Colors that are too bright or too dramatic can be distracting and can cause discomfort. Adjustments can be made by increasing or reducing the intensity, the amount, or the purity of a color. Adding white to a color reduces its brightness and changes its tint to a pastel that is soothing.

Variety is achieved by using contrasts between bright colors that stimulate and dark colors that relax. Variety is also achieved by using warm colors that excite and cool colors that soothe. For example, the blue (cool) end of the spectrum decreases arousal. Blue, violet, and green are cool, passive, and calming. Colors on the red end of the spectrum (warm) cause increased arousal. Red and its analogous hues are warm, active, and exciting. Contrary to the theory of warm colors being stimulating, certain pink hues have a tranquilizing effect. Bubble gum pink, called passive pink, creates an almost immediate reduction in aggressive behavior, making it particularly useful with agitated clients or prisoners (Schweitzer, Gilpin, & Frampton, 2004). Short-term exposure to a color does not necessarily have an effect.

Colors must be pleasing to be psychologically or physically therapeutic. Use of color can improve the way the body functions, deals with crises, and interacts with the environment. **Chromotherapy,** or photobiology, is the use of color to treat disease. Acceptance of chromotherapy as a means of healing and of maintaining a high level of wellness is growing.

In manipulating the environment through color, one must consider who will be affected and for how long, where it will be used, and why it is being used. For example, color in educational environments can affect children's performance. It was found that children with attention deficit hyperactivity disorder (ADHD) had better handwriting when writing on colored paper—an effect not found in children without ADHD (Imhof, 2004).

In a hospital lobby, visitors will be affected. Surroundings should be pleasant and cheerful. A variety of both warm and cool colors would be appropriate. In a maternity unit, where the client is not seriously ill, peach or rose would provide a comfortable environment. The cool tones of blues, greens, and grays would create a restful environment for chronically ill clients. Relaxation of the surgical client could be accomplished with the use of greens and blue-greens. Certain colors should be avoided in health care institutions such as those that cast unfavorable reflections on the human complexion—yellow-greens, yellow, and lavender.

When at home, people rest, relax, rejuvenate, and create. While on the job, the focus is on work. People produce, serve, and solve job-related problems, resting little if at all. Energy is therefore consumed more at work than at home. Using favorite colors can enhance a work environment. Maximum benefit from personal favorite colors is achieved if they are placed within three feet of a working space: on a table, a desk, or a chair; in a piece of art; as an accent color. Colors can act as strong energizers, improving mood and increasing productivity. The use of color for holistic health is further discussed in Chapter 20.

Scent and Health

People see only when there is enough light, touch only when contact is made with someone or something, and hear only sounds that are loud enough. But with every breath, the sense of smell is active. Smell is the mute sense, one without words. Smells are usually described in terms of other things such as smoke, fruit, flowers, and citrus or by the feelings they inspire as in disgusted, delighted, sickened, hypnotized, or intoxicated.

The sense of smell brings pleasure and it is also a protective device. Odors can elicit reactions of fear or a flight response (e.g., gas, ammonia, insecticides), alerting us to danger in our environment. The smells of spoiled food, smoke, and gas spell danger for those with a sense of smell. This protective device is missing for those with anosmia, placing them at risk. **Anosmia** means absence of the sense of smell.

Aromas form a direct link to emotions and memories. With the tripwire of smell, memories explode and complex visions are elicited by certain odors. When a scent enters the body, a message is sent to the cerebral cortex and into the limbic system, the emotional portion of the brain. The fragrance of roses may trigger the memory of a romantic moment or a special garden. What about the smell of fresh-baked cookies or bread? Evergreens, bayberry, and cinnamon? These aromas may elicit a relaxation response as they bring back memories of very special times. The smell of wood smoke may serve as a reminder of a fun-filled experience around a campfire or a devastating home fire.

The goals of aromatherapy include relaxation and healing. A therapeutically scented environment uses aromas that are associated with good past experiences. There is inconclusive evidence to support the use of aromatherapy in nursing practice other than for relaxation (Maddocks-Jennings & Wilkinson, 2004). Nurses who intend to incorporate aromatherapy in their plan of care should complete formal education in aromatherapy to obtain basic knowledge of the chemical and physical properties of essential oils as well as their safe application and evaluation of effects.

Workplace Safety and Health

A person's workplace is like a second home. Many employees spend 8–12 hours at work each day. The air, sound, space, and light in the work environment are therefore vital to employee job satisfaction, productivity, and safety. Smoke, noise, vibrations, crowded quarters, poor ventilation, and improper lighting can create undue stress. Temperature and humidity can cause physical uneasiness. Posture, reaching, and lifting all affect how the employee works.

Employers are required by law to provide training about potential exposure to hazardous materials. Prevention and control of exposures ensure a safe and healthy workplace. Controls fall into four major categories:

1. Substitution controls replace a hazardous substance or work process with a less hazardous one (e.g., substituting steam for gas sterilization or water-based paint for oil-based paint).

2. Engineering controls literally reengineer the work process or equipment to reduce the possibility of exposure or injury (e.g., installing an exhaust system to remove fumes or acoustic tiles to reduce noise levels).

3. Administrative controls reduce exposure through education, implementing safe work practices, and rotating jobs.

4. Equipment control provides personal protective equipment (e.g., goggles, gloves, or safety shoes) (OSHA, n.d.).

A combination of controls may be needed to control exposure and improve safety. For example, while using solvents to clean silkscreen, a woman became light-headed and noticed a rash on her hands. Installation of an exhaust fan to remove fumes (engineering control) and use of gloves and a respirator (equipment control) would reduce her exposure to the pollutants.

Ergonomics is the science of relationships of furniture and tools to the human body. Poor ergonomics can be connected to nonspecific aches, pains, and stresses. More specifically, ergonomic problems contribute to the following:

• lowered production and reduced quality of work

• increased lost time/absenteeism/turnover

• increased medical costs due to injuries and strains

• increased probability of errors and accidents

• increased workers' compensation costs

The two major goals of improving ergonomics are to provide a more effective workplace and to improve work conditions. Meeting these goals satisfies the needs of both employees and employers. Benefits of an ergonomics program include: greater comfort and higher morale, improved quality of work with fewer errors, greater efficiency, improved productivity with fewer errors, lower turnover, greater safety with fewer injuries, and reduced absenteeism.

An ergonomic specialist or team conducts a worksite analysis, recognizing, identifying, and prioritizing ergonomic hazards. More and more nurses are becoming ergonomic specialists. Information is gathered through observation, anthropometric data (human body measurements), an ergonomic checklist, videotapes, and analysis of tasks performed. The ergonomic checklist covers issues that relate to the use of hands, use of force, upper and lower body stress, work area, tool design, the pace of activity, and the number of repetitions. Findings are analyzed. Actions to reduce the number of repetitions, reduce the force required, and eliminate awkward positions are prioritized. A plan is developed and approved by management. Immediate actions usually include education and quick fixes. Many solutions are no cost or low cost (e.g., height adjustments, supports, training) and are highly visible to employees. Larger and more expensive design issues follow. Once the plan is in effect, a worksite team monitors progress, identifying continuing and new problems, taking necessary corrective action, and consulting with the ergonomic specialist as needed.

An ergonomic audit may take two to four weeks, depending on the complexity and the work area's size. Cost depends on the complexity of the area. Often the cost of doing nothing exceeds the cost of an extensive audit. An ergonomic audit often has a positive impact on employee morale simply because it proves that the company cares. Management often lacks information about ergonomic issues. Some managers believe that ergonomics assessments are not important because audits do not add value to their product. Therefore, there is a lack of interest and funding for ergonomic assessments.

Ergonomic interventions are most successful if affected individuals are included in discussions of action, prioritizing different available solutions, and making small improvements. People are motivated to make changes when presented with examples of similar situations in which improvements were successful.

Overall workplace injuries have decreased. However, the incidence of repetitive strain injury (RSI), or cumulative trauma, continues to rise. RSI is an umbrella term for several cumulative trauma disorders caused by low-intensity forces applied over a long period. Repetitive motions irritate specific anatomical structures. Tendons, tendon sheaths, muscles, ligaments, joints, and nerves are commonly affected. Microscopic damage, called microtrauma, occurs. Normally, healing of microtrauma occurs overnight. However, the healing process cannot keep pace with continued injury. Over time, tissues become inflamed and damaged, causing pain and limiting function. Carpal tunnel syndrome is an RSI resulting from overuse of the hands and arms, common among computer users. Tissues in the hand, arm, neck, and shoulders are involved.

Fatigue and sustained awkward posture may be as damaging as repetitive motion. Improper posture while working can bring the head position forward, increasing pressure on the muscles and nerves of the neck. Shoulders become stressed and fatigued, resulting in a nagging discomfort. Prolonged inappropriate posture can result in permanent physiological changes. Preventive and corrective measures reduce the risk of RSI. Work-site health can be improved using the ergonomic approaches summarized in Box 7-8.

Feng Shui

There are differences in Eastern and Western philosophies about human coexistence with the environment.

BOX 7-8 Tips to Prevent Back, Neck, and Joint Injuries

Lifting

1. Objects
   - Test weight first. Get help if needed.
   - Move close to object. Don't extend arms.
   - Form solid support by spreading feet apart to width of shoulders, bend your knees, and lift the object with the strength of your legs, not your back.
   - Never lift higher than your chest.
   - Break up heavy loads into smaller loads, use small steps, move slowly, and take frequent breaks from lifting.
2. Clients from bed
   - Raise bed to your level.
   - Ask for help if needed.
   - Safeguard transfers with use of a trapeze, sliding board, lateral assist device, transfer chair, or powered lift.

Ergonomics

1. Sitting
   - Get a quality desk chair with height adjuster.
   - Knees should be level with hips. Feet flat on floor.
   - Sit up straight. Use chair back for support (extra support with pillows if needed).
   - Hold in stomach muscles.
   - Balance head over shoulders, and avoid leaning forward.

2. Standing
   - Place one foot slightly in front of the other.
   - Wear low-heeled shoes with good arch supports.
3. Using computers
   - Place keyboard and mouse close to you.
   - Adjust top of computer screen to eye level.
   - Type with elbows at your side and forearms parallel to the floor.
   - Use armrests.
   - Relax shoulders and hands.
   - Vary work tasks.
   - Use wrist rest at base of keyboard.
   - Look away from screen every 10 minutes to avoid eyestrain.

Preventive Measures

- Stretch before you start. Keep muscles limber and warm.
- Exercise regularly and actively to keep fit, flexible, and strong.
- Wear properly fitting shoes allowing for "toe wiggle."
- Invest in a high-quality mattress (firm with numerous coils and thick padding), replace it every 10 years, and rotate it 180 degrees at least four times a year to prolong its life.

Adapted from No strain? No pain! by E. Santulli, 2004, Hospital Nursing, *34:(3).7–8; Public employers' ergonomics: Best practices, by C. A. Hamrick, 2004, April,* Journal of Occupational and Environmental Hygiene, *1(4), 42–46.*

To generalize, the Eastern philosophy believes nothing happens without consequence to something else. Western countries, by contrast, approach life and the environment with a philosophy of "I came, I saw, I conquered." The fundamental premise of feng shui is that *where* we are is as important as *who* we are. **Feng shui** (pronounced "fung shway") is an ancient Chinese practice of configuring one's environment to promote a healthy flow of chi, or vital energy, for health, happiness, and prosperity (Elioupoulis, 2004).

Feng shui is being used as an antidote to modern life, providing peace and serenity in a complex time of change, confusion, and stress. The Chinese believe that manipulating the environment can change fate. Feng shui teaches that a keen awareness of space can greatly improve circumstances.

Feng shui is a cross between art and science. Its roots are in ecology, aesthetics, philosophy, astrology, and interior design. It involves the use of geometric lines, colors, numbers, animal symbols, and the elements of fire, earth, metal, water, and wood to align furnishings, buildings, and the landscape (Santo Pietro, 2002). Though it transcends the confines of rational thought and the realm of logic, feng shui is firmly grounded in common sense and scientific observations.

In China, Indonesia, and other parts of Southeast Asia, feng shui is used in selecting building sites and in placement of buildings and furnishings. Building sites are selected to harmonize with the energies of the land. This is believed to attract good luck, health, and fortune. The totality of the location of the building, arrangement of its furniture and accessories, and the use of color within each room provides an environment that can be balanced, energizing, and positive or one that is unbal-anced, enervating, and negative. When inhabitants, buildings, and furnishings are in harmony with nature, good feng shui exists; serenity is evident.

The benefits of feng shui are being recognized in the West. Feng shui specialists were brought in to reorient parts of the Denver airport that had experienced many malfunctions during construction that had cost millions of dollars.

Many homeowners and business people alike would not consider beginning construction without consulting a geomancer, an expert who uses lines, figures, and geographic features in design. Working with the principles of feng shui, the geomancer assesses the geology and topography of a building's location. Land should not include harmful mineral deposits and should support vegetation but not be overgrown. There should not be stagnant water. The outdoor environment and view from the structure are also considered. An environment with a view of nature supports health if the scene contains healthy vegetation.

The traditional concepts of Asian life (Tao, chi, yin and yang) are incorporated into feng shui. **Tao** means to be connected. Each part of life is dependent on another to create a whole. Plants, pictures, and colors similar to outdoors provide a sense of connectedness with nature when used indoors. A connectedness should permeate the home as one moves from room to room.

Chi is invisible energy, or vitality. All living things are interrelated by cosmic chi that circulates through the earth and sky. In feng shui, efforts are made to encourage the flow of chi, echoing the gentle curves of nature in the environment. Poison arrows of straight lines and sharp edges or angles cause chi to move too swiftly or to be easily blocked. Straight lines can be broken by curves created by adding plants. Too much chi results in chaos. Too little chi results in lifelessness. **Sha** is bad chi and is believed to bring bad luck and poor health as well as family and business difficulties. Architectural elements and accessories in the home/office can be used to enhance or inhibit chi. Table 7-7 lists enhancers and inhibitors of chi which affect environmental balance.

Yin and yang represent opposites and the goal is to bring them into balance. Without balance there is danger of poor physical and mental health. An individual with a yin personality is quiet, reflective, introspective, and down to earth. An individual with a yang personality is outgoing and talkative, an extrovert, and always on the go. Each needs the other to maintain balance in their lives. The environment also contains the elements of yin and yang. Enhancers of yin and yang as related to elements in our environment are listed Table 7-8.

The exterior and the interior of a home work together. The exterior is like the shell of a crab, protecting the soft interior. The appearance of the exterior is a reflection of the interior, an indicator of the health and success of its inhabitants. Feng shui interventions include the following:

TABLE 7-7 The Environment and Chi

	Chi Enhancers	Chi Inhibitors
Architecture:	Curving pathways, open windows	Straight walls, closed doors
Space:	Uncluttered, open space	Clutter
Light:	Brightness and light	Darkness
Temperature:	Comfortable	Extremes
Shape:	Curves, undulating lines, rounded	Sharp angles,
Movement:	Swaying plants, wind chimes, prisms, fans	Stillness

Adapted from The Feng Shui Bible: The Definitive Guide to Improving Your Life, Home, Health, and Finances, *by S. Brown, 2005, New York: Sterling; and* Chic Living with Feng Shui: Stylish Designs for Harmonious Living, *by S. Stasney, 2004, New York: Sterling.*

TABLE 7-8 The Environment and Yin/Yang

	Yin Enhancers	Yang Enhancers
Light:	Muted light: less wattage, candles, closed drapes	Brighter lights, open drapes
Sound:	Create silence	Add music, ticking clocks, etc.
Color:	Muted, dark colors; monochromatic themes; cool, subdued, muted patterns	Bright, primary, contrasting colors; vibrant patterns
Humidity:	Increase: fountains	Decrease: dehumidifier
Fabrics:	Soft, silky, velvety	Solid colors, vertical stripes, shiny
Air movement:	Decrease	Increase: fans, wind chimes
Furnishings:	Low, heavy, solid furniture and accessories	Tall, thin, clear, light, firm, delicate, or irregular shapes
Space:	Increase flow of chi: remove clutter, open space	Decrease flow of chi: fill space with form (plants, friends)
Social:	Solitude	Company

From The Healing Home: Practical Ways to Harmonize Your Home and Energize Your Spirit, *by S. Ash, 2003, New York: Sterling;* The Feng Shui Bible: The Definitive Guide to Improving Your Life, Home, Health, and Finances, *by S. Brown, 2005, New York: Sterling; "Feng Shui Tips for Your Workspace," by H. G. Chissell, 2004, Lilipoh, 9(38), 17.*

1. Repositioning the furniture to change how living space is experienced.

2. Working with light (e.g., focusing attention on objects or people; varying amount; framing important areas; adding natural or artificial light).

3. Using color to alter the mood of persons entering a space.

4. Adding different colors, shapes, and textures of plants to unite people with outdoors and instill a sense of being connected.

5. Incorporating and maintaining a balance of movement (e.g., adding objects that initiate action, such as fans, chimes, cuckoo clocks).

6. Attending to placement of reflective surfaces (mirrors, metal) and heavy objects (tables, sofas, sculptures).

7. Incorporating sounds, both artificial (music) and natural (rustle of vegetation, water, rain, wind, critters).

8. Adding water, believed to be central to our existence.

9. Maintaining an uncluttered environment in the belief that cleaning up areas in your home can be a first step toward cleaning up parts of your life.

(Chissell, 2004; Schweitzer, Gilpin, & Frampton, 2004; San Pietro, 2002).

ENVIRONMENTAL DISASTERS

Environmental disasters can result from either natural, technological, or terrorist sources. In any event, environmental disasters unleash devastating forces. They are never expected. No community is immune to actual or potential threat to its health. In a world filled with technological advances, systems will fail and exposure to toxic materials will happen. Box 7-9 identifies major causes of disasters facing the world today.

Causes, occurrences of, and results from natural, technological, and terror-related disasters vary, but the effects of any disaster can cause acute stress followed by extended periods of uncertainty. Physical and psychological health of those involved can be altered for many years and sometimes for life. The following sections discuss major natural, technological, and terror-related disasters and associated health promotion aspects.

Natural Disasters

Individuals, communities, and health care systems are all affected by natural disasters. People living in areas prone to natural disasters may be lulled into a sense of complacency, suppressing the fact that these events often occur without warning. It is beyond the scope of this chapter to discuss all natural disaster causes. Those most recently experienced by the world, and those considered the most devastating, are discussed here.

Earthquakes

An earthquake is a sudden and rapid shaking of the earth caused by shifting of rock plates beneath the earth's surface. Fault lines are areas where plates meet and have the potential to break free and cause an earthquake, although earthquakes can occur in the middle of a plate as well. On average, there are about 70–75 earthquakes in the world each year. Injury and death from an

---

BOX 7-9   Causes of Disasters

- Broken or breached dams
- Earthquakes
- Extreme heat
- Fires
- Floods
- Hazardous materials
- Hurricanes
- Landslides

- Multihazard accidents
- Nuclear accidents
- Terrorism
- Thunderstorms
- Tornadoes
- Tsunamis
- Volcanoes
- Wildfires
- Winter storms

---

earthquake come not from the actual ground movement but from collapsing buildings, flying debris and glass, and panic by the people involved.

One of the world's worst natural disasters was the result of an earthquake. On December 26, 2004, an earthquake far out in the Indian Ocean produced a devastating tsunami that caused an estimated 223,000 deaths in India, Indonesia, Malaysia, Thailand, and other smaller countries (Wilder-Smith & Steffen, 2005; VanRooyen & Leaning, 2005). Tsunamis are ocean waves produced by earthquakes and by volcanic eruptions. Tsunamis are often incorrectly referred to as "tidal waves." Not all earthquakes produce tsunamis, but when they do, the waves may sweep ashore causing damage locally and at places thousands of miles from the earthquake epicenter.

In the United States, California experiences the most frequent damaging earthquakes and Alaska experiences the greatest number of large earthquakes—mostly in uninhabited areas. For populated earthquake-prone areas earthquake preparedness has become a way of life. In the event of a major earthquake, freeways and surface streets may be impassable and public services could be interrupted or taxed beyond their limits. Therefore, everyone must know how to provide for her or his own needs for an extended period of time, whether at work, at home, or on the road. Knowing how to prepare yourself for an earthquake in various areas is important to avoid serious injury. The following tips will help you be better prepared should an earthquake strike.

- **High-rise building**—Move against an interior wall and protect your head with your arms. Do not use the elevators. Do not be surprised if the alarm or sprinkler systems come on. Stay indoors to avoid falling debris and broken glass.

- **Outdoors**—Move to a clear area away from trees, signs, buildings, electrical wires, and poles.

- **Sidewalk near buildings**—Duck into a doorway to protect yourself from falling bricks, glass, plaster, and other debris.

- **Driving**—Pull over to the side of the road and stop. Avoid overpasses, power lines, and other hazards. Stay inside the vehicle until the shaking is over.
- **Crowded public place**—Do not rush for exits. Move away from display shelves containing objects that could fall.
- **Wheelchair**—Stay in it and move to a place of cover. If possible, lock your wheels, and protect your head with your arms.
- **Kitchen**—Move away from the refrigerator, stove, and overhead cupboards. (Appliances should have been prepared with anchors, and security latches should have been placed on cupboard doors.)
- **Stadium or theater**—Stay in your seat and protect your head with your arms. Do not try to leave until the shaking is over, and then leave calmly and in an orderly manner without rushing. (NEHRP, 2004; LAFD, 1997)

After an earthquake has passed, be prepared for aftershocks and plan to continue the tips just listed. Check for injuries, avoid broken glass, and watch for fires, gas leaks, and live electric wires. Communication is vital, and having access to a radio or television for emergency broadcasts is essential. Above all, remain calm and reassure others.

Hurricanes

Floyd, Ivan, Jeanne, Katrina, and Rita are all innocent-sounding names, but people who were in the paths of these devastating hurricanes can attest to their fury. According to FEMA (2005), a hurricane is a tropical storm with winds that have reached a constant speed of 74 miles per hour or more. Hurricane winds blow in a large spiral around a relatively calm center known as the "eye." The eye is generally 20 to 30 miles wide, and the storm may extend outward 400 miles. As a hurricane approaches, the skies will begin to darken and winds will grow in strength. As a hurricane nears land, it can bring torrential rains, high winds, and storm surges. A single hurricane can last for more than two weeks over open waters and can run a path across the entire length of the eastern seaboard. August and September are peak months during the hurricane season, which lasts from June 1 through November 30.

Advanced meteorological science has enabled the prediction and tracking of hurricanes for days and often weeks in advance. A hurricane "watch" is issued when there is a threat of hurricane conditions within 24 to 36 hours, and a "warning" is issued when there are winds of 74 miles per hour or greater or when dangerously high water and rough seas are expected in 24 hours or less. This system usually allows for adequate preparation and evacuation as needed. Even so, as seen with Hurricane Katrina, which made landfall on August 29, 2005, on the Gulf Coast of the United States, there can be cat-astrophic loss of life, injuries, exposure to toxins, widespread property damage, disease, and despair ("Norovirus Outbreak," 2005; "Surveillance for Illness," 2005). The cultural, psychological, social, economic, and political effects of the displacement of people from New Orleans to areas throughout the United States are still being felt.

Tornadoes

A tornado is a violently rotating column of air extending from a thunderstorm to the ground. It is estimated that over 800 tornadoes occur each year in the United States (National Weather Service, 2002). Box 7-10 provides additional facts about tornadoes, and Box 7-11 highlights important tornado terms.

Despite advanced warning, many people are killed or seriously injured by tornadoes. Those most at risk during a tornado include people in vehicles, the elderly, infants and children, people with disabilities, and mobile home dwellers. Language barriers also put people at risk if they do not understand warnings in a language unfamiliar to them.

Technological Disasters

With technological disasters, the threat of potential exposure precedes the threat created by actual exposure. Long-term uncertainty, chronic stress, and mental health problems are more likely to occur as a result of the psychophysiological processes associated with these disasters. Psychological processes may add to or exacerbate physiological effects on the body.

The Three Mile Island nuclear accident that occurred in 1979 in Pennsylvania provides a good example of the types of stressors involved with technological disasters.

BOX 7-10 Tornado Facts

- In the United States, tornadoes occur most frequently east of the Rocky Mountains during the spring and summer months.
- On average, 800 tornadoes are reported nationwide, resulting in 80 deaths and over 1,500 injuries.
- The most violent tornadoes are capable of tremendous destruction with wind speeds of 250 mph or more.
- Damage paths can be larger than one mile wide and 50 miles long.

Adapted from "Tornadoes . . . Nature's Most Violent Storms," National Weather Service, 2002, http://www.nssl.noaa.gov/NWSTornado/.

Radiation was actually released into the atmosphere. Additionally, radioactive wastewater and radioactive krypton gas were trapped in the containment building surrounding the reactor. People were concerned about current exposure and the threat of future exposure from the continuing sources of radiation in the plant. Fears escalated with continued leaks of the gas. Confusing and contradictory media reports destroyed credibility of key information sources.

A 20-year follow-up of residents near the Three Mile Island nuclear accident site concluded that there was no consistent evidence connecting the radioactivity released and deaths occurring during that time span (Talbott, Youk, McHugh-Pemu, & Zborowski, 2003). The psychological effects of technological disaster, however, regardless of cause, cannot be refuted.

Terror-Related Disasters

In recent years, the world has experienced terror-related disasters unparalleled in history. It has been reported that there were 12,216 individual terrorist bombings in the United States in the 10 years between 1980 and 1990, with each year becoming more destructive (Dickerson, Jezewski, Nelson-Tuttle, Shipkey, Wilk, & Crandall, 2002). On April 19,1995, the Alfred P. Murrah Federal Building, a U.S. government office complex in downtown Oklahoma City, Oklahoma, was destroyed, killing 168 people. This event was considered the largest domestic terrorist attack in the history of the United States and the largest terrorist attack of any kind in the nation's history until September 11, 2001.

On September 11, 2001, terrorists attacked the United States by flying two hijacked planes into the Twin Towers of the World Trade Center in New York City, result-

ing in 2,752 deaths, while a third plane flown into the Pentagon killed 189 people and another 44 were killed when a fourth hijacked jet crashed into a field in Pennsylvania. On July 7, 2005, a series of coordinated suicide bombings struck London's public transport system during the morning rush hour. The bombings killed 52 civilians and injured over 700 people. Box 7-12 provides a summary of these and other major terrorist events occurring within the last two decades.

According to the U.S. Federal Bureau of Investigation (FBI), **terrorism** is the "unlawful use of force and violence against persons or property to intimidate or coerce a government, the civilian population, or any segment thereof, in furtherance of political or social objectives" (Code of Federal Regulations Title 28). Although thousands of people have lost their lives in terrorist attacks, the goal of terrorism is to destroy the sense of well-being and trust in government (Hyams, Murphy, & Wessely, 2002). Terrorist-related disasters can result from the use of biological, chemical, or radiological (nuclear) weapons from national or international sources (Lee & Estes, 2003). These weapons, intended to cause death or serious bodily harm to a significant number of people, were deemed to be **weapons of mass destruction (WMDs)** by the U.S. Congress in 1996 (Mothershead, 2004). The U.S. Department of Homeland Security has recently used the term **weapons of mass effect (WMEs)** that more clearly denotes the motives of terrorists to cause widespread chaos and despair by whatever method used (Mothershead, 2004).

A detailed discussion of WMEs is beyond the scope of this chapter. *Terrorism and Disaster Management: Preparing Healthcare Leaders for the New Reality,* edited by K. Joanne McGlown, is an excellent resource for further study. It is important to realize, however, that there are things you can do to prepare for the unexpected. As was learned from the events of September 11, the following can happen after a terrorist attack:

- There can be significant numbers of casualties, damage to buildings and the infrastructure, or both. Employers need up-to-date information about any medical needs you may have and about how to contact your family or significant others.

- Heavy law enforcement involvement at local, state, and federal levels follows a terrorist attack due to the event's criminal nature.

- Health and mental health resources in the affected communities can be strained to their limits, perhaps even overwhelmed.

- Extensive media coverage, strong public fear, and international implications and consequences can continue for a prolonged period.

- Workplaces and schools may be closed, and there may be restrictions on domestic and international travel.

BOX 7-12 Summary of Major Terrorist Events Around the World

London, July 2005
A series of bombs were detonated on the capital's transit system, killing 52 and injuring 700.

Bali, Indonesia, October 2002
Two bombs ripped through a crowded nightclub, killing 200.

New York, Washington D.C., and Pennsylvania, September 11, 2001
Hijacked planes crashed into the World Trade Center, the Pentagon, and a field in Pennsylvania, killing a total of 2,985.

Yemen, October 2000
A bomb blast tore through the destroyer USS *Cole* in the Yemeni port of Aden, killing 17 sailors.

Kenya and Tanzania, August 1998
U.S. embassies in Kenya and Tanzania were bombed, killing 263 and injuring 5,000.

Lebanon, June 1998
Rocket-propelled grenades exploded near the U.S. embassy in Beirut without injuries.

Saudi Arabia, June 1996
A truck bomb killed 19 U.S. troops living at a base near Dhahran.

Oklahoma City, April 1995
A car bomb destroyed the Alfred P. Murrah Federal Building in downtown Oklahoma City, killing 168 people.

Japan, March 1995
Sarin, a deadly gas, was dispersed into the subways, killing 5 and injuring 275.

Scotland, December 1988
A terrorist bomb destroyed a Pan Am 747 over Lockerbie, killing 259 on board and 11 on the ground.

Greece, April 1986
Four people were killed in an explosion aboard a TWA passenger jet approaching Athens.

Germany, April 1986
A blast in a West Berlin disco killed 2 and injured 150.

Rome and Vienna, December 1985
Airport attacks at U.S. and Israeli airport check-in desks killed 16.

Mediterranean Sea, October 1985
Terrorists aboard the *Achille Lauro* cruise ship killed an American and tossed his body overboard.

Germany, August 1985
A car bomb at an American military base in Frankfurt killed 2 and injured 20.

El Salvador, June 1985
A machine gun attack at a cafe killed 13, including 6 Americans.

Spain, April 1985
An explosion at a restaurant near an American air base in Madrid killed 18 Spaniards.

Lebanon, October 1983
A car bomb killed 241 U.S. troops at the Beirut airport.

Lebanon, April 1983
A bombing at the U.S. embassy in Beirut killed 63.

- You and your family or household may have to evacuate an area, avoiding roads blocked for your safety.

- Recovery may take many months.

Successes of recent terrorist attacks have generated greater preparedness by government agencies. States have more responsibility and flexibility than ever before in providing public health protection. The Model State Emergency Health Powers Act reflects five basic public health functions to ensure the health of the people:

1. Preparedness/comprehensive planning for public health emergencies

2. Surveillance to detect and track public health emergencies

3. Management of property to ensure adequate availability of vaccines, pharmaceuticals, and hospitals, and to reduce public health hazards

4. Protection of persons, including mandatory vaccinations, testing, treatment, isolation, and quarantine when necessary

5. Communication to provide for clear and authoritative public information (Lee & Estes, 2003, p. 285).

Nurses are vital to the response effort and management of any disaster. After the September 11 attacks, state boards of nursing required that nurses complete continuing education on bioterrorism. Box 7-13 describes the nurse's role in bioterrorism preparedness. Sources for completing continuing education on bioterrorism are listed at the end of this chapter. Regardless of cause, all disasters involve risk assessment, preparedness, responsiveness, and recovery—the key principles in disaster planning and management.

Posttraumatic Stress Disorder

Victims of trauma are at risk for development of **posttraumatic stress disorder (PTSD).** PTSD is a constellation of continuing, long-term detrimental effects, including flashbacks, nightmares, insomnia, and concentration difficulties, resulting from exposure to trauma. The traumatic event may be a natural disaster (e.g., tornado, hurricane, flood, fire, earthquake, volcanic eruption), a technological or manmade disaster (massive toxic contamination from chemicals or radiation), a dramatic change in a work environment (restructuring, downsizing, reengineering), physical assault, or many other causes. It is estimated that one-third of the victims surviving the World Trade Center terrorist attack suffer from PTSD (Hyams, Murphy, & Wessely, 2002).

Responses to trauma, including specific symptoms of PTSD, are listed in Table 7-9.

Individuals experiencing PTSD may experience increased health problems, a decline in work/school performance, and a deterioration of family life. Symptoms of PTSD tend to decrease over the first several years. Interestingly, PTSD from natural disasters tends to disappear within two years of the event. However, effects of technological disasters seem to be more prolonged, lasting years (Hyams, Murphy & Wessely, 2002).

Much of the research of PTSD centers on combat veterans. Findings of these research studies correlate with those of victims of natural or technological disasters. The severity of the traumatizing event affects the development, extent, and duration of PTSD. Number of lives lost, amount of property damage, and effect on normal routines (e.g., school and work attendance) enter into the equation.

Effects of a disaster may last for years. Symptoms may develop months, even years later, after a period of no apparent symptoms. Many clients go undiscovered. A link is not made between the event and the current symptoms. Health care professionals are also at risk because of the nature of their work. They may experience vicarious traumatization even though they may not have been directly involved with the incident (Litz & Gray, 2002; Hyams, Murphy & Wessely, 2002).

Comorbidity, or coexisting disease, has been examined in stress research, with particular attention to the coexistence of psychiatric disorders and PTSD. The most frequent comorbid disorders are substance abuse, depression, generalized anxiety disorders, panic disorders and

TABLE 7-9 Responses to Trauma

Early symptoms of acute stress:	Fear, shock, anxiety, anger, irritability, insomnia, difficulty making decisions, inability to think creatively, forgetfulness, uncomfortable being alone, hyper-alert, easily startled, jumpiness, flashbacks, feeling loss of control, helplessness, loss of feeling secure in the world, sadness, increased use of alcohol and/or drugs, social withdrawal, physical discomfort, change in appetite, "emotional numbing," exhaustion
Symptoms of PTSD:	
1. Hyperarousal	Heightened startle response, irritability, insomnia, strong emotions rekindled by reminders of the trauma
2. Intrusion	Intrusive recollections, obsessing, flashbacks, nightmares
3. Constriction	Physical withdrawal, social isolation, avoidance of reminders, emotional numbing, depression, substance abuse

Adapted from "Clinical Outcomes of Gulf Veterans' Medical Assessment Programme Referrals to Specialized Centers for Gulf Veterans with Post-traumatic Stress Disorder," by H. A. Lee, R. Gabriel, and A. J. Bale, 2006, Military Medicine, 170(5), 400–405; and "Emotional Numbing in Posttraumatic Stress Disorder: Current and Future Research Directions," by B. T. Litz and M. J. Gray, 2002, Australian and New Zealand Journal of Psychiatry, 36, 198–204.

BOX 7-14   Emotional First Aid

Steps to Minimize the Psychological Effects of a Disaster

1. Provide precise instructions about dealing with an anticipated disaster.
2. Identify sources of accurate information.
3. Minimize exposure to death and injury.
4. Protect family members from unnecessary exposure to body parts, grotesque bodies, or the dead.
5. Initiate public education to normalize early stress responses.
6. Mobilize support systems and cross-linkages among professionals.
7. Participate in developing disaster-specific support systems.

Nurses can promote psychological health by helping the disaster victim to:
- Recognize symptoms of stress.
- Identify resources and activities.
- Recognize psychologically painful situations.
- Accept the reality of the situation.
- Develop an optimistic attitude.
- Avoid placing blame on others.
- Accept help and support.
- Resume activities of daily life.
- Connect with religious beliefs.

Adapted from "Unmet Need for Counseling Services by Children in New York City After the September 11th Attacks on the World Trade Center: Implications for Pediatricians," by G. Fairbrother, 2004, Pediatrics, 113, 1367–1374; "Terrorism, Posttraumatic Stress and Religious Coping," by J. B. Meisenhelder, 2002, Issues in Mental Health Nursing, 23(8): 771–782; and "Understanding Relationships Among Trauma, Post-traumatic Stress Disorder, and Health Outcomes," by P. P. Schnurr and B. L. Green, 2004, Advances in Mind-Body Medicine, 20(1): 18–29.

phobias, somatization disorders characterized by physical suffering, psychotic disorders, and personality disorders. Comorbid disorders may precede or create vulnerability to PTSD and may not be truly separate from PTSD (Schnurr & Green, 2004).

Health Promotion and Nursing Interventions for Environmental Disasters

The important role of health care professionals cannot be overemphasized in caring for those sick and injured as a result of natural technological, or terror-related disasters. Emergency and trauma care typically focuses on physical health. Little or no attention is given to preventing the long-term psychological effects.

Promoting both physical and psychological health for disaster victims is possible. Nurse therapists and clinical nurse specialists may fill key roles, especially in preventing PTSD, in working with people experiencing PTSD, and in educating others about the problem. The simplest approach to intervention should be used. Crisis intervention should be early, brief, and problem focused. Box 7-14 lists actions for "emotional first aid" for victims of trauma.

Certain individuals are at high risk for PTSD following a disaster. Elderly, psychologically disturbed, or mentally retarded persons or people with disabilities are dependent on a psychosocial stability. Turmoil surrounding a disaster places them at high risk. Others in high-risk categories include: traumatized survivors; children, particularly if separated from their parents; close relatives of those who died suddenly or traumatically; those responsible for removing the bodies of those who died;

and those living in communities that were devastated. At-risk groups must be identified as well as risk behaviors, symptoms, or signs that PTSD is developing.

Particular attention should be paid to young victims of traumatic stress such as the thousands of children directly affected by the events of September 11, 2001, and the hundreds of thousands more who were affected indirectly by the massive media coverage that followed. One recent report identified the following factors as important in understanding children's response to disaster:

1. Parental awareness of their reactions on their children: How parents respond affects how children respond.

2. Stages of children's response to disaster: Stage one is fright and disbelief followed by a desire to help, reflecting the resilience of children. Stage two manifests as regression with heightened emotional distress and other behaviors, including depression, sleep disturbances, play themes related to disaster, and others.

3. Developmental stage of children: Infants, toddlers, young children, and older children all respond differently according to their unique developmental stage.

4. Gender and ethnicity of children: Boys act out behaviorally while girls internalize reactions but are more vocal regarding their feelings.

5. Other factors: Poor social support, a history of psychological problems, introverted personality, and level of exposure to losses from a disaster are a few additional factors to consider (Hagan, 2005).

Preparation for Disasters

Nurses have been and will be committed to being on the front lines as caregivers and managers in natural, technological, and terror-related disasters. Completion of continuing education programs and participation in mock disaster drills can increase the efficiency and effectiveness of response to disaster in the community, hospital, or clinic setting. Nurses caring for families can help them to prepare for a disaster using the Family Disaster Planning Guide in Box 7-15. Recommended contents for a disaster supply kit can be found in Box 7-16.

Nurses also play key roles in environmental health through the use of assessment, collaborative, and political skills. Depending on the issue at hand and entities involved, processes in which nurses are involved can range from simple to complex, inexpensive to expensive, traditional to nontraditional, and short-term to long-range.

Nurses are important in identifying hazards, planning remedial or removal interventions, and educating the public. Community education is crucial. Methods of involvement include participating in community forums, giving or attending speeches at meetings of community organizations or events, making written and audiovisual materials available, and collaborating with mass media. Communicating problems, needs, and possible solutions to political representatives is also a responsibility that nurses have as professionals and as citizens. Public opinion and communication have tremendous influence on policy development for a healthier environment.

BOX 7-15 Family Disaster Planning Guide

I. Gather information about hazards. Contact your local National Weather Service office, emergency management or civil defense office, and American Red Cross chapter. Find out what types of disasters could occur and how you should respond. Learn your community's warning signals and evacuation plans.

II. Meet with your family to create a plan. Discuss the information you have gathered. Pick two places to meet: a spot outside your home for an emergency such as fire, and a place away from your neighborhood in case you can't return home. Choose an out-of-state friend as your "family check-in contact" for everyone to call if the family gets separated. Discuss what you would do if advised to evacuate. Don't forget special needs of the elderly and handicapped.

III. Implement your plan. Use the following steps in implementing your plan:
1. Post emergency telephone numbers by phones.
2. Install safety features in your house, such as smoke detectors and fire extinguishers.
3. Inspect your home for potential hazards (such as items that can move, fall, break, or catch fire) and correct them.

4. Have your family learn basic safety measures, such as CPR and first aid; how to use a fire extinguisher; and how and when to turn off water, gas, and electricity in your home.
5. Teach children how and when to call 911 or your local Emergency Medical Services number.
6. Keep enough supplies in your home to meet your needs for at least three days. Assemble a disaster supply kit (see Box 7-16) with items you may need in case of an evacuation. Store these supplies in sturdy, easy-to-carry containers, such as backpacks or duffel bags. Keep important family documents in a waterproof container. Keep a smaller disaster supply kit in the trunk of your car.
7. Plan for care of pets. Shelters do not usually accept pets nor do many hotels.

IV. Practice and maintain your plan. Ask questions to make sure your family remembers meeting places, phone numbers, and safety rules. Conduct drills. Test your smoke detectors monthly and change the batteries at least once a year. Test and recharge your fire extinguisher(s) according to the manufacturer's instructions. Replace stored water and food every six months.

From: American Red Cross, (n.d.). Terrorism—Preparing for the unexpected. *Retrieved December 22, 2005, from http://www.redcross.org/services/disaster/0,1082,0_589_,00.html; and Federal Emergency Management Administration (FEMA). (2005, December).* Hazards: Hurricanes. *Retrieved December 22, 2005, from http://www.fema.gov/hazards/hurricanes/; and Federal Emergency Management Administration (FEMA). (2006, July). Are you ready? An in-depth guide to citizen preparedness. Retrieved October 14, 2006, from www.fema.gov/areyouready/*

- a three-day supply of water (one gallon per person per day) and food that won't spoil
- one change of clothing and footwear per person
- one blanket or sleeping bag per person
- a first-aid kit, including prescription medicines

- emergency tools, including a battery-powered AA Weather Radio, a portable radio, a flashlight, and plenty of extra batteries
- an extra set of car keys and a credit card or cash
- special items for infants and family members who are elderly or disabled

From: American Red Cross, (n.d.). Terrorism—Preparing for the unexpected. Retrieved December 22, 2005, from http://www.redcross.org/services/disaster/0,1082,0_589_,00.html; and Federal Emergency Management Administration (FEMA). (2005, December). Hazards: Hurricanes. Retrieved December 22, 2005, from http://www.fema.gov/hazards/hurricanes/; and Federal Emergency Management Administration (FEMA). (2006, July). Are you ready? An in-depth guide to citizen preparedness. Retrieved October 14, 2006, from www.fema.gov/areyouready/

SUMMARY

Promoting environmental health is a complex, challenging task. Citizens and health care workers must continue to work together in the fight against environmental pollution. Researchers must continue to expand the knowledge base about the biological and psychosocial effects of environmental pollution. Community and environmental groups and legislatures must work together toward reduction of risk from environmental hazards and hold accountable those who place the environment at risk. Individuals and industries must be responsible in the use and disposal of potentially toxic products.

Key Concepts

1. Air, water, soil, sound, light, and space as well as environmental disasters influence environmental health.

2. The goals in environmental health are to minimize or eliminate pollutants in a threatening environment and to create an environment supportive of good health.

3. Psychological and physiological symptoms in every body system have been linked to occupational and environmental pollutants; however, determining the exact cause is difficult.

4. Reduction of or removal of pollutants is important to prevent chemical sensitization even in the absence of symptoms.

5. The nurse, using the nursing process and leadership skills, plays a key role in assisting individuals and communities to improve environmental health through personal and political action.

6. The alert nurse evaluates for potential environmental pollutants during assessments of individuals and their living and working areas.

7. Nursing interventions to improve environmental health may be simple or complex, inexpensive or expensive, traditional or nontraditional.

8. Natural, technological, or terror-related disasters create environmental risks and are associated with posttraumatic stress disorder.

9. All disasters involve risk assessment, preparedness, responsiveness, and recovery components.

10. Citizen groups have been successful in protecting their community's health. The nurse may be instrumental in forming and guiding these groups.

Learning Activities

1. Go to http://www.epa.gov/enviro/wme and enter your zip code to see a map of your region. Find out what emissions are being released into the air, where polluted waters exist, and what is being done (tracking, restoring, protecting) to aid the environment in your area.

2. Develop a family disaster plan for your family.

3. Participate in a mock disaster drill conducted by your educational facility, local hospital, or community organization and write down your experiences in a journal.

True/False Questions

1. T or F   The sense of smell is a reliable tool in detecting air pollution.

2. T or F   Radon gas is easily detected by its bluish tint and a pungent odor.

3. T or F   Outgassing is a technique for removing indoor pollutants.

4. T or F Olfactory adaptation is the ability to detect an odor regardless of its strength.

5. T or F The recommended humidity level for prevention of adverse effects of air pollution is between 30 and 50 percent.

6. T or F Noise-induced hearing loss can be reversed with surgery.

7. T or F Shades of green and blue-green can help in promoting relaxation.

8. T or F Dust from computer screens is electromagnetically charged and may cause skin problems.

9. T or F Chromotherapy is the science of relationships of furniture and tools to the human body.

10. T or F Weapons of mass destruction (WMDs) is a term that is synonymous with weapons of mass effect (WMEs).

Multiple Choice Questions

1. Which of the following terms is used to describe a diagnosable illness that can be directly linked to airborne building contaminants?
   a. Building-related illness
   b. Environmental health hazard
   c. SAD syndrome
   d. Sick building syndrome

2. The single most preventable source of indoor air pollution is:
   a. Carbon monoxide
   b. Natural gas
   c. Radon gas
   d. Tobacco smoke

3. Standards set by the Occupational Safety and Health Administration (OSHA) indicate that hearing impairment can occur with continued exposure to noise that is:
   a. 55 decibels or higher over 5 hours
   b. 65 decibels or higher over 6 hours
   c. 85 decibels or higher over 8 hours
   d. 95 decibels or higher over 10 hours

4. Ergonomics is best defined as
   a. Conservation of human energy
   b. Science of relationships of furniture and tools to the human body
   c. Study of work-related injury and disease
   d. Working with colors and sounds for improved work production

5. Which of the following is an appropriate action during an earthquake?
   a. If driving, keep driving and pull under an overpass for protection.
   b. If in a high-rise building, move against an interior wall.
   c. If in a stadium, leave your seat and move quickly to the nearest exit.
   d. If outdoors, move to the nearest tree for shelter and support.

Websites

http://www.epa.gov Contains an overview of the agency's mission, structure, strategic plan, budget, offices, and staff. Provides data on environmental laws, regulations, research, standards, compliance, and enforcement. Contains maps of specific regions accessible by zip code. Tells what facilities in the region release emissions into the air or if there are any polluted waters, among other information. Also tells what is being done (tracking, restoring, and protecting) to aid the environment in that area.

http://www.aapcc.org Lists poison control centers. Sources for continuing education on bioterrorism:

http://www.bt.cdc.gov Center for Disease Control and Prevention Training and Education

http://www.ceregistration.com Online Continuing Education for Nursing and Nursing Professionals

http://www.westernschools.com Nurses' Study Resource

http://www.healthceonline.com The CE Solutions Group

http://www.son.utmb.edu Texas Statewide Bioterrorism Continuing Education Project

Organizations

IAQ INFO
P.O. Box 37133
Washington, DC 20013-7133
Tel: (800) 438-4318; (703) 356-4020
Fax: (703) 356-5386
iaqinfo@aol.com
Operates Monday to Friday, 9 a.m. to 5 p.m. Eastern Standard Time (EST).
Indoor Air Quality Information Clearinghouse (IAQ INFO). Distributes EPA publications, answers questions on the phone, and makes referrals to other nonprofit and governmental organizations.

National Lead Information Center
Tel: (800) 424-LEAD (5323)
Operates 24 hours a day, seven days a week. Callers may order an information package and/or speak to an information specialist.

National Pesticide Information Center (NPIC)
Tel: (800) 858-PEST/(800) 858-7378
Sponsored by the Environmental Protection Agency, this center provides information about pesticides to the general public and the medical, veterinary, and professional communities.

National Radon Hotlines

Tel: (800) SOS-RADON/(800) 767-7236

Information recording on radon operates 24 hours a day.

Safe Drinking Water Hotline

Tel: (800) 426-4791

Provides information on regulations under the Safe Drinking Water Act and on lead and radon in drinking water, filter information, and a list of state drinking water offices.

Toxic Substances Control Act (TSCA) Assistance Information Service

Tel: (202) 554-1404

Provides information on regulations under the Toxic Substances Control Act and on the EPA's asbestos program.

U.S. Consumer Product Safety Commission (CPSC)

4330 East West Highway

Bethesda, MD 20814

Product Safety Hotline: (800) 638-CPSC

Teletypewriter for the hearing impaired (outside Maryland): (800) 638-8270

Takes complaints and answers questions about product safety.

U.S. Public Health Service

Division of Federal Occupational Health

Office of Environmental Hygiene, Region III, Room 1310

3535 Market St.

Philadelphia, PA 19104

Tel: (215) 596-1888

Fax: (215) 596-5024

Provides indoor air quality consultative services to federal agency managers.

Lead Poisoning Prevention Branch of the Centers for Disease Control and Prevention

4770 Buford Highway NE (F-42)

Atlanta, GA 30341-3724

Tel: (800) 488-7330

Resource for information on lead poisoning detection, prevention, and management.

Office on Smoking and Health of the Centers for Disease Control and Prevention

4770 Buford Highway NE (K-50)

Atlanta, GA 30341-3724

Tel: (404) 488-5701

Resource for information on smoking-related issues.

Occupational Safety and Health Administration (OSHA)

Office of Information and Consumer Affairs

Room N-3647, 200 Constitution Avenue NW

Washington, DC 20210

Tel: (202) 219-8151

Provides information and takes complaints on work-site health and safety issues, standards, and regulations.

References

American Federation of State, County, and Municipal Employees (AFSCME). (n.d.). *Health and safety fact sheet: Diesel exhaust.* Retrieved May 29, 2006, from http://www.afscme.org/health/faq-dies.htm

American Federation of State, County, and Municipal Employees (AFSCME). (2002, March). *Preventing back injuries in health care workers.* Retrieved June 5, 2006, from http://www.afscme.org/health/faq-back.htm

American Lung Association. (2005). *Asbestos.* Retrieved May 27, 2006, from http://www.lungusa.org

American Red Cross. (n.d.). *Terrorism: Preparing for the unexpected.* Retrieved December 22, 2005, from http://www.redcross.org/services/disaster/0,1082,0_589_,00.html

Ash, S. (2003). *The healing home: Practical ways to harmonize your home and energize your spirit.* New York: Sterling.

Beattie, A. (2003). *Feng shui garden design: Creating serenity.* North Clarendon, VT: Tuttle Publishing.

Better Hearing Institute. (2005). *Publication factoids.* Retrieved June 3, 2006, from http://www.betterhearing.org

Bioterrorism basics for nurses. (2005). Columbus, OH: The Bioterrorism Institute.

Brown, S. (2005). *The feng shui bible: The definitive guide to improving your life, home, health, and finances.* New York: Sterling.

California Air Resources Board. (2001). Indoor air pollution: A serious public health problem. Sacramento, CA: Research Division.

Caravati, E. M., & McCuigan, M. A. (2004). *Medical toxicology.* Philadelphia: Lippincott Williams & Wilkins.

Chissell, H. G. (2004, Winter). Feng shui tips for your workspace. *Lilipoh, 9*(38), 17.

Code of Federal Regulations Title 28, *Judicial administration*, Chapter I. Department of Justice, Part O, Subpart P, Federal Bureau of Investigation, Section 0.85, general functions.

Colls, J. F. (2002). *Air pollution.* London: Spon Press.

Coyle, A. J. (2005, February). "Nursing management models for response to bioterrorism." *Pulsepage,* 24–27.

Dangerous Decibels. (2005). *Information center: Hearing loss.* Retrieved December 20, 2005, from http://www.dangerousdecibels.org/hearingloss.cfm

Danielson, R. W. (2005). *Hearing loss prevention: Prevention of hearing loss from noise exposure.* Retrieved June 3, 2006, from http://www.betterhearing.org

Dickerson, S. S., Jezewski, M. A., Nelson-Tuttle, C., Shipkey, N., Wilk, N., & Crandall, B. (2002). Nursing at ground zero: Experiences during and after September 11 World Trade Center attack [Electronic version]. *Journal of the New York State Nurses Association, 33*(1), 1–10.

Elioupoulis, C. (2004). *Invitation to holistic health: A guide to living a balanced life.* Sudbury, MA: Jones and Bartlett.

Engel, L. S., Hill, D. A., Hoppin, J. A., Lubin, J. H., Lynch, C. F., & Pierce, J., et al. (2005, January). Pesticide use and breast cancer risk among farmers' wives in the agricultural health study. *American Journal of Epidemiology, 161*(2), 121-135.

Environmental Protection Agency (EPA). (2004, February). *Respiratory health effects of passive smoking: Lung cancer and other disorders.* Retrieved May 23, 2006, from http://www.epa.gov/smokefree/pubs/etsfs.html

Environmental Protection Agency (EPA). (2005a). *Asthma and indoor environments*. Retrieved December 11, 2005, from http://www.epa.gov/iaq/asthma/about.html

Environmental Protection Agency (EPA). (2005b). *Targeting indoor air pollution: EPA's approach and progress*. Retrieved December 11, 2005, from http://www.epa.gov/iaq/pubs/targetng.html

Environmental Protection Agency (EPA). (2005c). *Sources of indoor air pollution: Organic gases (Volatile Organic Compounds—VOCs)*. Retrieved December 11, 2005, from http://www.epa.gov/iaq/voc.html

Environmental Protection Agency (EPA). (2005d). *Sources of indoor air pollution: Biological pollutants*. Retrieved May 23, 2006, from http://www.epa.gov/iaq/biologic.html

Environmental Protection Agency (EPA). (2006a). *Indoor air facts no. 4 (revised): Sick building syndrome (SBS)*. Retrieved May 22, 2006, from http://www.epa.gov/iaq/pubs/sbs.html

Environmental Protection Agency (EPA). (2006b). *Indoor air pollution: An introduction for health professionals*. Retrieved May 27, 2006, from http://www.epa.gov/iaq/pubs/hpguide

Environmental Protection Agency (EPA). (2006c). *An office building occupant's guide to indoor air quality*. Retrieved May 29, 2006, from http://www.epa.gov/iaq/pubs/occupgd/html

Environmental Protection Agency (EPA). (2006d). *Particulate matter*. Retrieved May 23, 2006, from http://www.epa.gov/oar/particlepollution

Environmental Protection Agency (EPA). (2006e). *About EPA*. Retrieved May 21, 2006, from http://www.epa.gov/

Evans, G. W., & Kantrowitz, E. (2003). Socioeconomic status and health: The potential role of environmental risk exposure. In P. R. Lee and C. L. Estes (Eds.), *The nation's health* (pp. 93–119). Sudbury, MA: Jones and Bartlett.

Fairbrother, G. (2004, May). Unmet need for counseling services by children in New York City after the September 11th attacks on the World Trade Center: Implications for pediatricians. *Pediatrics, 113*, 1367–1374.

Federal Emergency Management Administration (FEMA). (2004, November). *Hazards: Tornados*. Retrieved December 22, 2005, from http://www.fema.gov/hazards/tornado/

Federal Emergency Management Administration (FEMA). (2005, December). *Hazards: Hurricanes*. Retrieved December 22, 2005, from http://www.fema.gov/hazards/hurricanes/

Federal Emergency Management Administration (FEMA). (2006, July). Are you ready? An in-depth guide to citizen preparedness. Retrieved October 14, 2006, from http://www.fema.gov/areyouready/

Freedman, J. (1975). *Crowding and behavior: The psychology of high-density living*. New York: The Viking Press.

Gerald, B. L. (2005, June). Water safety and disaster management procedures reported by Louisiana health care food service directors. *Journal of Environmental Health, 67*(10), 30–34.

Gibson, P. R., Elms, A. N., & Ruding, L. A. (2003). Perceived treatment efficacies for conventional and alternative therapies reported by persons with multiple chemical sensitivities. *Environmental Health Perspectives, 111*(12), 1498–1454.

Gordis, L. (2005). *Epidemiology*. Philadelphia: W.B. Saunders.

Guzzetta, C. E. (2005). Music therapy: Hearing the melody of the soul. In B. Dossey, L. Keegan, & C. Guzzetta (Eds.), *Holistic nursing: A handbook for practice* (4th ed., pp. 617–640). Sudbury, MA: Jones and Bartlett.

Hagan, J. F. (2005). Psychosocial implication of disaster or terrorism on children: A guide for the pediatrician. *Pediatrics, 116*(3), 787–795.

Hamrick, C. A. (2004, April). Public employers' ergonomics: Best practices. *Journal of Occupational and Environmental Hygiene, 1*(4), 42–46.

Hiss, T. (1990). *The experience of place*. New York: Alfred A. Knopf.

Hyams, K. C., Murphy, F. M., & Wessely, S. (2002). Responding to chemical, biological, or nuclear terrorism: The indirect and long-term health effects may present the greatest challenge. *Journal of Health Politics, Policy and Law, 27*(2), 273–286.

Imhof, M. (2004). Effects of color stimulation on handwriting performance of children with ADHD without and with additional learning disabilities. *European Child & Adolescent Psychiatry, 13*(3), 191–198.

Kleim, B., & Rock, B. (n.d.). *The New England region's changing climate*. Retrieved May 29, 2006, from http://www.necci.sr.unh.edu/necci-report/NERAch2

Kochkin, S. (2005a, July). MarkeTrak VII: Hearing loss population tops 31 million people. *The Hearing Review, 12*(7), 16–29.

Kochkin, S. (2005b). "Hearing loss: The prevalence of hearing loss." The Better Hearing Institute. Retrieved June 3, 2006, from http://www.betterhearing.org

Ledford, D. K. (2002, November 20). Building related illness: Your health and how it relates to your indoor environment. *The IEQ Review, 2*(20). Retrieved May 22, 2006, from http://www.imakenews.com/pureaircontrols/

Lee, H. A., Gabriel, R., & Bale, A. J. (2005, May). Clinical outcomes of Gulf Veterans' Medical Assessment Programme referrals to specialized centers for Gulf veterans with post-traumatic stress disorder. *Military Medicine, 170*(5), 400–405.

Lee, P. R., & Estes, L. E. (2003). *The nation's health*. Sudbury, MA: Jones and Bartlett.

Litz, B. T., & Gray, M. J. (2002). Emotional numbing in posttraumatic stress disorder: Current and future research directions. *Australian and New Zealand Journal of Psychiatry, 36*, 198–204.

Los Angeles Fire Department (LAFD). (1997). *Earthquake preparedness handbook*. Retrieved December 22, 2005, from http://www.lafd.org/eqtips.htm

Maddocks-Jennings, W., & Wilkinson, J. M. (2004, October). Aromatherapy practice in nursing: Literature review. *Journal of Advanced Nursing, 48*(1), 93–103.

Mayo Clinic. (2005, May 5). *Noise in the workplace: Safeguard your hearing*. Retrieved December 14, 2006, from http://www.mayoclinic.com/health/hearing-protection/WL00032

Mayo Clinic. (2006, July 24). *Eyestrain and your computer screen: Tips for getting relief*. Retrieved December 15, 2006, from http://www.mayoclinic.com/health/eyestrain/WL00060

McGlown, K. J. (Ed.). (2004). *Terrorism and disaster management: Preparing healthcare leaders for the new reality*. Chicago: Health Administration Press.

Meisenhelder, J. B. (2002, December). Terrorism, posttraumatic stress and religious coping. *Issues in Mental Health Nursing, 23*(8): 771–782.

Mella, D. L. (1988) *Language of color*. New York: Warner Books, Inc.

Mesolink.org. (2005). Retrieved May 27, 2006, from http://www.mesolink.org

Miller, A. (2005). Epidemiology, etiology, and natural treatment of seasonal affective disorder. *Alternative Medicine Review, 10*(1), 5–13.

Moran, E. (2002). *The complete idiot's guide to Feng Shui*. Indianapolis, IN: Alpha Books.

Mothershead, J. L. (2004). The new threat: Weapons of mass effect. In K. J. McGlown (Ed.), *Terrorism and disaster management* (pp. 27–49). Chicago: Health Administration Press.

National Earthquake Hazards Reduction Program (NEHRP). (2004, December 16). *Earthquake fact sheet*. Retrieved December 22, 2005, from http://www.fema.gov/hazards/earthquakes/nehrp/resources.shtm

National Weather Service. (2002, March 13). *Tornadoes: Nature's most violent storms; A preparedness guide*. Retrieved December 22, 2005, from http://www.nssl.noaa.gov/NWSTornado/

Norovirus outbreak among evacuees from Hurricane Katrina—Houston, Texas, September 2005. (2005, October 14). *Mortality and Morbidity Weekly Report, 54*, 1016–1018.

Occupational Safety and Health Administration (OSHA). (n.d.). *Diesel exhaust*. Retrieved May 29, 2006, from http://www.osha.gov/SLTC/dieselexhaust

Occupational Safety and Health Administration (OSHA). (2002). *Hearing conservation*. Retrieved December 19, 2005, from http://www.osha.gov/SLTC/noisehearingconservation/index.html

Papanek, V. (1995). *The green imperative: Natural design for the real world*. New York: Thames and Hudson.

Peterson, R. (2004, September 24). Answer to question #773 submitted to "Ask the Experts." *Health Physics Society.* Retrieved December 18, 2005, from http://hps.org/publicinformation/ate/q773.html

Pike-Paris, A. (2005). Indoor air quality: Part II—What it does. *Pediatric Nursing, 31*(1), 39–49.

Samet, J. M., & Spengler, J. D. (2003, September). Indoor environments and health: Moving into the 21st century. *American Journal of Public Health, 93*(9), 1489–1493.

SantoPietro, N. (2002, October). Better health with feng shui. *Bottom Line Health, 16*(10), 13–14.

Santulli, E. (2004). No strain? No pain! *Hospital Nursing, 34*(3), 7–8.

Schnurr, P. P., & Green, B. L. (2004). Understanding relationships among trauma, post-traumatic stress disorder, and health outcomes. *Advances in Mind-Body Medicine, 20*(1), 18–29.

Schweitzer, M., Gilpin, L., & Frampton, S. (2004). Healing spaces: Elements of environmental design that make an impact on health. *Journal of Alternative and Complementary Medicine, 10*(1), 71–83.

Spotts, P. N. (2004, August 5). "Blowing in the wind: Transatlantic pollution." *Christian Science Monitor.* Retrieved May 29, 2006, from http://www.csmonitor.com

Stasney, S. (2004). *Chic living with feng shui: Stylish designs for harmonious living.* New York: Sterling.

Surveillance for illness and injury after Hurricane Katrina—New Orleans, Louisiana, September 8–25, 2005. (2005, October 14). *Mortality and Morbidity Weekly Report, 54,* 1018.

Talbott, E. O., Youk, A. O., McHugh-Pemu, K. P., & Zborowski, J. V. (2003). Long-term follow-up of the residents of the Three Mile Island accident area: 1979–1998. *Environmental Health Perspectives, 111*(3), 341–348.

10 ways to reduce your exposure to chemicals. (2005, April). *Consumer Reports on Health, 17*(4), 1, 4–6.

Tseng, H., Chen, T., & Chou, S. (2005). SARS: Key factors in crisis management. *Journal of Nursing Research, 13*(1), 58–62.

VanRooyen, M., & Leaning, J. (2005). After the tsumani: Facing the public health challenges. *New England Journal of Medicine, 353*(5), 435–438.

"What is particulate matter?" (n.d.). Retrieved May 23, 2006, from http://www.airinfonow.org/html/ed_particulate.html

Wigle, D. T. (2003). *Child health and the environment.* New York: Oxford University Press.

Wilder-Smith, A., & Steffen, R. (2005, May 1). Tsunami and the role of the international travel health community. *Journal of Travel Medicine, 12*(3), 117–119.

Zeman, G. (2004). Health risks associated with living near high-voltage power lines. *Health Physics Society.* Retrieved December 18, 2005, from http://hps.org/hpspublications/articles/powerlines.html

Bibliography

Barrett, J., Coolidge, J., & Steenburger, M. (2003). *Feng shui your life.* New York: Sterling.

Bower, L. M. (1995). *The healthy household: A complete guide for creating a healthy indoor environment.* Bloomington, IN: Healthy House Institute.

Gibson, P. R. (2002). *Understanding and accommodating people with multiple chemical sensitivity in independent living.* Houston, TX: UIRU Publications.

Krohn, J., Taylor, F., Larson, E. M. (2000). *Allergy relief and prevention: A doctor's guide to treatment and self-care.* Vancouver, BC: Hartley & Marks.

Scaief, K. (2004). Womb pollution? *The Environmental Magazine, 15*(6), 12.

Serripo-Shaapiro, R. *A guide to detoxification for the chemically hypersensitive.* Albuquerque, NM: EIEIO Communications.

Chapter 8

THE MIND-BODY CONNECTION

Cheryl Levine, PhD, FNP-C, RN
Janice A. Maville, EdD, MSN, RN

KEY TERMS

coping strategies
crisis
general adaptation
   syndrome (GAS)
holistic medicine

hypnosis
immune modulation
immunoenhancement
mind-body dualism
perceptions

prospective studies
psychoneuroimmunology
   (PNI)
relaxation techniques
retrospective studies

social support
stress
stress response
stressor

OBJECTIVES

Upon completion of this chapter, the reader should be able to:

- Describe the ways by which the neural and endocrine systems modulate the immune function.

- List the outcome measurements used to determine changes in immune status.

- List five chemicals involved in the communication between the neural, endocrine, and immune systems.

- Describe how stress impacts the neural, endocrine, and immune systems.

- Discuss research findings on psychoneuroimmunology, stress, and illness.

- Identify normal lifetime stressors, emotional states, and diseases that can negatively impact the immune function.

- Describe at least three nursing interventions useful in promoting immunoenhancement.

INTRODUCTION

Behavioral scientists have long been aware of the impact of the mind on the development of and recovery from certain physical complaints such as headache, pain, and allergies. In fact, the belief in the interrelatedness of psychological states and illness can be traced to ancient times. The health beliefs of American Indians, such as the Navajo, include the need for harmony with nature and an integrated relationship with the earth and sky (Flowers, 2005). Galen, a physician living in about AD 200, noted that, compared to sanguine women, the more melancholy women had a higher susceptibility to breast cancer (Mailoo & Williams, 2004).

In spite of these ancient beliefs, modern medicine has functioned mainly on a Cartesian **mind-body dualism** philosophy. This separateness view of the mind and body, which has existed in medicine at least since the time of Descartes in 1619 (Moss, McGrady, Davies, & Wickramasekera, 2003), has allowed investigation and treatment to focus on the illness of the body with only a few diseases being thought to have a primary cause related to the mind. This view, however, has not been without criticism. Sir William Osler, the father of modern medicine, noted over 100 years ago that the patient's belief and the physician's belief are more important than what the physician actually does (Shealy, Norris, & Fahrion, 2002). Belief in the importance of a mind for a healthy body developed into the concept of **holistic medicine,** which uses social, psychological, and spiritual aspects to bring about wellness. Even though there are many clinical descriptions and cultural beliefs reflecting the mind-body connection, the development of health care standards for practice must be based upon rigorous experimental research.

The touting of numerous therapies, which were unproven and later shown ineffective, has caused many health care workers to be cautious of all mind-body treatments. During the last decade or two, however, the other half of the dualistic paradigm, the mind, has received more scientific attention and research.

Coming from the more recent research is an expanding body of knowledge about the influence of psychological factors on disease development, severity, and recovery. A model developed by Borysenko and Dveirin

(2005) postulates that there are three factors influencing disease susceptibility. These three factors are genetic predisposition, the environment, and the behavioral or psychological component. In this model, any one of the three components can be the primary cause of disease or the components can interact with one another. So genetics alone may be the cause of the disease as in hemophilia A, an environmental exposure may interact with a genetic predisposition as with smoking and emphysema, or a psychological stressor may interact with a genetic predisposition or environmental factor or both. This model fits very well with the belief that disease etiology is multifactorial. In addition, the model explains why some people get diseases and others do not even with apparently the same environmental exposures, or genetic predisposition, or both.

Although the study of the interrelationship of the mind and body has gone under several names in previous years, this field of study is now being called **psychoneuroimmunology (PNI).** PNI is concerned with the bidirectional communication between the brain and the immune system. Inherent in PNI is the information about how psychological factors may inhibit or enhance immune function. Psychological factors that suppress the immune system may result in disease. On the positive side, changes in the mind that enhance the immune system may reduce the symptoms of disease even if they do not cure the disease. Development of the PNI body of knowledge has many implications for nursing practice. It provides scientific foundation for many current and proposed nursing interventions in the areas of disease prevention, symptom modification, and health promotion. Nurses are responsible for assessing clients' emotional status, perceived stressors, and **coping strategies,** including **social support.**

Through PNI research, nursing will gain the knowledge needed to be able to give more holistic care and to support clients and their families in using effective coping strategies. Nurses can help diminish the negative effects of illness on clients and their families by including bio-psycho-social-spiritual aspects in their care.

THE PHYSIOLOGICAL BASIS

In order to understand the research on the mind-body interaction, a basic understanding of key systems is required. The nervous, endocrine, and immune systems can interact with one another in many unexpected ways to influence health.

The Nervous System

The nervous system (Figure 8-1) is divided into the central nervous system (CNS) and peripheral nervous system (PNS). These two major sections are further divided with the CNS being composed of the brain and spinal cord and the PNS consisting of the somatic nervous system and the autonomic nervous system (ANS). The somatic nervous system assists in interactions with the environment by controlling body movements and sending sensory messages related to pain, temperature, touch, sense of body position, vision, taste, hearing, and smell. The ANS helps regulate the internal organs through its two branches: sympathetic and parasympathetic nervous systems. The sympathetic branch is connected to the CNS along the thoracic and lumbar regions of the spinal cord. Its main function is to prepare the body for stress through the fight-or-flight response, and it innervates all major parts of the immune system. The chief messengers of the sympathetic nervous system are the two catecholamines: epinephrine and norepinephrine. The parasympathetic branch is connected through the cranial nerves and the sacral portion of the spinal cord and functions to maintain homeostasis and prepare the body for functions such as digestion and elimination.

Neurons are the specialized cells of the nervous system that transmit electrical impulses from their dendrite along their axon. These electrical impulses are then sent across the synapses to other neurons or cells of the organ systems by neurotransmitters.

The Neuropeptides

Over 100 molecules of amino acid called neuropeptides have been identified that carry messages between the brain, the endocrine system, and the immune system.

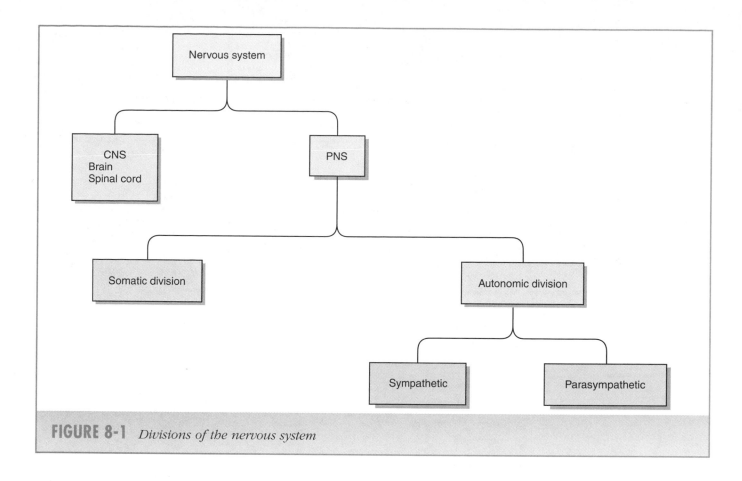

FIGURE 8-1 *Divisions of the nervous system*

Neuropeptides, therefore, act as a type of "informational connective tissue" that unite and coordinate all the cells, tissues, glands, organs, and systems of the body. Their unique ability to modulate chemical and physical responses in the body has earned them the title "healing molecule" (Glassey, 2001). Two examples of skin wound healing provide illustration. One study reported that neuropeptides were found to increase a substance called activin in the skin that causes pain, which, in turn, protects the skin from further injury (Cruise, Xu, & Hall, 2004). In another study, diminished neuropeptide levels were found to contribute to the impaired skin healing response associated with diabetes mellitus (Gibran et al., 2002).

Although neuropeptides play a major role in effecting responses in cells and tissues, they are generally considered to be mood specific. Components of the limbic system (the seat of the emotions), which include the thalamus, hypothalamus, hippocampus, amygdala, and parts of the basal ganglia, are concentration areas for neuropeptides. The hormone serotonin, which is responsible for our mood and feelings of well-being, is produced in the basal ganglia and projected into the hypothalamus from the brain stem, where it is also produced. Emotions, or feelings, that are produced are the result of a biochemical process that occurs between neuropeptides and receptor sites on cell membranes. Feelings are important pieces of information, and, like the information received from our sense of smell or touch, allow our bodies to make physiologic changes that affect the status of our health. The location of neuropeptide receptor sites on immune cells leads to the conclusion that they also influence healing.

The Endocrine System

The endocrine system is composed of glands that produce and secrete hormones that help the body maintain and regulate vital functions. Previously the organs considered part of the endocrine system were the pituitary, gonads, adrenal glands, thyroid, parathyroid, and pancreas. Other organs, however, have been identified as producers of hormones such as the kidney, liver, gastrointestinal tract, and salivary glands. Chiefly through the hypothalamic-pituitary-adrenal (HPA) axis, the endocrine system assists the body in response to stress, growth and development, and reproduction. In addition, the endocrine system maintains the electrolyte and acid-base balance and regulates energy metabolism. Figures 8-2 and 8-3 demonstrate the connection between the endocrine system structure and vital body functions such as growth and reproduction.

In the HPA axis, neurotransmitters such as serotonin, acetylcholine, and norepinephrine regulate the release of corticotropin releasing factor (CRF) from the hypothalamus. CRF causes the pituitary to secrete adrenocorticotropin hormone (ACTH) which stimulates the adrenal gland to release glucocorticoids. The level of glucocorticoids in the bloodstream serves as a negative feedback

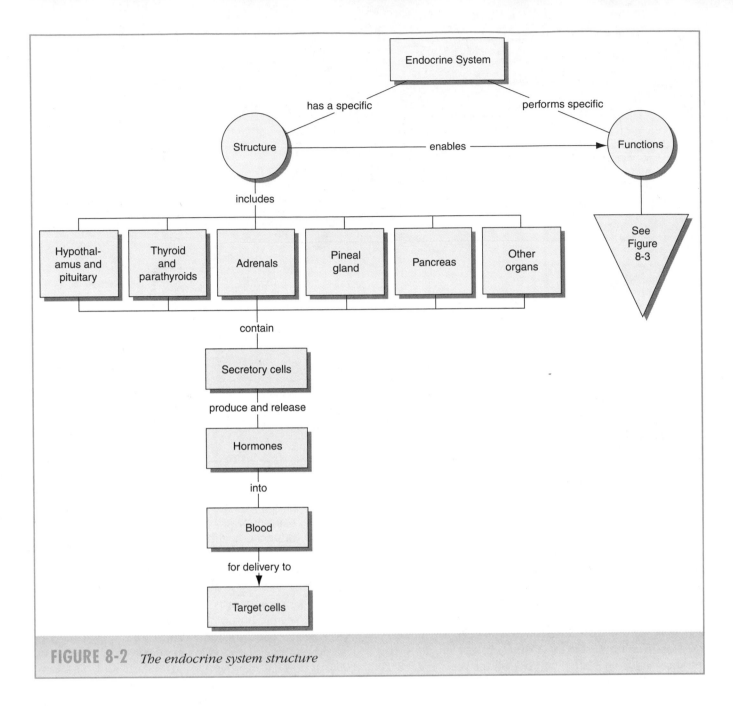

FIGURE 8-2 *The endocrine system structure*

loop to inhibit the release of further CRF. The glucocorticoids have a biphasic effect on the immune system. At low levels the immune system is activated, with the T lymphocytes being their most aggressive against antigens, and at high levels, like those released in response to stress, the T lymphocytes are damaged or destroyed.

The Immune System

The immune system operates as a surveillance system that is designed to protect the body from foreign substances. Responses to a foreign substance are either nonspecific or specific. Nonspecific responses result from phagocytosis, which is the body's first line of defense against viruses and bacteria. Phagocytic cells include monocytes and neutrophils that circulate in the blood and macrophages located in the tissues. These phagocytic cells engulf the foreign substance and, through the activation of chemicals, destroy it. These chemicals from the phagocytic cell also initiate the inflammatory process.

Specific responses are humoral (involving the B lymphocytes) and cell-mediated (involving the T lymphocytes). T lymphocytes and B lymphocytes represent the two broad classes of lymphocytes, and they differ in their function.

B lymphocytes, when activated by a pathogen, form plasma cells that produce antibodies or immunoglobulin: IgG, IgM, IgA, IgE, and IgD. Each immunoglobulin is designed to attack the specific pathogen that stimu-

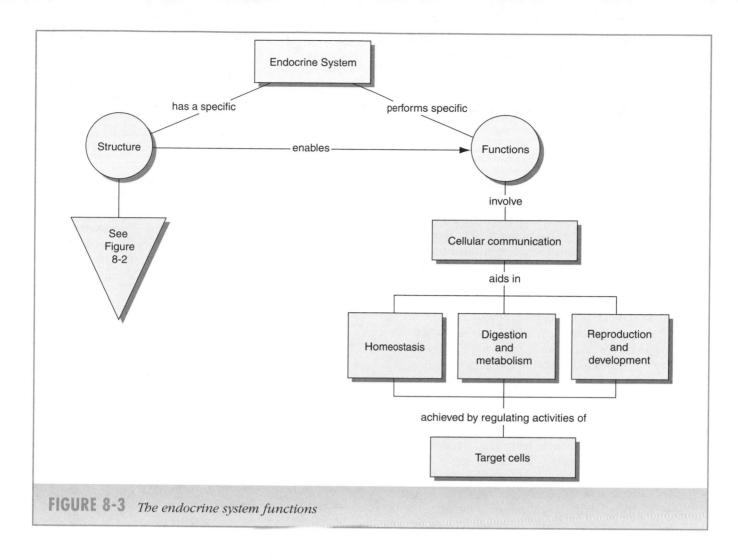

FIGURE 8-3 *The endocrine system functions*

lated its production. The antibodies function by combining with the antigen, activating the complement system, and stimulating phagocytosis, or pathogen cell destruction. The presence of antigens also stimulates the production of anti-idiotypic antibodies that interfere with the production and function of the immunoglobulin and help maintain the balance of the immune system.

T lymphocytes come in a variety of cells. Helper T cells produce lymphokines that facilitate the production of antibody from the B lymphocytes and produce interleukin-2, which stimulates the production of cytotoxic T cells and suppressor T cells. Cytotoxic T cells directly attack tumor cells and secrete cytokines that regulate other cells of the immune system. Suppressor T cells regulate the immune response by blocking the activation of B lymphocytes. Activation of both B and T lymphocytes produces some memory cells that can be activated rapidly in the future. Memory cells result in a more efficient system with the next exposure and can produce antibodies within 48 to 72 hours of exposure to the specific antigen.

Natural killer (NK) cells are another set of lymphocytes that have been identified. These NK cells have the ability to kill tumor cells and cells infected with microbes.

In contrast to other lymphocytes, the NK cells do not require prior exposure to the antigen for activation.

The protection of the body against pathogens is facilitated by both fever and sleep. Because of the importance of these two processes, the immune system is capable of initiating these responses. Fever can be produced by the effect of the cytokine interleukin-1 (IL-1) on the anterior hypothalamus. The resultant increase in temperature is lethal to many microorganisms and enhances most aspects of the immune system. In addition, IL-1 induces slow-wave sleep. Growth hormone is produced during this stage of sleep and further augments the immune system.

Laboratory methods used to measure immune response have improved over the years. Early studies have identified abnormalities in the peripheral blood smears. Levels of antibody production are used as a measure that the first-line defenses have failed or that a dormant infection has progressed to an active form as in reactivation of tuberculosis, Epstein-Barr virus, herpes virus, or cytomegalovirus infections. Conversely, high levels of antibody titer following immunization are a reflection of a functioning immune system. Many studies measure lymphocyte activation by stimulating lymphocytes with mitogens. More recently studies have added NK cell activity against tumor cells as a quantitative measure of the immune system's responsiveness.

Modulation Between the Neuroendocrine and Immune Systems

Through PNI research, various pathways by which the nervous and endocrine systems impact the immune system have been identified (Levy, 2002). Table 8-1 shows the chemical responses of specific hormones. A physical, emotional, or treatment variable facilitates enhancement or suppression of the degree of immune functioning. This process is called **immune modulation.**

Support for the interaction between the brain and the immune system comes from a variety of studies involving immune modulation. Examples of such studies include those demonstrating that: immune responses can be conditioned (Shealy, Norris, & Fahrion, 2002); stress alters the immune responses and healing in animal and human studies; and a correlation exists between immune and neuroendocrine correlates and repression in individuals following a series of natural disasters (Benight, Harper, Zimmer, Lowery, Sanger, & Laudenslager, 2004).

There is much evidence showing that innervation of the immune system can arise from glucocorticoids, catecholamines, neuropeptides, and hormones. The neuropeptides include endorphins, substance P, vasoactive intestinal polypeptide (VIP), and neuropeptide Y. Current studies indicate that the hormones may include prolactin and growth hormone (GH). A major communication pathway between the immune system and the brain is through cytokines such as interleukins, interferons, tumor necrosis factors, and growth-stimulating factors. These cytokines act on many different organ systems to produce the many physiological and behavioral responses to infection such as anorexia, fever, and sleepiness. The actions of these chemicals on the brain, endocrine system, and immune system indicate a much more complex process of bidirectional communication between the systems than was previously thought.

Evidence also exists that the immune system impacts the other bodily systems. Activation of the immune system produces a decrease in norepinephrine that will decrease the sympathetic stimulation. The exact mechanism, however, for this effect has not been demonstrated. The hormones secreted by the immune cells include ACTH, endogenous opioids, thyrotropin, VIP, GH, and luteinizing hormone. Leukocytes produce chemicals similar to pituitary hormones that stimulate the neuroendocrine systems. Monocytes secrete IL-1, which can increase ACTH and corticosterone levels.

THE ROLE OF STRESS

Stress is an emotional and physiological response to a stressor. In the 1940s, Hans Selye (1976) recognized the impact of stress on the body. A **stressor** was defined as a factor that placed a demand on the body necessitating an adaptational response. Three phases of the **general adaptation syndrome (GAS)** were noted: alarm reaction, resistance or adaptation phase, and exhaustion phase. The alarm reaction phase is initiated by an event or situation that requires some type of adaptive response by the individual. In response, the pituitary gland and the sympathetic branch of the autonomic nervous system are activated, sending a message to the central nervous system via epinephrine or norepinephrine that elicits the fight-or-flight reaction, otherwise known as the stress response, to the stressor. The resistance or adaptation phase is a coping mode whereby the body allows itself to return to a more normal state of functioning. Exhaustion occurs when the individual is exposed to long-term stress or stressors without adaptation.

GAS theory included the impact of modulators such as social support and coping ability. Outcomes of the stress could be psychological growth, no change, or an adverse health change. Selye's work identified the subjectivity of stress with individualized reactions of different people and different reactions at different times in the same person. However, there were many common features in response to similar stressors. These features were called the **stress response** and formed a set of physical changes the human body makes in response to a stressor or threat. It sometimes is called the "fight-or-flight" response. Immediate and prolonged effects of the stress response on selected body organs are identified in Table 8-2. Documented physiological responses to stress

TABLE 8-1	The Chemical Effects of Hormones on the Immune System
Hormone	**Chemical Effects**
ACTH	Suppresses T lymphocyte response Enhances NK cell activity
Glucocorticoids	Suppress T lymphocyte response
Norepinephrine	Suppresses T lymphocyte response Enhances NK cell activity
Growth hormone	Augments T lymphocyte cell activity Augments NK cell cytolytic activity
Thyroxin	May increase NK cell activity

TABLE 8-2 Immediate and Prolonged Effects of the Stress Response on Selected Body Organs, Systems, and Tissues

Body Organ, System, or Tissue	Response to Stress	Immediate Response/ Beneficial Effect	Prolonged Response/ Adverse Effect
Eyes	Pupils dilate	Greater acuity to see danger and escape routes	Unknown
Brain	Increased blood flow, increased metabolism of glucose	Greater focus and increased thought processes	"Thought" fatigue
Cardiovascular System	Increased heart rate and force of contractions	Increased cardiac output for more blood supply to muscles	Vasospasm leading to stroke or infarction
Pulmonary System	Increased respiratory rate and dilation of bronchi	Increased oxygen supply for energy	Fatigue; carbon dioxide retention and respiratory acidosis
Liver	Increased glucose production; increased gluconeogenesis; decreased glycogen synthesis	Increased energy	Depletion of energy reserve
Muscles	Increased breakdown of glycogen to glucose (gluconeogenesis) and increased muscle tension	Immediate energy	Nervous behavior, irritability, and discomfort
Fat Tissue	Increased breakdown of stored fat (lipolysis), more fatty acids in the bloodstream	Immediate energy	Increased risk for heart disease and stroke
Stomach	Increased acidity and decreased motility	Conserves energy for use by muscles and brain	Discomfort, nausea, ulceration
Salivary Glands	Decreased flow of saliva	Conserves energy	Thickened or lack of saliva, dry mouth, "cotton mouth"
Pancreas	Increased glucose production	Immediate energy	Stress-induced diabetes
Excretory System	Neuron stimulation of the bladder	Reduced urine flow and intestinal motility	Urge to urinate in spite of the fact that urine flow is reduced; possible constipation followed by diarrhea
Lymph Tissue	Increased release of T cells and natural killer cells	Heightened immune function	Reserve depletion; decreased immune function
Skin	Decreased blood flow	Conserves blood supply for use by muscles and brain	Cold hands/feet
Sweat Glands	Increased sympathetic nervous system response	Temperature regulation	Excessive sweating, blood plasma volume depletion, decreased blood pressure, weakness, fainting

Adapted from Pathophysiology: The Biologic Basis for Disease in Adults and Children *(5th ed.), by K. L. McCance & S. E. Huether, 2006, St. Louis: Mosby-Elsevier.*

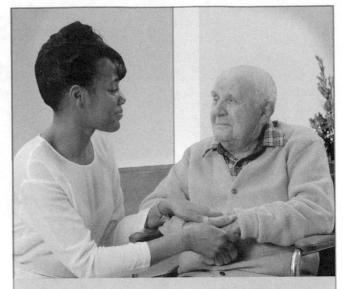

FIGURE 8-4 *Clasping the client's hand is one way to communicate through touch. What messages do you think are communicated by the nurse to the client in this situation?*

include activation of the sympathetic nervous system causing increased circulating catecholamines and stimulation of the HPA system with increased secretion of glucocorticoids and endorphins.

There are numerous effects on the immune system from the chemicals released in response to stress. T lymphocyte response is reduced by ACTH, glucocorticoids, epinephrine, and norepinephrine. Varying changes occur in the NK cell activity with inhibition produced by glucocorticoids and enhancement from other hormones. Growth hormone, which enhances both T lymphocyte and NK cell activity, may either increase or decrease in response to stress. In addition, neurohormones diminish the function of macrophages against tumor cells.

Factors that have been documented through research as impacting the individual's response to stressors include genetics, **perceptions,** environmental factors, and the type of stressor. Genetic factors include predisposition to disease, gender, and prior exposure with its physiological conditioning. A person's positive or negative perception about the stressor influences the impact on the body. Often if a person views a stressor as negative, then any positive aspects of the stressor are totally ignored (Jones, 2003). Coping strategies are part

of the perception factor allowing individuals to be trained to deal with stressors and overcome the negative perceptions. Environmental stressors have been shown to alter the immune status. Some of these factors are trauma, irradiation, malnutrition, drug and alcohol usage, temperature, and aging. The impact of the stressor is also influenced by its severity; timing, whether it be chronic, repetitive, or acute; escapability; and controllability. With chronic, repetitive stress, individuals may be trained not to continue to respond negatively. Stressors create a smaller response if they are perceived as something that can be avoided or controlled. Five categories of stressors, shown in Table 8-3, have been identified, distinguishing stressors according to duration and course (Segerstrom & Miller, 2004).

TABLE 8-3 Categories of Stressors

Stressor	Examples
1. Acute time-limited stressor	Public speaking, mental arithmetic
2. Brief naturalistic stressor	Academic exams, real-life short-term challenges
3. Stressful event sequences	Loss of a loved one, major natural disaster
4. Chronic stressors	Debilitating health condition, caregiver, refugee
5. Distant past stressors	Sexual assault in younger years, witness to traumatic event, prisoner of war

Adapted from Psychological Stress and the Human Immune System: A Meta-Analytical Study of 30 Years of Inquiry, by S. C. Segerstrom and G. E. Miller, 2004, Psychological Bulletin, 130(4), 601–630.

Massage Treatment and Immune Function in Children with HIV

Study Problem/Purpose: To investigate the effect of massage therapy on natural killer cytotoxic capacity and markers of HIV progress, CD4 and CD8 cell count in HIV-infected children.

Methods: The population consisted of children living in the Dominican Republic who lacked access to antiviral treatment and adequate nutrition, and who faced increased risks of developing opportunistic infections. A total of 24 children, 15 girls and 9 boys, were randomly assigned to one of two groups. One group received 20 minutes of massage twice a week for 12 weeks while the other group served as control and received a 20-minute friendly visit, including reading, conversation, and quiet games, without massage. During the first and last week of the 12-week study, blood tests were done to assess lymphocyte helper (CD4/T4) and suppressor (CD8/T8) counts.

Findings: The participants ranged in age from 2 to 8 years with 76 percent being under age 6. Immune parameters at baseline were similar in both groups. Postintervention laboratory reports revealed higher helper lymphocyte (CD4) counts in the treatment group and lower counts in the control group in addition to a greater loss of lymphocytes (T cells).

Implications: Although the sample size was small, the findings indicate that massage therapy has a positive effect on immune system functioning in HIV-infected children. Results of this research could be used to support the inclusion of massage therapy in the plan of care for HIV-infected individuals.

Shor-Posner, G., Miguez, M. J., Hernandez-Reif, M., Perez-Then, E., and Fletcher, M. (2004). Massage treatment in HIV-1 infected Dominican children: A preliminary report on the efficacy of massage therapy to preserve the immune system in children without antiretroviral medication. *Journal of Alternative and Complementary Medicine, 10*(6), 1093-1095.

PSYCHONEUROIMMUNOLOGY RESEARCH

The PNI literature includes much animal and human research. In the field of PNI it is more difficult and sometimes unethical to conduct the needed, tightly controlled, prospective studies on humans. **Prospective studies** are research studies that follow subjects without the disease (or outcome of interest) forward in time. Animal subjects are followed for enough person-years to establish incidence, morbidity, or mortality rates. Therefore there is currently much more animal than human research. Stress in animals has been induced through

Perceptions Alter Stress

Our everyday lives are often filled with stressors, and many of these we believe are out of our control. Projects or assignments may have been put off because of previous difficulties with similar tasks. As the due date for the project approaches, the stress level increases. Some of the problem may be in our thinking that we have to approach the task in the same manner that it was done the last time. Opening up our mind to other alternatives, changing our perceptions, gives us more control over the stressor. Perhaps it would be better to start writing a paper on a section that is known well rather than beginning with the introduction, or to make a game out of a nasty household chore. We could be increasing our own stress through our own negative perceptions.

such measures as overcrowding, noise, and electric shock. In general, the results of these studies have shown decreased immune function with increased susceptibility to cancer and infectious diseases. Studies have shown an impact of environmental stress on the development of cancer in rodents. Research in general has shown that mice in moderately stressed environments develop more cancer than those in low-stress environments. More recently, focus has shifted to studying behavioral and immunological reactions of mice in social conditions, with and without the added burden of cancer (Engler, Bailey, Engler, & Sheridan, 2004; Vegas, Beitia, Sánchez-Martin, Arregi, & Azpiroz, 2004). The major problem with these studies is the unknown generalizability of the results to humans.

Much of the research on humans is done using **retrospective studies** after the stressor or disease has occurred, preventing the researcher from controlling or manipulating the stressor. As highlighted in Box 8-1, human research in PNI has three areas of focus. These areas include (1) the effect of negative stressors such as examinations, bereavement, childbirth, depression, loneliness, and hopelessness; (2) the effect of stress on

BOX 8-1   PNI Research Focus Areas

The effect of negative stressors
The effect of stress on diseases
The effect of various stress management techniques

diseases such as tuberculosis, rheumatoid arthritis, Acquired Immunodeficiency Syndrome (AIDS), and herpes virus; and (3) the effect of various stress management techniques on **immunoenhancement** such as social support, **relaxation techniques,** biofeedback, and **hypnosis.** Because of the volume of research studies, only samples of the studies will be presented to illustrate the mind-body connection related to each of the three areas of PNI research. Chapter 18 provides a more in-depth discussion on various stress management techniques.

The Effect of Negative Life Stressors

Psychoneuroimmunology research has evaluated the changes in the immune function that occur with normal lifetime stressors such as academic examinations, bereavement over loss of a significant other, and childbirth. In addition, the effects of various emotional states like depression, loneliness, and hopelessness, and various types of stress like controllable and predictable stress have been evaluated.

Examination Stress

Stress is an emotional and physiological response to a stressor that triggers the sympathetic division of the autonomic nervous and endocrine systems into preparation for change or adaptation. For students, an impending examination could be identified as a stressor invoking emotional and physiological changes that could be described as examination stress. Research has documented the various emotional and immunological effects associated with students in academia. For example, one recent study found that college students have increased circulating monocytes, decreased CD4 and CD8 cells, and higher cortisol levels on exam days and increased antibody titers to latent viruses such as herpes simplex, Epstein-Barr virus, and cytomegalovirus (Segerstrom & Miller, 2004). Lower levels of T cells and higher self-reported incidences of health problems such as upper respiratory infections also have been found among students during exam times (Beaton, 2003).

Research studies such as this are significant in psychoneuroimmunology. It is important to note, however, that inherent in such research is the possibility of confounding factors that cannot be eliminated from influencing the subjects' health. As an example, researchers studying college freshmen found that lack of social support is a risk factor for depression in college students that is compounded by social isolation and feelings of loneliness resulting in weakened immunity (Pressman, Cohen, Miller, Barkin, Rabin, & Treanor, 2005). Nonetheless, regardless of its source, a clear connection is evident between stress, decreased immunity, and higher risk for alterations in the health of college students.

The examination stress model provides for understanding individual responses to other brief naturalistic stressors that result in stress. For example, preparing for

a speech or presentation to a group or organization may produce pressures similar to students' feelings of stress and anxiety as they prepare for exams.

Many instruments have been developed to assess stress. One in particular was developed especially to measure students' stress. It is the Hassles Assessment Scale for Students in College (HASS/COL) developed by Sarafino and Ewing (1999). The original scale listed 54 hassles, later revised to 57, with each to be rated according to frequency and unpleasantness in the past month and the degree to which it was dwelt upon (Pitt, 2005). Using valid instruments such as this one is important for college counselors and health professionals when determining interventions for stress reduction. Helping students manage stress early on may influence how they deal with stressful events in their adult lives. Box 8-2 offers some helpful tips to ease mental stress.

Bereavement

Bereavement is an indeterminate time of grieving the loss of a loved one, most likely through death, but it can also accompany separation or the severance of a rela-

BOX 8-2   Tips to Ease Mental Stress

- Take time out regularly, ideally outdoors, to improve circulation and delivery of nutrients and oxygen to the brain.
- Breathe. Deep breathing increases oxygen delivery to the brain.
- Keep away from stimulants. Avoid relying on stimulants such as caffeine, cigarettes, and drugs.
- Drink plenty of water (6–8 glasses a day). Dehydration negatively affects brain function.
- Eat healthy small meals regularly. This stabilizes blood sugar (glucose) levels, which is fuel for the brain.
- Use social support. Communicate with family members and friends who can be supportive.

tionship. Bereavement is a highly stressful event related to a variety of physical problems, including physical exhaustion, sleep disturbance, heart palpitations, shortness of breath, headaches, recurrent infections, high blood pressure, changes in weight and eating patterns, stomach upsets, hair loss, disruption of the menstrual cycle, irritability, worsening of any chronic condition such as diabetes or eczema, and susceptibility to opportunistic infections such as influenza.

The death of a spouse has been rated as the most stressful life event across all ages and cultural backgrounds (Holmes & Rahe, 1967). The loss of a loved one activates the stress response mechanism of the autonomic nervous system and immune system. Much research on bereavement and immune function, focused mainly on the elderly, has documented that individuals undergoing bereavement show reduced indicators of immune function, including suppression of lymphocyte stimulation, reduction of NK cell activity, T cell suppression, increased plasma cortisol levels, and altered response to antibody production (Segerstrom & Miller, 2004; Phillips, Carroll, Burns, Ring, Macleod, & Drayson, 2006).

Preexisting or chronic conditions often become worse, explaining, in part, why people are at higher risk of dying during the first year after the loss of a loved one. Several studies related to the mortality risk of the surviving spouse noted that survivors were at increased risk of death from any cause with an even greater risk for men (Christakis & Iwashyna, 2003). One study found that widowed non-caregivers have been reported to have increased depression symptoms and antidepressant medication use, significant weight loss, and maintenance of preexisting overall health risk behaviors (Dyer, 2002). A study on caregivers found that those with few symptoms of depression before bereavement tended to maintain these states afterward, but emotionally distressed caregivers tended to become more distressed, indicating that self-esteem and socio-emotional support play protective roles (Aneshensel, Botticello, & Yamamoto-Mitani, 2004).

Researchers have identified the caring for a spouse with dementia as a chronic uncontrollable stress. One study matched groups of caregiver spouses with non-caregiver spouses and concluded that an immune system pathway exists that links caregiver stress to serious health problems ("Research Reveals," 2003). In this study, caregivers had four times the amount of interleukin-6 (IL-6), a compound that circulates in the blood and helps regulate the immune system. Excess IL-6 contributes to muscle atrophy and several diseases of aging. It also promotes the production of C-reactive protein (CRP), a risk factor for cardiovascular disease. Both IL-6 and CRP are implicated in type 2 diabetes, osteoporosis, and arthritis. The IL-6 and CRP effects continued in caregivers for several years after the spouse had died, suggesting that chronic stress may have a lasting impact on the immune system. Unhealthy habits people develop in

response to stress, such as smoking, overeating, sleeping too little, and not exercising, are also linked to higher IL-6 levels.

Because of the multifactorial nature of the stress, the impact of other emotional states in addition to the bereavement has been evaluated. For instance, in a study of the impact of depression in bereaved caregivers, researchers found that immune function was only significantly decreased in subjects with high degrees of depression (Aneshensel, Botticello, & Yamamoto-Mitani, 2004).

Chronic Stress

Stress is useful to promote the adaptation of our bodies to events and conditions. Prolonged stress, however, results in wear and tear on the body. Box 8-3 lists many of the sources of chronic stress. Chronic activation of cortisol, the body's response to stress, can produce unhealthy physiological outcomes. Some of the results of chronic stress include the following:

- Aging

- Hypertension

- Diabetes

- Atherosclerosis

- Obesity

- Immune suppression

- Osteoporosis

- Muscle atrophy

- Brain atrophy

- Depression

- Skin disorders

- Cardiovascular disease (McEwen, 2004; Robles, Glaser, & Kiecolt-Glaser, 2005; Yehuda & McEwen, 2004; Velamoor & Mendonca, 2003).

BOX 8-3   Sources of Chronic Stress

Anger	Electromagnetic fields
Fear	Radiation
Worry	Geophysical stressors
Anxiety	Malabsorption
Depression	Low blood sugar
Guilt	Poor diet
Overwork	Nutritional deficiencies
Excessive exercise	Food allergies
Sleep deprivation	Inhalant allergies
Lifecycle disruption	Noise pollution
Late hours	Poor digestion
Surgery	Traumas (mental,
Gluten intolerance	emotional, physical)
Injury	Cortisol imbalance
Whiplash	Adult attention deficit
Inflammation	disorder (AADD)
Pain	Seasonal affective
Temperature	disorder (SAD)
extremes	Electromagnetic
Toxic chemical	sensitivity (from exten-
exposures	sive computer use)
Infections	Toxic personal
(chronic/acute)	relationships
Heavy metals	Perfectionism

From "Stress: The Mind-Body Connection," by M. Garrish, 2005, WebMed Live Events Transcript (October 6, 2005), retrieved January 16, 2006, from http:webcenter.health.webmd.netscape .com; "Stress Damages Immune System and Health," by R. Glaser and J. Kiecolt-Glaser, 2005, Discovery Medicine, 5(26), 165–169; and Biobehavioral Stress Response: Protective and Damaging Effects, by R. Yehuda and B. McEwen (Eds), 2004, New York: New York Academy of Science.

Crisis

Any stressful event has the potential to become overwhelming, resulting in crisis. A **crisis** is a situation of severe disorganization resulting when an individual's coping mechanisms are not effective, or when usual resources are lacking, or a combination of both (Schwecke, 2003). Crises are not limited to individuals alone, but can occur within families, groups, and communities. The discussion that follows focuses on crisis in the individual client but is applicable to families, groups, and communities.

Many clients seen by nurses are in some form of crisis. Crises may arise from events ranging from relatively minor, such as being late for an appointment or stuck in traffic, to major, such as the death of a loved one. It is not the stressor or event that is the crisis; it is the lack of effective coping skills that results in crisis. The ineffective ability to cope results in a state of distress often leading to panic. What results in crisis for one person

may not have the same effect on another person. Effects of crisis may be physical, psychological, cognitive, or relational distress. A person in crisis may become physically ill with nausea or vomiting, adopt dysfunctional coping patterns such as taking drugs, have irrational thoughts or ideas including suicide, or lose the ability to relate to others.

Crises are affected by culture, both that of the person or group experiencing the crisis and that of those intervening. Culture influences how situations are perceived and how they are responded to; perceptions and reactions vary according to how individuals and communities view and appraise their own responses (Dykeman, 2005). Understanding the cultural context of the crisis is paramount to its resolution.

It is important to note that crises create an opportunity for growth and development as well as for negative outcomes. Once a person learns how to cope with the crisis situation, that individual gains stability and self-confidence from learning new ways to cope or from garnering new resources (Schwecke, 2003). Research to support a crisis theory might establish a cause-effect relationship.

Crisis intervention requires immediate attention. It is a type of emotional first-aid (Rosenbluh, 2002). Basic intervention strategies for individuals or groups experiencing crisis are addressed in Box 8-4.

The Effect of Stress on Disease

Extensive research literature has shown a relationship between psychosocial stress and immune dysfunction in autoimmune diseases. Many other diseases have been studied with implications of similar psychological reac-

BOX 8-4   Basic Crisis Intervention Strategies

Intervene immediately to interrupt escalation and provide positive redirection.
Provide for physical and emotional safety.
Strive to understand and empathize, considering the cultural context of the victim.
Guide rational thought processes.
Avoid providing answers.
Help to identify personal coping skills, resources, and support systems.
Assist in developing a plan for action and commitment to the plan.

From "Anxiety, Coping, and Crisis," by L. H. Schwecke, 2003, in N. L. Keltner, L. H. Schwecke, and C. E. Bostrom (Eds.), Psychiatric Nursing (pp.120–129), St. Louis: Mosby; Guide to Crisis Intervention, by K. Kanel, 2006, Belmont, CA: Wadsworth; and "Emotional First-Aid," by E. Rosenbluh, 2002, retrieved June 12, 2006, from http://www.emotionalfirstaid.com.

tions, including the common cold, malignant melanoma, asthma, AIDS, and hypertension. However, there is still much variability in the individual's response to stress and perception of what is stressful. Additional factors considered in the stress reaction that may alter the response of an individual's immune function include personality and emotions, vulnerability, and perceptions of the stressful event, among others (Segerstrom & Miller, 2004). The effect of stress on disease has been extensively documented in the literature; therefore, examples related to depression, psychocutaneous disease, and cancer have been selected for brief discussion in the following sections.

Depression Factors

Clients with depression have been evaluated for response to mitogens and NK cell activity, which indicates decreased immune function. Depression frequently exists with other disease conditions. It is a potential risk factor for poor health and even death among individuals with numerous medical conditions such as heart disease and AIDS. There is strong evidence that depression is an independent risk factor for clients with congestive heart failure and coronary artery disease. There is no research, however, that shows that treating depression, either with therapy or antidepressant drugs, makes a difference in heart disease prognosis (Bachman, 2004).

The impact of depression on AIDS has been the focus of many studies. One study found that improvements in the diagnostic status of major depression were related to increases in NK cell activity among HIV-seropositive women (Cruess et al., 2005). Another study positively correlated depressive symptoms with viral load in clients with HIV infection (Evans et al., 2002).

Because of its effect on disrupting the anti-inflammatory process of the immune system, depression can influence several conditions associated with aging, including cardiovascular disease, osteoporosis, arthritis, type 2 diabetes, certain cancers, periodontal disease, frailty and functional decline, prolonged infection, and delayed wound healing (Bachman, 2004; Kiecolt-Glaser & Glaser, 2002; Tafet & Bernardini, 2003).

Psychocutaneous Disease

For many decades, psychological factors, including stress, have been implicated in the development and exacerbation of many skin disorders. Even some skin diseases have been noted to occur in certain personality types. However, because of the retrospective nature of such research, it is unclear if the psychological factors or the skin changes occur first. Some researchers have hypothesized that the emotional stressors occur first, reducing the time the person has to tend to the skin disease, and the result is an exacerbation of the disease.

Most clinicians and researchers agree that stress affects the course of dermatologic conditions such as psoriasis. Treating the condition should, therefore, include therapies aimed at reducing psychophysiological stress. Biofeedback training, psychotherapy, and hypnosis are examples of adjuncts to traditional medical treatment that can reduce stress levels and have been shown to have a positive effect on the course of psoriasis.

Many individuals with psoriasis use complementary and alternative modalities (CAM) as an adjunct to conventional treatment. One study found that as many as 62 percent of psoriasis clients used CAM (Ben-Arye, Ziv, Frenkel, Lavi, & Rosenman, 2003). The National Psoriasis Foundation (2005) endorses the supplemental use of practices that promote relaxation and stress reduction to manage stress and gain a sense of control over the disease, including massage, meditation, yoga, aromatherapy, guided imagery, progressive relaxation, tai chi, and reflexology.

Cancer

The relationship between stress and cancer has been demonstrated in animal studies with highly stressed mice having a higher incidence of cancer and faster growing tumors. In human studies, it is more difficult to control individual client variables and the type of stress. Therefore the results have been less consistent in humans.

The National Cancer Institute (NCI, n.d.) recognizes that, although studies have shown that stress factors (such as death of a spouse, social isolation, and medical school examinations) alter immune system functions, they have not provided definitive evidence of a direct cause-and-effect relationship between these immune system changes and the development of cancer. The NCI (n.d.) recommends more research to find if there is a relationship between psychological stress and the transformation of normal cells into cancerous cells.

For the past four decades, researchers have been evaluating the cancer personality. However, most of these studies have been retrospective with information about the prior personality based upon the cancer client's recall. The major weakness in these designs is that the client's current emotional state may be altering his or her perception of prior functioning. In addition, cancer has long latency periods during which the biological changes from the tumor could have been altering the client's emotional state long before the cancer was detected or diagnosed. Therefore the best study design would be a long-term prospective approach following healthy subjects.

There are, however, studies that have provided meaningful information regarding psychological factors reflecting perceptions and life events of individuals with cancer. One such study examined the perceived threat to life of the stage of cancer (stages are 1 to 4, with 1 being small tumor with no lymph node involvement and 4 being cancer spread to other organs) and found that the perception of the threat to life more than the stage of the cancer was significantly related to psychological distress and quality of life (Laubmeier & Zakowski, 2004). In another study, stressful life events, perceptions of global stress, and perceptions of cancer-related traumatic stress were studied in women with breast cancer (Golden-Kreutz & Andersen, 2004). The researchers found that each of these variables increased the risk for depressive symptoms and recommended the assessment of multiple sources of stress in order to promote health and well-being.

Spirituality and Psychoneuroimmunology

The subject of faith or spirituality and health and healing has become of great interest to researchers of complementary or alternative medicine (CAM) practice. In fact, the National Center for Complementary and Alternative Medicine (NCCAM) was created by the National Institutes of Health (NIH) to use rigorous research in CAM practices, train CAM researchers, and provide authoritative information to the public and professionals (NCCAM, 2005).

Mind-body medicine is one of five major areas of research focus for NCCAM, with spirituality among the top areas of research. The NCCAM sponsored one of the largest and most comprehensive surveys to date on Americans' use of complementary and alternative medicine. Surveying more than 31,000 adults, this study found that within the preceding 12 months of the survey, 36 percent of those surveyed had used complementary and alternative medicine (CAM) exclusive of prayer as part of the definition; when prayer was included in the definition of CAM, 62 percent had used CAM (Barnes, Powell-Griner, McFann, & Nahin, 2004). Among all complementary methods used (massage, chiropractic, yoga, etc.), prayer for health was the method used most often.

There is a growing body of research supporting the possibility that religious involvement might affect physical health via the neuroendocrine and immune mechanisms (Koenig & Cohen, 2002; Seeman, Dubin, & Seeman, 2003). Studies have credited spirituality with lowering blood pressure, lowering mortality rates from heart disease, reducing stress, increasing sense of well-being, prolonging life, and reducing costs through shorter hospital stays (Etnyer et al., 2005; Koenig & Cohen, 2002; NCCAM, 2005). Such research is problematic in that there is lack of consensus on how to quantify spirituality or spiritual well-being in order for rigorous research to occur (Burkhardt & Nagai-Jacobson, 2005). In general, researchers are consistent on two points: (1) religiosity/spirituality is linked to health-related physiological processes, including cardiovascular, neuroendocrine, and immune function; and (2) more solid evidence is needed. Nonetheless, recognizing the importance of spirituality in the lives of clients is important as nurses provide holistic care. Understanding the relevance of spirituality for both the nurse and the client enhances the compassion that is fundamental to the practice of nursing.

Controversies Related to PNI Research

Even though there are volumes of research in the field of PNI, the findings are still considered controversial. In general the issues concerning the studies are related to the use of animals for study, the retrospective nature of human studies, the multifactorial nature of stress and illness, and measurement problems. The problem with interpreting animal and retrospective studies has been addressed previously.

Multiple factors are related to stress and contribute to the illnesses, making it difficult to pull out one factor for study. The multifactorial aspects include the many different types of stress, different perceptions about the stressor, different genetic predispositions, and different coping strategies. Added to this are the different psychological functioning, age, nutritional status, sleep patterns, physical activity, use of alcohol or medications, and menstrual phases. With all of the factors involved, the sample sizes need to be much larger to be able to statistically evaluate the variables involved.

Measurement has been a problem in relation to immune function, stress, and symptomology of disease. Use of only one measurement of immune function has been known to miss important relationships that do exist. The use of peripheral blood for samples may be inaccurate because cortisol may result in changes in the migration of the peripheral cells. Also stress and personality variables have been included in some instruments to assess disease. This is especially true of diseases that are thought to have a psychological factor and diseases that have fatigue and pain as symptoms, such as AIDS, chronic fatigue syndrome, and cancer.

NURSING IMPLICATIONS

Even Florence Nightingale recognized the importance of nursing's role in producing a state of body and mind that would be conducive to healing (Hood & Leddy, 2006). Nightingale noted that healing could be promoted by paying attention to promoting comfort, hygiene, nutrition, and sleep. Recommended changes in the environment that were important in promoting adequate sleep were to reduce noise and client anxiety. The current PNI research gives further support to these beliefs of Nightingale and encourages further endeavors to reduce the negative effects of stress.

It is important for nurses to assess the client's level of stress, type of stress, sources of stress, perception of the stress, and effectiveness of coping strategies. Attention must be directed toward assisting the client in modulating the stress through measures like increasing social support, maintaining open communication in expressing emotions, using humor, and regaining control.

Many times with illness, people lose control over their environment. Regaining control, even if only in a limited way, can help ameliorate the stress. Clients need to be allowed to participate in their own care and to decide what parts they want control over, even if they are able to control only a small fraction of the care. For hospitalized clients who have been removed from their familiar home environment, nurses can still allow choices in the daily schedule, type of food within limits, type of music in the room, and timing and amount of visiting hours for family.

Clients undergoing stressful situations can be offered complementary and alternative stress reduction therapies. Such alternative methods should not be used to replace the standard medical treatments, but can be used to reduce anxiety and depression and to ameliorate the negative effects of stress. Interventions that can be tried include the following:

- relaxation techniques, including progressive muscular relaxation, meditation, and yoga
- selective awareness, including hypnosis and guided imagery
- biofeedback
- cognitive distraction involving hobbies or video games
- movement, including exercise and dance
- humor
- prayer

Because the responses to these therapies vary with individual clients, nurses should be able to guide clients in selecting an appropriate therapy or therapies. Further information about these interventions and how to use them is presented in Chapter 18.

SUMMARY

The nervous, immune, and endocrine systems are in constant biochemical communication using their chemical signals. These same chemical signals can also affect individual behavior and the response to stress. Disruption of this communication network in any way by factors related to the environment, existence of multiple diseases, or psychological state can exacerbate the infectious, inflammatory, autoimmune, and mood diseases that these systems guard against.

Health care professionals can no longer ignore current research in the field of psychoneuroimmunology associating the impact of the mind, the emotions, or the spirit on the health or well-being of the body or on the disease and healing processes (Dyer, 2002). Even though the studies do not always have consistent results, there is enough evidence to support the use of complementary and alternative therapies by health care providers to reduce the negative effects of stress and promote health of the body and mind.

Nursing theorists such as Florence Nightingale (Environmental Theory of Nursing), Martha Rogers (Science of Unitary Human Beings), Madeleine Leininger (Cultural Care Diversity and Universality), and others discussed in Chapter 2 reflect the rich tradition of nursing that incorporates a holistic philosophy of mind-body interconnectedness (Hood & Leddy, 2006). Lynn Keegan, leader in holistic nursing practice and education, has philosophized that "disease and distress can be viewed as opportunities for increased awareness of the interconnectedness of body, mind and spirit" (Bright, 2002, p. 42).

Objectives/Goals: Through participation in discussion of this case study, participants will have the opportunity to:

1. Identify stressors and conditions that contribute to stressors
2. Relate symptoms to the physiological effects of stress
3. Apply the General Adaptation theory
4. Discuss measures to cope with stress

Health Promotion Concern, History and Physical, Present Health Status, Past Health Status, Family History, and Social History

Doug Cunningham is a 38-year-old, white, non-Hispanic male returning to the university to study for a degree in architecture. He began college immediately after graduating from high school and completed two years, but dropped out after marrying his high school girlfriend. He is now a newly divorced father of three children ages 16, 12, and 7. He changed from working full time to part time at the construction company where he has been employed as a roofer for the past eight years. Child support payments take most of his paycheck, and he struggles financially each month. He was an only child, and the recent death of his parents has left him with a very small inheritance that he is using to finance his return to school. Returning to school was a decision he made in order to become more financially secure and to reach his dream of becoming an architect. Doug is 6 feet 2 inches tall and weighs 190 pounds. He had hepatitis during his sophomore year in high school and is at risk for hypertension because both his parents had it. His mother died after having a stroke and his father passed away following a massive myocardial infarction. Doug lives in a small three-room apartment and has his children with him every other weekend. He enjoys socializing with friends from work, eats out every day at fast-food restaurants, drinks one or two beers on the weekend, and has from six to eight cups of regular coffee per day. He stopped smoking after the birth of his first child, but began again during his first semester back in college. He exercises daily by doing sit-ups and push-ups. He studies every night for at least five hours and sleeps only four or five hours nightly compared to his usual seven hours. He admits to feeling exhausted and "on edge." Although he says that he does his best when he "pushes" himself, he reveals that he feels extremely anxious about taking exams and feels pressured to make all A's because he is the oldest in all his classes. He takes one multivitamin daily (seven per week) and two full-strength aspirin for headaches (about 14 per week). Doug is concerned about the effect that stress is having on him and wants to know how to better manage it.

Review of Pertinent Domains

Biological Domain

Physical examination reveals a well-developed and generally physically healthy middle-aged male. Vital signs were: blood pressure 126/74, pulse 88, respirations 18. A two-inch healing abrasion (scratch) is noted behind his right ear.

Neurological: Experiences dull headaches about three times weekly, especially in the evening while studying.

Gastrointestinal: Reports upset stomach usually two days prior to a major exam. Before an exam last week, he had two episodes of vomiting. He eats irregularly, and his diet is high in carbohydrates, sugars, and caffeine and is void of fruits.

Cardiovascular: Reports having a "pounding heart" several hours before an exam and during the night when he tries to sleep.

Integumentary: Has been noticing a fine rash on his neck, face, and arms that goes away after an exam. Rash is accompanied by itching, and he finds himself unconsciously scratching behind his right ear.

Nose and throat: Complains of "always getting a cold" after an exam, with scratchy throat, cough, stuffy nose.

Diagnostic testing: All of Doug's blood tests are within normal range.

Psychological Domain

Cognitive: Has maintained a 4.0 grade point average during the first semester back in college. Is aware that he is experiencing stress, stating that he has trouble concentrating and that his mind seems to "jump from one thing to another."

Psychological: States that he feels "good" about himself and that he is trying to better himself to make life better for his children. He commented that he is "afraid to fail."

Social Domain

Doug is alert, oriented, and able to communicate verbally with appropriate affect. He enjoys being with his children and friends. He admits having a strained relationship with ex-wife.

(continues)

Environmental Domain

Doug lives alone, interacting daily with fellow students or friends or both. He does not cook for himself and eats at fast-food restaurants.

Questions for Discussion

1. Identify two major stressors in Doug's life. Identify at least five conditions contributing to the stressors.

2. Doug knows that his symptoms are connected to stress, but wants to know how stress causes them. Explain this to him using the General Adaptation Syndrome theory and factors from psychoneuroimmunology.

3. Doug wants to know how he can manage stress. What are some ways that you can suggest?

4. What other risks to health are apparent in Doug's life that indicate a need for health promotion?

Key Concepts

1. The nervous system impacts the immune system through the neurotransmitter receptor sites on immune cells.

2. The sympathetic nervous system stimulates the secretion of catecholamines and encephalins from the adrenal glands, which modulate the immune system.

3. The HPA axis inhibits the immune function through secretion of glucocorticoids.

4. Immune function can be measured through antibody levels, lymphocyte activation by mitogens, and NK cell activity against tumor cells.

5. Communication between the neural, endocrine, and immune systems is done through chemicals such as catecholamines, glucocorticoids, serotonin, interleukins, interferons, endorphins, and encephalins.

6. Stress activates the sympathetic nervous system, causing increased circulating catecholamines and stimulation of the HPA system with increased secretion of glucocorticoids and endorphins.

7. Normal life stressors that can have negative effects on the immune system include examinations, bereavement, childbirth, depression, loneliness, and hopelessness.

8. Immunoenhancement has been demonstrated through the use of social support, relaxation therapy, movement, biofeedback, guided imagery, cognitive distraction, humor, hypnosis, exercise, and prayer.

Learning Activities

1. Find three nursing research studies focusing on the influence of stress on illness and identify their implications for nursing practice.

2. Reflect on stress management techniques you use to manage your personal stress. Make a list of these.

3. Share and compare your stress management strategies with fellow nursing students.

True/False Questions

1. T or F Mind-body dualism is a harmonious blending of the mind and body, where one is affected by the other.

2. T or F The chief messengers of the sympathetic nervous system are the two catecholamines epinephrine and norepinephrine.

3. T or F NK cells are lymphocyte cells that do not require prior exposure to the antigen for activation.

4. T or F The three major areas of research in psychoneuroimmunology include the effect of negative stressors, the effect of microorganisms and disease, and the effect of medication on stress levels.

5. T or F Chronic activation of cortisol can result in cardiovascular disease.

6. T or F Researchers have found that there is a direct link between stress and the development of cancer in humans.

Multiple Choice Questions

1. Which of the following characterizes the alarm stage in Selye's General Adaptation Syndrome theory?
   a. Decreased cortisol levels in the circulatory system
   b. Decreased pituitary gland activity
   c. Increased parasympathetic nervous system activity
   d. Increased sympathetic nervous system activity

2. Which of the following is not a characteristic of the stress response?
   a. Increased urine flow
   b. Decreased pupil size
   c. Decreased muscle tone
   d. Increased gastric motility

3. Which one of the following is the amino acid responsible for major communication that unites and coordinates all the cells, tissues, glands, organs, and systems of the body?
   a. Cortisol
   b. Epinephrine
   c. Neuropeptides
   d. T lymphocytes

4. Which of the following would be the most immediate nursing action for appropriate crisis intervention?
   a. Assist in developing a plan for action and commitment to the plan.
   b. Guide rational thought processes.
   c. Help to identify personal coping skills, resources, and support systems.
   d. Provide for physical and emotional safety.

Websites

http://www.stress.org American Institute of Stress. A nonprofit organization established in 1978 at the request of Hans Selye to serve as a clearinghouse for information on all stress-related subjects. The Institute publishes a monthly newsletter, *Health and Stress.*

http://www.cmbm.org Center for Mind-Body Medicine. Includes a list of online resources and training programs sponsored by the Center, including Mind-Body-Spirit Medicine.

http://www.healthy.net HealthWorld Online offers a general overview of mind-body medicine, including articles such as Introduction to Mind/Body Medicine, Mind/Body Therapies, and Mind/Body Approaches to Health Disorders. Includes links to interviews with Larry Dossey, MD, Deepak Chopra, MD, and James Gordon, MD.

http://www.nicabm.com/ National Institute for Clinical Applications of Behavioral Medicine. Offers continuing education on mind-body topics for health care practitioners.

Organizations

American Holistic Nurses Association
P.O. Box 2130
Flagstaff, AZ 86003-2130
Tel: (800) 278-2462
Email: info@ahna.org

American Holistic Nurses Association (AHNA) is a nonprofit educational organization open to nurses and other individuals interested in holistically oriented health care practices throughout the United States and the world. AHNA supports the education of nurses, allied health practitioners, and the general public on health-related issues.

National Institute for Clinical Applications of Behavioral Medicine
P.O. Box 523
6D Ledgebrook Drive
Mansfield Center, CT 06250
Tel: (203) 456-1153
http://www.nicabm.com/

This group offers training for mind-body practices and techniques for health practitioners.

Videos

1. **An Introduction to the Mind/Body Medical Institute** (Herbert Benson, MD). Introduces the field of mind-body medicine and the work of the M/BMI. Tapes can be ordered online at http://www.mbmi.org/shop/.

2. **The Biophysiology of Stress** (Richard Friedman). Describes the psychological, behavioral, and biological consequences (acute and chronic) of exposure to stress. Emphasizes ways in which the perception of stress changes internal physiology and the way these changes can affect the development of physical illnesses. Tapes can be ordered online at http://www.mbmi.org/shop/.

3. **Body, Mind and Soul** (Deepak Chopra, MD). Provides an introduction to the practice of Ayurveda, a system of health care that treats the whole person, operating on the guiding principle that the mind exerts the deepest influence on the body. Dr. Chopra addresses such questions as: What are the mechanics of perception? What is the body and what is the mind? Does the soul really exist?

4. **Energetics of Healing** (Caroline Myss, PhD). Sounds True, Boulder, CO. Using computer graphics created especially for this program, Dr. Myss pulls back the body's energy anatomy and discusses the chakra centers and correlates them with daily practices for learning the physical language of the spirit—and the spiritual language of the body.

5. **Recovering the Soul: A Scientific and Spiritual Search** (Larry Dossey, MD). Dr. Dossey details scientific data that suggest a spiritual dimension of the individual person and of the person in relation to others. He suggests ways in which we might honor our soul-based dimensions.

Audiotapes and CDs

1. **Basic Relaxation/Mindfulness Meditation** (Olivia Hoblitzelle). Reviews the relaxation response and key techniques such as breath awareness, body scan relaxation, and the use of a focus word. Provides breath and awareness as "primary tools" that enable relaxation response to be incorporated into daily activities. Tapes can be ordered online at http://www.mbmi.org

2. **Nurturing Your Immune System** (Lynn W. Brallier, RN, MSN, PhD). Addresses immune functioning and stress. Selections can be ordered by calling (888) 553–4010.

3. **Why People Don't Heal: Spiritual Madness, Spiritual Power, Spiritual Practice** (Caroline Myss). Discusses the connection between the mind, body, and healing. Audiotapes can be ordered online at http://www.amazon.com or http://www.amazon.ca

4. **Self-Empathy/Nurturing Change** (Peg Baim, RN, MS, NP). Uses peaceful and rhythmic music with guided meditation to counter anxiety, enhance self-awareness, and enhance total well-being. Tapes can be ordered online at http://www.mbmi.org

5. **Sound Body, Sound Mind** (Andrew Weil, MD). One-hour tape that includes eight meditations for optimum health. Tapes can be ordered online at http://www.amazon.com or http://www.bn.com

References

Aneshensel, C. S., Botticello, A. L., & Yamamoto-Mitani, N. (2004). When caregiving ends: The course of depressive symptoms after bereavement. *Journal of Health & Social Behavior, 45*(4), 422–440.

Bachman, J. (2004, June). Depression in disease management practices for chronic conditions. *Depression in Primary Care.* Retrieved January 16, 2006, from http://www.wpic.pitt.edu/dppc/downloads/Depression

Barnes, P. M, Powell-Griner, E., McFann, K., & Nahin, R. L. (2004, May 27). Complementary and alternative medicine use among adults: United States, 2002. *CDC Advance Data Report #343.* Retrieved June 13, 2006, from http://www.nccam.nih.gov/news/report.pdf

Beaton, D. (2003, November). Effects of stress and psychological disorders on the immune system. Retrieved December 16, 2006, from http://www.personalityresearch.org/papers/beaton.html

Ben-Arye, E., Ziv, M., Frenkel, M., Lavi, I., & Rosenman, D. (2003). Complementary medicine and psoriasis: Linking the patient's outlook with evidence-based medicine. *Dermatology, 207*(3), 302–307.

Benight, C. C., Harper, M. L., Zimmer, D. L., Lowery, M., Sanger, J., & Laudenslager, M. L. (2004). Repression following a series of natural disasters: Immune and neuroendocrine correlates. *Psychology & Health, 19,* 337–352.

Borysenko, J., & Dveirin, G. (2005). *Say yes to change.* Carlsbad, CA: Hay House.

Bright, M. A. (2002). *Holistic health and healing.* Philadelphia: F. A. Davis.

Burkhardt, M. A., & Nagai-Jacobson, M. G. (2005). Spirituality and health. In B. M. Dossey, L. Keegan, & C. E. Guzzetta (Eds.), *Holistic nursing: A handbook for practice* (4th ed.). Sudbury, MA: Jones & Bartlett.

Christakis, N., & Iwashyna, T. (2003). The health impact of health care on families: A matched cohort study of hospice use by descendents and mortality outcomes in surviving widowed spouses. *Social Science and Medicine, 57,* 465–475.

Cruess, D. G., et al. (2005). Association of resolution of major depression with increased natural killer cell activity among HIV-seropositive women. *American Journal of Psychiatry, 162*(11), 2125–2130.

Cruise, B. A., Xu, P., & Hall, A. K. (2004). Wounds increase activin in skin and a vasoactive neuropeptide in sensory ganglia. *Developmental Biology, 271*(1), 1–10.

Dyer, K. A. (2002). *Psychoneuroimmunology (PNI).* Retrieved January 15, 2006, from http://www.journeyofhearts.org

Dykeman, B. F. (2005). Cultural implications of crisis intervention. *Journal of Instructional Psychology, 32*(1), 45–48.

Engler, H., Bailey, M. T., Engler, A., & Sheridan, J. F. (2004). Effects of repeated social stress on leukocyte distribution in bone marrow, peripheral blood and spleen. *Journal of Neuroimmunology, 148*(1–2), 106–115.

Etnyer, A., Rauschhuber, M., Gilliland, I., Cook, J., Mahon, M., Allwein, D., et al. (2005). Cardiovascular risk among older Hispanic women. *American Association of Occupational Health Nurses Journal, 54*(3), 120–128.

Evans, D. L., Ten Have, T. R., Douglas, S. D., et al. (2002). Association of depression with viral load, CD8 T lymphocytes, and natural killer cells in women with HIV infection. *American Journal of Psychiatry, 159,* 1752–1759.

Flowers, D. L. (2005). Culturally competent nursing care for American Indian clients in a critical care setting. *Critical Care Nursing, 25*(1), 45–50.

Garrish, M. (2005). Stress: The mind-body connection. *WebMed Live Events Transcript (October 6, 2005).* Retrieved January 16, 2006, from http://www.webcenter.health.webmd.netscape.com

Gibran, J. S., et al. (2002). Diminished neuropeptide levels contribute to the impaired cutaneous healing response associated with diabetes mellitus. *Journal of Surgical Research, 108*(1), 122–128.

Glaser, R., & Kiecolt-Glaser, J. (2005). Stress damages immune system and health. *Discovery Medicine, 5*(26), 165–169.

Glassey, D. J. (2001). *Body work and neuropeptides: The molecules of healing.* Retrieved January 14, 2006, from http://www.healtouch.com/csft/bodywork.html

Golden-Kreutz, D. M., & Andersen, B. L. (2004). Depressive symptoms after breast cancer surgery: Relationships with global, cancer-related, and life event stress. *Psycho-Oncology, 13,* 211–220.

Holmes, T. H., & Rahe, R. H. (1967). The social readjustment rating scale. *Journal of Psychosomatic Research, 11*(2), 213–218.

Hood, L., & Leddy, S. (2006). *Leddy and Pepper's conceptual bases of professional nursing.* Philadelphia: Lippincott Williams & Wilkins.

Jones, J. (2003). Stress responses, pressure ulcer development and adaptation. *British Journal of Nursing, 12,* 17–23.

Kanel, K. (2006). *Guide to crisis intervention.* Belmont, CA: Wadsworth.

Kiecolt-Glaser, J. K., & Glaser, R. (2002). Depression and immune function: Central pathways to morbidity and mortality. *Journal of Psychosomatic Research, 53,* 873–876.

Koenig, H. G., & Cohen, H. J. (Eds.). (2002). *The link between religion and health: Psychoneuroimmunology and the faith factor.* Oxford, England: Oxford University Press.

Laubmeier, K. K., & Zakowski, S. G. (2004). The role of objective versus perceived life threat in the psychological adjustment to cancer. *Psychology and Health, 19*(4), 425–437.

Levy, E. (2002). Psychophysiology of mind-body healing. In M. A. Bright (Ed.), *Holistic health and healing* (pp. 55–69). Philadelphia: F. A. Davis.

Mailoo, V. J., & Williams, C. J. (2004). Psychoneuroimmunology: A theoretical basis for occupational therapy in oncology? *International Journal of Therapy & Rehabilitation, 11*(1), 7–12.

McCance, K. L., & Huether, S. E. (2006). *Pathophysiology: The biologic basis for disease in adults and children* (5th ed.). St. Louis: Mosby-Elsevier.

McEwen, B. (2004). Protection and damage from acute and chronic stress: Allostasis and allostatic overload and relevance to the pathophysiology of psychiatric disorders. *Annals of the New York Academy of Sciences, 1032*, 1–7. Retrieved January 16, 2006, from http://www.annalsnyas.org/cgi/content/abstract/1032/1/1

Moss, D., McGrady, A., Davies, T. C., & Wickramasekera, I. (2003). *Handbook of mind-body medicine for primary care*. Thousand Oaks, CA: Sage.

National Cancer Institute (NCI) (n.d.). Psychological stress and cancer. *National Cancer Institute Fact Sheet*. Retrieved January 16, 2006, from http://www.cancer.gov/cancertopics/factsheet/Risk/stress

National Center for Complementary and Alternative Medicine (NCCAM). (2005). *Prayer and spirituality in health: Ancient practices, modern science, 12*(1). Retrieved June 13, 2006, from http://www.nccam.nih.gov

National Psoriasis Foundation. (2005). Alternative approaches to psoriasis treatment. Retrieved January 16, 2006, from http://www.psoriasis.org/treatment/psoriasis/alternative/mind_body.php

Phillips, A. C., Carroll, D., Burns, V. E., Ring, C., Macleod, J., and Drayson, M. (2006). Bereavement and marriage are associated with antibody response to influenza vaccination in the elderly. *Brain, Behavior, and Immunity, 20*(3), 279–289.

Pitt, M. A. (2005). Development and psychometric evaluation of the revised university student hassles scale. *Educational and Psychological Measurement, 65*(6), 984–1010.

Pressman, S. D., Cohen, S., Miller, G. E., Barkin, A., Rabin, B. S., & Treanor, J. J. (2005). Loneliness, social network size and immune response to influenza vaccination in college freshmen. *Health Psychology, 24*(3), 297–306.

Research reveals biology of harmful stress. (2003). *Harvard Women's Health Watch, 11*(1), 1.

Robles, G. F., Glaser, R., & Kiecolt-Glaser, J. K. (2005). Out of balance: A new look at chronic stress, depression, and immunity. *Current Directions in Psychological Science, 14*(2), 111–115.

Rosenbluh, E. (2002). Emotional first-aid. Retrieved June 12, 2006, from http://www.emotionalfirstaid.com.

Sarafino, E. P., & Ewing, M. (1999). The hassles assessment scale for students in college: Measuring the frequency and unpleasant-ness of and dwelling on stressful events. *Journal of American College Health, 48*(2), 75–83.

Schwecke, L. H. (2003). Anxiety, coping, and crisis. In N. L. Keltner, L. H. Schwecke, & C. E. Bostrom (Eds.), *Psychiatric nursing* (pp.120–129). St. Louis: Mosby.

Seeman, T. E., Dubin, L. F., & Seeman, M. (2003). Religiosity/spirituality and health: A critical review of the evidence for biological pathways. *American Psychologist, 58*(1), 53–63.

Segerstrom, S. C., & Miller, G. E. (2004). Psychological stress and the human immune system: A meta-analytical study of 30 years of inquiry. *Psychological Bulletin, 130*(4), 601–630.

Selye, H. (1976). *Stress in health and disease*. Boston: Butterworth-Heinemann, Ltd.

Shealy, N. C., Norris, P. A., & Fahrion, S. L. (2002). *Mind-body medicines*. Retrieved January 14, 2005, from http://www.amsa.org/humed/camresources/C2.doc

Shor-Posner, G., Miguez, M. J., Hernandez-Reif, M., Perez-Then, E., & Fletcher, M. 2004, *The Journal of Alternative and Complementary Medicine, 10*(6), 1093–1095.

Tafet, G. E., & Bernardini, R. (2003). Psychoneuroendocrinological links between chronic stress and depression. *Progress in Neuropsychopharmacology, Biology, and Psychiatry, 27*(6), 893–903.

Vegas, O., Beitia, G., Sánchez-Martin, J. R., Arregi, A., & Azpiroz, A. (2004). Behavioral and neurochemical responses in mice bearing tumors submitted to social stress. *Behavioural Brain Research, 155*(1), 125–134.

Velamoor, R., & Mendonca, J. (2003, May). Chronic stress due to job strain. *Workplace Safety and Insurance Appeals Tribunal*. Retrieved January 16, 2006, from http://www.wsiat.on.ca/english/mlo/chronic_screen.htm

Yehuda, R., & McEwen, B. (Eds.). (2004). *Biobehavioral stress response: Protective and damaging effects*. New York: New York Academy of Science.

Bibliography

Benson, H. (1975). *The relaxation response*. New York: Avon.

Block, S., & Block, C. B. (2005). *Come to your senses: Demystifying the mind-body connection*. Hillsboro, OR: Beyond Words Publishing.

Mailis-Gagnon, A., & Israelson, D. (2005). *Beyond pain: Making the mind-body connection*. Ann Arbor: University of Michigan Press.

O'Brien, M. E. (2003). *Prayer in nursing: The spirituality of compassionate caregiving*. Boston, MA: Jones & Bartlett.

Roberts, A. (2005). *Crisis intervention handbook: Assessment, treatment, and research* (3rd ed.) Oxford, England: Oxford University Press.

Sorajjakool, S., & Lamberton, H. H. (2004). *Spirituality, health, and wholeness: An introductory guide for the health care professional*. New York: Hawthorne Press.

SECTION III

PROMOTING HEALTH THROUGHOUT THE LIFE CYCLE

CHAPTER 9
The Mother, Infant, and Toddler

CHAPTER 10
The Child

CHAPTER 11
The Adolescent and Young Adult

CHAPTER 12
The Middle-Aged Adult

CHAPTER 13
The Older Adult

Chapter 9

THE MOTHER, INFANT, AND TODDLER

Barbara A. Tucker, PhD, FNP, APRN-BC

KEY TERMS

amniocentesis
attachment
bruising
constipation
couvade

diarrhea
embryo
fetus
gestational diabetes
infant

isoimmunization
morbidity
mortality
pica
postpartum

screening
sexuality
teratogens
urinary incontinence

OBJECTIVES

Upon completion of this chapter, the reader should be able to:

- Examine health promotion strategies in the biological domain for mothers, infants, and toddlers.

- Identify nursing responsibilities for screening to promote the health of mothers, infants, and toddlers.

- Relate theories of cognitive and emotional development to health promotion strategies in infants and toddlers.

- Identify social networks and their importance in maternal and infant health.

- Describe occurrence, signs and symptoms, and nursing responsibilities relating to child abuse and neglect.

- Identify legislative actions designed to improve the health of mothers and infants.

- Describe parental and nursing responsibilities for promoting infant and toddler safety.

- Relate normal sexual development to strategies designed to promote sexual health in infants.

- Describe spiritual influences on health promotion in pregnant women, infants, and toddlers.

INTRODUCTION

Ideally, health promotion for the mother and infant should begin prior to conception. As the focus of health care moves from a disease focus to a preventive focus, preconception education and screening provide the opportunity to promote a healthy beginning for the infant and the mother. Attention to the health of the mother- and father-to-be prior to conception has the potential to dramatically reduce infant **mortality** (death rate) and **morbidity** (illness rate). Education for conception and parenting should begin in high school with information about promoting development of a healthy fetus, such as proper nutrition and avoidance of substance abuse and of anything that can lead to abnormal development of embryonic structures **(teratogens).** Information about the physiology of conception, maternal changes during pregnancy, fetal growth and development, and the psychological preparation for parenthood is also important. Counseling prior to conception can facilitate the identification and reduction of known risks. Appropriate preconception counseling helps promote physically and emotionally healthy parents, resulting in optimal prenatal, intrapartum, and postpartum maternal and fetal health and, ultimately, a healthy child and family.

Planned pregnancies occur less frequently than unplanned pregnancies. According to the latest statistics available, over 50 percent of pregnancies for adult women are unplanned, and 95 percent of teenage pregnancies are unplanned (Henshaw, 1998). This makes preconception counseling and advisement all the more important for teens as well as adult women. Health care providers should take advantage of every health care visit to discuss the potential for pregnancy and how women can protect themselves and their potential fetuses. The time of greatest vulnerability to environmental insult for a fetus is the first 17 to 56 days postconception (Brundage, 2002); however, many women will not even realize they are pregnant during this time. Almost 20 percent of pregnant women will not seek prenatal care before the end of the third month of pregnancy.

Although there have been major improvements in access to prenatal care, there has been little change in the incidence of a host of conditions affecting children and their families, such as congenital anomalies, preterm births, low birth weight, and maternal mortality. Once a pregnancy is established, some health promotion interventions may not be as effective. Preconception care has the potential to make a significant impact.

This chapter will cover health promotion for the mother, the infant, and the toddler. The biological, psychological, social, political, environmental, and sexual domains will provide a guiding framework.

THE MOTHER

A woman's health status, lifestyle, and history are important determinants of a healthy pregnancy outcome. Maternal health promotion strategies for preconception, pregnancy, and postpartum are discussed in the following sections.

Biological Domain

Knowledge of the biologic factors and physiologic processes involved in the functioning of the body before, during, and after pregnancy are of primary importance. Nutrition, screening, immunization, and activity will be covered in this domain.

Preconception

Prior to conception, access to safe, effective birth control and knowledge of the availability and safety of emergency contraception are critical to reducing the incidence of unplanned pregnancies. Table 9-1 discusses available birth control method choices, their effectiveness, and how they are used. Health care providers have the opportunity to provide preconception counseling each time women come in for personal care (annual exams or sick visits) or for care of their children (well child visits or sick visits).

Evaluation of present dietary habits and preferences is an important part of preconception nutritional counseling. The potential mother's diet should include good sources of iron, calcium, and B vitamins. The diet should be low in fat, but have sufficient calories to maintain her normal weight. Lean meats, dried beans, whole grain cereals and breads, and dairy products should be included in the diet. Vigorous dieting, eating disorders, and extreme exercise may lead to irregular or anovulatory menstrual cycles, making it difficult to conceive. There is an increased risk of developing pregnancy-induced hypertension, preeclampsia, and gestational diabetes in women who are overweight or obese at the start of a pregnancy (Goldberg, 2003). Underweight or overweight conditions should be managed prior to trying to become pregnant. The diet should be supplemented with 0.4 mg of folic acid per day to reduce the risk of having an infant with a neural tube disorder, such as spina bifida or anencephaly. This supplementation is in addition to a diet rich in folic acid sources such as fortified grains and dark green, leafy vegetables. In fact, all women capable of pregnancy should be encouraged to take folate supplementation. If a woman has a history of having an infant with a neural tube disorder, she should be instructed to take 4 mg per day beginning at least one month before conception and continuing through the first three months of pregnancy.

A healthy diet is important for potential fathers-to-be, too. The minerals zinc and selenium are important to improving sperm production, and the diet should include foods that contain adequate amounts of these nutrients, such as whole grain breads and cereals, beans, broccoli, and lean meats.

Genetic history screening is important for the prospective mother and father, including a review for previous preterm or low birth weight babies, children with significant malformations, sickle-cell or thalassemic anemias, Tay-Sachs disease, cystic fibrosis, any syndromes or associations, and congenital hearing loss. Genetic counseling should be recommended when any of these conditions is present in the background of either potential parent. Older couples need counseling about a potential chromosomal abnormality causing Down Syndrome and education about the availability of testing.

The prospective mother should be screened for medical conditions such as diabetes mellitus, seizure disorders, anemia, hypertension, renal disease, deep vein thrombosis, phenylketonuria (PKU), depression, and psychiatric disorders. These conditions can potentially put both mother and fetus at risk both because of the disease and the teratogenic effects of the medications used to treat them. Women with documented diabetes need preconception counseling because the most common anomalies in infants born to diabetic women are to organs that develop in the first seven to eight weeks of gestation. Controlling blood glucose both prior to and during the first months of pregnancy can help reduce these anomalies (Korenbrot, Steinberg, Bender, & Newberry, 2002). Women with PKU need to begin dietary restrictions at least three months prior to conception. All prescription and over-the-counter medications and supplements should be reviewed for potential teratogenic effects. Medications for seizure disorders have a potential for being teratogens. The decision whether to continue or discontinue them should be made by the potential mother and her health care provider after weighing the risks to the fetus versus the benefits to the mother. Dental work should be done prior to the initiation of the pregnancy in order to avoid unnecessary exposure to x-rays and medications.

Additional screening should include evaluation of immunizations and infectious disease risk. Women planning pregnancy should be up-to-date on the rubella,

TABLE 9-1 Birth Control Methods

Method	Choices	Effectiveness	How to Use
Hormonal contraceptives prevent pregnancy by:	Transdermal patch	99%	Apply once a week for three weeks in a row; Week four without patch.
• Preventing the ovary from releasing an egg into a fallopian tube	Oral contraceptive (The Pill)	99%	Take daily, at approximately the same time.
• Thickening cervical mucus, making it difficult for sperm to enter the uterus to fertilize the egg	Contraceptive injection	99%	Injected monthly or every three months.
• Thinning the lining of the endometrium to prevent implantation	Progestin-releasing device (IUD)	99%	Inserted by health care provider into the uterus.
	Vaginal ring	99%	Worn in vagina for three weeks in a row; Week four without ring
Nonhormonal contraceptives prevent pregnancy by:	Male condom	97%	Use a new one every time before sex.
• Providing a barrier against sperm	Female condom	95%	Use a new one every time before sex.
• Interfering with sperm movement	Intrauterine device (IUD)	99%	Inserted by health care provider into the uterus
• Creating a difficult environment for sperm to travel	Spermicides (foams, jellies, creams, suppositories)	94%	Inserted no more than one hour before sex. Use with vaginal barrier increases effectiveness.
	Diaphragm	94%	Inserted up to six to eight hours before sex. Spermicide must be applied each time.
	Cervical cap	84–91%	Inserted up to 48 hours before sex Spermicide must be applied each time.
Nonhormonal permanent methods prevent pregnancy by:	Microinsert	99%	Insert placed into each fallopian tube.
• Providing a barrier against sperm	Surgical sterilization	99%	Surgical interruption of fallopian tubes.
• Interfering with sperm movement	Vasectomy	99%	Surgical interruption of vas deferens.

varicella, and hepatitis B immunizations, because these viruses are known to place a fetus at risk (Gottesman, 2004). A tetanus booster is necessary every 10 years. Women also should be screened for human immunodeficiency virus (HIV) and for syphilis to decrease the risk of transmission to the fetus.

Potential mothers-to-be should be encouraged to have an exercise program that can be continued during pregnancy. Aerobic and strength-conditioning exercises that produce a better state of fitness prior to conception will help reduce risks of obesity, gestational diabetes, pregnancy-induced hypertension, and physical complaints during pregnancy.

Women and men who are considering pregnancy should avoid alcohol or have no more than two drinks a week. Binge drinking should be strictly avoided. Prenatal exposure to alcohol can cause a range of physical, mental, behavioral, and/or learning disabilities. Alcohol also affects the absorption and utilization of folate, which is necessary to prevent neural tube disorders.

Avoidance of tobacco and illegal drugs should also be stressed for both the mother- and father-to-be because these substances can affect both fertility and fetal development. The dangers to the fetus from smoking—impaired fetal growth and low birth weight—are well documented. Cessation strategies can be discussed along with the benefits of quitting. Even reducing smoking as much as possible can be of benefit. Cocaine, heroin, marijuana, and other illegal drugs have a negative impact on the developing fetus and the newborn. Pregnant women with drug addictions may suffer from poor nutrition or altered immunity and can expose their unborn babies to hepatitis B and HIV infection, placing newborns at risk for drug withdrawal and low birth weight as well as other complications.

Pregnancy

Pregnancy (gestation) normally lasts approximately 40 weeks, nine calendar months, 10 lunar months, or three trimesters. Gestational age is calculated from the first day of the last normal menstrual period, assuming the woman has a 28-day cycle. From conception to eight weeks, the product of pregnancy is termed an **embryo.** From the eighth week until delivery, it is a **fetus.** An **infant** is the live-born individual from the moment of birth until one year of life. The diagnosis of pregnancy is usually made on the basis of a history of amenorrhea (cessation of menses), an enlarging uterus, and a positive pregnancy test. The approximate date of labor onset can be estimated by using Naegele's Rule: counting back 90 days (three months) from the first day of the last menstrual period and adding seven days and one year to that date.

Over 4 million women give birth each year in the United States. Two to three pregnant women die of pregnancy complications each day (Jones, 2004). Some of the leading causes of pregnancy-related deaths are hemorrhage, blood clot, hypertension, and infection. Box 9-1 lists the most common complications of pregnancy. Better access to health care, better quality of prenatal care, and health and lifestyle changes could help prevent over half these deaths. The following health promotion strategies discuss some of the interventions to help reduce pregnancy-related complications and deaths.

BOX 9-1 Common Complications of Pregnancy

- Ectopic pregnancy
- High blood pressure
- Complicated delivery
- Premature labor
- Depression
- Infection
- Diabetes
- Hemorrhage

Nutrition Pregnant women should eat a well-balanced, varied diet with an increase of 350 to 450 kcal per day in the second and third trimesters. Adolescents need nutrition for both the pregnancy and their own physical growth. Adolescents and vegetarians may benefit from the additional counseling of a registered dietitian. For women with a normal body mass index, a weight gain of 25 to 35 pounds during the pregnancy is recommended by the U.S. Institute of Medicine. Weight gains of less than 25 pounds have been associated with low birth weight and preterm birth, while larger weight gains have been associated with increased risk of overly large infants, cesarean delivery, and postpartum weight retention (Kirkham, Harris, & Grzybowski, 2005a). A multivitamin is recommended for pregnant women who are adolescents or who have poor diets or nutritional status. Individuals who feel their diets are not as good or varied as recommended also should take a multivitamin. In addition, pregnant women should have a daily intake of 1,000 to 1,300 mg of calcium, 1 to 4 mg of folic acid, and 30 mg of iron. Some multivitamin supplements are especially formulated for pre-pregnant and pregnant women and meet all the preceding requirements. High levels of vitamin A and D should be avoided (Goldberg, 2003).

Aspartame (Nutrasweet) and sucralose (Splenda) are probably safe during pregnancy, but saccharin should be avoided because it is known to cross the placenta and remain in fetal tissue (Goldberg, 2003). Small to moderate amounts of caffeine (150 to 300 mg per day) are safe. The average caffeine content of six ounces of the following common beverages is: coffee, 100 mg; tea, 30 mg; and soft drinks, 30–48 mg. Limiting caffeine is frequently advised due to a potential association with spontaneous abortion and low birth weight infants. Pregnant women should avoid raw eggs, raw or undercooked meat, unwashed fruits and vegetables, and unpasteurized milk and milk products as well as soft and blue-veined cheeses such as feta, Brie, and queso fresco because there is a risk of contamination with a bacteria that can cause spontaneous abortion, preterm delivery, or stillbirth. Delicatessen foods and liver/meat spreads have the same bacteria risk. According to the National Center for Complementary and Alternative Medicine, use of teas from herbal products such as chamomile, licorice, peppermint, and raspberry leaf may be unsafe in pregnancy. The FDA urges caution with all herbal products during pregnancy.

Many pregnant women experience nausea and vomiting, food aversions, and food cravings. Changes in hormone levels, intestinal motility, and a heightened sense of taste and smell have been suggested as possible causes (Goldberg, 2003). The majority of pregnant women experience nausea or vomiting or both, generally from the fourth to the sixteenth weeks of pregnancy. Health care providers are reluctant to prescribe antinausea medications except in cases of uncontrollable nausea and vomiting (hyperemesis gravidarum). Nausea or vomiting or both without additional pathological symptoms indicating illness (fever, abdominal pain, jaundice, etc.) is usually associated with a positive pregnancy outcome. See Table 9-2, Common Complaints of Pregnancy, for strategies to control nausea and vomiting in pregnancy. Food cravings and food aversions are unlikely to have an adverse effect on the mother's nutritional status or weight as long as the overall diet is nutritionally balanced and sufficient.

Pica (the ingestion of substances that have no food value) sometimes occurs during pregnancy. Clay and laundry starch are two common examples. Contrary to popular myth, this practice does not derive from physiologic craving, but seems to be a folk custom, especially in the southeastern United States. The major concern with pica is that it may substitute nonnutritious bulk for good nutrition.

In addition to nausea and vomiting, pregnant women experience numerous other discomforts such as constipation, hemorrhoids, fatigue, backache, muscle cramps, edema, and heartburn. Table 9-2 provides recommendations to help alleviate or reduce these common discomforts.

Substance Use Pregnant women should avoid or significantly limit alcohol use. Alcohol intake of more than two drinks a day has been associated with fetal mental retardation, malformation, growth retardation, spontaneous abortion, and behavioral disorders. Many women develop an aversion to the taste and smell of alcoholic drinks during pregnancy and find it easy to avoid use.

Smoking during pregnancy carries the risk of spontaneous abortion, low birth weight, and attention deficit disorder (Brundage, 2002). Stopping smoking by 16 weeks of gestation reduces the risks to the fetus. Adverse effects are dose related (the higher the number of cigarettes consumed, the more nicotine gets into the system); therefore, even reducing the number of cigarettes to fewer than 10 per day is helpful. Behavioral techniques, support groups, and bupropion (Zyban) may be used in smoking cessation efforts during pregnancy. Nicotine patches or gums are not recommended during pregnancy because they contain nicotine.

Use of illegal drugs during pregnancy can lead to severe problems for the infant. Spontaneous abortion, prematurity, growth retardation, and congenital defects are associated with maternal cocaine use. Intrauterine growth restriction, hyperactivity, and severe withdrawal syndrome are associated with maternal heroin use. Prematurity and jitteriness in the newborn may result from maternal use of marijuana (Brundage, 2002).

Screening Couples should be screened for potential genetic issues if they did not receive screening prior to conception. Areas to investigate should include family history of genetic disorders, previous fetus or child with a genetic disorder, or a history of recurrent miscarriage.

Testing for neural tube defects and chromosomal abnormalities such as trisomy 21 (Down Syndrome) and trisomy 18 (Edward Syndrome) is available through serum marker screening (human chorionic gonadotropin, unconjugated estriol, and α-fetoprotein levels), usually done between 15 and 20 weeks of gestation (Kirkham, Harris, & Grzybowski, 2005b). Newer, noninvasive screening for Down Syndrome can be conducted at 10 to 13 weeks of gestation and involves a combination of ultrasound and blood tests. Women should be counseled that there is approximately 87 percent sensitivity for these tests; therefore, some false positives and false negatives may occur. Pregnancies at increased risk for chromosomal abnormalities (see Box 9-2) should be offered **amniocentesis** (sampling of the amniotic fluid through a transabdominal puncture with ultrasound guidance) or chorionic villus sampling (obtaining a sample of the chorionic villi through the vagina). Amniocentesis can be performed after 15 weeks of gestation and CVS is performed at 10 to 12 weeks of gestation. Each procedure carries a small risk of spontaneous abortion. Testing for these abnormalities provides pregnant women the option of terminating the pregnancy at a safe time. If they choose not to abort, it provides the opportunity to prepare for an infant with possible physical or mental disabilities.

Health promotion requires early pregnancy screening for asymptomatic bacteriuria, syphilis, rubella, hepatitis B, and HIV infection. Testing for gonorrhea, chlamydia, and bacterial vaginosis may also be indicated. History of chicken pox and genital or orolabial herpes should be ascertained. A vaginorectal culture screening for group B streptococcal infection should be done at 35 to 37 weeks of gestation. Each of these infectious diseases has a potential for severe, if not fatal, complications for the fetus or newborn.

All pregnant women should be tested for immunity to rubella. Use of the vaccine for measles, mumps, and rubella (MMR) is contraindicated during pregnancy; therefore, women who are not immune should be cautioned to avoid anyone with a rash or viral illness. If a woman contracts rubella, administration of rubella serum

---

BOX 9-2   Risk Factors for Chromosomal Abnormalities

Mother older than 35 with a singleton pregnancy
Mother older than 32 with multiple fetus pregnancy
Fetus with an identified structural anomaly
Fetus with ultrasound showing increased fetal neck thickness
Mother with a previously affected pregnancy
Couple with chromosomal abnormalities
Mother with a positive maternal serum screen

TABLE 9-2 Common Complaints of Pregnancy

Problem	Recommendations
Nausea/Vomiting	Eat small, frequent, easily digested meals. Eat crackers upon arising. Drink fluids between meals, rather than with meals. Sip ginger tea or take ginger tablets. Take vitamin B6 supplement 25 mg three times daily. Avoid sights and smells that trigger nausea. Use acupressure or acupuncture.
Constipation	Use bulk-forming, nonnutritive laxatives. Use a stool softener, such as docusate sodium. Exercise regularly. Drink six to eight glasses of water daily.
Hemorrhoids	Avoid constipation. Apply topical anesthetics, witch hazel pads, and ice packs. Rest and sleep on the side. Avoid straining while defecating.
Fatigue	Get adequate sleep and rest. Make sure diet is nutritionally adequate.
Backache	Practice exercises of pregnancy (pelvic tilt, rocking back arch, etc). Avoid prolonged sitting or standing. Take warm tub baths. Use massage and relaxation techniques. Sleep on a firm, supportive mattress, in a side lying position, and use pillows to support back and legs.
Calf/Thigh/Buttock Muscle Cramps	Avoid stretching legs, pointing toes, excessive walking. Do calf stretching exercises. Ensure adequate (not excessive) intake of dairy and calcium products.
Edema	Lie in a lateral recumbent position one to two hours per day. Avoid constrictive clothing on legs and arms. Get regular exercise.
Dyspepsia (Heartburn)	Consume calcium carbonate, one to two tabs as needed. Avoid lying down, bending, or stooping for two hours after eating. Avoid restrictive clothing around waist. Avoid hot, spicy, fatty, gas-forming foods. Eat small, frequent meals.

immunoglobulin will reduce her symptoms, but will not alter the risk or the severity of congenital rubella syndrome in the infant. Immunization for rubella should be given postpartum.

All pregnant women should be vaccinated against poliomyelitis if not already immune. Diphtheria and tetanus toxoid should be administered if exposure to pathogens is possible. Women at risk also can be given the hepatitis B vaccine series. Immune globulin is recommended for pregnant women exposed to hepatitis A,

hepatitis B, tetanus, chicken pox, or rabies. Live virus vaccines should be avoided during pregnancy because of possible effects on the fetus.

Mothers-to-be should have blood type, Rh status, and atypical antibody titer screening early in pregnancy. Rh status refers to presence (Rh-positive) or absence (Rh-negative) of Rh antigen on the red blood cells. Rh-negative mothers can be sensitized (**isoimmunization**) through exposure to blood or blood products that contain an antigen not found in their blood cells, prompting production of antibodies to that antigen. If the fetus is Rh positive, the potential exists for maternal antibodies to cause severe damage to fetal blood cells, resulting in anemia, liver failure, and ultimately fetal death. The incidence of maternal isoimmunization has decreased due to the administration of Rh immune globulin (Rhogam). Rhogam is given to nonsensitized Rh-negative women during pregnancy at 28 weeks of gestation, following any procedure where a potential for mixing Rh-positive fetal and Rh-negative maternal blood exists, and after delivery if the infant is Rh positive.

Pregnant women should be monitored for **gestational diabetes** (diabetes that occurs during pregnancy as a result of hormonal changes). Approximately 2 to 5 percent of women develop gestational diabetes. Increased rates of hypertensive disorders, large infants, and cesarean delivery are associated with this disorder. Women should be screened at 24 to 28 weeks of gestation using an oral glucose tolerance test. Treatment may be dietary intervention or dietary intervention with insulin injection. The diabetes usually ceases with the end of the pregnancy; however, the mother is at increased risk to develop diabetes later in life.

Pregnant women with chronic diseases require more frequent monitoring. Poorly controlled insulin-dependent diabetes increases the rate of spontaneous abortion and fetal anomalies. It also increases the incidence of stillbirth. Uncontrolled chronic hypertension increases the risk of preeclampsia, renal insufficiency, and fetal growth retardation.

Additional screening for pregnant women involves exploring the risk of exposure to hazards in the workplace or at home. Working pregnant women must be aware of any possible job-related exposure to hazardous substances or ionizing radiation. At home, prolonged exposure to pesticides and to solvents such as paint thinners and strippers must be avoided.

Exercise, Activity, and Sleep Exercise recommendations during pregnancy have become less restrictive over the last decade. Physically fit women are encouraged to maintain a good fitness level throughout their pregnancy, but to avoid trying to reach peak fitness or train for competition. Aerobic and strength-conditioning exercises with a low risk of loss of balance or fetal trauma are recommended. Previously inactive women are encouraged to start a program of moderate exercise. Pregnant women who do not participate in some form of exercise are at increased risk for loss of muscular and cardiovascular fitness, excessive weight gain, gestational diabetes, pregnancy-induced hypertension, development of varicose veins, difficulty breathing, and low back pain. Table 9-3 lists other counseling issues during pregnancy.

Women may work during pregnancy as long as the pregnancy is uncomplicated and there are no known hazards in the job or workplace. Some modifications may need to be made, such as avoiding overtime hours, exhaustion, extreme temperatures, and noxious odors or fumes; taking breaks from constant standing or sitting; and avoiding strenuous work or lifting over 25 pounds.

Sleep is important during pregnancy. Many pregnant women complain of sleep difficulties, frequent urination, and fatigue, especially toward the end of pregnancy. Women who sleep seven to eight hours nightly with few disruptions have a shorter duration of labor, approximately 18 hours, as compared to 29 hours for women who sleep less than six hours or who awaken frequently (Lee & Gay, 2004). Women with decreased sleep time or frequent wakenings may be three to four times more likely to have cesarean deliveries. Health promotion includes encouraging women to schedule at least eight hours in bed at night and reminding them that they are "sleeping for two."

Postpartum

The **postpartum** period is defined as the time between delivery and the return of a woman's reproductive organs to the nonpregnant state, generally about six weeks. Just as in pregnancy, the woman is faced with enormous physiological changes necessary to accomplish physical restoration. Postpartum health promotion strategies in

TABLE 9-3 Counseling Issues During Pregnancy

Concern	Client Teaching
Exercise	Get 30 minutes of moderate exercise daily. Avoid activities with risk of falls or abdominal injuries. Scuba diving is not recommended.
Workplace	Avoid prolonged standing or sitting.
Travel	Air travel is generally safe until four weeks prior to expected delivery. On lengthy trips, walk for 5–10 minutes every two hours; urinate every two hours. Have a list of obstetricians in the area and a copy of prenatal records. Avoid travel to high altitudes or in unpressurized airplanes. Discuss additional precautions for foreign travel with health care provider.
Hot tubs, saunas	Avoid due to high temperature and possible fainting.
Hair treatments	Avoid hair dyes and treatments during first trimester.
Medications, supplements, herbal remedies	Check with health care provider before taking any medications (prescribed or over-the-counter), supplements, or herbal remedies.
Sex	Safe at any time during pregnancy except when membranes have ruptured or there is vaginal bleeding.
Constipation	Stool softeners may be needed to avoid constipation.

Ask Yourself

Cesarean Section Trend

The rate of cesarean sections in the United States is at an all-time high. According to the National Center for Health Statistics (2002), approximately 29.1 percent, or one in three, of all births, even those involving healthy, first-time pregnancies with full-term, single babies, are by cesarean section. The increase is attributed to fears of malpractice lawsuits if a vaginal delivery goes wrong, the preferences of mothers and physicians, and the decreasing use of vaginal births after cesarean section. What is your opinion of this trend? What are the potential consequences for the mother? For the baby? On the cost of having a baby?

the biological domain include nutrition, rest/sleep/activity, contraception, screening, and immunizations.

Postdelivery, the new mother should continue a well-balanced diet that includes protein foods, fruits, vegetables, milk products, and a high fluid intake. Continuation of a daily vitamin and mineral supplement is advisable. Caloric intake should remain about the same as during pregnancy. High fluid intake is especially important if the mother is breast feeding her infant. Lactation uses about 500 calories a day in the making of the milk and the energy contained in the protein, fat, and carbohydrates of the milk itself (Goldberg, 2003), but should not be touted as a magic way to lose weight following childbirth. The more weight gained during the pregnancy, the more the mother will need to lose following the pregnancy. Women who gain excessive weight during pregnancy are more likely to be overweight or obese following delivery.

Early ambulation following delivery provides a sense of well-being and promotes return of the reproductive organs to their prepregnancy state. This does not mean that the new mother should resume all her previous activities immediately after delivery. Rest is essential as the new mother adjusts to her new responsibilities. Many new mothers do not sleep well at night and should be encouraged to relax and possibly nap during the times that the infant is sleeping.

An exercise program to strengthen the muscles of the back, pelvic floor, and abdomen can be started within the first week postpartum; however, strenuous exercise should be postponed until approximately three weeks after delivery. New mothers can begin with a single exercise performed five times and repeated several times daily. Additional exercises can be added one at a time. Moderate exercise during lactation does not adversely affect breast milk production.

Pregnancy and childbirth are major risk factors for the development of **urinary incontinence** (the involuntary leakage of urine). Women with antenatal urinary incontinence, obesity, significant perineal trauma during delivery, large infants, and multiple pregnancies may be at increased risk for urinary incontinence. Urinary incontinence after childbirth may be temporary, but over 60 percent of women experiencing incontinence during pregnancy still have the problem 15 years later (JBI, 2005). Pelvic floor muscle exercises (also known as Kegel exercises) to strengthen the perivaginal and perianal musculature are recommended immediately postpartum to reduce or resolve the occurrence of urinary leakage.

Contraceptive methods should be discussed prior to discharge from the hospital following birth. Breast-feeding is not an effective birth control method. A woman may become pregnant even if her menses haven't resumed. The potential for pregnancy increases dramatically in breast-feeding women who have resumed their menstruation. Table 9-1 discussed birth control options.

Nonimmune women should be given the rubella vaccine prior to hospital discharge. Breast-feeding is not a contraindication. If the mother is Rh negative and non-sensitized, the Rh status of the infant should be checked and Rhogam immune globulin given if indicated.

Psychological and Sociological Domains

The psychological domain involves individual feelings, behavior, and changes in behavior. The social domain encompasses social networks such as families, social groups, organizations, and communities.

A significant psychosocial development in the life of a woman is the decision to parent. In an ideal world, every pregnancy would be a planned and wanted pregnancy, resulting in a loved and wanted child. Pregnancy, whether planned or unplanned, brings with it enormous emotional upheavals, adjustments, and consequences. Having a child will have a significant impact upon the individual as well as the social networks with whom the individual has a bond or maintains contact.

Preconception

Preconception care should include psychosocial evaluation and counseling. Couples should be encouraged to discuss the decision to attempt a pregnancy and how this will affect their lives and relationship. The couple's social, financial, and psychological readiness for pregnancy and commitment to parenthood should be assessed. In some communities, preconception classes are available through adult education programs. Preconception education has the potential to improve parenting skills and pregnancy outcomes. Providing knowledge about fetal growth and development promotes intrauterine bonding between parent and child. Preconception counseling gives prospective parents the opportunity to

make informed decisions and lifestyle adjustments to promote a successful pregnancy outcome.

Pregnancy

Psychological issues during pregnancy can include depression, emotional liability, and self-esteem and body image disturbances. The fluctuation of hormone levels during pregnancy can lead to feelings of anxiety, depression, sadness, elation, and confusion. Many women are unable to discuss their negative emotions and feelings for fear of being perceived as not wanting the pregnancy. Most women have self-esteem and body image issues as they go through a period of emotional adjustment to the bodily changes that are occurring. The main health promotion strategy is to help women realize that the feelings, emotions, and changes that are occurring are normal and will resolve following the pregnancy. Health care providers need to be able to recognize the spectrum of emotions that are normal as well as common mental health problems during pregnancy.

All pregnant women experience stress; however, high-level physical or emotional stress can be harmful for pregnant women, causing fatigue, sleeplessness, anxiety, poor appetite or overeating, headaches, and backaches. Pregnancy-related discomforts (nausea, fatigue, frequent urination, swelling, and backache) are temporary sources of stress which can be reduced with a healthy diet, regular exercise, and adequate rest and sleep. Expectant mothers should not expect to accomplish everything that they did before pregnancy. Seeking support and assistance from the partner, family members, relatives, or friends is important. The quality of social support given to a woman during pregnancy has been positively correlated with maternal-fetal attachment, later parenting skills, and children's intelligence (Slykerman et al., 2005). Health care providers may be able to find resources in the community as well as discuss stress reduction/relaxation techniques. The majority of women are able to adjust to the physical and psychological changes of pregnancy; however, some women need additional assistance.

Approximately 10 to 20 percent of pregnant women experience major depressive symptoms during pregnancy (Seehusen, Baldwin, Runkle, & Clark, 2005). Box 9-3 lists symptoms associated with depression. Identification of risk factors such as personal and/or family history of mood disorder, marital conflict, limited social support, and substance abuse should lead health care providers to screen for depression (Marcus, Flynn, Blow, & Barry, 2003). Behavioral therapy in the form of support groups, counseling, or psychotherapy is recommended for first-line treatment. There is limited data on the effect of antidepressant medications on the fetus (Dolan, 2005).

Screening should also include assessment for domestic violence. Domestic violence—also called domestic abuse, intimate partner violence, or battering—may include coercion, threats, intimidation, isolation, and emotional, sexual, and physical abuse. Screening questions can

Depressed mood lasting for two weeks or longer with five or more of the following:
- Sleep disturbances
- Lack of interest
- Feelings of guilt
- Loss of energy
- Difficulty concentrating
- Changes in appetite
- Restlessness or slowed movement
- Suicidal thoughts or ideas

From Diagnostic and Statistical Manual of Mental Disorders–TR *(4th ed.) by American Psychiatric Association, 2000, Washington, DC: Author.*

be found in Box 9-4. Violence in pregnancy is a serious health care issue and is associated with an increased risk of miscarriage, infection, preterm labor, placental abruption, and low birth weight babies. Unintended pregnancy increases the likelihood of violence two to four times. Abuse during pregnancy is linked with delay in getting prenatal care, depression, substance abuse, smoking, anemia, less than optimal weight gain, and unhealthy eating patterns (Saltzman, Johnson, Gilbert, & Goodwin, 2003).

Cultural and psychological factors (and possibly hormone changes) may cause the father-to-be to experience symptoms of pregnancy, too. It is estimated that

BOX 9-4   Screening for Domestic Violence

Preliminary Questions:
- Do you ever feel unsafe at home?
- Are you in a relationship in which you have been physically hurt or felt threatened?
- Have you ever been or are you currently concerned about being harmed by your partner or someone close to you?

Additional Questions for Positive Responses:
- Have you ever felt afraid of your partner or ex-partner?
- Has a partner or ex-partner currently or ever:
  - Pushed, grabbed, slapped, choked, or kicked you?
  - Forced you to have sex or made you do sexual things you didn't want to do?
  - Threatened to hurt you, your children, or someone close to you?
  - Stalked, followed, or monitored you?

from 11 to 65 percent of expectant fathers experience pregnancy symptoms such as nausea, weight gain, and difficulty sleeping (Polinski, 2005). **Couvade** is the medical term for sympathetic pregnancy. First used to describe the practice in which a father simulates labor and childbirth, the term now includes the sharing of pregnancy symptoms. Couvade seems to be a universal phenomenon and occurs across cultures.

Postpartum

Rapid hormonal changes, lack of sleep, and meeting the demands of the new infant frequently cause the new mother to experience mood swings, depression, difficulty concentrating, and lack of appetite. These "baby blues" usually start about three to four days after delivery and may last for several days. Baby blues is considered a normal part of early motherhood and usually

Research Note

Screening for Domestic Violence in Pregnant Women

Study Problem/Purpose: To examine the correlates of domestic violence during pregnancy.

Methods: A total of 197 pregnant women, ages 14 to 41, recruited from an inner-city clinic, were assessed for partner interaction during conflict, anxiety, depression, perceived stress, social support, negative interactions with the baby's father, and domestic violence. The sample was 49 percent African American, 45 percent Latina, and 6 percent White. Sixty-five percent were unmarried, and 59.6 percent were living with the baby's father. Median annual income was $10,000–$20,000 with 49.4 percent less than $10,000.

Findings: Seventeen percent experienced some form of violence within the last year and 13.3% experienced violence from their partner, with 4.8 percent commencing with the pregnancy. Those reporting violence were significantly younger and with lower incomes. African American women reported more verbal aggression than did Latinas. More frequent violence was associated with less social support and more negative interactions with the baby's father, rather than with cultural subgroup.

Implications: This study supports the need to screen pregnant women for domestic violence in medical settings and indicates that screening for psychosocial variables such as negative interactions may also help detect whether violence is occurring.

Sagrestano, L., Carroll, D., Rodriguez, A., and Nuwayhid, B. (2004). Demographic, psychological, and relationship factors in domestic violence during pregnancy in a sample of low-income women of color. *Psychology of Women Quarterly, 28,* 309–322.

goes away within about 10 days after delivery. Health promotion strategies for dealing with these normal feelings are found in Box 9-5.

Women who have more severe symptoms or whose symptoms last longer have postpartum depression. Box 9-3 lists common symptoms of depression. Risk factors for the development of this more serious depression include previous postpartum depression, previous diagnosis of depression not related to pregnancy, relationship problems, lack of social support, and stressful life events. Postpartum depression develops in 10 to 20 percent of women in the first six months after delivery (See-husen et al., 2005) and can have harmful effects on maternal-infant bonding, child development, and family functioning. Postpartum depression is considered a medical emergency that, left untreated, can lead to suicide and infanticide.

Postpartum depression affects the entire family. Approximately 25 to 50 percent of fathers will develop mild to moderate depression if the mother has postpartum depression. Paternal symptoms usually start later in the postpartum period and may last for up to a year (Goodman, 2004). Risk factors for paternal depression include a personal history of depression, maternal depression, and changes in the couple's relationship and functioning. Children of depressed parents are more likely to develop social, physical, and psychological impairments (Lewinsohn, Olino, and Klein, 2005).

The most important health promotion strategy is screening for and/or recognizing postpartum depression as early as possible—at the mother's postpartum visit or the infant's checkup. Postpartum depression is treated much like any other depression with support, counseling, and medication. Some women feel better within a few weeks, but others feel depressed for several months. Women must be counseled that help is available and that they can get better.

BOX 9-5   **Health Promotion Strategies for the Baby Blues**

1. Talk to someone about your feelings—a friend, relative, or health care provider.
2. Find someone to help you with child care, household chores, and errands.
3. Take 15 minutes a day for yourself—read, exercise, take a bath, or meditate.
4. Keep a diary and write down your emotions as a way of letting them out.
5. Don't be upset if you can't get everything done. Don't try to be a super mom.
6. Recognize that it's OK to feel overwhelmed with the changes and challenges.

Another psychosocial issue that may occur during the postpartum period relates to sibling rivalry. Parents can encourage older children to verbalize their emotions, role-play safe handling of a newborn with a doll, tolerate some regression, and give the older children individual attention each day. Encouraging grandparents and other visitors to pay attention to the older children first is also helpful.

Political Domain

The political domain in health promotion encompasses governmental efforts in legislating environmental and behavioral changes that promote health. Laws affecting the mother's mental and physical health during the preconception, pregnancy, and postpartum periods are discussed in the following sections.

Preconception

Women should have the right and the knowledge to make reproductive decisions about themselves. These rights include access to infertility care as well as contraception and abortion. There has not been any assault on access to infertility care, but contraception and abortion continue to generate controversy in the political and social arenas. It was not until 1965 that the use of contraception by married individuals was deemed legal. The 1965 Supreme Court decision in *Griswold v. Connecticut* struck down many state laws (albeit rarely enforced) against contraception. This right to privacy was extended to unmarried people in 1972. Today, 23 states mandate some form of contraceptive equity laws to impose requirements on insurers to provide coverage of FDA-approved prescription contraceptive drugs and devices on terms comparable to those of other prescription drugs. The equity law may contain a loophole or "refusal clause" which allows some entities or individuals that can demonstrate a religious objection to contraception to escape the requirements.

The availability and use of emergency contraception (EC) also has been a subject of political and legal controversy. EC is a safe, effective way to prevent pregnancy using the same hormones found in birth control pills. EC must be used shortly after unprotected sex. EC is best known for women who have been raped, but the methods are appropriate for women who have experienced condom breaks, women who did not use any method of contraception because they were not planning on having sex, or women who had unprotected intercourse for any other reason. Unfortunately, not all women are aware of the availability of emergency contraceptives and not all health care providers routinely inform women about the option. Although all the research and expert opinion have shown EC to be both safe and effective, the FDA decision to allow EC to be available without prescription has been delayed due to political pressure. Health promotion demands that women be informed about emergency contraception, which could prevent as many as a million unwanted pregnancies annually in the United States. A toll-free hotline and a website with information about emergency contraception are listed at the end of this chapter.

Throughout the centuries, unwanted and unplanned pregnancies worldwide have resulted in abortion, whether legal or illegal. In 1973, the right to privacy was extended to abortion in the *Roe v. Wade* Supreme Court decision, which legalized abortion. Recent legislation has reduced access and availability of safe, confidential abortions and reduced women's control over their own reproduction.

Pregnancy

Pregnant women are provided certain protections under the law during pregnancy. Although working women are not guaranteed paid maternity leave or insurance reimbursement during pregnancy, pregnant women do have protection against discrimination and, in many cases, are allowed unpaid leave. They also have protection against the risk of exposure to hazards in the workplace that might injure the fetus.

The Pregnancy Discrimination Act of 1978 requires employers with 15 or more employees to treat pregnant workers as any other employees with medical or disability conditions. It prevents an employer from firing a pregnant woman based on her pregnancy or a pregnancy-related illness or from forcing her to take a mandatory pregnancy or maternity leave. Pregnant women have the right to modified work tasks, to work as long as they are able, and to have their jobs protected during maternity leave.

Postpartum

The Family and Medical Leave Act of 1993 requires companies with 50 or more employees to allow a pregnant mother or her partner to take up to 12 weeks of unpaid leave in the 12-month period following the birth of their baby. Pregnant women may take this leave intermittently or for the full 12 weeks at one time. Typically, an employee must have worked a minimum of one full year with the company to quality for benefits under the Family Leave Act. Information about pregnancy rights and family leave can be obtained through the U.S. Department of Labor.

Environmental Domain

The environmental domain is defined as the external conditions and influences on an individual. A woman can be exposed to various chemicals in her work setting, her home, or other environments.

Preconception and Pregnancy

Exposure to chemicals should be avoided during the preconception period and during the first trimester, during which organogenesis occurs. Work areas should be

Nursing Alert

Seat Belt Use During Pregnancy

Motor vehicle crashes account for up to 70 percent of traumatic injury and death in pregnant women (Beck, Gilbert, & Shults, 2005). All pregnant women should use shoulder and lap belts when traveling in a car. The lap portion should be placed below the abdomen, across the upper thighs. The shoulder portion should rest between the breasts. Both belts should be worn snugly. Health care providers should discuss the consistent, proper use of seat belts periodically throughout the pregnancy.

well ventilated and protective gloves should be worn when dealing with chemicals such as household cleaning items. Chemical fumes, particularly from paint or turpentine, should be avoided and any chemical spills on the skin immediately washed.

Lead poisoning can cause mental retardation and central nervous system anomalies in the fetus. Homes built before 1980 may have lead-based paint on walls. Houses should be checked for lead before home improvements are done. Other sources of lead may be drinking water from lead pipes, unwashed fruits and vegetables, and solder from cans. Hobbies such as pottery making and leaded glass work may also expose the pregnant woman to an increased amount of lead.

There are environmental safeguards for the working pregnant woman. The Occupational Safety and Health Administration requires that employers provide either a workplace free of hazards likely to cause fetal death or serious harm or a written Material Safety Data Sheet, listing hazardous substances or ionizing radiation that might be encountered in the workplace. See the end of the chapter for additional information about teratogens.

Postpartum

A breast-feeding mother must remember that any environmental exposure that affects her may also affect her infant. Chemicals, medications, radiopharmaceuticals, and illegal drugs have all been shown to be transmitted in breast milk, sometimes in highly increased concentrations.

Sexual Domain

The sexual domain encompasses all the characteristics that differentiate the male and the female as well as the individual's expression of those differences. **Sexuality** is a broad term which includes not only the dimensions of sexual desire and sexual response but also the individual's view of self and presentation of self. The expression of an individual's identity and reflection of the basic need for emotional and physical closeness with another is a uniquely human quality.

Preconception

Health promotion prior to conception involves assessing the individual's knowledge and practice regarding sexuality as well as the health care provider's personal attitudes and values about sex and sexuality. Health care providers should be able to provide information about the effect of various health problems and diseases on sexuality and sexual functioning. Education about sexual functioning, safe sex practices, and the dynamics of a sexual relationship can enhance the positive aspects of sexuality. Individuals with sexual dysfunction should be referred to experts in sex therapy.

Pregnancy

Sexual desire and sexual response during pregnancy are affected by physical, hormonal, and psychosocial factors. Some women and men have increased sexual desire, while others may have less. Sexual activity during pregnancy is perfectly safe for women experiencing a normal pregnancy. Only women with a history of miscarriage or with a high-risk pregnancy may need to abstain. Many couples continue to have sex up to the time of delivery; however, different positions may be necessary due to the enlarging uterus (e.g., side lying, woman on top). Sex during pregnancy will not hurt the fetus. The pregnant woman may experience strong contractions during orgasm, but these should not be painful and are safe unless the woman is at risk for preterm labor. Toward the end of the third trimester, these contractions may help stimulate or strengthen labor and the semen deposited has chemicals that can help the cervix prepare for labor. Health promotion strategies include education for the couple about the nature of sexual response, the need for communication, and alternative forms of sexual expression during pregnancy.

Postpartum

Sexual relations may be resumed approximately two weeks following delivery; however, a return to prepregnant sexual response patterns may be delayed for up to 12 weeks postpartum because of decreased genital vasocongestion, vaginal lubrication, and orgasmic intensity. Interest in sexual activity varies considerably during the early postpartum period. Most women report low or absent sexual desire due to fatigue, weakness, painful intercourse, vaginal irritation, and fear of injury; however, the majority of women resume sexual relations six to eight weeks postpartum. A well-rested, emotionally supported mother may feel more interest in resuming the sexual relationship. Sharing of family tasks and responsibilities, sharing of child and infant care, alone time for parents, and loving communication will facilitate readjustment to the marital relationship. Other health promo-

tion strategies include use of water-soluble gels for lubrication, lubricated condoms, and positions to reduce depth of penetration. Breast-feeding mothers can nurse the baby prior to sexual intimacy if milk ejection during sex is a concern. Counseling about the fluctuations of sexual interest, strategies to reduce discomfort, the importance of sleep and rest, the value of emotional support and sharing of tasks, and contraceptive methods should be done before the new mother leaves the hospital.

Spiritual Domain

For some women, spirituality may be heightened during pregnancy and may be a source of personal support. Spirituality affects behavior. Religious beliefs, as part of spirituality, may become more important and can affect decision making, such as selection of the type of birthing experience or the naming of the newborn. If unresolved earlier in the relationship, conflicts may occur or become heightened in couples who have different religious faiths. Professional counseling may be needed to assist the couple to accommodate differences or accept differing religious beliefs or spiritual orientation in order to enhance the experience of pregnancy and parenthood. See Chapters 11 and 12 for information on spirituality related to young and middle-aged adults. Table 9-4 summarizes health promotion in pregnancy according to pertinent domains.

THE INFANT AND TODDLER

The infant mortality rate (the rate at which babies less than one year of age die) in the United States has declined more than 3 percent per year since 1950. The infant mortality rate for the year 2000 was 6.9 infant deaths per 1,000 live births (NCHS, 2002), the lowest ever recorded. This decline has been primarily attributed to decreased deaths from causes such as pneumonia and influenza, respiratory distress syndrome, prematurity and low birthweight, congenital anomalies, and accidents. Infant mortality rates are used to compare health and well-being of populations across and within countries.

Unfortunately, the United States ranks 28th in the world in infant mortality. This is largely due to disparities which exist among various racial and ethnic groups in this country, particularly African Americans, whose infant mortality rate for 2000 was 11.4 infant deaths per 1,000 live births. The increasing emphasis in the health care system on reducing disparities in health promotion and preventive care should lead to significant decreases in infant mortality in coming years.

There are numerous health promotion needs between infancy and age 3, many of which offer a significant opportunity to make an impact on the lifetime health of an individual. Because the infant is totally dependent

TABLE 9-4 Health Promotion in Pregnancy

Related Domain	Risk Assessment	Health Promotion Action
Biological	Nutrition	Well-balanced, varied diet with increased calories, calcium, and vitamin C and a folic acid supplement
	Exercise	Daily exercise
	Substance use	Avoidance of tobacco, alcohol, and unprescribed or illegal drugs or medications
	Genetic abnormalities	Screening for neural tube disorders and chromosomal abnormalities
	Infection	Screening for asymptomatic bacteriuria, syphilis, rubella, hepatitis B, HIV, and group B streptococcal infection
	Isoimmunization	Assessment of blood type, Rh status, and atypical antibody titer
Psychological and Sociological	Pregnancy complications	Assessment for gestational diabetes, pregnancy-induced hypertension, and growth abnormalities
	Psychological and physical well-being	Screening for depression and intimate partner violence
Political	Legal protection	Education about the Pregnancy Discrimination Act and the Family and Medical Leave Act
Environmental	Environmental hazards	Avoidance of exposure to toxic chemicals, fumes, lead, and ionizing radiation
Sexual	Sexual response	Education about the nature of sexual response and alternative forms of sexual expression

upon caregivers, health promotion strategies are carried out by the parents or other caregivers. The term caregiver here is used interchangeably with parent.

Biological Domain

The biological domain encompasses all the biologic factors and physiologic processes involved in the functioning of the body. The areas of nutrition, elimination, sleep and activity, immunization, and screening are addressed for the infant and toddler.

Nutrition

The most important nutrition health promotion strategy is to encourage the mother to breast-feed her infant (see Figure 9-1). Breast milk is the preferred source of nutrition for almost all babies for at least the first year of life. Breast milk contains the correct percentages of fat, protein, carbohydrate, and minerals needed for optimum

growth as well as immunoglobulins, antibodies, and enzymes to help protect the infant. Breast-fed infants have reduced rates of otitis media, respiratory infection, gastroenteritis, and atopic eczema (USPSTF, 2003).

National data from 1998 showed that approximately 64 percent of all mothers breast-fed postpartum, but only 29 percent were still breast-feeding by six months (USPSTF, 2003), even though it is recommended for the first year. One reason for quitting is concern about adequate milk supply. At 10 to 14 days postpartum, there is a normal transition from firm, dramatically full breasts to softer, less-engorged breasts. Many women assume this transition means a reduced supply; however, inadequate milk supply is usually a factor of an underlying health problem in the infant, ineffective suckling capability, or infrequent feedings (Page-Goertz, 2005). Maternal contraindications to breast-feeding are uncommon (maternal HIV infection and taking selected medications), but there are several risk factors for insufficient milk supply:

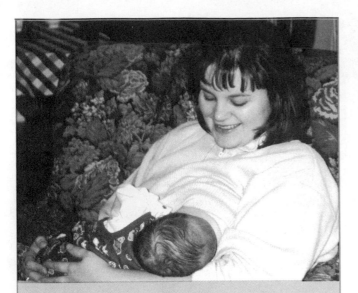

FIGURE 9-1 *Breast-feeding gives an infant the optimal start for growth and development. It is the preferred source of infant nutrition.*

BOX 9-6   How to Promote Breast-Feeding

Provide structured breast-feeding education and behavioral counseling programs led by specially trained nurses or lactation specialists during the prenatal period.

Encourage early maternal contact with the newborn through rooming-in and feeding on demand.

Avoid formula supplementation and provision of commercial discharge packs that contain samples of infant formula.

Encourage mothers to provide frequent, round-the-clock feedings.

Discuss the importance of adequate rest, diet, and fluid intake.

Teach mothers who are returning to work how to use an electric pump to maintain a sufficient milk supply.

Provide resources on breast-feeding and information about support groups in the area.

previous breast surgery, breast radiation, and endocrine disorders. Health promotion strategies to encourage initiation and continuation of breast-feeding are found in Box 9-6. The breast-fed infant does not get fluoride through the breast milk; therefore, regular supplementation is recommended after 6 months of age.

Cow's milk is not an appropriate nutritional source for any infant under 1 year of age. Cow's milk–based formulas with adjusted nutrient percentages and reduced mineral content provide appropriate, relatively inexpensive nutrition when the mother cannot or does not breast-feed. Infants who are fed formula should be on an iron-fortified infant formula. There is no scientific evidence that iron in the formula increases diarrhea, constipation, or colic. Breast-fed infants may need iron supplementation beginning at 6 months of age. This is why the American Academy of Pediatrics recommends screening of all infants for iron-deficiency anemia between 6 and 9 months of age. Infants fed premixed formula need fluoride supplementation just as breast-fed infants do. If powdered or concentrated formula is mixed with fluoride-containing water, no supplementation is needed.

Infants with an allergy or intolerance to cow's milk protein may also have an allergy to soy protein. A casein or whey hydrolysated formula is recommended instead of a soy-based formula. Table 9-5 compares the contents of breast milk, cow's milk, and prepared cow's milk–based formula.

Infants are not physiologically or developmentally ready for solid foods until about 6 months of age when they have sufficient control of their heads and necks to sit up with only a little help. A total milk diet of breast milk or formula is nutritionally adequate until that time.

Nursing Alert

No Sweet Treats for Infants

Honey in food or on pacifiers should be avoided during the infant's first year. Honey is an uncooked food and a known source of bacterial spores that produce a toxin which can cause infant botulism. Signs of infant botulism include constipation, weak suck and cry, generalized weakness, and apnea.

Solid foods should be introduced one at a time with new foods spaced several days apart to be able to assess for food intolerances. The sequence of food additions is largely a matter of preference; however, delaying the introduction of egg whites, wheat, corn, shellfish, and peanuts for at least the first year may reduce the development of allergies to these foods. Infants do not need sugar or salt added to foods to enhance flavor. The caregiver should read the labels of all prepared foods before feeding them to the infant. Unnecessary food additives should be avoided.

Toddlers usually consume "table" food. An important nutrition health promotion strategy for this age group is to serve a wide variety of fruits, vegetables, and meats, enabling the toddler to experience different tastes and textures. Toddlers may be at risk for inadequate

Nutrient	Breast Milk (percentage of total)	Cow's Milk (percentage of total)	Formula (percentage of total)
Protein			
Calories	7%	20%	20%
Casein	40%	80%	40–80%
Whey	60%	20%	18–60%
Fat			
Calories	50%	50%	30–54%
Linoleic Acid	7%	1%	10%
Carbohydrate			
Calories	42%	30%	40–50%
Minerals per 100 kcal			
Calcium (mg)	50	186	75
Phosphorous (mg)	25	145	65
Sodium (mEq)	1	3.3	1.7
Chloride (mEq)	2.1	6	2.7
Potassium (mEq)	1.6	4.6	2.3
Iron			
Content	0.3 to 0.5 mg/L	0.5 mg/L	0.5 mg/L
Absorption	50%	10%	4%

Adapted from Bowe's and Church's food values of portions commonly used *(18th ed.), by J. A. T. Pennington and J. S. Douglass, 2004, Philadelphia: Lippincott Williams & Wilkins.*

nutrition if the family does not eat a balanced diet with a wide variety of foods. A diet consistent with MyPyramid developed by the U.S. Departments of Agriculture and Health and Human Services is nutritionally sound. Chapter 14 has a detailed discussion of the role of nutrition in health promotion. Toddlers should not have a fat limitation in their diets because fat is needed during this time for the completion of brain development. Whole milk, rather than reduced-fat milk, should be used until 2 years of age. Toddlers eating a balanced diet with a variety of foods do not need supplementary vitamins; however, a "poor eater" may benefit. Fluoride supplements are needed if not supplied in the local water.

Elimination

Renal development is not complete until the end of the first year of life; therefore, an infant's urine is usually very pale with little odor. An infant who voids 6 to 12 times a day is getting sufficient fluid intake. Urination increases as fluid intake increases. The infant begins life with a relatively small bladder that gradually increases in size, resulting in increasingly longer periods of dryness. Prevention of dehydration is an important health promotion strategy. Promoting healthy renal functioning requires an awareness of conditions that lead to dehydration: fever, vomiting, diarrhea, elevated environmental temperatures, reduced fluid intake, and prolonged periods without fluid intake. Caregivers should be made aware of the need for increased fluids when these conditions occur.

Infant stools vary in consistency, color, and frequency, depending upon whether the infant is breast-fed or formula-fed. Breast-fed infants tend to have bright yellow, loose stools anywhere from five or six times a day to once every three to four days. Formula-fed infants tend to have lighter yellow, firmer stools anywhere from two or three times a day to once every three to four days. Health promotion involves educating caregivers about normal stooling patterns, diarrhea, and constipation. **Diarrhea** is defined as the frequent passage of watery, unformed fecal material. **Constipation** is defined as difficult or infrequent passage of hard, dry fecal material. Counseling caregivers about the wide variety of stooling patterns should help eliminate anxiety over whether the infant is having diarrhea or constipation. The knowledge that diarrhea stools are watery and may contain mucus, blood, or pus and that constipated stools are small, hard, and dry should also reduce unnecessary concern.

Toilet training is a developmental task of toddlerhood. Brain and spinal cord maturation takes approximately two years. The toddler is relatively unaware of body functions until about 18 to 24 months of age; therefore, attempting to initiate toilet training prior to readiness will certainly meet with less than satisfactory results. As a rule, boys are not ready to toilet train as soon as girls and they tend to take longer to toilet train than girls. Counseling caretakers to be aware of the physiological and developmental signs of readiness (or lack of readiness) for toilet training is a health promotion strategy which may positively influence an individual's elimination practices and concerns throughout the life span.

The majority of childhood constipation is functional, a result of the interaction between the child's development, gastrointestinal physiology, nutritional intake, and parental expectations. Organic or anatomic problems cause only 5 percent of constipation in children. Difficulty with expulsion and drying of the fecal mass in the colon are the most common causes of functional constipation (Mason et al., 2004). If the stool is hard and dry, then passing the stool becomes painful, and the child attempts to withhold the stool. As larger amounts of stool collect in the rectum, passage causes even more pain and even more withholding. A diet with adequate fiber intake (high-fiber breakfast cereals, breads, and crackers as well as fresh fruits and vegetables), a toilet-sitting schedule following meals, and positive reinforcement for stooling are health promotion strategies to prevent or treat constipation or both before it becomes chronic.

Sleep and Activity

Sleep patterns of the infant are related to the nervous system and growth. As the nervous system matures and the infant's rate of growth slows, the infant will have shortened sleep times and longer awake times. The infant goes from sleeping 80 percent of the 24-hour day at birth to 50 percent at 1 year of age through toddlerhood.

The major health promotion strategy in this area has to do with the recommended sleeping position for infants. Sudden Infant Death Syndrome (SIDS) is the leading cause of death in infants (CDC, 2004). Studies examining the incidence of SIDS found that sleeping in a prone (stomach down) position increased the occurrence. Infants sleeping on their sides also have an increased incidence; therefore, the American Academy of Pediatrics recommends that infants be placed in a fully supine (on the back) sleeping position (AAP, 2005). In addition, AAP recommends that infants sleep in the same room as adults (but not in the same bed) and that a pacifier be offered at naptime and bedtime for at least the first year. Soft bedding and soft objects in the infant's sleeping environment should be avoided. This "back to sleep" position recommendation only refers to infants during sleep.

Awake and observed infants should be allowed and encouraged to have some time on their stomachs for muscular and neurological development and to prevent flat spots on the occiput. As the infant matures and is able to turn from the supine to the prone position, the recommendation is that caregivers continue to place the infant in the supine position when putting the infant to sleep, but allow the infant to adopt whatever position is preferred. The benefit of the nonprone sleeping position has been significant. Within the first two years following publication of the recommendation, the rate of SIDS in the United States decreased by 15 to 20 percent and has declined by 57 percent since 1990 (CDC, 2004).

The toddler usually sleeps about 12 hours at night and takes one daytime nap. As the toddler matures, she or he may give up the daytime nap. The toddler's increasing independence may be exerted in resisting bedtime. The nurse should recommend a quiet bedtime routine to reduce physical and emotional stimuli. Reading a favorite story and taking a favorite blanket or soft toy to bed should help establish the structure and security needed by the toddler. A nightlight may also increase feelings of security.

Research Note

Pacifiers Prevent SIDS Deaths

Study Problem/Purpose: To examine differences in babies who died of Sudden Infant Death Syndrome (SIDS) and those who did not.

Methods: Researchers interviewed mothers or people who cared for 185 infants who had died of SIDS and 312 control subjects in 11 California counties. Those interviewed provided information about pacifier use during the baby's final sleep or the sleep the night before the interview, as well as details on other environmental factors related to sleep and SIDS risk factors.

Findings: Use of a pacifier during sleep was associated with a 90 percent reduced risk of SIDS, compared with babies who did not use pacifiers. Many of the babies who died of SIDS were not using pacifiers at the time of death. The reduction in risk of death held true across an interracially diverse population in every socio-demographic category and in every category of risk factors.

Implications: Use of a pacifier to quiet and comfort newborns can also reduce the risk of SIDS. The bulky handle of the pacifier may change the airway passage around the nose and mouth and prevent accidental suffocation by creating a way for air to pass around the baby's face.

From *Pacifiers Prevent SIDS Deaths: Study*, by A. Gardner, 2005, retrieved January 9, 2006, from http://www.medicinenet.com/script/main/art.asp?articlekey=55615&pf=3&page=1.

Infants receive their activity during play with themselves, with their caretakers, and with toys or other objects. Caretakers may need to be educated as to the importance to physical development of frequent stimulation through play; however, structured infant exercise programs have not been shown to be therapeutically beneficial for healthy infants. The infant's bones are susceptible to trauma, and the infant lacks the strength and reflexes for protection from external forces. Opportunities for touching, holding, face-to-face contact, and the use of safe toys will provide sufficient activity and motivation for infant physical development.

Obtaining sufficient activity and exercise is rarely a problem for the toddler. The ability to walk independently is only the first of many motor skill accomplishments. Toddlers, such as the ones pictured in Figure 9-2, seem to be constantly in motion as they learn, practice, and refine their motor skills. The health promotion strategy during this time is encouraging and reinforcing skill development by providing opportunities for safe new learning while understanding the toddler's sometime frustration with the new learning.

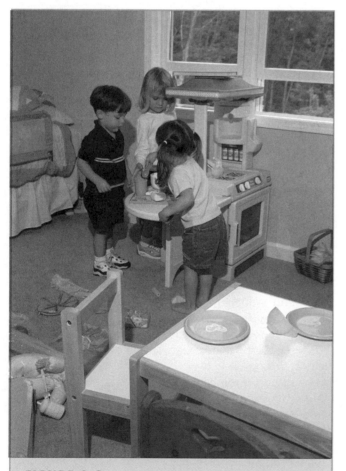

FIGURE 9-2 *Toddlers are in constant motion and need an appropriate place to expend their energy.*

Immunization

The first disease for which an immunization was discovered was smallpox, a disease from which approximately 20 percent died, and those who survived suffered from disfigurement and sometimes blindness. Edward Jenner successfully tested an immunization against smallpox in 1796. The discovery that certain infectious diseases could be prevented was a significant disease prevention strategy. Until this time, human beings were subject to sudden, devastating epidemics of infectious diseases.

The advent of immunizations changed the major cause of death from infectious diseases such as diphtheria, smallpox, and yellow fever to chronic diseases associated with aging. Vaccines, antibiotics, and improved sanitation are responsible for making infectious diseases a relatively minor cause of death in the United States. In fact, the global eradication of smallpox was certified by the World Health Organization in 1980 following a worldwide program of immunization and case hunting.

Immunization decreased the incidence of childhood diseases such as measles, diphtheria, rubella, and pertussis to such an extent that the general public became complacent about following immunization schedules. These common childhood diseases, which were almost gone during the 1970s, are coming back. Encouraging caregivers to follow the recommended immunization schedule depicted in Table 10-2 as closely as possible is a significant health promotion strategy in preventing the spread of preventable illnesses as well as potential life-threatening complications which may result from the disease.

In addition to the vaccines listed in Table 10-2, other immunizations are available. A vaccine for rotavirus, the major cause of viral diarrhea in infants and young children, has been developed; however, the Centers for Disease Control and Prevention postponed routine use of the vaccine in July 1999 due to an increased incidence of intestinal complications in infants receiving the immunization. Further data collection and analysis may enable it to be added to the immunization recommendation list at a future date.

The yearly influenza vaccination is especially important for all children with neurological conditions that can cause breathing or swallowing difficulties. The flu vaccine can be administered to infants as young as 6 months (CDC, 2006). Hepatitis A immunization has now been expanded to include all children beginning at 1 year of age. Finding a vaccination for respiratory syncytial virus, the most common cause of bronchiolitis and pneumonia in infants under 1 year of age, is a high research priority, but none is available at present.

Immunization practices and recommendations change frequently. It is the nurse's responsibility to know the most up-to-date information for administration. This information can be obtained through the Centers for Disease Control and Prevention and the American Academy of Pediatrics Advisory Committee on Immunization Practices.

Many individuals consider the common childhood diseases to be relatively mild and a part of growing up; however, there are serious complications as well as mortality associated with these diseases.

Screening

Screening is the use of a diagnostic procedure such as a laboratory test or an evaluation tool to determine the presence of a particular disease or risk factors known to be associated with a health problem. Screening is a secondary intervention strategy that has the potential to provide cost-effective preventive care. Screening is done for conditions which have significant effects on the quality and quantity of life and, if found before symptoms begin, treatment can reduce morbidity and mortality. Significant for the infant and toddler is screening for newborn metabolic defects, anemia, hearing problems, abnormal growth patterns, and developmental delays.

Determination of which diseases are included in the newborn screening is a function of each individual state, thus explaining the lack of uniformity throughout the United States. Each state analyzes the cost-benefit ratio of performing the testing versus not performing the testing. There are substantial costs associated with newborn screening, including the actual cost of the test, false negatives, parental anxiety, and confirmatory testing. The ethical and financial dilemma that then arises relates to the availability and assumption of treatment costs and follow-up services for those treatable disorders identified in the screening. Although it is recognized that the financial cost of screening for a selected group of treatable devastating disorders is certainly less than the financial cost of long-term care of individuals not identified and treated, the human costs have not been fully analyzed.

An additional concern associated with newborn screening relates to the timing of the tests. Tests to identify the congenital conditions of phenylketonuria, hypothyroidism, homocystinuria, and galactosemia measure concentrations of analytes in the blood that increase over time. With early hospital discharge, specimens are sometimes collected before the newborn is 24 hours old. The primary health promotion strategy is to avoid false-negative test results. A second specimen should be collected within two weeks if the first specimen was collected before the newborn was 24 hours old.

Defects of Metabolism The primary purpose of screening newborns for metabolic defects is to detect infants with treatable metabolic illnesses that may result in severe mental retardation and institutionalization if undetected and untreated. All 50 states plus the District of Columbia, Puerto Rico, and the U.S. Virgin Islands screen for phenylketonuria and hypothyroidism. Galactosemia is included in the screening for all states and territories except Arkansas, Hawaii, Louisiana, Nebraska, Pennsylvania, Washington, and Puerto Rico. Screening for maple syrup urine disease, homocystinuria, and biotinidase deficiency occurs in more than 20 states and territories.

Anemia Iron deficiency is the most common cause of anemia in infants and toddlers. Any infant with a history of low birth weight, consumption of cow's milk starting before 6 months of age, or consumption of a non-iron-fortified formula should have a measurement of the hemoglobin or hematocrit level between 6 and 9 months of age. Prevention of untreated anemia is an important health promotion strategy to enhance normal growth and development and resistance to infection.

Hearing Deficits The ability to hear is essential to the infant and toddler for development of speech and language as well as emotional, social, and intellectual development. Assessment of the infant's startle or turning response to a noise produced outside the infant's field of vision should be conducted as a minimum at birth and at 6 months. Although the observation of the startle or turning response is at best subjective and imprecise, the absence of babbling at 6 months coupled with any parental reports of lack of response warrants evaluation by an audiologist. The health promotion strategy to promote sensory development is to conduct hearing screening at every well-child visit. A child whose hearing impairment is not discovered within the first three years of life may have his or her communication ability permanently hampered.

Growth Retardation The measurement of height, weight, and head and chest circumferences is a health promotion strategy to assess growth patterns. Every individual will have an individual pattern, but comparison to known average patterns as well as the infants or toddler's own past pattern enables the identification of any dramatic changes. Pattern changes may be the result of genetic, nutritional, emotional, or disease influence or all of these.

Developmental Delays Early screening and identification of developmental disabilities in children results in effective therapy for treatable problems and accessing resources for nonreversible problems. Although early detection and intervention for developmental delays has substantial benefits, a large portion of healthy children are not routinely screened. Use of direct screening tools can be costly because they require both time and a person trained specifically in the administration and interpretation of the test. Periodic screening for delays or deviations should be conducted on every child; however, at a minimum, screening should occur when there is expressed parental concern about infant or toddler development. Additionally, children at high risk for developmental delays should be routinely screened. This includes infants who were premature, had a low birth weight, or had other abnormalities at birth.

The most widely used screening tool for developmental delays is the Denver Developmental Screening Test (DDST) II, which was revised and restandardized in 1990. The DDST II is a brief, validated test with a high rate of sensitivity. It screens for a variety of mental, language, and social items as well as sensory and motor achievements. It can be used from birth to 6 years of age to provide mean ages and normal ranges of variation in the accomplishment of fine and gross motor tasks. The predictive value in culturally and economically diverse populations has been improved with the addition of norms for subgroups based on place of residence, ethnicity, and mother's education.

Psychological Domain

The psychological domain involves application of theories of individual behavior and changes of behavior. For the infant and toddler, Jean Piaget's stages of cognitive development and Erik Erikson's stages of emotional development are the most applicable.

Cognitive Development

Jean Piaget's interest in intellectual development led to his belief that each child had a biological blueprint for cognitive development. He believed that the brain does not just mature on its own, but that it is stimulated by experiences the child has in the environment. He postulated a framework to describe the evolution of learning and adaptation which demonstrates the processing of interactions (or experiences) between the child and the environment (Brainerd, 1978). This cognitive development theory (see Table 9-6) provides an explanation of how the child learns.

Children pass through definite stages of cognitive growth demonstrated by changes in behavior or thought. The infant in the sensorimotor period is attempting to coordinate simple motor activities to adapt to and interact with the environment. Health promotion strategies during this period involve teaching the caregivers to stimulate the infant's cognitive development through use of patterns on toys or crib attachments that encourage gazing. Observing moving objects helps develop the infant's ability for visual pursuit. Having safe, brightly colored toys within reach encourages reaching, grasping, and cause-effect development ("If I can reach it, I can bring it closer").

The toddler begins to depend less on physical manipulation and more on mental problem-solving. Exploratory behavior continues, with the toddler demonstrating curiosity about everything in his or her environment. The toddler touches, samples, and moves everything within reach: food, objects, and even people. The toddler can complete simple tasks, such as putting away one or two toys or obtaining a requested object. Toddlers are great mimics of observed behaviors, both in humans and nonhumans. Health promotion strategies involve encouraging this safe exploration and the verbal development that will be the basis for representational thoughts and symbols.

Emotional Development

Erik Erikson studied the psychological development of the child (see Table 9-7). He felt that psychological growth was the result of resolution of developmental crises from infancy through older adulthood. Without crisis resolution at each stage, the individual does not have a firm foundation for succeeding in the following stages (Erikson, 1950).

Resolution in the first stage of trust versus mistrust occurs when the infant learns that basic needs for food and comfort will be met. Infants should be fed whenever they show signs of hunger: alertness, activity, and mouthing. Crying is considered a late-stage indicator of hunger. Quick attention to the infant's needs helps develop the infant's belief that the world is a safe and predictable place to be. An infant that does not get sufficient food or comforting attention may always have a sense of deprivation and lack of trust in caregivers. Health promotion strategies at this stage involve teaching the parents or caregivers about the nutritional needs and feeding patterns of infants and encouraging them to hold and comfort the infant as much as possible.

Resolution of the second stage, autonomy versus shame and doubt, occurs for the toddler as he learns that he can control his own behavior. A toddler whose independent behavior is restricted will doubt his ability. If his efforts are greeted with a lack of acceptance, he

TABLE 9-6 Stages of Cognitive Development According to Jean Piaget

Age	Cognitive Stage	Characteristics
Birth to 2 years	Sensorimotor	Moves from pure reflex adaptations to having a beginning grasp of cause and effect Able to complete small goal-directed tasks Realizes objects only if in sight
2 to 7 years	Preoperational	Has representational thoughts of past, present, and future Able to use and understand symbols such as language Makes simple classifications Has difficulty differentiating real from not real Believes he or she can influence reality through thought—magical thinking Sees world only from egocentric point of view
7 to 11 years	Concrete operations	Able to perform concrete, action-oriented logical reasoning for familiar situations Increases use of symbols to represent reality Groups, sorts, and orders objects and concepts Analyzes relationships Able to reverse mental operations Understands concepts of reversibility, conservation, and transformation
11 to 15 years (and possibly up to 18–20)	Formal operations	Has true logical thinking Has capacity for abstract thought Able to predict and formulate hypotheses

Adapted from Piaget's theory of intelligence, *by C. J. Brainerd, 1978; Englewood Cliffs, NJ: Prentice Hall.*

will develop shame. Health promotion strategies at this stage involve encouraging appropriate independent behaviors for the toddler so that he can develop confidence in his own abilities.

Social Domain

Issues within the social domain for the infant and toddler include the use of day-care facilities, child abuse and neglect, and cultural influences.

Family

For the infant, the social network is the family and caregivers. It is this social network that creates the growth-promoting environment necessary for infant well-being. The basis for this growth-promoting environment is the development of attachment between parents and infants. **Attachment** is a unique, specific, and enduring relationship involving mutual trust, responsiveness, and caring (Klaus & Kennel, 1985). It starts with development of a unilateral relationship (called bonding) initiated by the parents and then develops into attachment, which is a reciprocal relationship where the infant is able to respond to and elicit responses from the parents. During attachment building, parents use eye contact, touching, and talking to get to know their infant. An important health promotion strategy is to facilitate and encourage this acquaintance behavior as early and as frequently as possible. Extreme stress or illness may interfere with development of attachment. Nurses must observe for negative patterns of parenting behaviors such as verbal expressions of dissatisfaction with the baby, failure to respond to the infant's crying, and reduced touching or holding of the infant. Parental support, education, role modeling, and encouragement may assist the parent-infant relationship to progress in a positive manner.

By the time the infant becomes a toddler, a reciprocal relationship with the parents and any older siblings has developed; however, the addition of a new infant to the family may cause jealousy and regression in interactive social skills if parents do not devote some attention to preparation for the event. Including the toddler (as much as appropriate) in preparatory activities, reading books on anticipating a new baby, and spending special time alone with the toddler following the arrival of the

TABLE 9-7 Stages of Psychological Development According to Erik Erikson

Level	Conflict	Definition	Behaviors
Infant	Trust Mistrust	Optimism, warmth Sense of deprivation	Smiling, responsive to interactions Feeding disorders, failure to thrive
Toddler	Autonomy Shame and doubt	Self-control, adequacy Sense of inner failure	Curiosity, assertiveness, self-feeding Extreme separation anxiety, sleep distur- bances, toilet training disturbances
Preschool	Initiative Guilt	Ability to direct own actions Anxiety about being bad	Independence Temper tantrums, withdrawal
School age	Industry Inferiority	Skill competence Sense of inadequacy	Self-confident, cooperative Perseveres, completes tasks Passive, moody, depressed Incomplete tasks, isolated
Adolescent	Identity Role confusion	Image of self as unique Doubt about identity	Confident Develops loyal friendships Delinquent behavior Sense of futility Psychotic episodes
Young adult	Intimacy Isolation	Close relationships Distance from others	Committed in relationships Self-abandonment Loner in relationships Avoids social situations
Middle-aged adult	Generativity Stagnation	Concern for future generations Self-concern	Involved in family and community Self-absorbed, loner, depression
Old adult	Ego integrity Despair	Satisfaction with life Nonacceptance of life	Dignified, shows pride Sees death as part of life Fear of death, anger, depression

Adapted from Childhood and society, *by E. Erikson, 1950, New York: Norton.*

new baby may assist the toddler in adjusting to a new social position.

Day Care

In many families, all available caregivers are working outside the home and must place their children in day-care settings. There are two types of day-care facilities. One is the center-based facility (private, church, or community-center–related), which is staffed by professional child-care workers and aides and may care for a large number of children. The second is the family day-care center which is licensed to care for a limited number of children in the home. The health promotion strategy for children of working parents is to educate the parents about how to evaluate the safety and quality of a day-care facility. The nurse should encourage parents to visit facilities when there are children in the facility. They should be encouraged to observe the cleanliness and safety of the facility as well as the interaction between the children and the staff. Repeated, unannounced visits should be conducted both before and after enrolling the infant or toddler.

Child Abuse and Neglect

Based on reported incidents, almost one million children were victims of child abuse and neglect in 2003 (ACF, 2003). Unfortunately, many cases are unknown or not reported. More children suffer neglect than any other form of maltreatment. The investigations by child protective services revealed that about 60 percent of victims suffered neglect, 20 percent physical abuse, 10 percent sexual abuse, 5 percent emotional maltreatment, and 17 percent other forms of maltreatment. The highest rate of abuse involved children from birth to 3 years of age—

approximately 16.4 per 1,000 children of the same age group. Girls were slightly more likely to be abused than boys (ACF, 2003).

Any child may be abused. Child abuse occurs in both genders and in all levels of society. Factors which tend to increase a child's risk of abuse include being premature or having low birth weight; being perceived as looking "unusual" or "different"; having a disease or congenital abnormality; being physically, emotionally, or developmentally disabled; having a high level of motor activity or being fussy and irritable; living in poverty; and living in environments with substance abuse, high crime, and violence.

An important health promotion strategy for this issue is for health care providers to be alert for signs of abuse. **Bruising** (the leakage of blood into skin tissue damaged by a direct blow or a crushing injury) is the earliest and most visible sign. Other signs the nurse should be alert for include: abrasions, hematomas, poor skin care, burns on the lower extremities, malnutrition, bite marks, retinal hemorrhage, and discrepancies between the reported cause of the injury and the injuries seen. Parental behaviors may also alert the nurse. Typically, when a child has an accident, the parents seek help quickly, offer consistent details about the accident, are concerned about the child's status, have difficulty leaving the child, and may express guilt over not preventing the accident. Abusing parents, however, seem evasive about the injury, offer fewer or even conflicting details about the accident, appear inconvenienced or angry, and are not as solicitous about the child or his or her progress.

Bruises seen in infants, especially on the face and buttocks, are suspicious. In toddlers, injuries to the upper arms, trunk, front of the thighs, sides of the face, ears, neck, genitalia, stomach, and buttocks are more likely associated with intentional, nonaccidental injuries. Bruising on the shins, hips, lower arms, forehead, hands, or bony prominences are more consistent with accidental injuries.

Cultural Influences

The infant is profoundly influenced by the culture/ethnicity of the parents or caregivers or both. The family's perceptions of illness, the cause of illness, childrearing practices, nutrition, and behavior reflect the cultural heritage. Because the infant is totally dependent upon these individuals for nutrition, health care, affection, and safety, it is vital that the nurse plan health promotion strategies with a knowledge of and sensitivity to the family's culture/ethnicity as well as her or his own. Knowledge of previous encounters with the health care community and any problems which might have occurred due to language barriers, religious values, family lines of authority, family roles, or use of traditional (folk) medicine will form the basis for collaboration with the family in planning health promotion strategies for the infant.

Family cultural beliefs, values, and practices continue to mold the toddler, who is now able to participate in some of the family's cultural activities such as celebrations and religious observances. Culturally sensitive collaboration continues to be key to developing health promotion strategies.

Political Domain

Two initiatives have an impact on health promotion for the infant and toddler. One is the Supplemental Food Program for Women, Infants, and Children (WIC), and the other concerns safety legislature on requiring car safety seats.

WIC Program

The Supplemental Food Program for Women, Infants, and Children is a grant program administered by the Food and Nutrition Service of the U.S. Department of Agriculture. It provides nutrition assessment and education, breast-feeding guidance and support, food supplements, and referral for health and social services to low-income pregnant, breast-feeding, and postpartum women, infants, and children under age 5 who are at nutritional risk. Eligibility is based on income and nutritional need.

Safety Legislation

The key safety legislation that affects the health of the infant and toddler is the mandate for the use of car safety seats. All 50 states require infants traveling in cars to be restrained in a car safety seat. A properly used car safety seat can reduce the risk of dying in a crash for an infant by 71 percent and for a toddler by 54 percent, according to the National Highway Traffic Safety Administration. The health promotion strategy for this issue is parental education about the proper size, placement, and use of car safety seats. Tips for infant and toddler car safety are listed in Box 9-7.

Although airbags save hundreds of lives each year, the high-speed deployment of passenger-side airbags

- Place the infant/toddler in the car safety seat, even for short trips.
- Ensure that the car's seat belt holds the safety seat firmly without sliding.
- Use rear-facing safety seats for infants/toddlers under 20 pounds.
- Place the safety seat in the center of the back seat.
- Never place an infant or toddler in a front seat with an airbag.
- Never use an infant carrier instead of a safety seat.
- Ensure that straps lie flat and are held on shoulders with a harness retainer clip.
- Watch for product recalls of car safety seats.

has resulted in the deaths of children placed in the front seat of cars. Infants in rear-facing safety seats are too close to the airbag housing and have been injured or killed by the force of the deployment. Toddlers, restrained or not restrained, have also been injured or killed by passenger bags. Only infants and toddlers who must be constantly within reach of the driver should be placed in the front seat, and then only after the airbag is turned off or disabled.

Environmental Domain

Accidents are responsible for the deaths of thousands of infants and toddlers annually. Over 90 percent are preventable. Specific environmental safety tips for infants and toddlers are listed in Table 9-8. Educating parents and caregivers on how to prevent accidents is the primary health promotion strategy. Reminding parents that toddlers are great mimics is also important. Children may learn dangerous or harmful activities from watching parents and caregivers ("monkey see, monkey do"). Therefore, parents should refrain from doing anything in front of the toddler that they don't want the toddler to imitate, such as taking medicine, holding pins or nails in the mouth, smoking, not wearing seat belts, using lighters or matches, and the like.

Parents should be instructed to keep all important numbers by every phone in the house: ambulance, doctor, police, poison control center, and so on. They need appropriate medical supplies in the house, such as bandages, syrup of ipecac (to induce vomiting), and antibiotic ointment. Knowing cardiopulmonary resuscitation may be vital in an instance where the infant is choking or not breathing. And last, parents should be cautioned to be especially vigilant away from home. The toddler's natural curiosity in an unfamiliar place may lead to tragedy.

Sexual Domain

Although full expression of one's sexuality is an adult phenomenon, its development begins in infancy. An infant's sex (or gender) is determined at conception and developed prenatally through hormones. After birth, the infant's sexuality continues developing through the influence of hormones and by parental (or caregiver) interactions. The infant develops gender-specific responses influenced by the caregiver's responses. If the caregiver, either consciously or unconsciously, believes that boys should be treated differently from girls, then a sex role differentiation is being taught and learned.

An important health promotion strategy involving the sexual domain in infants is to educate caregivers about an infant's natural exploration of the body. By 5 or 6 months, infants will locate their genital area during bathing or diaper change. Just as these infants explored and manipulated their hands and feet, they will manipulate their genitals. Males will often experience an erection and females may have some lubrication. Assuring caregivers of this natural sequence of events may prevent undue concern about this activity and set the stage to promote healthy development of the infant's self-image and sexuality.

The gender-specific differences caused by gender-specific caregiving practices become apparent in the toddler. Toddlers can identify themselves as a boy or a girl and usually display the behaviors expected of their gender. They observe and imitate their same-sex parent. Children of both genders should be allowed to play with dolls, trucks, and other toys formerly considered gender-specific without parents being concerned that such play is "sissy" or "tomboyish." By toddlerhood, self-concept as a girl or boy is completed.

Toddlers have increasing control over their own bodies (running, jumping, toileting, self-feeding) and may increase their genital stimulation. Caregivers who are comfortable with their own sexuality will be able to view this exploration as a natural extension of the toddler's curiosity.

Spiritual Domain

The spiritual domain relates to the essence of life, encompassing religious values and practices. The outward expression of spirituality is often through an organized church or religious institution. An individual's daily interactions with others, goals, and feelings of self-worth come from spiritual beliefs. These beliefs affect the individual's definition of health, life, quality of life, and health care practices.

Spiritual and religious values are shown to infants and toddlers through helping them to develop a sense of trust and a belief in the security of their environment. The foundation begun in these early years is the initial step in the development of self-esteem and self-love. The health promotion strategy for this domain is to encourage

TABLE 9-8 Environmental Safety for Infants and Toddlers

Accident	Prevention Strategies
Falls	Place infant in crib for sleeping. Never leave toddler unattended in high chair or shopping cart. Use safety gates to block stairways. Be sure scatter rugs don't slip. Always light a room when entering. Teach safe use of stairs when walking.
Suffocation/choking	Place infant on back or side to sleep. Avoid soft bedding, pillows, sheepskins under infants. Be sure window blind or curtain cords are out of reach. Be sure crib rails are no wider spaced than $2\frac{1}{2}$ inches and there are no broken or missing rails. Keep small objects out of reach. Check floors and countertops for small objects daily.
Electrocution	Plug unused electrical outlets with clear covers (no cartoon characters). Fill all empty light sockets with bulbs. Don't keep unused extension cords plugged in.
Poisoning	Lock up household cleaning products. Keep medicines out of reach. Don't take adult medicine in front of toddlers. Keep liquor cabinets locked. Keep poison control number by phone.
Drowning	Never leave infant/toddler alone in the bathtub or near any water (pool, mop bucket, washing machine). Close toilet lids.
Burns	Check bath water temperature before putting infant/toddler in it. Use back burners on stove most often. Turn pot handles toward back of stove. Never leave an iron unattended. Install smoke detectors and check regularly. Never leave a cigarette burning.
Cuts	Don't let toddlers use glass tumblers. Use decals on glass doors at toddler's eye level. Put breakable objects out of reach. Keep scissors and knives out of reach.

parents to show love and comfort to their infants and toddlers. Table 9-9 summarizes health promotion for infants and toddlers according to pertinent domains.

SUMMARY

Promoting the health of mothers, infants, and toddlers begins prior to conception with the education of potential parents, ideally beginning in high school. Educational programs focusing on personal health and wellness, conception, fetal development, and infant care can reduce infant mortality and morbidity.

There are many health promotion and preventive care interventions for the mother. This chapter grouped health promotion strategies into three opportunities for intervention: preconception, pregnancy, and postpartum. Each period of intervention was viewed through the biological, psychological and sociological, environmental, political, sexual, and spiritual domains.

Health promotion strategies for the infant and toddler were viewed through the biological, psychological and sociological, environmental, political, sexual, and spiritual domains. These provided a comprehensive look at health promotion in the infant and toddler years of life.

TABLE 9-9 Health Promotion for Infants and Toddlers

Related Domain	Risk Assessment	Health Promotion Action
Biological	Nutrition	Breast-feeding for the first year of life
	Elimination	Education about identification and management of diarrhea and constipation
	Sleep	Back sleeping only until infant can turn alone Establishment of bedtime ritual for toddlers
	Play	Frequent stimulation for infants Provision of a safe learning environment for toddlers
	Immunization	Maintenance of recommended immunization schedule
Psychological	Screening for abnormalities	Assessment for defects of metabolism, anemia, hearing deficits, growth retardation, and developmental delays
Social	Development	Assessment for appropriate cognitive and emotional development
Political	Abuse and neglect	Assessment for child abuse and neglect
Environmental	Protection	Education about availability of supplemental food program and about car safety seats
	Safety	Anticipatory guidance about potential for accidents such as falls, suffocation/choking, electrocution, poisoning, drowning, burns, and cuts

CASE STUDY Mary Grace Sullivan: At Risk for Preterm Labor

Objectives/Goals: Through participation in discussion of this case study, participants will have the opportunity to:
1. Define preterm or premature labor.
2. Discuss risk factors for preterm labor and delivery.
3. Discuss lifestyle and environmental changes to reduce preterm labor risk.

Health Promotion Concern, History and Physical, Present Health Status, Past Health Status, Family History, and Social History

Mary Grace Sullivan is a 38-year-old Irish American female who is being seen in the prenatal clinic. She is an elementary school teacher and has been married for approximately eight years. She has been unable to conceive for the last six years, and this pregnancy is a result of in vitro fertilization. She has been taking prenatal vitamins for the last six months.

She is very concerned about this pregnancy because a year ago her sister had a premature baby who was in the neonatal intensive care unit for two months. Mary Grace does not smoke or drink and is up-to-date with all her immunizations. She works out at the gym three days a week after work, using the treadmill, stationary bike, and universal weight machine.

Review of Pertinent Domains
Biological Domain

Physical examination reveals a 5'4" Caucasian female weighing 116 pounds. Her BMI is 20, which puts her in the normal category. Blood pressure is 98/68. Breasts are firm, without dominant masses. Abdomen is soft, nontender, without masses, hernias, or organomegaly. External genitalia are normal. Vagina is pink, moist, without excessive discharge. Cervix is bluish, closed, without lesions. All other systems are unremarkable.

Genitourinary: In vitro fertilization was six weeks ago. She has not had a menstrual period for two months. Breasts are tender bilaterally.

Diagnostic testing: Urine pregnancy test is positive. Hemoglobin, hematocrit, urinalysis, TSH, metabolic profile, and fasting serum glucose are within normal limits.

Psychological Domain

Mary Grace and her husband are both very excited about the pregnancy, but apprehensive about the possibility of preterm labor.

Social Domain

Her husband's parents live in town, but her parents and siblings live in a town approximately two hours' drive away.

Educational Issues

Mary Grace and her husband need education about the risks for preterm labor: personal, lifestyle, environmental, and medical. They also need information about the signs and symptoms of preterm labor as well as the treatments that are available.

Questions for Discussion

1. What risk factors does Mary Grace have for preterm labor?
2. What lifestyle or environmental risks may need to be addressed?
3. What signs and symptoms of preterm labor should Mary Grace know?

Key Concepts

1. Health promotion for mothers-to-be begins prior to conception. They need education about the physiological and psychological changes of pregnancy as well as fetal development. An exercise program, a healthy, well-balanced diet with folate supplementation, and avoidance of substances known to be harmful to the fetus should be initiated prior to pregnancy. Potential parents should have genetic history screening for inheritable abnormalities, and mothers should have screening for chronic diseases that might adversely affect the fetus.

2. During pregnancy, the mother-to-be should continue with a healthy lifestyle. Screening during this time is for gestational diabetes, isoimmunization, and congenital anomalies. Health promotion involves helping the mother reduce common discomforts that occur during pregnancy.

3. Following delivery, the mother undergoes as many physiological and psychological changes as she did during pregnancy. Health promotion involves encouraging the mother to get adequate rest and nutrition, helping the mother to find social and emotional support, and screening for postpartum depression.

4. Health promotion for infants and toddlers in the biological domain includes strategies related to nutrition, elimination, sleep and activity, and immunizations.

5. Screening for actual or potential health problems in infants and toddlers is vital for promoting the quality and quantity of life. Nurses assist in screening for metabolic defects, anemia, hearing problems, abnormal growth, and developmental delays.

6. Promoting health in the psychological domain requires an understanding of normal cognitive and emotional development for infants and toddlers. Theoretical frameworks developed by Jean Piaget and Erik Erikson provide a foundation for evaluating development of infants and toddlers.

7. Health promotion in the social domain for infants and toddlers evolves from the family to include daycare networks.

8. Child abuse and neglect affect more than 1 million children annually. Nurses need to look for physical signs, including bruising, hematomas, poor skin care, malnutrition, bite marks, and retinal hemorrhage. Parental behavior and discrepancies between the reported cause of injury and the injury seen can also be important keys to identifying abuse. Any suspicion of abuse or neglect must, by law, be reported to the appropriate authorities.

9. In addition to legislation mandating reporting of suspected child abuse, there are other social actions for health promotion from the political domain. These include the Supplemental Food Program for Women, Infants, and Children (WIC) and car safety seat requirement laws.

10. Nurses and parents share responsibility for promoting safety of infants and toddlers. Safety strategies, including foods appropriate for age, immunizations, and car seats, are important. Preventing physical and psychological trauma is vital to ensure healthy development throughout the life span.

11. Important in the sexual domain is the education of parents and caregivers about normal sexual development of infants and toddlers.

12. Spiritual beliefs and practices of the parents and caregivers influence health promotion in the spiritual domain.

Learning Activities

1. Observe an infant's behavior and compare to Erikson's stages of psychological development.

2. Use local or Internet sources or both to find the infant mortality rate for your area. With classmates, discuss approaches to reduce infant mortality.

3. List the immunization schedule for an infant through childhood.

4. Develop a pamphlet for a new mother that addresses the symptoms of depression.

True/False Questions

1. T or F   A cervical cap is a nonhormonal permanent method of birth control.

2. T or F   One out of three births in the United States is by cesarean section.

3. T or F   According to the recommended immunization schedule, initial immunization for measles, mumps, and rubella (MMR) should occur just before a child enters first grade.

4. T or F   Children with mild illnesses such as a cold or flu should not receive their scheduled immunization.

Multiple Choice Questions

1. The best time to discuss breast-feeding with an expectant mother is:
   a. During prenatal visits.
   b. Immediately before birth.
   c. During her postpartum hospital stay.
   d. At the first infant check-up.

2. All women capable of getting pregnant should take:
   a. Extra calcium.
   b. Folate.
   c. Iron supplements.
   d. Multivitamins.

3. The safest place for an infant under 20 pounds in an automobile is in an approved infant car seat placed:
   a. Behind the driver's seat.
   b. In the center of the back seat.
   c. Facing the rear in the front seat.
   d. Behind the passenger's seat.

Websites/Hotline

http://www.acf.hhs.gov Site for the Administration for Children and Families that provides information about services, policies, and programs affecting children, including child maltreatment.

http://www.marchofdimes.com March of Dimes organization site that provides information about pregnancy, infants, and preventing birth defects; also has a health information center about pregnancy and caring for newborns.

http://www.mayoclinic.com Contains a section titled Domestic Violence Toward Women: Recognize the Patterns and Seek Help, written to help victims of domestic violence, with description of an abusive relationship, signs of abuse, how to break the cycle, and options/resources.

http://www.not-2-late.com Provides information about emergency contraception and resources for EC. Can be accessed in English, Spanish, and Arabic.

National Domestic Violence Hotline (800) 799-SAFE or (800) 799-7233. Provides crisis intervention and referrals to in-state or out-of-state resources such as women's shelters or crisis centers.

References

Administration for Children and Families (ACF). (2003). *Child maltreatment*. Retrieved January 10, 2006, from http://www.acf.hhs.gov/programs/cb/pubs/cm03/index.htm

American Academy of Pediatrics (AAP). 2005. The changing concept of sudden infant death syndrome: Diagnostic coding shifts, controversies regarding the sleeping environment, and new variable to consider in reducing risk. *Pediatrics, 116*(5), 1245–1255.

American Psychiatric Association. (2000). *Diagnostic and statistical manual of mental disorders-TR (4th ed)*. Washington, DC: Author.

Beck, L., Gilbert, B., & Shults, R. (2005). Prevalence of seat belt use among reproductive-aged women and prenatal counseling to wear seat belts. *American Journal of Obstetrics and Gynecology, 192*(2), 580–585.

Brainerd, C. J. (1978). Piaget's theory of intelligence. Englewood cliffs, NJ: Prentice Hall.

Brundage, S. (2002). Preconception health care. *American Family Physician, 65*, 2507–2514.

Centers for Disease Control and Prevention (CDC). (2006). Recommended childhood and adolescent immunization schedule. *MMWR, 54*(52), Q1–Q4.

Centers for Disease Control and Prevention (CDC). (2004). *Safe motherhood: Promoting health for women before, during, and after pregnancy*. Atlanta: CDC.

Dolan, S. (2005). Medication exposure during pregnancy: Antidepressants. *Medscape Ob/Gyn & Women's Health, 10*(1).

Erikson, E. (1950). Childhood and society. New York: Norton.

Gardner, A. (2005). Pacifiers prevent SIDS deaths: Study. Retrieved January 9, from http://www.medicinenet.com/script/main/art.asp?articlekey= 55615&pf=3&page=1

Goldberg, G. (2003). Nutrition in pregnancy: The facts and fallacies. *Nursing Standard, 17*(19), 39–42.

Goodman, J. (2004). Paternal postpartum depression, its relationship to maternal postpartum depression, and implications for family health. *Journal of Advanced Nursing, 45*, 26–35.

Gottesman, M. (2004). Preconception education: Caring for the future. *Journal of Pediatric Health Care, 18*(1), 40–44.

Henshaw, S. (1998). Unintended pregnancy in the United States. *Family Planning Perspectives, 30*(1), 24–29, 46.

JBI. (2005). The effectiveness of a pelvic floor muscle exercise program on urinary incontinence following childbirth. *Best Practice, 9*(2), Blackwell Publishing Asia, Australia.

Jones, W. (2004). *Safe motherhood: Promoting health for women before, during, and after pregnancy*. Centers for Disease Control and Prevention. Atlanta, GA: U.S. Department of Health and Human Services.

Kirkham, C., Harris, S., & Grzybowski, S. (2005a). Evidence-based prenatal care: Part I. General prenatal care and counseling issues. *American Family Physician, 71*, 1307–1316, 1321–1322.

Kirkham, C., Harris, S., & Grzybowski, S. (2005b). Evidence-based prenatal care: Part II. General prenatal care and counseling issues. *American Family Physician, 71*, 1555–1562.

Klaus, M. H., & Kennel, J. H. (1985). Parent-infant bonding. St. Louis: Mosby Press.

Korenbrot, C., Steinberg, A., Bender, C., & Newberry, S. (2002). Preconception care: A systematic review. *Maternal and Child Health Journal, 6*(2), 75–88.

Lee, K., & Gay, C. (2004). Pregnant women with good sleep patterns have shorter labors and fewer cesarean deliveries. *American Journal of Obstetrics and Gynecology, 191*, 2041–2046.

Lewinsohn, P. M., Olino, T. M., & Klein, D. N. (2005). Psychosocial impairment in offspring of depressed parents. *Psychological Medicine, 35* (10), 1493–1503.

Marcus, S., Flynn, H., Blow, F., & Barry, K. (2003). Depressive symptoms among pregnant women screened in obstetrics. *Journal of Women's Health, 12*(4), 373–380.

Mason, D., Tobias, N., Lutkenhoff, M., Stoops, M., & Ferguson, D. (2004). The APN's guide to pediatric constipation management. *Nurse Practitioner, 29*(7), 13–21.

National Center for Health Statistics (NCHS). (2002). Infant, neonatal, and postneonatal mortality rates. *National Vital Statistics Report, 50*(15), 100.

Page-Goertz, S. (2005). Weight gain concerns in the breastfed infant. *Advance for Nurse Practitioners, 13*(2), 45–48.

Pennington, J.A.T., & Douglass, J. S. (2004). Bowe's and Church's food values of portions commonly used (18th ed.). Philadelphia: Lippincott Williams & Wilkins

Polinski, M. (2005). *Feeling her pain: The male pregnancy experience*. Retrieved January 2, 2006, from http://pregnancytoday.com

Sagrestano, L., Carroll, D., Rodriguez, A., & Nuwayhid, B. (2004). Demographic, psychological, and relationship factors in domestic violence during pregnancy in a sample of low-income women of color. *Psychology of Women Quarterly, 28*, 309–322.

Saltzman, L., Johnson, C., Gilbert, B., & Goodwin, F. (2003). Physical abuse around the time of pregnancy: An examination of prevalence and risk factors in 16 states. *Maternal and Child Health Journal, 7*, 31–42.

Seehusen, D., Baldwin, L., Runkle, G., & Clark, G. (2005). Are family physicians appropriately screening for postpartum depression? *Journal of the American Board of Family Practice, 18*(2), 104–112.

Slykerman, R., Thompson, J., Pryor, J., Becroft, D., Robinson, E., Clark, P., Wild, C., & Mitchell, E. (2005). Maternal stress, social support and preschool children's intelligence. *Early Human Development, 81*(10), 815–821.

U.S. Preventive Services Task Force (USPSTF). (2003). Behavioral interventions to promote breastfeeding: Recommendations and rationale. *American Journal for Nurse Practitioners, 7*(11), 23–32.

Bibliography

Pilliteri, A. (2006). *Maternal and child health nursing: Care of the childbearing and childrearing family*. Philadelphia: Lippincott Williams & Wilkins.

Potts, N., & Mandleco, B. (2002). *Pediatric nursing: Caring for children and their families*. Albany, NY: Thomson Delmar Learning.

Speroff, L., & Darney, P. D. (2005). *A clinical guide to contraception* (4th ed.). Philadelphia: Lippincott Williams & Wilkins.

Yost, N. P., Bloom, S. L., McIntire, D. D., & Leveno, K. J. (2005). Prospective observational study of domestic violence during pregnancy. *Obstetrics & Gynecology, 106*, 61–65.

Chapter 10

THE CHILD

Barbara A. Tucker, PhD, FNP, APRN-BC

KEY TERMS

acanthosis nigricans
attention-deficit/
   hyperactivity disorder
body mass index (BMI)

egocentric
encopresis
enuresis
incontinence

metabolic syndrome
night terror
nightmare
overweight

peer
scoliosis

OBJECTIVES

Upon completion of this chapter, the reader should be able to:

- Examine health promotion strategies in the biological domain for children.

- Identify nursing responsibilities for screening to promote the health of children.

- Relate theories of cognitive and emotional development to health promotion strategies in children.

- Identify social networks and their importance in child health.

- Describe occurrence, signs and symptoms, and nursing responsibilities relating to child abuse and neglect.

- Identify legislative actions designed to improve the health of children.

- Describe parental and nursing responsibilities for promoting child safety.

- Relate normal sexual development to strategies designed to promote sexual health in children.

- Describe spiritual influences on health promotion in children.

INTRODUCTION

Childhood is typically divided into two periods: the preschool years and the school-age years. The preschool years include ages 3 to 6. Physical growth has slowed, but significant social, emotional, and cognitive growth is occurring. Preschool children are learning how to get along with others and understand another's feelings and needs. They enjoy playing games, reading books, and being with other children, and they can be away from parents and caregivers for longer periods. Preschoolers are beginning to gain mastery over their bodies with toileting, feeding, and dressing by themselves. They are gaining mastery over language and can often be great conversationalists, talking about all sorts of subjects, asking innumerable questions, and expressing their own ideas about things. All these developments help prepare the preschooler for entrance into formal education.

The school-age years include ages 6 to 12, where development is focused on mental abilities, competence, and self-esteem. Although growth in height and weight is slower, growth in learning and motor skills is impressive. School-age children learn to read, write, do mathematics, and understand a wide variety of other subjects such as geography, history, and music. Their world is no longer focused on themselves and the family unit, but expands to include peers and the school environment. The major developmental tasks are achievement in school and acceptance by peers. The school-age years are often called the "calm before the storm" of adolescence.

THE PRESCHOOL AND SCHOOL-AGE CHILD

The enormous physical and psychological development of the preschool and school-age years makes health promotion critical. Health promotion strategies can begin to involve the child in a more active role.

Biological Domain

The biological areas of nutrition, elimination, sleep and activity, immunization, and screening will be discussed in this section as they relate to health promotion for the preschool and the school-age child. The health promotion strategies recommended are largely the responsibility of the parents/caregivers and the nurse.

Nutrition

Both the preschool and the school-age child need a balanced diet that includes a wide variety of foods. MyPyramid (see Chapter 14) serves as a guide to planning the diet. In contrast to infants and toddlers, children of this age benefit from a diet low in total fat (30 percent or less of total calories). Saturated fat, cholesterol, sugar, and salt should also be monitored. The nurse needs to encourage a diet of poultry, fish, lean meat, low-fat and skim milk products, dried peas and beans, whole grain breads and cereals, vegetables, and fruits.

The first step in assessing a child's weight and nutrition is to determine the **body mass index (BMI).** The BMI is a number that shows body weight adjusted for height and can be calculated using inches and pounds or meters and kilograms. The child's weight in pounds is divided by height in inches squared and multiplied by 703; alternately, the child's weight in kilograms is divided by height in meters squared. The CDC provides a calculator at http://www.cdc.gov, then search for "bmi calculator." In children, BMI is used to assess underweight, overweight, and risk for overweight. Because body fat changes in children as they grow older and differences exist between boys and girls, BMI should be plotted on a gender-specific growth chart that uses percentiles to show how the child's BMI compares to that of children of the same gender and age. Nurses use the established percentile cutoff point in Table 10-1 to identify underweight and overweight in children. BMI is a useful tool for assessment because it provides a reference for adolescents that can be used beyond puberty, it compares well to laboratory measures of body fat, and it can be used to track body size throughout life.

Assessing a child's weight should also include a review of the child's growth pattern—weight-for-height before the age of 2 and BMI after the age of 2. Development of a weight problem can be noted if the child moves either up or down across percentile lines. Asking about the child's eating habits and activity levels is also important.

Parents of preschoolers often become concerned with their child's food preferences and lack of interest in eating. The preschooler's emerging ability to control her or his environment is frequently demonstrated by adamant food preferences and rejections. Many reject cooked vegetables, mixed foods, and new foods. Frustrated parents may be helped by the nurse to review the overall nutritional adequacy of the diet, to evaluate for the presence of pressure and stress during mealtimes, and to learn a variety of ways to introduce adequate nutrition to the diet. Suggestions for managing the "picky eater" are presented in Box 10-1.

Parents have a major influence over the nutritional adequacy of the child's diet that goes beyond the purchasing and preparing of the food. Providing the child with role models who eat and enjoy a wide variety of nutritious foods is essential. The child's food preferences generally reflect those of the parents. Parents should seek to make mealtime a comfortable, social experience without coaxing, threatening, or bribing. Making food an issue is certain to make the child more adamant about not eating. Parents should be reassured that the appetite and the acceptance of new foods usually increases as the child gets older.

Vitamins may be a good supplement to the preschooler's diet, especially during periods of increased food fussiness. Fluoride supplements are needed if there is

---

TABLE 10-1 Weight Classification by Body Mass Index (BMI)

Underweight	BMI-for-age < 5th percentile
Normal	BMI-for-age 5th to < 85th percentile
At risk of overweight	BMI-for-age 85th to < 95th percentile
Overweight	BMI-for-age ≥ 95th percentile

BOX 10-1 Managing the "Picky Eater"

1. Serve vegetables raw and cut into finger-sized pieces. Use for snacks.
2. Provide a sauce for dipping vegetables such as melted cheese, salad dressing, or yogurt.
3. Serve foods plain and separated, rather than in casseroles, in stews, or creamed.
4. Serve small portions arranged attractively and separately on the plate.
5. Cut easily chewable meat into bite-sized pieces.
6. Continue to introduce new foods even if met with rejection at first.
7. Serve one food on the child's "like list" at each meal.
8. Incorporate pureed vegetables (carrots, squash, spinach) into sauces for pizza or spaghetti.
9. Avoid allowing excessive eating between meals.
10. Encourage participation with meal planning and preparation (selecting a nutritious menu, setting the table, stirring an instant pudding).

none in the local water supply. Calcium and vitamin D intake needs to be assessed. National data show that many children do not get enough calcium, increasing their risk for developing osteoporosis in adulthood. Children need calcium for bone formation and weight-bearing exercise to strengthen bones. Drinking sodas instead of milk or calcium-fortified juice and increased time in sedentary activities place bones at risk. Screening for calcium intake and bone health should occur at age 2 to 3 after weaning from breast milk or formula, at age 8 to 9 before the adolescent growth spurt, and again during puberty when the peak rate of bone mass growth occurs.

The school-age child may continue to display some food preferences, occasionally only eating one specific food. Health promotion strategies are similar to those for the preschool child, but need to include assessment of those meals eaten at school. Although the majority of schools use the USDA school lunch guideline of less than 30 percent of calories from fat, many schools also sell or have vending machines with high-fat, high-calorie, and high-sugar items. Schools use these vending machines as a source of income and may be reluctant to remove them or restrict their use. Soft-drink vending machines are found in 58 percent of elementary schools and 94 percent of high schools (Holcomb, 2004). Most school-age children drink at least one high-sugar soft drink daily, with some consuming three or more.

Although the majority of parents of preschoolers are concerned about children who won't eat, an increasing minority are concerned about overweight children. Obesity has become epidemic in the United States. It has now reached down from adults to children and can even be found among preschool children as young as 4. Overweight in 4-and 5-year-old girls has increased from 5.8 percent in the 1970s to over 10 percent, almost doubling (Ogden, Flegal, Carroll et al., 2002). Overweight for boys has also increased, but not as much as for girls. This increase in overweight has been seen in all races and ethnicities. Hispanic children have the highest prevalence, followed by Black children, and White children have the lowest.

To assess for overweight in children, the BMI should be plotted on gender-specific growth charts. Plotting weight-for-age and weight-for-height percentiles instead may result in failure to recognize almost 75 percent of overweight children (Louthan et al., 2005). In children, risk of being overweight is defined as being between the 85th and 94th percentiles for age/sex-specific BMI. **Overweight** is defined as being at or above the 95th percentile for age/sex-specific BMI. A red flag for development of a weight problem is moving up across percentiles. Family history, eating habits, activity levels, and social relationships are also important. Laboratory studies include fasting serum glucose, lipoprotein panel, and insulin levels as well as a serum ALT.

The increase in preschool obesity has serious implications for future child health because it affects physiologic measures such as blood pressure and cholesterol and jeopardizes mental health. Childhood obesity affects self-esteem, peer relationships, inclusion in social events, and participation in sports. Influenced by the media and societal attitudes, even preschoolers develop negative attitudes toward obesity and avoid picking an obese child for a playmate (Rich et al., 2005).

Twenty percent of overweight 4-year-olds will be obese as adults (Holcomb, 2004). And if the condition persists into adolescence, 70 to 80 percent will be overweight or obese as adults. Adults who were overweight as children have increased morbidity and mortality rates independent of their adult weight (Holcomb, 2004).

The percentage of overweight children age 6 through 11 has doubled since the 1960s, overshadowing all other diseases in its frequency in the pediatric population. Childhood obesity is associated with increased risk of hyperlipidemia, hypertension, insulin resistance, diabetes mellitus, and arteriosclerosis later in life (Henry, 2005). Recognizing and reducing childhood obesity is important not only because of its relationship with adult obesity and the associated medical complications but also because these same complications are now being demonstrated by children. Overweight children are developing type 2 diabetes mellitus and hypertension, diseases formerly found almost exclusively in adults. There is also an increase in asthma and obstructive sleep apnea. Overweight children have orthopedic problems, especially in weight-bearing joints, and psychosocial problems related to poor self-esteem. In addition, overweight girls may have an early menarche.

Several risk factors are associated with childhood obesity. High birth weight, maternal diabetes, and family history of obesity pose known risks. Infants of diabetic mothers born with a high birth weight (Large for Gestational Age) are at significant risk of developing **Metabolic Syndrome,** an association of obesity, insulin resistance, glucose intolerance, hypertension, and dyslipidemia that predisposes the individual to diabetes and cardiovascular disease (Boney, Verma, Tucker, & Vohr, 2005). When one parent is obese, the child is three times more likely to become obese in adulthood; if both parents are obese, the child is more than 10 times as likely (Holcomb, 2004). Parental weight is more of a risk factor before age 3 than is the child's actual weight. Maternal obesity in early pregnancy more than doubles the risk of overweight at 2 to 4 years of age (Whitaker, 2004). Other risk factors include low income, low education, absence of family meals, and lack of physical activity. In some immigrant or poor populations, the fear of starvation can lead parents to believe that overweight children are healthy.

Interventions to prevent childhood obesity should be initiated before school age and continue throughout the school years. Nursery schools, Head Start centers, and day-care centers could initiate comprehensive health education programs which can continue into the school years. In addition, schools can promote physical activity. Unfortunately, many schools are reducing or cutting physical education from the curriculum, just as the obesity epidemic is being documented.

Prevention and treatment must involve the whole family making healthful lifestyle changes. Parental education is essential. Parents are in control—they buy the food, cook the food, and decide where food is eaten. Box 10-2 lists ways parents can help their overweight children. Primary prevention health promotion strategies include altering food preferences by introducing children to a wide variety of fruits and vegetables and reducing television and computer time, which will limit snacking and exposure to food advertising and will provide an opportunity for more active behaviors.

Obesity treatment programs for children do not have weight loss as a goal. The aim is to halt weight gain so the child will grow into his or her body weight over a period of months to years. Programs for the school-age child should have three components: physical activity, diet management, and behavior modification.

Adopting a formal exercise program, or simply becoming more active, is valuable to burn fat, increase

Ask Yourself

Preventing Childhood Obesity

Prevention of childhood obesity should begin as early in life as possible. Nurses are in a position to teach parents so that they can guide their children. Health promotion strategies involve the parents, the children, and the schools. How can the nurse be involved personally, professionally, politically, or all three to promote prevention of childhood obesity?

energy expenditure, and maintain lost weight. Even if body weight and body fat percentage do not change, 50 minutes of aerobic exercise three times per week results in improvement in blood lipid profiles and blood pressure. Diet management must be combined with physical activity to be effective.

Fasting or extreme caloric restriction is not advisable for children. This approach not only is psychologically stressful but may adversely affect growth and the child's perception of "normal" eating. Changes in metabolism from severe calorie restriction followed by binge eating may cause children to gain rather than lose weight (AAP, 2003). Helping children to adopt good eating habits without severe calorie restriction is a better health promotion choice. Balanced diets with moderate caloric restriction, especially reduced dietary fat, have been successful in treating obesity. Nutritional education is also beneficial.

Behavioral modification such as self-monitoring and recording food intake and physical activity, slowing the rate of eating, limiting the time and place of eating, and using nonfood rewards and incentives for desirable behaviors have been successful. Including parents in behaviorally based treatments is particularly effective. Parents should be taught to avoid using food as a reward and to allow children to leave food on their plates when their appetites are satisfied.

Elimination

The majority of preschool children have attained independent toileting with only occasional "accidents." These lapses are usually due to not wanting to interrupt play activities. The school-age child usually has an elimination pattern similar to that of an adult, urinating every three to four hours with a bowel movement every one to two days. Some children, however, may have a problem with elimination.

Enuresis is involuntary urinary incontinence in a child 5 years of age or older who has no physical abnormality causing the incontinence. **Incontinence** is defined as the inability to retain urine or feces. Enuresis refers to urine. Over 90 percent of children with enuresis have primary nocturnal enuresis, or "bedwetting." These chil-

BOX 10-2 Parents' Guide to Promoting Normal Weight in Children

- Be a good role model—be more active and improve your own diet.
- When grocery shopping, choose fruits and vegetables over convenience foods high in sugar and fat.
- Have healthy snacks available (fresh fruit, low-fat popcorn, low-fat frozen yogurt) and eliminate high-fat, high-sugar foods from the home (chips, pizza, cookies, ice cream, etc.).
- Limit sweetened beverages, including those containing fruit juices.
- Select recipes and methods of cooking that are lower in fat (baking, broiling instead of frying).
- Put colorful foods on the table: green and yellow vegetables, fruits of various colors, brown whole grain breads. Limit white carbohydrates: rice, pasta, white bread, sugar (desserts).
- Sit down together for family meals.
- Limit television and computer time to fewer than two hours daily.
- Encourage physical activity such as riding a bike 20 minutes a day, scheduling regular family walks, using the stairs rather than the elevator, parking far back in the mall lot.
- Ask your health care provider to plot your child's growth curve on the BMI gender-specific chart.

Research Note

A Dietary-Behavioral-Physical Activity Intervention for Childhood Obesity

Study Problem/Purpose: To examine the short- and long-term effects of a three-month combined dietary-behavioral-physical activity intervention on anthropometric measures, body composition, dietary and leisure-time habits, fitness, and lipid profiles among obese children.

Method: In a randomized prospective study, 24 obese subjects completed a three-month nutritional, behavioral, and exercise intervention. Subjects and parents heard four evening lectures: childhood obesity, general nutrition, therapeutic nutrition for obesity, and exercise for obesity. Subjects met with a dietitian six times during the three months, reviewing nutritional information and receiving a reduced-calorie diet. They participated in a twice-weekly exercise program as well as 30–45 minutes of extra activity once a week.

Findings: When compared to a control group of 22 obese, age- and gender-matched control subjects at the end of three months, the participants demonstrated significant decreases in body weight, body fat percentage, and total cholesterol levels. In a one-year follow-up, 20 of the participants continued to demonstrate a lower BMI and body fat percentage. Body weight was maintained among the participants as compared with a significant increase among the control subjects. In addition, habitual physical activity was significantly increased among the intervention participants.

Implications: Obese children show short-term and long-term benefits from interventions that include nutrition, behavioral modification, and physical activity. They are able to incorporate health promotion principles into their daily activities and lifestyles, thus improving their chances of becoming healthy adults.

Nemet, D., et al. (2005). Short- and long-term beneficial effects of combined dietary-behavioral-physical activity intervention for the treatment of childhood obesity. *Pediatrics*, 115(4), 443-449.

dren wet only at night during sleep, and they have never had a sustained period of nocturnal dryness. The occurrence of primary enuresis is common and decreases with age: 15 percent in 5-year-olds, 9 percent in 10-year-olds, and 1 percent in 15-year-olds (Sethi, Subhash, & Shipra, 2005). Boys are more likely than girls to be enuretic, and there is frequently a family history of enuresis, especially in the father.

Less common is secondary enuresis which develops after a child has a sustained period of bladder control. This development is frequently associated with a stressful event in the child's life: birth of a sibling, loss of a significant person, or extreme family disharmony.

The major health promotion strategy for families with an enuretic child is to help prevent low self-esteem and decreased self-confidence in the child. The nurse should be sure the child has been evaluated for a possible organic problem causing the enuresis such as bladder infection, neurologic abnormality, seizure disorder, diabetes mellitus, and urinary tract abnormality. Once an organic cause is ruled out, the nurse may recommend a bladder exercise program, pharmacologic therapy, or a wet alarm system. The nurse is able to provide support through sharing information about the condition, the treatment modalities, and the emotional distress enuresis causes.

Encopresis is fecal incontinence in a child 4 years of age or older who has no physical abnormality causing the incontinence. Incontinence in this case refers to the inability to retain feces. Functional encopresis affects 1 to 1.5 percent of school-age children, with males affected four times more commonly than females. Many are also enuretic. The health promotion strategy for this condition involves support by the nurse for the family and child as they undergo a bowel training program and professional counseling.

Sleep and Activity

The preschool child typically sleeps 8 to 12 hours at night. Napping behavior and need varies among children. Many preschoolers do not need a period of sleep during the day, but benefit from a time of quiet in the afternoon. Others do better with approximately one-half hour to one hour of sleep to supplement their nighttime sleep.

Bedtime becomes a time of ritual. Preschoolers may resist bedtime and attempt to prolong the bedtime ritual. Box 10-3 lists ways to facilitate preschooler bedtime.

Getting the child to stay in bed is not always easy. One innovative method is to give preschool and school-age children a free pass to get out of bed once each night. A card embossed with the child's name can be turned in for one brief visit out of the bedroom for a specific purpose—a drink of water, a hug, or a bathroom visit. If the child cries or leaves the room after the pass has been used, parents should ignore the crying and return the child to bed without eye contact and without a word. Many children save the pass for later and then fall asleep, secure in the knowledge that they had the pass. Also, knowing that leaving the bedroom is no longer forbidden removes some of its allure.

Preschoolers commonly waken during the night. Providing reassurance without restarting the bedtime ritual is usually sufficient. If awakening is due to a **night terror** (where child screams out, cries, and does not respond to parents), the parent should understand that the child is not fully awake and the terror will abate in 10 to 15 minutes. The child will fall back asleep without remembering the dream. **Nightmares** (or anxiety dreams) are more common than night terrors. The child will fully

BOX 10-3 Helping the Preschooler
at Bedtime

1. Develop a bedtime ritual of 30–45 minutes (stories, prayers, music, sitting quietly).
2. Adhere to the ritual as much as possible.
3. Be firm about bedtime.
4. Allow the child to take a special soft toy or blanket to bed.
5. Try putting a night-light in the child's room if not already using one.
6. If the child awakens during the night, reassure the child but keep the child in her or his own bed.
7. Avoid vigorous activity, sweet treats, and frightening stories or television before bedtime.

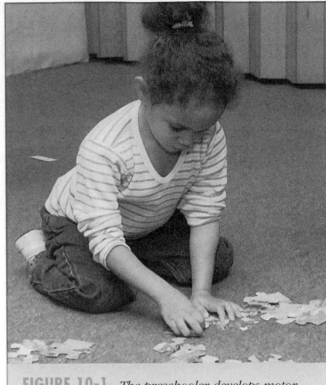

FIGURE 10-1 *The preschooler develops motor skills through repetition and trial and error.*

awaken and can describe the dream to the parents. Calm reassurance is helpful to the child at this time.

The school-age child usually sleeps between 8 and 12 hours at night. Most do not take naps during the day. Bedtime is not usually a source of struggle between the school-age child and the parents. Parents who establish an agreed-upon bedtime with the child and allow flexibility when appropriate usually receive cooperation from the child. Nightmares and night terrors may still occur, but sleepwalking and sleeptalking are more common. The health promotion strategy is to reassure parents that these sleep disturbances will tend to be outgrown. Parents should protect the sleepwalking child from injury and gently guide the child back to bed.

The preschool child receives exercise through play. The natural tendency of a preschooler to explore the environment should provide enough motor activity to achieve an adequate level of physical fitness. As shown in Figure 10-1, motor skill development occurs best in an unstructured, noncompetitive environment, allowing the preschooler to experiment and learn by trial and error. The primary health promotion strategy is to provide a safe environment for this play and exploration. The majority of children are not ready to participate in organized sports before 6 years of age.

School-age children need 20 to 30 minutes of vigorous physical activity at least three times a week as a minimum. The nurse should assess the activity level of the child through questions about interest and participation in active and sedentary hobbies, time spent watching television, participation in organized physical activity programs, and family exercise habits. Encouraging physical activity habits that would form a lifelong behavior important to improving general well-being and prevention of illness is the primary health promotion strategy for this age group. The promotion of physical activity habits in

early childhood may be the initial step in developing lifelong behaviors.

Immunization

Immunizations for the preschooler or school-age child include a booster for diphtheria-pertussis-tetanus and for polio. The trivalent oral polio vaccine is normally used except in an immune-compromised child or a child with an immune-compromised individual in the home. In those instances, the injectable vaccine may be used. Table 10-2 provides the recommended immunization schedule for children under age 7 who were not immunized in infancy. It also outlines a catch-up vaccination schedule for children ages 7–18 (Tables on pages 206–208).

Since the advent of the varicella vaccine in 1995, severe cases of chicken pox are rare; however, mild to moderate cases are being found in children who received the vaccine more than three years earlier. CDC investigators are researching whether a second dose (booster) of the vaccine will be necessary. If so, it will not add to the number of injections that the child must receive because a vaccine combining measles, mumps, rubella, and varicella is expected in the next few years.

There are additional immunizations which should be considered for at-risk preschool or school-age children. Hepatitis A is an acute, self-limiting virus which is transmitted from person to person, usually by the fecal-oral route. Children living in communities with high infection rates of hepatitis A or traveling to areas with known hepatitis A infections should be immunized with the two-dose series. Children with chronic pulmonary or cardiovascular disease should be immunized for pneumococcal diseases such as pneumonia and meningitis as well as annually for influenza. Children with immune system deficiencies need immunization against bacterial meningitis. Prevention of contagious diseases for which immunization is available is a key health promotion strategy.

Screening

Annual health maintenance visits are opportunities to screen for disease as well as to provide health teaching and anticipatory guidance. The preschooler is mature enough to cooperate with objective vision and hearing screening using standardized pictures and pure-tone audiometry. Screening for anemia and blood abnormalities such as sickle cell anemia and thalassemia should be accompanied by screening for lead. Explaining these tests gives the nurse the opportunity to discuss ways to prevent lead ingestion.

Screening blood cholesterol levels is only recommended when there is a family history of hyperlipidemia or early myocardial infarction. Blood pressure screening is begun during the preschool years. Hypertension in children less than 10 years of age usually has an organic cause. The preschooler should be screened for tuberculosis (TB) around 4 years of age. Children at high risk for TB should be screened annually. High-risk groups include medically underserved low-income populations, foreign-born children from high-prevalence countries, children in close contact with infectious TB cases, and children with compromised immune systems. Some schools require TB screening prior to enrolling.

The preschooler should have the first visit to the dentist by age 3. Follow-up discussions about proper dental care and toothbrushing can be done at each health maintenance visit along with encouraging regular visits to the dentist.

The school-age child should have vision screening prior to entry into school and periodically during the school years. Vision problems such as accommodation problems, strabismus, and astigmatism are common during the school-age years. Vision screening should also include testing for color blindness. Warning signs for vision problems in children are listed in Box 10-4.

BOX 10-4   Warning Signs for Vision Problems in Children

- Squinting
- Tilting the head to look at something
- Reluctance to do close work
- Complaining of frequent headaches

Recurrent or chronic ear infections are common in school-age children, making periodic hearing tests an important screen for hearing loss. Blood pressure screening is important for all school-age children and especially those in identified groups at high risk: obese, premature or low birth weight, and those with hypertensive parents.

The spine should be assessed for **scoliosis** (a lateral curvature of the spine), which begins during the school-age years and is aggravated by the adolescent growth spurt. Extreme curvature can impinge on lung expansion and cardiac action.

The skin should be assessed for **acanthosis nigricans,** a skin condition associated with insulin resistance and type 2 diabetes. Acanthosis nigricans (AN) is characterized by symmetrical, velvety, light brown to black, poorly marginated plaques with accentuation of skin markings (Figure 10-2). AN usually develops in flexural

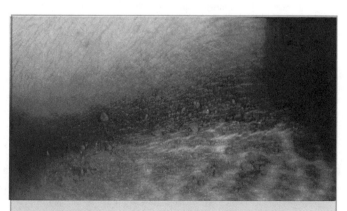

FIGURE 10-2 *This photo shows acanthosis nigricans on the back area of a child's neck.*

DEPARTMENT OF HEALTH AND HUMAN SERVICES • CENTERS FOR DISEASE CONTROL AND PREVENTION

Recommended Immunization Schedule for Persons Aged 0–6 Years—UNITED STATES • 2007

Vaccine ▼ Age ▶	Birth	1 month	2 months	4 months	6 months	12 months	15 months	18 months	19–23 months	2–3 years	4–6 years
Hepatitis B[1]	HepB	HepB		see footnote 1	HepB					HepB Series	
Rotavirus[2]			Rota	Rota	Rota						
Diphtheria, Tetanus, Pertussis[3]			DTaP	DTaP	DTaP		DTaP				DTaP
Haemophilus influenzae type b[4]			Hib	Hib	*Hib*[4]	Hib		Hib			
Pneumococcal[5]			PCV	PCV	PCV	PCV				PCV / PPV	
Inactivated Poliovirus			IPV	IPV		IPV					IPV
Influenza[6]						Influenza (Yearly)					
Measles, Mumps, Rubella[7]						MMR					MMR
Varicella[8]						Varicella					Varicella
Hepatitis A[9]						HepA (2 doses)				HepA Series	
Meningococcal[10]										MPSV4	

Range of recommended ages

Catch-up immunization

Certain high-risk groups

This schedule indicates the recommended ages for routine administration of currently licensed childhood vaccines, as of December 1, 2006, for children aged 0–6 years. Additional information is available at http://www.cdc.gov/nip/recs/child-schedule.htm. Any dose not administered at the recommended age should be administered at any subsequent visit, when indicated and feasible. Additional vaccines may be licensed and recommended during the year. Licensed combination vaccines may be used whenever any components of the combination are indicated and other components of the vaccine are not contraindicated and if approved by the Food and Drug Administration for that dose of the series. Providers should consult the respective Advisory Committee on Immunization Practices statement for detailed recommendations. Clinically significant adverse events that follow immunization should be reported to the Vaccine Adverse Event Reporting System (VAERS). Guidance about how to obtain and complete a VAERS form is available at http://www.vaers, hhs.gov or by telephone, 800-822-7967.

1. Hepatitis B vaccine (HepB). *(Minimum age: birth)*
At birth:
- Administer monovalent HepB to all newborns before hospital discharge.
- If mother is hepatitis surface antigen (HBsAg)-positive, administer HepB and 0.5 mL of hepatitis B immune globulin (HBIG) within 12 hours of birth.
- If mother's HBsAg status is unknown, administer HepB within 12 hours of birth. Determine the HBsAg status as soon as possible and if HBsAg-positive, administer HBIG (no later than age 1 week).
- If mother is HBsAg-negative, the birth dose can only be delayed with physician's order and mother's negative HBsAg laboratory report documented in the infant's medical record.

After the birth dose:
- The HepB series should be completed with either monovalent HepB or a combination vaccine containing HepB. The second dose should be administered at age 1–2 months. The final dose should be administered at age ≥ 24 weeks. Infants born to HBsAg-positive mothers should be tested for HBsAg and antibody to HBsAg after completion of ≥ 3 doses of a licensed HepB series, at age 9–18 months (generally at the next well-child visit).

4-month dose:
- It is permissible to administer 4 doses of HepB when combination vaccines are administered after the birth dose. If monovalent HepB is used for doses after the birth dose, a dose at age 4 months is not needed.

2. Rotavirus vaccine (Rota). *(Minimum age: 6 weeks)*
- Administer the first dose at age 6–12 weeks. Do not start the series later than age 12 weeks.
- Administer the final dose in the series by age 32 weeks. Do not administer a dose later than age 32 weeks.
- Data on safety and efficacy outside of these age ranges are insufficient.

3. Diphtheria and tetanus toxoids and acellular pertussis vaccine (DTaP). *(Minimum age: 6 weeks)*
- The fourth dose of DTaP may be administered as early as age 12 months, provided 6 months have elapsed since the third dose.
- Administer the final dose in the series at age 4–6 years.

4. *Haemophilus influenzae* type b conjugate vaccine (Hib). *(Minimum age: 6 weeks)*
- If PRP-OMP (PedvaxHIB® or ComVax® [Merck]) is administered at ages 2 and 4 months, a dose at age 6 months is not required.
- TriHiBit® (DTaP/Hib) combination products should not be used for primary immunization but can be used as boosters following any Hib vaccine in children aged ≥ 12 months.

5. Pneumococcal vaccine. *(Minimum age: 6 weeks for pneumococcal conjugate vaccine [PCV]; 2 years for pneumococcal polysaccharide vaccine [PPV])*
- Administer PCV at ages 24–59 months in certain high-risk groups. Administer PPV to children aged ≥ 2 years in certain high-risk groups. See *MMWR* 2000;49(No. RR-9):1–35.

6. Influenza vaccine. *(Minimum age: 6 months for trivalent inactivated influenza vaccine [TIV]; 5 years for live, attenuated influenza vaccine [LAIV])*
- All children aged 6–59 months and close contacts of all children aged 0–59 months are recommended to receive influenza vaccine.
- Influenza vaccine is recommended annually for children aged ≥ 59 months with certain risk factors, health-care workers, and other persons (including household members) in close contact with persons in groups at high risk. See *MMWR* 2006;55(No. RR-10):1–41.
- For healthy persons aged 5–49 years, LAIV may be used as an alternative to TIV.
- Children receiving TIV should receive 0.25 mL if aged 6–35 months or 0.5 mL if aged ≥ 3 years.
- Children aged <9 years who are receiving influenza vaccine for the first time should receive 2 doses (separated by ≥ 4 weeks for TIV and ≥ 6 weeks for LAIV).

7. Measles, mumps, and rubella vaccine (MMR). *(Minimum age: 12 months)*
- Administer the second dose of MMR at age 4–6 years. MMR may be administered before age 4–6 years, provided ≥ 4 weeks have elapsed since the first dose and both doses are administered at age ≥ 12 months.

8. Varicella vaccine. *(Minimum age: 12 months)*
- Administer the second dose of varicella vaccine at age 4–6 years. Varicella vaccine may be administered before age 4–6 years, provided that ≥ 3 months have elapsed since the first dose and both doses are administered at age ≥ 12 months. If second dose was administered ≥ 28 days following the first dose, the second dose does not need to be repeated.

9. Hepatitis A vaccine (HepA). *(Minimum age: 12 months)*
- HepA is recommended for all children aged 1 year (i.e., aged 12–23 months). The 2 doses in the series should be administered at least 6 months apart.
- Children not fully vaccinated by age 2 years can be vaccinated at subsequent visits.
- HepA is recommended for certain other groups of children, including in areas where vaccination programs target older children. See *MMWR* 2006;55(No. RR-7):1–23.

10. Meningococcal polysaccharide vaccine (MPSV4). *(Minimum age: 2 years)*
- Administer MPSV4 to children aged 2–10 years with terminal complement deficiencies or anatomic or functional asplenia and certain other high-risk groups. See *MMWR* 2005;54(No. RR-7):1–21.

The Recommended Immunization Schedules for Persons Aged 0–18 Years are approved by the Advisory Committee on Immunization Practices (http://www.cdc.gov/nip/acip), the American Academy of Pediatrics (http://www.aap.org), and the American Academy of Family Physicians (http://www.aafp.org).

SAFER • HEALTHIER • PEOPLE™

DEPARTMENT OF HEALTH AND HUMAN SERVICES • CENTERS FOR DISEASE CONTROL AND PREVENTION

Recommended Immunization Schedule for Persons Aged 7–18 Years—UNITED STATES • 2007

Vaccine ▼ Age ►	7–10 years	11–12 YEARS	13–14 years	15 years	16–18 years
Tetanus, Diphtheria, Pertussis[1]	*see footnote 1*	Tdap	Tdap		
Human Papillomavirus[2]	*see footnote 2*	HPV (3 doses)	HPV Series		
Meningococcal[3]	MPSV4	MCV4	MCV4[3] MCV4		
Pneumococcal[4]		PPV			
Influenza[5]		Influenza (Yearly)			
Hepatitis A[6]		HepA Series			
Hepatitis B[7]		HepB Series			
Inactivated Poliovirus[8]		IPV Series			
Measles, Mumps, Rubella[9]		MMR Series			
Varicella[10]		Varicella Series			

Range of recommended ages

Catch-up immunization

Certain high-risk groups

This schedule indicates the recommended ages for routine administration of currently licensed childhood vaccines, as of December 1, 2006, for children aged 7–18 years. Additional information is available at http://www.cdc.gov/nip/recs/child-schedule.htm. Any dose not administered at the recommended age should be administered at any subsequent visit, when indicated and feasible. Additional vaccines may be licensed and recommended during the year. Licensed combination vaccines may be used whenever any components of the combination are indicated and other components of the vaccine are not contraindicated and if approved by the Food and Drug Administration for that dose of the series. Providers should consult the respective Advisory Committee on Immunization Practices statement for detailed recommendations. Clinically significant adverse events that follow immunization should be reported to the Vaccine Adverse Event Reporting System (VAERS). Guidance about how to obtain and complete a VAERS form is available at http://www.vaers.hhs.gov or by telephone, 800-822-7967.

1. **Tetanus and diphtheria toxoids and acellular pertussis vaccine (Tdap).**
   (Minimum age: 10 years for BOOSTRIX® and 11 years for ADACEL™)
   • Administer at age 11–12 years for those who have completed the recommended childhood DTP/DTaP vaccination series and have not received a tetanus and diphtheria toxoids vaccine (Td) booster dose.
   • Adolescents aged 13–18 years who missed the 11–12 year Td/Tdap booster dose should also receive a single dose of Tdap if they have completed the recommended childhood DTP/DTaP vaccination series.

2. **Human papillomavirus vaccine (HPV).** *(Minimum age: 9 years)*
   • Administer the first dose of the HPV vaccine series to females at age 11–12 years.
   • Administer the second dose 2 months after the first dose and the third dose 6 months after the first dose.
   • Administer the HPV vaccine series to females at age 13–18 years if not previously vaccinated.

3. **Meningococcal vaccine.** *(Minimum age: 11 years for meningococcal conjugate vaccine [MCV4]; 2 years for meningococcal polysaccharide vaccine [MPSV4])*
   • Administer MCV4 at age 11–12 years and to previously unvaccinated adolescents at high school entry (at approximately age 15 years).
   • Administer MCV4 to previously unvaccinated college freshmen living in dormitories; MPSV4 is an acceptable alternative.
   • Vaccination against invasive meningococcal disease is recommended for children and adolescents aged ≥ 2 years with terminal complement deficiencies or anatomic or functional asplenia and certain other high-risk groups. See *MMWR* 2005;54(No. RR-7):1–21. Use MPSV4 for children aged 2–10 years and MCV4 or MPSV4 for older children.

4. **Pneumococcal polysaccharide vaccine (PPV).** *(Minimum age: 2 years)*
   • Administer for certain high-risk groups. See *MMWR* 1997;46(No. RR-8):1–24, and *MMWR* 2000;49(No. RR-9):1–35.

5. **Influenza vaccine.** *(Minimum age: 6 months for trivalent inactivated influenza vaccine [TIV]; 5 years for live, attenuated influenza vaccine [LAIV])*
   • Influenza vaccine is recommended annually for persons with certain risk factors, health-care workers, and other persons (including household members) in close contact with persons in groups at high risk. See *MMWR* 2006;55 (No. RR-10):1–41.
   • For healthy persons aged 5–49 years, LAIV may be used as an alternative to TIV.
   • Children aged < 9 years who are receiving influenza vaccine for the first time should receive 2 doses (separated by ≥ 4 weeks for TIV and ≥ 6 weeks for LAIV).

6. **Hepatitis A vaccine (HepA).** *(Minimum age: 12 months)*
   • The 2 doses in the series should be administered at least 6 months apart.
   • HepA is recommended for certain other groups of children, including in areas where vaccination programs target older children. See *MMWR* 2006;55 (No. RR-7):1–23.

7. **Hepatitis B vaccine (HepB).** *(Minimum age: birth)*
   • Administer the 3-dose series to those who were not previously vaccinated.
   • A 2-dose series of Recombivax HB® is licensed for children aged 11–15 years.

8. **Inactivated poliovirus vaccine (IPV).** *(Minimum age: 6 weeks)*
   • For children who received an all-IPV or all-oral poliovirus (OPV) series, a fourth dose is not necessary if the third dose was administered at age ≥ 4 years.
   • If both OPV and IPV were administered as part of a series, a total of 4 doses should be administered, regardless of the child's current age.

9. **Measles, mumps, and rubella vaccine (MMR).** *(Minimum age: 12 months)*
   • If not previously vaccinated, administer 2 doses of MMR during any visit, with ≥ 4 weeks between the doses.

10. **Varicella vaccine.** *(Minimum age: 12 months)*
    • Administer 2 doses of varicella vaccine to persons without evidence of immunity.
    • Administer 2 doses of varicella vaccine to persons aged <13 years at least 3 months apart. Do not repeat the second dose, if administered ≥ 28 days after the first dose.
    • Administer 2 doses of varicella vaccine to persons aged ≥ 13 years at least 4 weeks apart.

The Recommended Immunization Schedules for Persons Aged 0–18 Years are approved by the Advisory Committee on Immunization Practices (http://www.cdc.gov/nip/acip), the American Academy of Pediatrics (http://www.aap.org), and the American Academy of Family Physicians (http://www.aafp.org).

SAFER • HEALTHIER • PEOPLE™

Catch-up Immunization Schedule
for Persons Aged 4 Months–18 Years Who Start Late or Who Are More Than 1 Month Behind

UNITED STATES • 2007

The table below provides catch-up schedules and minimum intervals between doses for children whose vaccinations have been delayed. A vaccine series does not need to be restarted, regardless of the time that has elapsed between doses. Use the section appropriate for the child's age.

CATCH-UP SCHEDULE FOR PERSONS AGED 4 MONTHS–6 YEARS

Vaccine	Minimum Age for Dose 1	Minimum Interval Between Doses			
		Dose 1 to Dose 2	Dose 2 to Dose 3	Dose 3 to Dose 4	Dose 4 to Dose 5
Hepatitis B[1]	Birth	4 weeks	8 weeks (and 16 weeks after first dose)		
Rotavirus[2]	6 wks	4 weeks	4 weeks		
Diphtheria, Tetanus, Pertussis[3]	6 wks	4 weeks	4 weeks	6 months	6 months[3]
Haemophilus influenzae type b[4]	6 wks	4 weeks if first dose administered at age < 12 months / 8 weeks (as final dose) if first dose administered at age 12–14 months / No further doses needed if first dose administered at age ≥ 15 months	4 weeks[4] if current age < 12 months / 8 weeks (as final dose)[4] if current age ≥ 12 months and second dose administered at age < 15 months / No further doses needed if previous dose administered at age ≥ 15 months	8 weeks (as final dose) This dose only necessary for children aged 12 months–5 years who received 3 doses before age 12 months	
Pneumococcal[5]	6 wks	4 weeks if first dose administered at age < 12 months and current age < 24 months / 8 weeks (as final dose) if first dose administered at age ≥ 12 months or current age 24–59 months / No further doses needed for healthy children if first dose administered at age ≥ 24 months	4 weeks if current age < 12 months / 8 weeks (as final dose) if current age ≥ 12 months / No further doses needed for healthy children if previous dose administered at age ≥ 24 months	8 weeks (as final dose) This dose only necessary for children aged 12 months–5 years who received 3 doses before age 12 months	
Inactivated Poliovirus[6]	6 wks	4 weeks	4 weeks	4 weeks[6]	
Measles, Mumps, Rubella[7]	12 mos	4 weeks			
Varicella[8]	12 mos	3 months			
Hepatitis A[9]	12 mos	6 months			

CATCH-UP SCHEDULE FOR PERSONS AGED 7–18 YEARS

Vaccine	Minimum Age for Dose 1	Dose 1 to Dose 2	Dose 2 to Dose 3	Dose 3 to Dose 4	Dose 4 to Dose 5
Tetanus, Diphtheria/ Tetanus, Diphtheria, Pertussis[10]	7 yrs[10]	4 weeks	8 weeks if first dose administered at age < 12 months / 6 months if first dose administered at age ≥ 12 months	6 months if first dose administered at age < 12 months	
Human Papillomavirus[11]	9 yrs	4 weeks	12 weeks		
Hepatitis A[9]	12 mos	6 months			
Hepatitis B[1]	Birth	4 weeks	8 weeks (and 16 weeks after first dose)		
Inactivated Poliovirus[6]	6 wks	4 weeks	4 weeks	4 weeks[6]	
Measles, Mumps, Rubella[7]	12 mos	4 weeks			
Varicella[8]	12 mos	4 weeks if first dose administered at age ≥ 13 years / 3 months if first dose administered at age < 13 years			

1. Hepatitis B vaccine (HepB). *(Minimum age: birth)*
- Administer the 3-dose series to those who were not previously vaccinated.
- A 2-dose series of Recombivax HB® is licensed for children aged 11–15 years.

2. Rotavirus vaccine (Rota). *(Minimum age: 6 weeks)*
- Do not start the series later than age 12 weeks.
- Administer the final dose in the series by age 32 weeks. Do not administer a dose later than age 32 weeks.
- Data on safety and efficacy outside of these age ranges are insufficient.

3. Diphtheria and tetanus toxoids and acellular pertussis vaccine (DTaP). *(Minimum age: 6 weeks)*
- The fifth dose is not necessary if the fourth dose was administered at age ≥ 4 years.
- DTaP is not indicated for persons aged ≥ 7 years.

4. *Haemophilus influenzae* type b conjugate vaccine (Hib). *(Minimum age: 6 weeks)*
- Vaccine is not generally recommended for children aged ≥ 5 years.
- If current age < 12 months and the first 2 doses were PRP-OMP (PedvaxHIB® or ComVax® [Merck]), the third (and final) dose should be administered at age 12–15 months and at least 8 weeks after the second dose.
- If first dose was administered at age 7–11 months, administer 2 doses separated by 4 weeks plus a booster at age 12–15 months.

5. Pneumococcal conjugate vaccine (PCV). *(Minimum age: 6 weeks)*
- Vaccine is not generally recommended for children aged ≥ 5 years.

6. Inactivated poliovirus vaccine (IPV). *(Minimum age: 6 weeks)*
- For children who received an all-IPV or all-oral poliovirus (OPV) series, a fourth dose is not necessary if third dose was administered at age ≥ 4 years.
- If both OPV and IPV were administered as part of a series, a total of 4 doses should be administered, regardless of the child's current age.

7. Measles, mumps, and rubella vaccine (MMR). *(Minimum age: 12 months)*
- The second dose of MMR is recommended routinely at age 4–6 years but may be administered earlier if desired.
- If not previously vaccinated, administer 2 doses of MMR during any visit with ≥ 4 weeks between the doses.

8. Varicella vaccine. *(Minimum age: 12 months)*
- The second dose of varicella vaccine is recommended routinely at age 4–6 years but may be administered earlier if desired.
- Do not repeat the second dose in persons aged <13 years if administered ≥ 28 days after the first dose.

9. Hepatitis A vaccine (HepA). *(Minimum age: 12 months)*
- HepA is recommended for certain groups of children, including in areas where vaccination programs target older children. See *MMWR* 2006;55(No. RR-7):1–23.

10. Tetanus and diphtheria toxoids vaccine (Td) and tetanus and diphtheria toxoids and acellular pertussis vaccine (Tdap). *(Minimum ages: 7 years for Td, 10 years for BOOSTRIX®, and 11 years for ADACEL™)*
- Tdap should be substituted for a single dose of Td in the primary catch-up series or as a booster if age appropriate; use Td for other doses.
- A 5-year interval from the last Td dose is encouraged when Tdap is used as a booster dose. A booster (fourth) dose is needed if any of the previous doses were administered at age <12 months. Refer to ACIP recommendations for further information. See *MMWR* 2006;55(No. RR-3).

11. Human papillomavirus vaccine (HPV). *(Minimum age: 9 years)*
- Administer the HPV vaccine series to females at age 13–18 years if not previously vaccinated.

Information about reporting reactions after immunization is available online at http://www.vaers.hhs.gov or by telephone via the 24-hour national toll-free information line 800-822-7967. Suspected cases of vaccine-preventable diseases should be reported to the state or local health department. Additional information, including precautions and contraindications for immunization, is available from the National Center for Immunization and Respiratory Diseases at http://www.cdc.gov/nip/default.htm or telephone, 800-CDC-INFO (800-232-4636).

DEPARTMENT OF HEALTH AND HUMAN SERVICES • CENTERS FOR DISEASE CONTROL AND PREVENTION • SAFER • HEALTHIER • PEOPLE

areas, especially the axillae, nape of the neck, the groin, and the anogenital areas. Obesity is the most common abnormality associated with AN between the ages of 12 and 30. Individuals with AN usually exhibit fasting plasma insulin levels markedly higher than those in other obese individuals without these cutaneous changes. Obese children with insulin resistance are at a high risk of developing type 2 diabetes. Screening for AN can lead to health promotion strategies that reduce obesity in children with AN. Weight loss and daily exercise can reverse the pathophysiological process responsible for AN by reducing both insulin resistance and compensatory hyperinsulinemia, thereby reducing the risk of type 2 diabetes mellitus.

Psychological Domain

Preschool children are in Piaget's preoperational stage of cognitive development in which they are able to perform symbolic functioning—making and verbalizing mental images (Brainerd, 1978). Symbolic functioning is especially noted during play when children use symbolic games to represent reality. They use play objects to represent real objects in their environment, such as using a popsicle stick to represent a spoon to eat a make-believe lunch, or a rock to represent a cookie. The social rules and interactions of society are imitated during play, sometimes with an imaginary friend or pet. Thought processes are very concrete and **egocentric,** concentrating upon themselves with little or no regard to others or the external world. The preschoolers have difficulty concentrating on more than one aspect of a situation and cannot fathom a point of view other than their own. It is through play that preschoolers experience and learn about their environment, learn social roles, and develop both fine and gross motor skills. The primary health promotion strategy for this cognitive development is having a loving caretaker for the child to imitate who encourages safe exploration of the real world and development of imagination, logical thinking skills, and creative activities.

Emotional assessment of the preschooler finds the child in Erikson's third stage of development, wrestling with resolution of the initiative versus guilt conflict. Resolution of this developmental crisis finds the child becoming more assertive and exuberantly initiating new tasks using his or her developing physical and mental mastery. This quest for power may bring with it feelings of guilt for being too forceful. Health promotion strategies seek to promote the development of physical and mental mastery in situations over which the child has control. Achieving mastery of new actions and situations encourages the preschooler to continue exploration and experimentation. Criticism or ridicule promotes feelings of guilt and inadequacy, inhibiting further initiative.

The school-age child moves into Piaget's concrete operational stage of cognitive development (Brainerd,

1978). In this stage, the child demonstrates cooperative rather than egocentric interactions, the ability to classify and order objects, and an understanding of the concepts of reversibility, transformation, and conservation. A school-age child begins to be able to see another's point of view, even requesting another's advice or including another person in conversation. The ability to classify and order objects forms the basis for learning mathematics and understanding relationships. Realizing that objects and activities can be reversed, changed, or remain the same despite a slight change in form is an important development in the child's ability to understand the world. The concept of time also develops during this period.

Although the preschool child may participate in a formal type of educational experience, it is the school-age child who faces the prospect of the next 12 years in the institution of school. The changes in personal and social relationships encountered with entry into school often present a developmental crisis for both the child and the family. The school-age child is under constant pressure to learn new skills. The developmental task according to Erikson is industry versus inferiority (Erikson, 1950). The mastery of both personal and social tasks gives children a sense of industry—the belief that they can learn, solve problems, and be a part of the real world.

Health promotion strategies involve giving the child an opportunity to learn competence without excessive fear of the consequences of failure. The child who is given no cushion for the experience of learning will become fearful and withdrawn and resist trying new skills or activities. Occasionally these children will seek attention in an inappropriate manner through acting-out behaviors: bossiness, lying, and destructive activities.

Attention-Deficit/Hyperactivity Disorder

Attention-deficit/hyperactivity disorder (ADHD) is a neurobehavioral disorder found in approximately 9 percent of boys and 3 percent of girls (Maharaj & Call-Schmidt, 2005). Increased impulsivity, inability to concentrate, hyperactivity, and difficulties in school and family relationships are the most common symptoms. The majority of children with this disorder do not have a learning disability, but they usually have difficulty with schoolwork and may have a three- to five-year developmental delay as compared to their peers. Children with ADHD should be evaluated by a multidisciplinary team to determine the need for assistance. Sometimes medications are needed to allow the students to more fully participate in their education, improve their academic and social skills, and decrease their impulsivity. Parent education classes, advocacy group conferences, support groups, social skill classes, and counseling for both the child and the family may also help with behavioral management. In the classroom, there are numerous strategies to help the child with ADHD (see Box 10-5).

- Seat the child in the front of the room, away from sources of distraction like doors or windows.
- Seat the child near a task-focused child.
- Teach the child to make a list and cross off completed tasks.
- Provide frequent bathroom breaks and allow the child to move around the classroom as needed.
- Allow the child to leave the room for a few minutes if frustrated.
- Develop consistent routines.
- Help the child keep the work space neat and uncluttered.

Communicate regularly with the parents about the child's behavior and progress.

Children diagnosed with ADHD are entitled to a free and appropriate public education as well as special education programs as needed (see the Political Domain section later in this chapter). The health promotion strategy for this condition is to educate parents and teachers about the symptoms of ADHD, so that the condition can be recognized earlier in the child's educational career with methods and strategies implemented to prevent developmental delays.

Social Domain

The social domain for the preschool and school-age child is focused on relationships with the family, peers, and the community. Significant social influences also include television and culture.

Relationships

Exploring their own roles as well as trying out others helps preschoolers understand who they are in relation to their families and the world. The ability to imagine how others feel and behave moves the child from total egocentrism toward cooperation in the world. Most preschoolers have a sibling—older, younger, or both. The health promotion strategy recommended in this area is observing and guiding the social relationship between the siblings.

Preschoolers with an older sibling may find themselves envious of all the attention the older sibling receives and frustrated at being unable to do similar things. Praising the preschooler for her or his own accomplishments will help the child have positive feelings about herself or himself, thus building self-esteem.

Preschoolers who have been presented with a younger sibling may display jealousy plus regressive demanding behaviors. Parents who inform the preschooler about the upcoming addition to the family, involve the preschooler in preparations, and encourage the preschooler to express her or his personal opinions will experience a less difficult period of transition. Once the new arrival is in the home, spending special time alone with the preschooler, encouraging the preschooler to help the parents in caring for the baby, and giving the preschooler a doll to promote role play as a caregiver may also assist in the transition.

People outside the immediate family may begin to influence the child if they are in contact frequently enough. Grandparents, aunts and uncles, and peers provide the child with insights into different social situations, preparing the child to interact in group situations, cooperate with others, and increase personal independence. All these social accomplishments help prepare the child for school. Again, praise for the child's accomplishments and positive reinforcement for cooperative behaviors are the needed strategies to promote the child's social health.

The broadening of social contacts outside the home continues for the school-age child. **Peers** (individuals of the same age) play a central role in the development of the child's identity, often competing with that of the parents. During the first half of the school-age years (6 to 9), same-gender peers are preferred. This preference changes as the child moves toward adolescence. Interactions with peers often lead to testing of rules and values learned from the parents. Peer acceptance helps build the child's self-esteem and feelings of self-worth, but the lessening of parental influence may cause anxiety in some parents. Parents with high self-esteem who have demonstrated an affectionate, supportive relationship with the child will continue to be the primary role models and support for the developing child. Health promotion strategies for the child involve approval and reinforcement of appropriate behaviors and accomplishments. For the parents of the school-age child, strategies involve exploring parental concerns and guiding or validating supportive parental behaviors.

Television

Outside the family, the most significant social influence on the preschool and school-age child is television. In the United States, children watch an average of 25 hours of television weekly (Strasburger & Wilson, 2002). By the time they graduate from high school, they will have spent less time in the classroom than watching television. Children who watch three to four hours of television daily tend to perform poorer in school, read and exercise less, be obese, play less well with friends, have fewer hobbies, and view the world as a dangerous and scary place. In addition, these children tend to have an increased potential for alcohol and drug use as well as earlier involvement in sexual activity (Gidwani et al., 2002).

Watching of television advertisements may be as harmful as television programs such as soap operas, adult sitcoms, adult talk shows, and violent shows. Although preschoolers do not understand that the purpose of advertising is to sell a product, school-age children who watch a lot of television are more likely to believe the advertising claims. A review of advertisements during typical Saturday morning children's programming finds that 90 percent are selling sugary cereals, candy, salty snacks, fatty foods, junk food, and toys. Children see tens of thousands of alcohol commercials before they reach the legal age to consume such beverages. There is approximately one hour of commercials for every five hours of programming.

Not all television watching is detrimental. With guided program selection, the preschooler can develop imagination and learn letters, numbers, colors, and shapes. The school-age child, with appropriate guidance in program selection, can learn historical information, geography, and positive behaviors such as cooperation and friendship. Box 10-6 describes the health promotion strategies that can be recommended to parents and caregivers who want to use television watching in a healthy and positive way.

Cultural Influences

As the preschooler takes a more active role in family practices, rituals, and holidays, she may begin to notice differences between her cultural heritage and that of playmates or neighbors. The natural curiosity about the world demonstrated by this age group provides an excellent opportunity to begin education about diversity in cultures, races, and individuals. Health promotion strategies involve imparting an appreciation for the contribution diversity brings to the world. Prejudices demonstrated by the parents, caregivers, or playmates will be rapidly adopted by the preschooler.

The school-age child has increased opportunities to interact with individuals from different cultures. Parents and teachers can promote respect and appreciation for cultural differences through reading assignments, classroom interactions, and participation in various cultural events. Knowledge of the beliefs, values, and practices of diverse cultures reduces the development of ethnocentrism and prejudice.

Political Domain

Political initiatives that have had a direct impact on the preschool and school-age child include Medicaid, the State Children's Health Insurance program, and the National School Lunch Program. Each of these federal initiatives addresses child health through health promotion. In addition, the Individuals with Disabilities Education Act and Section 504 of the Rehabilitation Act have had a strong impact on the education provided for preschool and school-age children.

Medicaid and the State Children's Health Insurance Program

Although children birth to 18 years made up 29 percent of the population in 1999, they accounted for only 12 percent of spending on personal health care (Keehan, Lazenby, Zezza, & Catlin, 2004). Two-thirds of their health care is financed through private health insurance and Medicaid. Title XIX of the Social Security Act (Medicaid) provides federal matching funds for states to provide comprehensive preventive, acute, and chronic care services for eligible low-income children. Title XXI, the State Children's Health Insurance Program (SCHIP), was passed in 1997 to expand public health insurance coverage for low-income children in families that cannot afford private health insurance but make too much money to qualify for Medicaid. In its first year, 1999,

---

BOX 10-6 Guide to Healthy Use of Television

Preschool Children	School-Age Children
1. Limit TV viewing to one–two hours daily.	1. Limit TV viewing to one–two hours daily.
2. Choose shows and videos developed especially for preschoolers.	2. Select developmentally appropriate shows.
3. Make a weekly plan for appropriate shows.	3. Discuss unrealistic role models and values when viewed on a program.
4. Discuss what is fantasy and what is real on TV shows.	4. Encourage activities other than television watching: sports, hobbies, play.
5. Prohibit watching of violence.	5. Prohibit watching of violence.
6. Turn off TV during family mealtime.	6. Turn off TV while completing homework.
7. Set an example for responsible TV watching.	7. Do not allow child to have a TV in her or his bedroom.

SCHIP spending was $1.6 billion, or less than 1 percent of children's total health spending. As the program grew, spending reached $5.7 billion in 2002 (Keehan et al., 2004). Children with greater health service needs tend to participate in Medicaid/SCHIP at higher rates than other children do (Dubay, Kenney, & Haley, 2002). Reaching the millions of children who are eligible but who remain uninsured continues to be an important health promotion challenge and strategy.

National School Lunch Program

Another federal benefit that has a significant impact on the health of school-age children is the National School Lunch Program. Enacted in 1946 to provide the opportunity for children to receive at least one healthy meal every school day, the program reimburses schools for providing a nutritious meal to eligible children. Over 29 million children participated in the lunch program in 2004 through 92,000 participating schools.

The Individuals with Disabilities Education Act

Two federal laws entitle children diagnosed with ADHD to get assistance with their educational needs. The Individuals with Disabilities Education Act (IDEA) provides funding to guarantee 3- to 21-year-olds a free and appropriate education, based on assessment of individual needs, in the least restrictive environment that is racially and culturally unbiased, as well as an individualized education program (IEP) prepared by a team of professionals (Maharaj & Call-Schmidt, 2005). The act requires school systems to pay for related services such as transportation, audiology, recreation, psychological services, and social work services. It requires a written IEP for each child with parental input in educational planning and decision making.

Section 504 of the Rehabilitation Act was passed to end discrimination against any person with a handicap. When a child has emotional or behavioral problems in school, Section 504 protects the child from discrimination and provides interventions in the classroom. If a child with a disability has been identified and confirmed by school testing, accommodations must be made to assist the child to succeed in the classroom. If a child does not qualify for special education (IDEA), he or she can be evaluated for a Section 504 accommodation, so that behavior and curriculum modification can be implemented.

Environmental Domain

The accident rate for preschoolers is less than that for toddlers; however, preschoolers are still impulsive and lack sufficient maturity to recognize all potential dangers. Table 10-4 lists common sources of injury for preschool children and health promotion strategies to help prevent accidental injury. Two areas of health promotion should be emphasized: street safety and firearm safety.

The preschool child is not mature enough to play close to streets or cross streets without adult supervision. Use of riding toys should be confined to sidewalks and other protected areas, with particular care being used if there are driveway intersections. Firearm safety has been receiving needed attention, especially with the passage of some recent state laws allowing the personal carrying of handguns. Many of these states have also passed laws holding the gun owners responsible for accidents or injuries caused by their guns. There is no truly safe place for a loaded gun in any household where a child might be living or visiting. The only safe gun is unloaded, with the gun and the ammunition stored separately under lock and key.

An environmental hazard that affects both the preschool and the school-age child is exposure to tobacco smoke. Approximately 43 percent of children from 2 months to 11 years of age live in homes with at least one smoker. Epidemiologic studies have associated increased rates of lower respiratory illness and increased rates of middle ear effusion, asthma, and SIDS with exposure of children to environmental smoke. Childhood exposure may also increase rates of cancer development in adulthood. Promoting a smoke-free environment is a health promotion strategy that would benefit individuals across the life span.

Bicycle riding is responsible for a large majority of accidents to school-age children. The use of helmets has been shown to reduce the risk of head injury by 85 percent (Clements, 2005). Helmets must be properly fitted and meet the standards developed by the Snell Memorial Foundation and the American National Standards Institutes. The American Pediatrics Association has recommended that retail stores sell inexpensive approved helmets as a "package deal" to individuals buying bicycles. Positive factors that influence a child's compliance with wearing a bicycle helmet include parental ownership and use of a helmet while cycling, parental rules enforcing helmet use, and peers and siblings who use a helmet. Children were 100 times more likely to own and use a helmet if their parents used one (Clements, 2005). Negative factors include cost, appearance, comfort, inconvenience, and not seeing a need because of riding close to home.

The potential for injuries from contact sports and playground equipment for this age group makes adult supervision during these activities imperative.

Sexual Domain

The preschool child recognizes gender differences and has a developing sexual curiosity. Negative reactions from caregivers toward this curiosity will make the child repress these feelings and may be detrimental to the child's developing body- and self-image. The preschool age is the age of "1,000 questions," and some of those questions will be about sex. Parents need accurate infor-

TABLE 10-4 Environmental Safety for Preschool and School-Age Children

Source of Injury	Prevention Strategies
Automobiles	Supervise children younger than 10 when crossing streets. Teach street-crossing techniques. Use a booster seat if child is under 70 lb. Always use both lap and shoulder restraints. If shoulder restraint crosses child's face, place it behind the child. Encourage riding in the back seat. Keep car doors locked when moving. Do not allow child to ride in the cargo area of a pick-up, van, or station wagon. Provide a good role model.
Sports/play	Participate in a bicycle training course. Use a bicycle helmet for rider and passenger. Use bike lanes if available. Watch traffic and encourage off-peak riding times. Use safety helmet and pads when skating. Use safety lenses for indicated sports and hobbies. Provide adequate adult supervision for playground and team sports activities. Watch for exhaustion and heat exposure. Restrict play around stairs and windows or on furniture.
Poison	Keep medicines and dangerous chemicals in a locked cabinet. Buy vitamins and other over-the-counter medications in small quantities. Keep a bottle of ipecac syrup available to induce vomiting when necessary.
Water	Teach children to swim. Never let children swim alone. Use a personal flotation device in boats and around lakes and rivers.
Fire/burns	Always supervise children cooking. Keep hot water heater set at 120–130 degrees. Install smoke detectors and test regularly. Use flame-retardant clothing around stoves, fires, and adults who smoke.
Firearms	Keep all firearms unloaded and locked up.

mation in order to give factual responses. The ability to supply age-appropriate information with honesty is essential to helping the child develop. Choosing the right time and place and taking advantage of "teachable moments" may help parents deal with the barrage of questions more comfortably. The questions that naturally arise when the child notices that the mother has breasts or that father has a penis, or sees a sexually oriented program or advertisement on television, may create a teachable moment. Parents can also use books, pamphlets, or situations to stimulate teachable moments.

Sexuality education (factual information about anatomy, physiology, birth control, and sexually transmitted diseases) should occur during the school-age years. Although school-age children are at the height of their sexual curiosity, their sexual urges are dormant, making this the ideal time to prepare them for the upcoming changes of puberty. Age-appropriate information about

puberty and reproduction can be presented before the child becomes self-conscious about his or her emerging sexuality. The understanding of the information should be evaluated, because the child can misinterpret, pick up on limited parts, or be influenced by misinformation from peers. A vital health promotion strategy for the nurse is to encourage parents and schools to collaborate in providing factual, complete sexuality information for the school-age child.

Spiritual Domain

The preschool child begins more active participation in the spiritual and religious life of the family. Reading books, saying simple prayers, and participating in the celebration of religious holidays and family rituals are appropriate methods for developing the spiritual health of young children. Both the preschool and the school-age child should be taught the value of kindness, goodness, patience, faithfulness, gentleness, and self-control.

The school-age child is mature enough for reading, study, and discussion about the family's religious and spiritual beliefs. In addition to participation in celebrations and rituals, the school-age child can observe and understand the application of religious principles to everyday life.

SUMMARY

Promoting the health of the preschool and school-age child recognizes the significant social, emotional, and cognitive growth that is occurring. Providing adequate nutrition without causing overweight or obesity requires education about wholesome diets and the need for regular physical activity. Screening for immunization status, vision and hearing problems, delayed development, and learning and behavior problems as well as physical problems is essential. Keeping preschool and school-age children safe and preventing accidents play a crucial role in helping them grow up healthy.

This chapter grouped health promotion strategies into sections for the preschool and the school-age child. Each age group was viewed through biological, psychological, social, political, environmental, sexual, and spiritual domains for a comprehensive look at health promotion in the early years of life. Table 10-5 provides suggested health promotion actions related to areas of risk assessment for these domains that specifically apply to children.

TABLE 10-5 Health Promotion in Children

Related Domain	Risk Assessment	Health Promotion Action
Biological	Nutrition	Varied, well-balanced diet with reduced fat and empty calories.
		Identify underweight, at-risk for overweight, and overweight children through Body Mass Index.
	Elimination	Assessment for enuresis, encopresis, or both with appropriate follow-up.
	Sleep and activity	Bedtime routines and rituals. Regular physical activity (30 minutes at least three to four times weekly).
	Immunization	Adherence to immunization schedule and catch-up if needed.
Psychological	Cognitive and emotional development	Assessment for appropriate cognitive and emotional development according to age and stage.
Social	Relationships	Approval and reinforcement of appropriate behaviors with family and peers. Supervised and guided television watching.
Environmental	Accidents	Anticipatory guidance to prevent accidental injury.
Sexual	Knowledge	Encourage factual, age-appropriate information from parents and schools.
Spiritual	Values Beliefs	Encourage application of religious principles to everyday life.

Objectives/Goals: Through participation in discussion of this case study, participants will have the opportunity to:

1. Discuss the assessment of a child for weight and nutrition.
2. Investigate the relationship between overweight and development of type 2 diabetes.
3. Discuss dietary and activity changes to prevent childhood obesity.

Health Promotion Concern, History and Physical, Present Health Status, Past Health Status, Family History, and Social History

Shauney Williams is a 10-year-old Black female who was referred for evaluation of grade 2 acanthosis nigricans on the nape of her neck. She is in the fourth grade in a local elementary school and is making As and Bs in her school work. She is the youngest of three children in the family. Her birth was a spontaneous vaginal delivery, and she weighed 8 pounds 12 ounces. Her mother is 5'4" and weighs approximately 180 pounds. She weighed about the same before Shauney's birth. Shauney has always been above the 75th percentile in the weight-for-age and height-for-age charts. She is up-to-date with her immunizations.

Review of Pertinent Domains

Biological Domain

Physical exam: Reveals a 4'10" female weighing 108 pounds. Her BMI is 22.6, which puts her at risk for overweight. Thyroid is without enlargement or nodules.

Genitourinary: Shauney reports no problems in this area. She has regular bowel movements and urinates with no problems.

Integumentary: Shauney noticed the darkening on the back of her neck approximately one year ago. She says she also has it under her arms. She has a velvety, hyperpigmented brown plaque with accentuated skin markings on the nape of her neck. The hyperpigmentation is a lighter brown in her axillae.

Cardiovascular: Her blood pressure is normal for her age.

24-Hour Diet Recall: Sugar Frosted Flakes and whole milk for breakfast. School lunch plus ice cream bar from vending machine for lunch. After-school snack of cookies and cola drink. Fried chicken, green beans, corn, and mashed potatoes with gravy for dinner. Bedtime snack of small piece of cake and whole milk.

Activity Recall: Played softball in physical education at school. Watched TV and played video games on the computer during the afternoon after school. Watched TV after dinner with family until bedtime.

Diagnostic Testing: Shauney's hematocrit, urinalysis, TSH, ALT, and fasting serum glucose and lipid panel are within normal limits. Her fasting serum insulin level is slightly elevated.

Psychological Domain

Shauney's grades are above average, and she has no trouble completing assignments on time. Shauney's and the family's readiness to make lifestyle changes needs to be assessed.

Social Domain

Shauney is a bright, sociable child who makes friends easily.

Environmental Domain

Shauney's family is upper middle-class and surrounds her with love, but as the youngest in the family, she is always rewarded with lots of candies and rich foods, which she likes to eat in abundance. No limits are placed on Shauney's eating habits and, as a consequence, she is considered big for her age. Shauney and her family need education about the presence of acanthosis nigricans as a marker for insulin resistance, the relationship between overweight and development of type 2 diabetes, and the need for a wholesome, low-fat diet and daily exercise.

Questions for Discussion

1. What risk factors does Shauney have for being overweight?
2. Why should Shauney's mother be concerned about her daughter having acanthosis nigricans?
3. What changes in lifestyle should be recommended for Shauney and her family?

Key Concepts

1. Health promotion for infants and children in the biological domain includes strategies related to nutrition, elimination, sleep and activity, and immunization.

2. Screening for actual or potential health problems in children is vital for promoting the quality and quantity of life. Nurses assist in screening for hypertension, TB, vision and hearing problems, scoliosis, and acanthosis nigricans for school-age children.

3. Promoting health in the psychological domain requires an understanding of normal cognitive and emotional development. Theoretical frameworks developed by Jean Piaget and Erik Erikson provide a foundation for evaluating development of children.

4. Health promotion in the social domain for children evolves from the family to include day-care networks, school, and the community. The influence of television should be consistently evaluated and regulated.

5. Child abuse and neglect occur in more than 1 million children annually. Nurses need to look for physical signs including bruising, hematomas, poor skin care, malnutrition, bite marks, and retinal hemorrhage. Parental behavior and discrepancies between the reported cause of injury and the injury seen can also be important keys to identifying abuse. Any suspicion of abuse or neglect must, by law, be reported to the appropriate authorities.

6. In addition to legislation mandating reporting of suspected child abuse, there are other social actions for health promotion from the political domain. These include the Supplemental Food Program for Women, Infants, and Children (WIC), car occupant safety requirement laws, Medicaid, SCHIP and IDEA programs, and the National School Lunch Program.

7. Nurses and parents share responsibility for promoting safety of children. Safety strategies include providing foods appropriate for age; giving immunizations; using seatbelts, car seats, and protective helmets; and teaching behaviors for healthy lifestyles. Preventing physical and psychological trauma is vital to ensure healthy development throughout the life span.

8. Important in the sexual domain is the education of parents and caregivers about normal sexual development of children. The provision of complete, accurate sexuality education is critical for the development of sexual health.

9. Spiritual beliefs and practices of the parents and caregivers influence health promotion in the spiritual domain.

Learning Activities

1. Plan an educational program designed to assist parents with management of the preschooler or school-age child who is a "picky eater."

2. Develop a brochure for parents related to the prevention of overweight in children.

3. List positive findings for acanthosis nigricans. Participate in a screening for acanthosis nigricans.

True/False Questions

1. T or F   The first step in assessing a child's weight and nutrition is to determine the child's body mass index (BMI).

2. T of F   The USDA school lunch guideline recommends that less than 20 percent of calories should come from fat.

3. T or F   A high birth weight, maternal diabetes, and a family history of obesity pose known risks for childhood obesity.

4. T or F   Children with mild illnesses such as colds, flu, and ear infections (either with or without fever) should still get their immunizations on schedule.

Multiple Choice Questions

1. The average weekly amount of time a 10-year-old watches television is approximately:
   a.   8 hours.
   b.   15 hours.
   c.   25 hours.
   d.   36 hours.

2. Strategies to help a preschooler adjust to the addition of a new sibling to the family include which of the following?
   a.   Assure the preschooler that she or he will love the new baby.
   b.   Give the preschooler a doll to promote role play as a caregiver.
   c.   Avoid discussion about the new baby until one or two weeks before its arrival because of the short attention span of most preschoolers.
   d.   Wait until the new baby arrives to move the preschooler to a new room.

3. Which of the following is a significant influence on whether a child uses a bicycle helmet?
   a.   The helmet fits properly.
   b.   The parent uses a helmet while cycling.
   c.   The child has had a previous accident with a head injury.
   d.   The bicycle will be ridden over one mile from home.

Websites

http://www.smallstep.gov U.S. Department of Health and Human Services. Site at which you can subscribe to a newsletter and download a comprehensive book, *A Parent's Guide to Healthy Eating and Physical Activity*.

http://www.diabetes.org American Diabetes Association. Offers a wealth of information on diabetes for all ages.

http://www.eatright.org American Dietetic Association. Offers a current search engine to help locate useful nutrition-related content accurately and quickly.

http://www.cdc.gov CDC on BMI. Has a link to explain and calculate body mass index.

http://www.aap.org American Academy of Pediatrics. An excellent resource for topics related to children and adolescents.

Organizations

Department of Child and Adolescent Health and Development (CAH)
World Health Organization
Avenue Appia 20, CH-1211
Geneva 27, Switzerland
Email: cah@who.int
Provides resources for child and adolescent health and development.

Partnership for Children's Health and the Environment
1646 Dow Road
Freeland, WA 98249
Tel: (360) 331-7904
E-mal: emiller@iceh.org
Provides information and networking for children's health.

Children's Safety Network (CNS) National Injury and Violence Prevention Resource Center
Main Office: Education Development Center, Inc.
55 Chapel Street
Newton, MA 02458-1060
Tel: (617) 618-2230
E-mail: csn@edc.org
Washington Office: Education Development Center, Inc.
1000 Potomac St., Suite 350
Washington, DC 20007
Tel: (202) 572-3734
E-mail: eschmidt@edc.org
Provides information for children's safety.

References

American Academy of Pediatrics (AAP). (2003). Prevention of pediatric overweight and obesity. *Pediatrics, 112*(2), 424–430.

Boney, C., Verma, A., Tucker, R., & Vohr, B. (2005). Metabolic syndrome in childhood: Association with birth weight, maternal obesity, and gestational diabetes mellitus. *Pediatrics, 115*(3), e290–296.

Brainerd, C. J. (1978). Piaget's theory of intelligence. Englewood Cliffs, NJ: Prentice Hall.

Clements, J. (2005). Promoting the use of bicycle helmets during primary care visits. *Journal of the American Academy of Nurse Practitioners, 17*(9), 350–354.

Dubay, L., Kenney, G., & Haley, J. (2002). Children's participation in Medicaid and SCHIP: Early in the SCHIP era. *New Federalism: National Survey of America's Families*, Number B-40. Washington, DC: The Urban Institute.

Erikson, E. (1950). Childhood and society. New York: Norton.

Gidwani, P., Sobol, A., DeJong, W., Perrin, J., & Gortmaker, S. (2002). Television viewing and initiation of smoking among youth. *Pediatrics, 110*(3), 505–508.

Henry, L. (2005). Childhood obesity: What can be done to help today's youth? *Pediatric Nursing, 31*(1), 13–16.

Holcomb, S. (2004). Obesity in children and adolescents: Guidelines for prevention and management. *Nurse Practitioner, 29*(8), 9–15.

Keehan, S., Lazenby, H., Zezza, M., & Catlin, M. (2004). Age estimates in the national health accounts. *Health Care Financing Review/Web Exclusive, 1*(1), 1–16.

Louthan, M., Lafferty-Oza, M., Smith, E. et al. (2005). Diagnosis and treatment frequency for overweight children and adolescents at well child visits. *Clinical Pediatrics, 44*, 57–61.

Maharaj, G., & Call-Schmidt, T. (2005). Advocating for children with ADHD. *Advance for Nurse Practitioners, 13*(2), 53–56.

Nemet, D., Barkan, S., Epstein, Y., Friedland, O., Kowen, G., & Eliakim, A. (2005). Short- and long-term beneficial effects of a combined dietary-behavioral-physical activity intervention for the treatment of childhood obesity. *Pediatrics, 115*(4), e443–449.

Ogden, C. I., Flegal, K. M., Carroll, M. D., et al. (2002). Prevalence and trends in overweight among U.S. children and adolescents, 1999–2000. *Journal of the American Medical Association, 288*, 1728–1732.

Rich, S., DiMarco, N., Huettig, C., Essery, E., Andersson, E., & Sanborn, C. (2005). Perceptions of health status and play activities in parents of overweight Hispanic toddlers and preschoolers. *Family and Community Health, 28*(2), 130–142.

Sethi, S., Subhash, B., & Shipra, M. (2005). Nocturnal enuresis: A review. *Journal of Pediatric Neurology 3*(1), 11–18.

Strasburger, V., & Wilson, B. (2002). *Children, adolescents, and the media*. Thousand Oaks, CA: Sage.

Whitaker, R. (2004). Predicting preschooler obesity at birth: The role of maternal obesity in early pregnancy. *Pediatrics, 114*(1), e29–36.

Chapter 11

THE ADOLESCENT AND YOUNG ADULT

Barbara A. Tucker, PhD, FPN, APRN-BC

KEY TERMS

abuse
acne
alpha brain waves
anorexia nervosa
bulimia nervosa
cohabitation

dental caries
intimate partner violence
gonads
gynecomastia
homosexuality
hypothalamus

incest
masturbation
meditation
melanoma
menarche
Papanicolaou (Pap) test

premenstrual
  syndrome (PMS)
puberty
substance abuse

OBJECTIVES

Upon completion of this chapter, the reader should be able to:

- Examine health promotion strategies in the biological domain for adolescents and young adults.
- Identify nursing responsibilities for screening to promote health of adolescents and young adults.
- Relate theories of cognitive and emotional development to health promotion strategies in adolescents and young adults.
- Describe occurrence of, signs and symptoms of, nursing responsibilities for, and strategies to reduce or prevent abuse and domestic violence.
- Identify political influences on the adolescent and young adult.
- Describe strategies to reduce accidental deaths in adolescents and young adults.
- Relate normal emotional and sexual development to strategies designed to promote sexual health in adolescents and young adults.
- Describe spiritual development in adolescents and young adults.

INTRODUCTION

Individuals in the adolescent and young adult period of their life span are generally the healthiest they have ever been or will be. Their mortality rates are among the lowest of all age groups, and they have the lowest morbidity rates for chronic medical conditions of the entire population. This healthy condition may lessen the adolescent's or young adult's perceived need for health promotion. It is important to note, however, that the major causes of death for older adults have their roots in the behaviors adopted during the adolescent and young adult stages. Unhealthy eating patterns and low levels of physical activity are important factors in later development of cardiovascular disease. An equal threat to health are the social morbidities of unintended pregnancy, sexually transmitted infections, homicide, suicide, injuries related to violence, and substance abuse. The prevention of health-risk behaviors and the development of health-promoting behaviors during the adolescent and young adult period will have a lifelong positive effect on health status.

This chapter is divided into two sections: the adolescent and the young adult. Health promotion strategies are viewed through the biological, psychological, social, political, environmental, sexual, and spiritual domains to provide a guiding framework for organization.

THE ADOLESCENT

The period between childhood and adulthood is called adolescence. It is characterized by physical, sexual, and psychological maturation. This maturation signals the transference of health promotion responsibilities from the caregivers, or parents, to the individual.

Biological Domain

In chronological terms, adolescence is generally a period of 10 to 12 years beginning with the onset of puberty. By definition, **puberty** is the period in life during which members of both genders become capable of reproduction. This period of change usually occurs between the ages of 11 and 15 in boys and 9 and 16 in girls, ending in the attainment of sexual maturity (Kaplan and Love-Osborne, 2003). In addition, the physical growth to the adult stature is also completed.

Puberty

Puberty is a dynamic biological process which is determined by highly organized mechanisms intrinsic to each individual. It depends on a complex interaction between the hypothalamus, anterior pituitary, the **gonads** (ovaries and testes), and the body's muscles and skeleton.

Control over these events is primarily in the **hypothalamus**, the gland in the brain responsible for control of metabolic activities, regulation of body temperature, integration of sympathetic and parasympathetic activities, and secretion of releasing (stimulating) and inhibiting hormones (Guyton & Hall, 2006). The hypothalamus

secretes two releasing hormones to stimulate the anterior pituitary gland. One stimulates the pituitary gland to release sex steroids and the other stimulates the pituitary to release growth hormones. The sex steroids (follicle-stimulating hormone and luteinizing hormone) stimulate maturation of the gonads. The hormones produced by the gonads are responsible for the development of the secondary sex characteristics. The estrogenic activity of the ovaries causes growth and development of the vagina, uterus, Fallopian tubes, and breasts. The androgenic activity of the testes causes growth and development of the penis, scrotum, prostate, and larynx. Figure 11-1 illustrates the hormone stimulation in puberty.

The hypothalamus also plays a part in stimulating the maturation of the adrenal glands. This adrenal and gonadal maturation provides the hormones which are responsible for development of pubic hair.

Musculoskeletal growth is controlled by the hypothalamus with each individual having his or her own

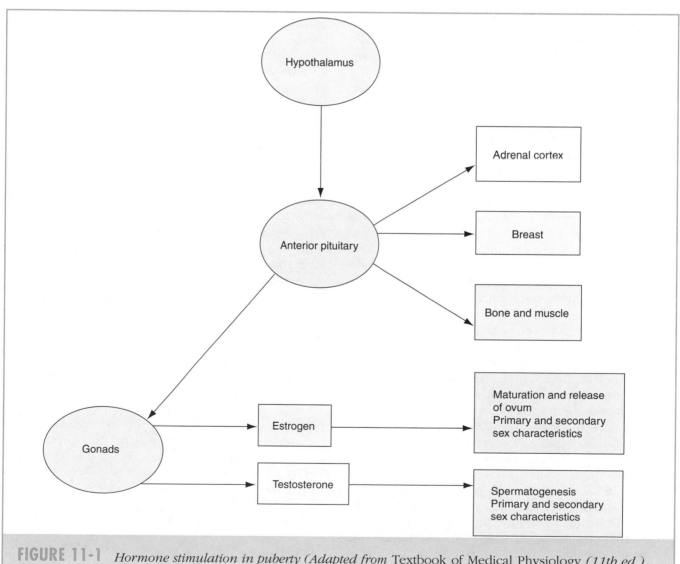

FIGURE 11-1 *Hormone stimulation in puberty (Adapted from* Textbook of Medical Physiology *(11th ed.), by A. C. Guyton and J. E. Hall, 2006, Philadelphia: Saunders.)*

maturation and growth schedule. Adolescents will grow at varying rates, and the rate of growth is not related to ultimate size. Unless there is a pathologic condition, the boy who gets his height early will fall into the same average adult height range as the boy who gets his height later (Kaplan and Love-Osborne, 2003). The primary health promotion strategy is educating adolescents and their parents about the normal variation among individuals. Applying the standardized growth charts used for younger age groups is not appropriate for normal individual adolescents in puberty. Early developers may jump from the 75th percentile to the 95th percentile and then plateau, while late developers may fall from the 25th percentile to the 10th percentile and have a late spurt. In general, tall children will tend to be tall adults and short children will tend to be short adults. Key factors in eventual height are genetics and nutrition, not growth tempo.

The disturbance in the androgen-estrogen balance found in puberty is one of the causes of acne, the "bane of existence" in 85 percent of adolescents. **Acne** is an inflammatory process of the sebaceous follicles of the skin, characterized by papules, comedones, and pustules (Morelli & Weston, 2003). The increased secretion of androgen in both males and females increases the size and activity of the sebaceous glands, primarily on the face, chest, and upper back. Acne can be treated both topically and systemically, depending on its severity. The nurse needs to encourage parents of adolescents with severe acne in which there are pustules, cysts, and nodules to seek treatment to prevent scarring. Severe acne may require systemic antibiotics, oral retinoids, or both to decrease sebum production and inflammation (Morelli & Weston, 2003). Moderate acne responds to topical antibiotics and topical keratolytic agents to relieve follicular obstruction. Adolescents with mild acne can reduce its effects by following the guidelines found in Box 11-1. Restricting dietary intake of certain substances such as chocolate has not proven to affect acne formation; however, a hereditary tendency toward development of acne has been noted. Providing emotional support and understanding is a key health promotion strategy for adolescents with acne.

Early or late physical maturation can put adolescents at risk. Early-maturing girls may be unprepared for the emotional and social demands placed on them. They may not have the social maturity to handle advances from older males, putting them at risk for unwanted pregnancies and sexually transmitted diseases. They are also at risk for depression and substance abuse. Late-maturing boys whose development is out of sync with their peers are at increased risk for depression and being bullied. In order to prove their maturity, they may be tempted to participate in high-risk behaviors such as sexual activity, smoking, or delinquency. Helping parents understand that adolescent autonomy should be determined by the teen's chronological age and social and emotional devel-

BOX 11-1   Self-Care for Adolescent Acne

1. Wash the skin thoroughly at least twice a day.
2. Wash after vigorous activity that causes sweating.
3. Use a mild soap.
4. Apply a benzoyl peroxide preparation (5–10 percent) once or twice daily to lesions.
5. Avoid intense scrubbing and skin abrasion while washing.
6. Avoid squeezing or picking at lesions.
7. Use non-oil-based cosmetics and moisturizers.
8. Avoid touching the face or other acne sites with hands.
9. Avoid external factors that may obstruct follicles at the hairline, such as headbands, hats, and hairspray.

opment and not by the level of physical maturation is an important health promotion strategy.

Female Puberty Breast development in girls is one of the earliest observable signs of female puberty. The average age for beginning breast development is 11 years with a range of 9 to 13 years (Anderson, Dallal, and Must, 2003). Late developers may gain reassurance from the knowledge that there is no relationship between timing of breast development and eventual breast size (Kaplan and Love-Osborne, 2003). It is not unusual for one breast to be noticeably larger than the other during early development. The nurse should make it a point to discuss this potential asymmetry with the adolescent in order to reassure her of its normalcy. Boys may also have some breast development, called **gynecomastia,** during early puberty. They need reassurance that it is a transient condition that will regress within a year or two.

Menarche (the initiation of menstruation) usually occurs about two and one-half years after breast development begins (Kaplan and Love-Osborne, 2003). Ninety-five percent of females will begin menstruation between 11 and 15 years of age. This wide variation in mean age appears to be influenced by ethnic, socioeconomic, and possibly athletic factors. The time between cycles is frequently irregular in the first year or two and should not be a cause for alarm if there is no other evidence of organic pathology. The primary health promotion strategy is to prepare the adolescent and her parents for menarche through education. This anticipatory guidance can help the participants to view the experience in a significantly healthier and more positive manner.

Male Puberty In male puberty, testicular growth and development begins prior to penile growth. The mean age for initiation of testicular growth is 11 years with about four years needed to attain full development (Kaplan and Love-Osborne, 2003). The left testicle will hang lower than the right once puberty begins. Penile growth begins around 12 years of age and takes about three years to complete. Release of sperm generally begins between 12 and 14 years of age. Erections occur more frequently and are common upon awakening. Preparing and reassuring the adolescent male of the normalcy of frequent erections and release of sperm during sleep (nocturnal emissions or wet dreams) is an important health promotion strategy.

Nutrition

It is well recognized that an adolescent in the midst of a growth spurt needs adequate nutrition; however, adolescence tends to be the time when nutrition receives less than optimal attention. Skipping meals, snacking, and eating at fast-food restaurants are frequent occurrences. Adolescents on average get 34 percent of calories from fat and 53 percent from carbohydrates (Mandleco, 2004). Calcium, iron, and protein intake are frequently less than adequate to support growth in males and females. National data show that the highest iron deficiency anemia prevalence rates are found in adolescent girls from 12 to 19 years of age (Mandleco, 2004).

The home environment can be a positive influence on healthy eating behavior; however, current trends show that only about 50 percent of adolescents eat with their families every day (CDC, 2006). The school environment attempts to offer nutritionally adequate foods, but a large portion of adolescents choose nutritionally empty, high-calorie, high-fat foods from vending machines or fast-food sources. A primary prevention strategy is dietary modification for youth at risk of chronic diseases such as coronary artery disease before atherosclerotic lesions can cause irreparable damage. The need to promote the benefits of a low-fat eating pattern in youth has been supported by the finding of atherosclerotic occlusions on the aorta and right coronary arteries when adoles-

cents who died in accidents were autopsied The most important health promotion strategy for achieving adequate adolescent nutrition is educating adolescents and their families about the immediate effect of eating behaviors on health and the long-term effect of eating behaviors on adult eating patterns. Lifestyle changes may be easier to make before lifelong habits are established.

Both malnutrition and obesity are found in the adolescent age group. Malnutrition (an inadequate intake of calories) may be a result of lack of access to food due to poverty, a result of poor eating habits, or a result of anorexia nervosa or bulimia nervosa or both (Sigel, 2003). **Anorexia nervosa** is an eating disorder in which the individual voluntarily refuses to eat because of excessive concern over body shape or weight. **Bulimia nervosa** is related to anorexia and is characterized by binge eating followed by purging through self-induced vomiting, laxatives, diuretics, or excessive exercise. Both conditions result in inadequate nutritional support for the rapid physiological development of adolescence. The most prominent signs and symptoms of anorexia nervosa and bulimia nervosa are listed in Table 11-1. Disordered eating can be seen in both genders, across socioeconomic levels, and in most ethnic groups. There is an increasing incidence of very young girls with obsessive concern over dieting, fitness, weight loss, and body image. A partial listing of risk factors for the development of eating disorders can be found in Box 11-2. Even though the symptoms of eating disorders are physical, the cause is psychiatric, and treatment needs to be sought from a mental health practitioner (Sigel, 2003). The longer the duration of the eating disorder, the harder it is to achieve recovery; therefore, patients need to be diagnosed early in the disease process (Rome, et al., 2003). Parents, educators, and coaches can help with early recognition of the first signs of disordered eating, such as a preference for eating alone, severe limitation in food choices, ritualized eating habits, excessive fluid intake, excessive chewing of ice or gum, or recent vegetarianism. Health care practitioners

---

TABLE 11-1 Signs and Symptoms of Anorexia Nervosa and Bulimia Nervosa

Anorexia Nervosa	Bulimia Nervosa
1. Refusal to eat	1. Binge eating followed by purging
2. Plays with food and eats only very small amounts	2. Loss of tooth enamel, especially on posterior front teeth
3. Perceives body or body part as being fat even though thin	3. Calluses on dorsum of fingers or scars on dorsum of hand
4. Dry skin, fine downy body hair	4. Reddened knuckles
5. Absent menses	5. Enlarged parotid gland
6. Hypothermia, hypotension, bradycardia	6. Increased peristalsis, rectal bleeding, or constipation

BOX 11-2 Major Risk Factors for Eating Disorders

Biological
- History of excessive dieting, skipped meals, compulsive exercise
- Obesity
- Depression

Psychological
- Body image distortion or dissatisfaction
- Low self-esteem
- Personality traits such as perfectionism
- Physical or sexual abuse

Family
- Family history of eating disorder or obesity
- Parental attitudes, behaviors, or comments regarding appearance
- Affective illness or alcoholism in first-degree relatives

Sociocultural
- Participation in "visual sports" such as ballet, gymnastics, modeling
- Peer pressure
- Media influence: TV, magazines

Adapted from "The Prevention of Eating Disorders: A Review of the Research on Risk Factors with Implications for Practice" by J. H. White, 2000, Journal of Child and Adolescent Psychiatric Nursing, 13*(2), 76–88; and "Parental Factors, Mass Media Influences, and the Onset of Eating Disorders in a Prospective Population-based Cohort," by M. A. Martinez-Gonzalez et al., 2003,* Pediatrics, 111*(2), 315–321.*

should screen for body image, changes in diet or dietary habits, and alterations of growth patterns (Rome et al., 2003). Lack of treatment may result in numerous complications throughout the body, including death.

The prevalence of obesity in adolescence has increased by 39 percent in the last 20 years (Kaplan and Love-Osborne, 2003). This increase in prevalence has been related to a decrease in physical activity coupled with the typical high-fat, high-carbohydrate diet consumed by youths. Eight out of 10 obese adolescents will continue to be obese in adulthood. Medical risks of adolescent obesity include hypertension, atherosclerosis, cerebrovascular accidents, diabetes mellitus, gallbladder disease, and degenerative arthritis. Of equal importance are the psychosocial hazards. Obese adolescents may experience isolation, distorted peer relationships, poor self-esteem, and depression (Mandleco, 2004). The most effective health promotion strategy for reducing or preventing adolescent obesity or both is encouraging parents and youths to combine an increase in physical activity with eating behavior changes.

Activity

The physical condition of adolescents is steadily declining. Today's adolescents have less muscle tone, poorer endurance, and a higher body fat percentage than their parents had (Mandleco, 2004).

The majority of actual physical activity for the adolescent centers around organized sports. Teenage boys and girls should be encouraged to participate in team-centered or individual physical activities or both to promote bone and muscle development as well as enhance psychosocial development and self-esteem. Adolescent physical activity has many positive long-term effects, such as helping control weight, promoting psychological well-being, and reducing depression and anxiety. In addition, regular physical activity reduces the risk of dying from cardiovascular disease and developing diabetes, hypertension, colon cancer, and osteoporosis. Health promotion strategies should focus on improving opportunities for recreation and play and promoting fitness through appropriate role models. It only takes moderate physical activity on a daily basis to produce the desired benefits and to establish a pattern for lifelong fitness.

Screening

Although screening is classified as secondary prevention, it is an important health promotion strategy. Screening for presence of disease or risk factors during adolescence may include assessment for signs and symptoms of hypertension, dental caries and periodontal disease, substance use, and sexually transmitted infections.

Blood Pressure As blood pressure determination has become more routine in children, systemic hypertension has become more widely recognized in this age group. Blood pressure should be routinely measured at any office visit because hypertension is a known risk factor for heart disease. To obtain an accurate blood pressure reading, use the widest cuff that will fit between the axilla and the antecubital fossa. Using too large a cuff may decrease the readings by 5 mm Hg, while too small a cuff will increase readings by 10 to 50 mm Hg. Health promotion for adolescents with hypertension starts with losing weight if obese, avoiding excessive salt intake, starting a regular exercise program, and avoiding cigarette smoking and oral contraceptives.

Dental Caries and Gum Disease Although the addition of fluoride to municipal water supplies and the emphasis on daily tooth brushing have reduced the prevalence of **dental caries** (progressive decalcification of the enamel of a tooth), the majority of adolescents will have at least one cavity in their permanent teeth by the age of 17. In addition, up to one-third will have gum disease. Dietary habits may increase the incidence of cavities. Snacking, unbalanced diets with low levels of calcium, and high intake of carbonated beverages place the adolescent at risk for tooth decay. Carbonated beverages reduce the pH of the mouth to 2.5, a level conducive to tooth decay. In addition, hormones, orthodontic appliances, and the natural rebellion and desire for independence may contribute to poor adolescent oral hygiene. Oral screening should also include observation for malalignment, crowding of teeth, and mismatching upper and lower dental arches. Adolescents with any of these problems need a dental referral. The oral health status of adults is dependent upon their preventive care as adolescents. Daily flossing, brushing after meals, and maintaining a regular schedule for dental cleaning and screening are all part of health promotion activities for oral health. Peer pressure and the developmental focus of adolescents on appearance often provide the motivation for good oral hygiene. The minimum goal should be one thorough cleaning with brushing and flossing teeth before bedtime.

Substance Use Screening for dental caries provides the nurse with an excellent opportunity to provide health promotion counseling about the hazards of tobacco use. The average age at which smokers first try a cigarette is 14 (American Lung Association, 2006). Ninety percent of all adult smokers started habitual tobacco use by age 21. The 2003 Youth Risk Behavior Surveillance System (YRBSS) surveys of high school students conducted by the Centers for Disease Control and prevention found that 71 percent of White students, 66 percent of Black students, and 76 percent of Hispanic students had used tobacco at some time (CDC, 2004). Once an adolescent is a regular smoker, the effectiveness of recruitment and retention in a smoking cessation program is extremely low. Approximately 40 percent of adolescents who try

cigarettes become regular smokers (CDC, 2004). Risk factors related to the initiation of tobacco use are found in Box 11-3.

BOX 11-3 Tobacco Use Risk Factors

Sociodemographic Factors
- Low socioeconomic status
- Early adolescence (11–15 years)

Environmental Factors
- Accessibility
- Parental and sibling use
- Peer use

Behavioral Factors
- Poor academic achievement
- Rebelliousness and risk taking
- Alcohol use

Personal Factors
- Perceived acceptability
- Perceived benefits
- Low self-esteem
- Depression

Research Note

Tobacco Product Marketing and Smoking Behaviors in Adolescents

Study Problem/Purpose: To determine whether adolescents' exposure to tobacco marketing was associated with self-reported smoking.

Method: The Survey of Teen Opinions About Retail Environments was administered to 2,125 middle school students.

Findings: There was a 50 percent increase in the odds of ever smoking in the students who reported visits to a small grocery, convenience, or liquor store daily or at least weekly. Boys and Latino youth had more exposure to retail tobacco marketing as did students who reported low maternal supervision, high risk-taking, and exposure to social influences to smoke.

Implications: The unregulated proliferation of tobacco marketing in stores may influence smoking behaviors in adolescents as much as having a parent or household member who smokes.

Henriksen, L., Feighery, E., Yang, Y., and Fortman, S. (2004). Association of retail tobacco marketing with adolescent smoking. *American Journal of Public Health, 94*(12).

Adolescents are knowledgeable about the long-term health problems of cardiovascular disease and lung cancer associated with tobacco use; however, this knowledge is not a sufficient deterrent to keep them from smoking. The most effective health promotion strategy is to concentrate on the short-term effects. Emphasizing the detrimental cosmetic effects of yellowed teeth and bad breath as well as the health effects of decreased stamina and athletic performance is an important health promotion strategy to discourage tobacco use. Personal appearance is highly important in adolescence, and knowledge about long-term detrimental effects of smoking such as facial wrinkles and nicotine-stained fingers can also be a deterrent to smoking. Adolescents from lower socioeconomic groups and those with lower academic achievement have higher tobacco use rates and should be targeted for tobacco prevention strategies. In addition, adolescents with low self-image, poor social skills, or other risk-taking behaviors need skills to identify and resist the social influences to smoke.

The adolescent also should be asked about the use of smokeless tobacco products such as dip and chewing tobacco. The YRBSS found that over 7.6 percent of White, 2 percent of Black, and 4 percent of Hispanic students used smokeless tobacco (CDC, 2004). Smokeless tobacco can be more addicting than cigarettes since nicotine is easily absorbed by the oral mucosa. The intensity of the withdrawal symptoms makes quitting use of smokeless tobacco difficult. Again, emphasis on cosmetic effects of bad breath, discoloration of teeth, dental caries, and gum recession is more effective than emphasis on the potential danger for the development of oral cancer.

There is an association between tobacco use and the use of alcohol and other drugs (Elliott & Erickson, 2002); therefore, screening for use of other substances is also essential. The pressure produced by the tremendous physical and emotional growth and development experienced by adolescents may cause them to experiment with substances that make them feel less insecure, more confident, or simply different. Substances may also be used to reduce the stress of transitioning through the developmental tasks of adolescence. Drinking is viewed as normal experimental behavior by society, but adolescents are at increased risk because of their limited experience with alcohol, their smaller body size, and the more rapid progression toward dependence. This may lead to **substance abuse,** frequently defined as the habitual use of alcohol or illegal substances such as marijuana, cocaine, methamphetamine, and numerous others. The 2003 YRBSS found that over 75 percent of White, 73 percent of Black, and 79 percent of Hispanic high school students had used alcohol at some time. Over 40 percent of all three groups had used marijuana with over 22 percent continuing its use. Box 11-4 illustrates the percentage of high school students who reported drug-related behaviors.

BOX 11-4 Substance Use by High School Students

Smoked a whole cigarette	Percentage
• White	58.1%
• Black	58.4%
• Hispanic	61.9%
Drank alcohol	
• White	75.4%
• Black	71.4%
• Hispanic	79.5%
Tried marijuana	
• White	39.8%
• Black	43.3%
• Hispanic	42.7%
Tried cocaine	
• White	8.7%
• Black	3.2%
• Hispanic	12.5%

Adapted from "Surveillance Summaries," by CDC, 2004, MMWR, 53 (No. SS-2).

The pressures generated by the tremendous changes occurring during adolescence do not account for all adolescent substance abuse; therefore, in order to prevent substance abuse, the risk factors for substance use must be examined. The nurse who is aware of the influence of all these factors on the adolescent's potential for alcohol and substance abuse can assist the individual and the family in developing health promotion strategies to reduce the potential. An individual adolescent's potential for alcohol or drug abuse is most likely influenced by genetic, familial, environmental, and/or developmental factors. Twin and sibling studies on alcoholism have revealed a genetic vulnerability in some individuals. Children of alcoholics have a 25 percent chance of becoming alcoholics themselves (AACAP, 2002). There is also an increased vulnerability in individuals from dysfunctional families, especially if parents are substance abusers themselves. These adolescents may have low self-esteem, decreased feelings of belonging, high levels of frustration and anger, and a reduced ability to negotiate the social environment. The school and peer environments form an important social environment for adolescents. Belonging to a substance-using peer group is one of the strongest predictors of substance use. Excessive use of alcohol usually starts in the home, but may be reinforced by the peer group.

The use of alcohol is widely advertised and frequently seen on television and in movies by adolescents.

Other substance use is also common in movies. Advertising portrays alcohol use as sophisticated and a natural part of life, essential to social acceptance, and a reward after work, at a sporting event, or for relaxing. The risks of alcohol are minimized or totally omitted. The home is the primary source of alcohol for adolescents; however, parental attitudes and behaviors may vary drastically. Families who do not use alcohol or who do not drink excessively usually reinforce appropriate alcohol use. Families who accept and encourage excessive drinking or who have a history of antisocial behavior and poor parenting skills increase the risk of having children who use alcohol and other substances inappropriately. An assessment of the adolescent's genetic heritage, level of family support, educational environment, and freedom to experiment with new role development forms the basis for developing health promotion strategies to prevent alcohol and substance abuse. Table 11-2 describes risk factors and prevention strategies for adolescent alcohol use.

Adolescents who do not abuse alcohol or other substances have been found to have social competence, problem-solving skills, autonomy, and a sense of purpose and future. Adolescents who are depressed, or those who have been physically or sexually abused, may use alcohol or other substances to help cope with their psychological distress.

There is a relationship between substance abuse and sexual activity. Drugs and alcohol can lower an adolescent's inhibition against sexual activity, or sex can be a means to obtain drugs or alcohol. The 2003 YRBSS found that up to 21 percent of females and 30 percent of males reported using alcohol or drugs at their last sexual intercourse.

Sexually Transmitted Infections The adolescent period is characterized by sexual curiosity, experimentation, and risk-taking behavior, increasing the adolescent's risk of exposure to sexually transmitted infections. Approximately 46.7 percent of high school students have engaged in sexual intercourse, with 7.4 percent reporting intercourse before age 13, and 14.4 percent reporting more than four sex partners (CDC, 2004). Screening for sexually transmitted infections is a health promotion strategy for all sexually active adolescents, especially those with a history of substance abuse.

Over 3 million persons age 15 to 24 get a sexually transmitted disease annually. In a single act of unprotected sexual intercourse, an adolescent female has a 1 percent risk of acquiring HIV/AIDS (human immunodeficiency virus/Acquired Immunodeficiency Syndrome), a 30 percent chance of getting genital herpes, and a 50 percent chance of contracting gonorrhea. Adolescents as a whole have higher rates of gonorrhea than sexually active men and women age 20 to 44. Screening for sexually transmitted diseases is critical to prevent transmission and later problems with infertility and cancer.

Sexually active adolescents should receive complete information on their risk for acquiring sexually transmitted infections. Counseling about the effective measures to reduce risk includes abstaining from sexual activity,

TABLE 11-2 Risk Factors and Prevention Strategies for Adolescent Alcohol Use

Source	Risk Factor	Prevention Strategies
Society/Community	Acceptability of alcohol use behavior as portrayed through media. Availability of alcohol.	Reduce alcohol advertising and media portrayal of unacceptable alcohol use. Enforce minimum legal drinking age.
School	Decreased commitment and involvement in school. Presence of behavioral or attention problems or both.	Promote academic involvement and achievement. Refer students with problem behavior.
Family	Family role models use alcohol inappropriately. Poor family nurturing, communication, or both. Decreased familial interaction.	Family role models avoid inappropriate alcohol use. Parent communication and parenting training. Parent involvement in school and home activities.
Peers	Peers are alcohol users. Rejection by peers.	Monitor alcohol use by peers. Supervise recreational outlets.
Individual	Genetic susceptibility. Decreased social or problem-solving skills.	Teach about hereditary potential for susceptibility to alcoholism. Foster self-esteem and use of life skills.

maintaining a mutually faithful monogamous relationship with an uninfected partner, using condoms regularly, and avoiding casual sexual contact with high-risk individuals. Guidelines for effective condom use are found in Box 11-5.

Psychological Domain

The psychological domain for the adolescent includes both cognitive and emotional development. In addition to cognitive development, the concepts of invulnerability, body image, and moral development are discussed. Depression and suicide are discussed with emotional development.

Cognitive Development

According to Jean Piaget, as adolescents mature, they move beyond using concrete, actual experience as the only basis for their thought processes to using abstract, logical, and hypothetical processes (Brainerd, 1978). Cognitively mature adolescents are able to think in abstraction and demonstrate logical analyses. They are able to "think about thinking," which enables them to become more introspective. This permits reflections on self, prior relationships, and future interactions. Adolescents spend a great deal of time contemplating the limitless variety of roles, situations, or both which might arise in their lives. Their world has numerous partly developed theories about themselves and life. Thoughts

---

BOX 11-5   Guidelines for Effective Condom Use

- Handle condoms carefully to avoid damaging with fingernails or sharp objects.
- Use a new condom in good condition for each act of intercourse.
- Check the expiration date on the package. Do not use condoms beyond the date of expiration.
- Place the condom on an erect penis before any intimate contact and unroll completely to the base.
- Leave a space at the tip of the condom and remove air pockets in the space.
- Ensure adequate lubrication during intercourse. Water-based lubricants (e.g., K-Y jelly, spermicidal foam or gel) should be used. Petroleum jelly, mineral oil, hand lotion, baby oil, cold cream, massage oil, and other oil-based lubricants should not be used because they may damage latex condoms.
- Hold condom firmly against base of penis during withdrawal, and withdraw while the penis is still erect so that the condom remains in place.

---

go beyond immediate situations and current interpersonal relationships to personally relevant future possibilities. Increased cognitive maturity enables the adolescent to think hypothetically and to anticipate the possible consequences of actions on such things as selection of an occupation, a marriage partner, and future lifestyle. Health promotion strategies promote this introspection, reflection, and projection.

Invulnerability It has been hypothesized that younger adolescents exhibit a cognitive egocentrism characterized by an exaggerated sense of uniqueness (Elkind, 1967). This egocentrism is demonstrated by a belief in their invulnerability and lack of susceptibility to the natural laws that pertain to others. Elkind felt that this belief was one of the causes of adolescent risk-taking behaviors; however, studies have demonstrated that adolescents do not underestimate their vulnerability any more than adults (Millstein & Igra, 1995). The expectation that adolescents move toward adult decision making and self-determination may push the adolescent toward experimentation and risk-taking as a means to accomplish autonomy and mastery. Other proposed reasons for adolescent risk-taking behaviors include curiosity, resentment of authority, anxiety, low self-esteem, and feelings of inadequacy or isolation. A health promotion strategy in this psychological domain is to determine the most likely etiology of a particular risk-taking behavior and which developmental processes may be contributing factors before proposing solutions or behavior changes.

Body Image The rapid changes in physical appearance occurring during the adolescent period cause adolescents to constantly evaluate and reevaluate their own bodies. They compare and contrast their bodies with those of their peers as well as some imaginary ideal. Judgments are influenced by reactions from others, their own level of self-esteem, and prevailing standards of attractiveness. Young adolescents are often self-critical. They believe that others are constantly evaluating them and are as critical of them as they are of themselves. The belief in an "imaginary audience" helps explain the adolescent self-consciousness, need for privacy, and fear of scrutiny. This egocentrism also helps explain the development of tight peer groups which seek to diminish individual differences among themselves by promoting extreme conformity. Cognitive egocentrism is less evident as the adolescent undergoes advanced cognitive development.

Moral Development The development of a sense of values and ethical behavior is a cognitive process which develops through maturation and changing social relationships. Lawrence Kohlberg, a psychologist, presented various ethical dilemmas to males of school age through young adulthood and then compiled their responses and the reasons for their choices. He found three distinct levels of moral development, each having two types of motivation, represented as stages. The levels were sequential and depended significantly on cognitive development; however, only a small percentage of individuals progress to the most mature stages (Kohlberg, 1981).

Working with Kohlberg was Carol Gilligan, whose research focused on moral development in females. She found a difference in responses provided by women, indicating that women approach moral dilemmas from a different perspective than men (Gilligan, 1982). Women define the moral problem by relationships with others, emphasizing caring and concern, while men have a justice perspective, emphasizing the preservation of rules, rights, and principles.

Understanding the different levels of development as well as individual perspectives will help the nurse in planning health promotion strategies reflective of individual differences. Parents can help facilitate moral development by modeling altruistic and caring behavior toward others. Identifying issues involving fairness and morality and initiating conversations about concepts such as racism, sexism, homophobia, ageism, and biases against persons with disabilities helps adolescents to take the perspective of others, express themselves, ask questions, clarify their values, and evaluate their reasoning. Encouraging adolescents to volunteer in the community promotes a sense of purpose and meaning and enhances moral development.

Emotional Development

According to Erik Erikson (1950), the central developmental task of adolescence is to develop a sense of identity. The adolescent attempts to discover who he or she is. The adolescent must leave behind childhood beliefs and fantasies and assume the responsibilities and decision making of adulthood. To do this, the adolescent explores various roles and beliefs in an attempt to develop an individual identity separate from the family. Adolescents have the task of integrating themselves into society through confronting the potential for role confusion in order to establish an equilibrium in which a firm identity is developed (Erikson, 1950).

Helping an adolescent raise her or his self-esteem is a significant health promotion strategy for parents and health professionals. Identifying specific areas that are important to the adolescent and finding resources to enable the adolescent to succeed in those areas help improve self-concept, contributing to self-esteem. Providing support and encouragement to help an adolescent face a problem instead of avoiding it also enhances self-esteem.

Promoting emotional health must be considered a significant strategy in reducing morbidity and mortality in adolescents. Mental health problems are occurring more frequently and earlier in life (Hagman and Bechtold, 2003). Problems range from behavioral disorders such as depression, eating disorders, and substance abuse to severe depression, suicide, and schizophrenia.

Depression There is a relationship between adolescent depression and abuse of alcohol or substances. The risk for substance abuse and subsequent mental health problems increases with a family history of substance abuse, early initiation of substance use, and association with peer group users.

One in 10 high school students suffer from clinical depression (Hagman & Bechtold, 2003). Stress in relationships at school or home, decreased social support due to divorce or moving, and the presence of learning, conduct, or attention disorders place adolescents at risk for depression. Warning signs for adolescent depression and suicide are found in Box 11-6. The depressed adolescent may progress to thoughts or actions relating to suicide. Feelings of hopelessness and anger, social isolation, overt family conflict, and poor communication have also been associated with adolescent suicide.

Suicide In 2002, suicide was the third leading cause of death in males 10 to 24 years of age and females 15 to 19 years of age. White and Native American adolescents have suicide rates twice as high as other racial/ethnic groups. Adolescent suicide rates reflect a threefold increase in the last 30 years, an increase which has risen at twice the rate of adult suicide. Even so, these statistics only reflect suicide attempts that result in death. Nonfatal attempts are often unreported. Risk factors for suicidal behaviors are found in Box 11-7. Depressed adolescents who are planning to commit suicide may write about suicide, talk about suicide or not being around much longer, clean out their rooms or school lockers, give or throw away important possessions, become suddenly cheerful, or all of these. Families of depressed adolescents should be made aware of these warning signs.

Prevention strategies focus on programs to develop social skills, self-esteem, communication, problem solving, crisis/stress management, and anger control. This support should come from the family, the school, and the community. Positive communication and social support from the family encourages interaction between the parents and the adolescents. Parental involvement in the school provides

---

BOX 11-6 Warning Signs for Adolescent Depression

- Noticeable sadness, hostility, or irritability
- Decreased interest in or withdrawal from usual family, school, or peer activities
- Changes in eating, sleeping, personal hygiene, or activity patterns
- Decline in school performance or refusal to attend school
- Drug and alcohol use

a bridge of support between the two places adolescents spend the majority of their time. Communities that have useful roles for adolescents in providing community service reinforce the support provided by parents and schools, thus increasing adolescent self-efficacy.

Social Domain

The adolescent is seen by much of society as a source of concern. Rising rates of adolescent substance abuse, pregnancy, suicide, and violence reflect the social change being experienced. Many have blamed changes in the structure of families for the unhealthy and maladaptive functioning in troubled adolescents, and cite the lack of character development in adolescents who are deprived of the stabilizing influence of familial experiences.

Family

The major social role of the family of an adolescent is to provide support for the adolescent's search for identity and independence. As the adolescent begins to spend more time away from home with peers, the family may overreact by either imposing strict rules on the adolescent's behavior or by discarding all rules. Neither of these options provides the support needed by adolescents as they strive to develop their own identity and independence. The health promotion strategy to be recommended to the family by the nurse is emotional support of the adolescent accompanied by encouragement of the adolescent's movement toward autonomy. Regardless of the family form—single parent, shared custody, adoptive, traditional—adolescents need warm, involved adults who provide firm guidelines and limits, have appropriate developmental expectations, and encourage development of individual beliefs. Using reasoning and persuasion, explaining rules, discussing issues, and listening respectfully are hallmarks of effective parenting practices.

Peers

The expanded peer life and increased social activities of adolescents enable their movement toward personal identity formation and autonomy. The intense relationships in peer groups facilitate this movement. By identifying with peers, adolescents are able to individuate from parents and family. Peers provide the bridge of support between being a child in the family and being an autonomous adult in society. Although the intense pressure to conform and suppress individual personality may result in risk-taking behavior, the maturing cognitive development allows adolescents to consider the consequences of possible actions. Peer influence tends to be strongest in issues such as dress, music, language, and sexual behavior, while parental influence is more notable in issues of underlying moral and social values. The types of peers with whom an adolescent affiliates is a stronger predictor of behavior than family, school, or community characteristics. Affiliating with deviant peers is associated with a growth in delinquent behavior such as drug use, high-risk sexual behavior, antisocial actions, and violent offenses (Urberg, Luo, Pilgrim, & Degirmencioglu, 2003).

The health promotion strategy during this time is to assure parents that peer influence tends to concern external issues and be short-lived, while parental influence affects long-range goals, values, and attitudes. Parents should be cautioned that it is important to monitor and control with whom their adolescents affiliate. Parents can be reassured that peer influence is strongest during early adolescence. Not all peer influence is negative. Peers can influence positive, health-promoting behaviors through peer education and counseling programs available in many communities. The relationship with peers offers an opportunity for acceptance and a feeling of belonging, for trying different roles and behaviors within the safety of the group, for observing role models and developing a sense of identity, and for integrating a new body image and self-concept.

Abuse

Infants and toddlers are the most common victims of abuse, with adolescents ranking second. **Abuse** is defined as physical, emotional, or sexual maltreatment. Although the exact numbers of adolescents who have been abused or neglected cannot be known, there are almost a million cases of abuse that are substantiated or indicated annually.

The dynamics of families with adolescents may make the adolescents more vulnerable to maltreatment and make the parents more likely to abuse. A disequilibrium is created by the interaction of the adolescent's emerging physical, cognitive, emotional, and sexual potential with the midlife readjustments being faced by parents. Parents may feel threatened by the adolescent's ability to find flaws in the parents' reasoning, to retaliate or leave home, and to make autonomous relationships outside the family. Adolescent abuse also has been linked to multiple problems within the family, such as divorce and separation, financial stress, and overt conflict. Adolescents with developmental problems and decreased social competency are at increased risk for maltreatment.

Abuse may also take the form of **incest**, defined as sexual contact with the adolescent by any member of the family or household. Girls are at highest risk, but boys are also victimized. In addition to creating psychological difficulties for the adolescent in the area of sexuality, incest puts the adolescent at risk for pregnancy, sexually transmitted infections contracted during the relationship, or both. The prevalence of incest is underestimated due to underreporting. Adolescents may be in a state of denial or may have been threatened with severe consequences for reporting the abuse.

When there is abuse, intense family conflict, or identity problems, adolescents may decide to leave home. Runaway youth are adolescents under 18 years of age who leave home without permission and whose whereabouts are unknown. Walkaway youth leave home but their whereabouts are known. Thrownaway youth have been told to leave, have been abandoned, or have been runaways not allowed to return home. Homeless youth have no place for shelter and are in need of care, services, and supervision. Many runaway or homeless youth in shelters report being physically or sexually abused. Runaway or homeless adolescents have little or no economic support and are at high risk for further abuse, illness, unintended pregnancy, sexually transmitted diseases, substance abuse, and violence.

Health promotion for these adolescents includes both prevention strategies and identification of maltreatment. Mandatory child abuse and neglect reporting laws have been in effect since 1968. Teens should be encouraged to report abuse or incest. Health care providers need to be educated as to the signs of abuse. Box 11-8 lists both the physical and the behavioral signs of abuse. Intervention and prevention strategies must focus on providing age-appropriate and culturally sensitive counseling for adolescents, providing family education and training programs, and promoting positive sociocultural values which make family violence unacceptable. In addition, programs providing street outreach, shelter, food, education and job training, substance abuse rehabilitation, and health care services need to be made available.

Culture

The primary cultural influence in adolescence is the culture of peers. Childhood ethnic and cultural influences are less obvious as the adolescent attempts to conform to the predominant adolescent culture. Conflicts may arise as the adolescent tries to look like or act like the model being promoted in the latest media advertising campaign. When the minority adolescent attempts to emulate the majority adolescent culture, the family may feel that the adolescent is rejecting his or her cultural heritage or values. The primary health promotion strategy is to help parents recognize the limited influence peer culture has on long-term adolescent values. Supporting adolescent efforts at conformity in external

issues while recognizing personal identities will enable the adolescent to move through this developmental stage more easily.

Political Domain

Legislation affecting adolescents primarily deals with minimum age requirements for assuming adult responsibilities such as driving, using alcohol and cigarettes, marrying, and purchasing firearms. This legislation reflects society's belief that adolescents lack experience, adequate perspective, and the judgment needed to recognize and avoid danger. Knowledge of the significant diversity in maturational level diversity among 16-year-old adolescents illustrates the need to deal with adolescents on an individual basis, especially in matters of health care.

Encouraged by the National Highway Traffic Safety Administration, licensing systems that prolong the learning process for young, novice drivers now exist in 38 states. Graduated driver's licensing eases younger drivers into driving through a phased approach. It sets a minimum age for a learner's permit, requires a licensed adult in the vehicle and certification of practice hours, restricts teenage passenger numbers, and restricts nighttime driving hours. States implementing these restrictions have found up to a 25 percent decrease in crashes by teenage drivers overall and approximately a 50 percent reduction in nighttime crashes (National Highway Traffic Safety Administration, 2003).

The establishment of school-based clinics has brought health care to children and adolescents who did not typically have access to care. Approximately one in eight children under the age of 18 have no health insurance. Although school-based clinics were initially developed

---

BOX 11-8 Signs of Abuse

Physical Signs
- Bruising
- Muscle or bone injury
- Recurrent abdominal pain
- Frequent urinary tract infections
- Sexually transmitted infection
- Pregnancy

Behavioral Signs
- Withdrawal, guilt, or depression
- Sleep disturbances
- Appetite disturbances
- School problems
- Substance abuse
- Promiscuity

to prevent adolescent pregnancies, most have expanded their roles to include primary health care, referral, health and nutrition education, preventive care, and substance-abuse counseling. Parental consent for treatment is generally required; however, some clinics provide services to mature adolescents without parental consent. Some adolescents are economically and emotionally independent from their families and are recognized as "emancipated minors," fully authorized to take responsibility for many aspects of their lives.

Adolescents are more likely to seek services where they can be guaranteed confidentiality, especially for contraception and sexually transmitted disease treatment. Conservative groups fear that confidential services usurp parental authority and are currently seeking to require parental consent for all services. Although it is to be wished that every adolescent had the type of relationship with his or her parents which promoted communication on all issues affecting the adolescent, the reality is that many would risk emotional or physical harm in seeking permission for contraceptive care, pregnancy determination or termination, and sexually transmitted disease treatment. The primary health promotion strategy is to encourage appropriate communication between parents and adolescents while keeping confidential health care services available.

Environmental Domain

Accidents and violence are two important environmental factors influencing the health of adolescents. An accident is an unforeseen or unplanned event or happening, leading to an unintentional injury. Violence, however, is intentional. Violence can be defined as behaviors that threaten, attempt, or inflict physical harm on others.

Accidents

Traumatic injury is a serious health concern for adolescents, with motor vehicle accidents being the leading cause of death in 16- to 20-year-olds. The risk for accidents is high due to the enormous changes adolescents are undergoing physically, cognitively, emotionally, and socially. The characteristics of adolescent development such as challenging adult authority, desiring autonomy, experimenting in risky situations, seeking peer approval, and seeking to enhance self-esteem contribute to the numbers of adolescent injuries. Driving habits and the tendency to take risks may be influenced by emotions, peer group pressure, and other stresses. Adolescents are more likely than adult drivers to report that they speed, run red lights, make illegal turns, and do not wear seat belts. When compared on a per-mile-driven basis with the general population, 16-year-old drivers are 20 times more likely to have an accident. Although nighttime driving is challenging for all age groups, adolescents have a disproportionately greater rate of nighttime accidents and fatalities. They are four times more likely to be killed while driving at night than during the day.

The National Center for Health Statistics notes that 36 percent of all deaths for 15- to 19-year olds are from motor vehicle crashes (Kochanek, Murphy, Anderson, & Scott, 2004). Younger drivers are more likely to speed, tailgate, and engage in other dangerous behavior and are less likely to recognize or respond to hazards due to inexperience (McKnight & McKnight, 2003). Sixteen-year-old drivers have crash rates three times higher than those of 17-year-olds and five times higher than those of 18-year-olds. Contributing to these higher crash rates are lack of driving experience and inadequate driving skills; excessive driving during higher-risk nighttime hours; risk-taking behaviors; poor driving judgment and decision making; drinking and driving; and distractions from teenage passengers. A 16-year-old is three times more likely to die in a car crash when carrying three passengers than when transporting one passenger (McKnight & McKnight, 2003).

The availability of alcohol and the legal ability to drive a car interact with the adolescent's developmental characteristics to produce one of the greatest hazards to adolescent health—motor vehicle–related injuries. Drivers between the ages of 16 and 20 who are involved in fatal accidents are more likely to be alcohol-impaired than drivers in any other age group.

Many adolescents seek part-time jobs to earn money and to gain experience. Approximately 200,000 of these young workers suffer work-related injuries each year (New York Committee on Safety and Health, 2005). Reasons for these injuries include insufficient training; inexperience; dangerous and/or inappropriate jobs in high-risk areas such as restaurants, fast food, and construction; and lack of supervision. Health promotion strategies include assuring appropriate education, training, and supervision for young workers. Education should include body mechanics, hazardous chemicals, and proper use of equipment. Other leading causes of unintentional injury are drowning, firearms, poisoning, and burns. Table 11-3 discusses injury risks and strategies for prevention.

Violence

Violence is a major contributor to deaths, disabilities, and injuries of adolescents. Adolescents age 12 to 19 experience violent crimes at rates higher than other age groups. The National Center for Victims of Crime found that almost 40 percent of American adolescents witnessed violence, 17 percent were victims of physical assault,

TABLE 11-3 Environmental Safety for Adolescents and Young Adults

Accident	Prevention Strategies
Motor vehicle injury	Never drive after drinking. Never ride with anyone who has been drinking. Always use seat belts—both in front and in back. Encourage loss of driving privileges for driving rule infractions. Avoid night driving for adolescents when possible.
Firearm injury	Never keep a loaded gun unsecured in the house. Require gun safety courses before gun use. Wear bright clothing when hunting. Avoid alcohol use when using firearms.
Poisoning	Identify problems with alcohol and substance abuse. Discard all prescription drugs not used during the illness. Check labels of over-the-counter medications for expiration dates.
Sports injury	Wear proper safety equipment—bike helmets, knee and elbow protectors, football helmets and pads. Observe proper safety practices during training as well as during competition. Confine bike riding to approved bike lanes and trails. Warm up before vigorous exercise. Do not combine alcohol and sports activities.
Drowning	Avoid swimming alone. Use a personal flotation device while sailing. Require supervised experience and training for boat driving. Do not combine alcohol and water sports. Dive only where water has sufficient depth.
Burns	Install smoke detectors and check regularly. Never leave an iron unattended. Never leave a cigarette burning. Never smoke in bed or when sleepy. Check bath water or shower temperature before entering.

9 percent were victims of physically abusive punishment, and 8 percent were victims of sexual assault (National Institute of Justice, 2003). Factors associated with the rising incidence of adolescent violence are media influence, drug and alcohol use, peer influence through gangs, availability of firearms, family violence, and poverty. Violence has moved into the schools. Incidents involving fights, guns, alcohol, vandalism, and sexual assaults are commonly reported. Minority rates of homicide, especially for Black males, are an important problem. Firearms are involved in the majority of homicidal deaths which are characteristically intraracial and among acquaintances. Gun control has been proposed as a health promotion strategy to prevent injury to adolescents; however, there are no specific data available to support this strategy. Programs to deal with conflict may have a more immediate and far-reaching impact on adolescent health. Violence prevention must include cooperative programs involving schools, law enforcement, health care providers, parents,

and adolescents. Issues which should be considered include poverty, health care access, abuse, racial/ethnic inequities, gun availability, alcohol and other substance use, and the influence of the media.

Sexual Domain

Although humans are sexual beings from birth, it is during the adolescent period that the individual develops his or her sexual identity. The accomplishment of a stable sexual role and self-image is a significant developmental task of adolescence.

During early adolescence, males, more than females, express their sexuality through masturbation. **Masturbation** is defined as self-manipulation of the genitals for the purpose of sexual pleasure. This activity in either gender is considered normal sexual behavior unless it becomes so time consuming that it interferes with activities of daily living or is conducted publicly.

Sexual curiosity and experimentation characterize the adolescent period. Males are more sexually active than females, possibly due to the prominence of their sexual organs which are more easily manipulated, the increased levels of sexual aggressiveness caused by testosterone levels, and the female focus on love and affection rather than sexual gratification (Sahler & Kreipe, 1991). Information gathered about adolescent sexuality shows that the majority of adolescents begin having sex in their mid to late teens. Fifty-six percent of females and 73 percent of males have had sexual intercourse before age 18 (Kaplan & Love-Osborn 2003). One in five adolescents does not have intercourse. Use of contraception (usually a condom) at first intercourse has increased to approximately 78 percent. Nine out of 10 sexually active females and their partners use a contraceptive method, although not always consistently or correctly.

Predictive factors for early sexual intercourse are early puberty, sexual abuse, poverty, poor parental support, lack of school or career goals, and poor school performance (AAP, 2005). Delayed initiation of sexual intercourse is associated with living in a stable two-parent home, religious involvement, and increased family income.

Sexual exploration among same gender adolescents is common, perhaps because it is less threatening than heterosexual relationships. The health promotion strategy is to acknowledge that this behavior is a variant of normal sexual development and not a definite homosexual orientation; however, sensitive and thorough discussion with the adolescent can help the adolescent analyze this behavior. The adolescent struggling with his or her sexual identity needs confirmation of personal worth and acceptance.

Many homosexuals first become aware of their sexual orientation during adolescence. **Homosexuality** is defined as the sexual orientation of a person who is sexually attracted to a person of the same sex. Both males and females can be homosexual. Male homosexuals are sometimes designated as gay, while female homosexuals are designated as lesbian. Although the cause is unknown, homosexuality may be a result of a combination of genetic, physiological, and environmental factors. Gay and lesbian adolescents, like their heterosexual counterparts, have the same developmental tasks of establishing a sexual identity and deciding on sexual behaviors. Health promotion for homosexual adolescents includes care that is confidential, nonjudgmental, and without heterosexual bias. Regardless of sexual orientation, all adolescents need encouragement to practice abstinence as well as information and anticipatory guidance about the seriousness of sexually transmitted infections.

Adolescent Pregnancy

The society of the United States has changed from agricultural and manufacturing occupations to occupations dependent upon technology and education. This has extended the time required for the educational process and has delayed the time when individuals become independent with adult responsibilities. Adolescents become sexually mature long before they are ready or able to assume the responsibilities of adulthood. This has led to a significant increase in the percentage of adolescents who are sexually active. Despite the increased use of contraceptives, many adolescents have been sexually active for a year or more before seeking information or prescriptions for contraception. Fifty percent of adolescent pregnancies occur within the first six months of sexual intercourse (AAP, 2005). Early onset of sexual activity with subsequent pregnancies, abortions, childrearing, and parenting responsibilities presents a significant and complex societal problem.

Pregnant adolescents have a higher incidence of medical complications for both mother and child than do adult women (AAP, 2005). The risk for low infant birth weight, premature birth, increased infant and maternal death rates, pregnancy-induced hypertension, anemia, and sexually transmitted infections is greater in the adolescent population. Psychosocial complications include not completing school, increased levels of poverty, limited vocational opportunities, and repeat pregnancies.

Health promotion strategies need to directly address prevention of adolescent pregnancy. Abstinence counseling to postpone early sexual activity lays the foundation for pregnancy prevention. Accurate and comprehensive education about sexuality starts in childhood and continues during adolescence. Assuring access to contraception for sexually active adolescents is imperative. When prevention has not been successful, confidential access to abortion services or comprehensive pregnancy programs can assure improved outcomes.

Spiritual Domain

Adolescent psychological development forms the basis for addressing the spiritual domain. As adolescents strive to discover who they are and what their role is, they question every aspect of themselves and their world. They attempt to reconcile the values, roles, and responsibilities learned from parents with the world they observe. Feelings and emotions are frequently labile and unexplainable. Parents need reassurance that this time of conflict and rebellion is a necessary activity by which the adolescent searches for her or his own identity and purpose in life. Group contact and interaction with peers from a church or synagogue provide support, influence, and affirmation for the adolescent, strengthening commitment to his or her religious belief. For many adolescents, churches serve as both a spiritual resource and a source of social support.

Health promotion strategies include frankly and accurately discussing the relationship between sexuality and religious beliefs; encouraging involvement with youth groups and activities which provide spiritual, social, and peer support; involving the whole family in religious activities and recreation; and providing a mechanism for communication and sharing within the family. The spiritual health and well-being of the family provides the support needed for the adolescent to feel he is able to explore and discover who he is and what his role in life will be. Adolescents whose families place importance on church or synagogue attendance and prayer are less likely to participate in substance abuse and risky sexual behaviors (Hendricks, 2005).

THE YOUNG ADULT

Individuals are considered to be in the young adult stage from about ages 18 through 35. Many of the physical and emotional changes which were initiated during the adolescent years continue through the early years of the young adult stage. Knowledge of these changes continues to focus health promotion and disease prevention strategies. The biological, psychological, social, political, environmental, sexual, and spiritual domains are the guiding framework for organization of these strategies.

Biological Domain

Generally, physical growth is complete by age 20 to 25; therefore, health promotion strategies in the biological domain continue to focus on building and maintaining the body's health through appropriate nutrition, exercise, and rest. Intervention for common health problems such as obesity and stress may be needed. Secondary prevention activities include screening for substance abuse, sexually transmitted infections, and malignancies.

Nutrition

The health of an individual is based on a balanced and nutritious diet. Young adults understand this concept; however, knowledge alone is unlikely to influence their nutritional habits. Food choice is shaped by ethnic heritage, financial status, religious beliefs, and personal likes and dislikes. Food preferences and behaviors are developed from childhood through adolescence and by the time individuals are young adults, these habits and preferences have become an integral part of their perception of themselves as sociocultural beings. Chapter 14 discusses the components of a balanced and nutritious diet in depth.

Approximately one-third of adults 20 years of age and older are estimated to be overweight. The relationship between being overweight and developing adult-onset diabetes, hypertension, and cardiac disease has been well documented. In addition, obesity has been associated with an increased risk of certain cancers, gallbladder diseases, sleep disorders, venous blood clots, and osteoarthritis. Quality of life issues affected by obesity are mobility and physical endurance, as well as social, academic, and vocational functioning.

Spotlight On

To Eat or Not to Eat, That Is the Question

Every few weeks, newspapers and magazines publish articles about the benefits or dangers of different foods. What is the nurse's responsibility in relation to this dietary information and concerns discussed in the media?

The health promotion strategy to promote intake of a balanced and nutritious diet is to appeal to the young adult's sense of social approval and self-esteem. Dietary modification is the most commonly used weight-loss strategy. Dietary information should be provided that is ethnically and religiously sensitive, as well as relevant to individual lifestyle and financial status. Recommending routine physical activity has been shown to increase the long-term effects of weight loss.

Dietary calcium intake by many young women is less than recommended and required for building and maintaining bones. This reduced calcium intake may be a risk factor in bone mineral loss and weakening of bones in later life. The primary health promotion strategy for adolescents and young women is to encourage eating foods that have a high calcium content and taking calcium supplements in order to obtain 1,200 to 1,500 milligrams per day. Common foods high in calcium include broccoli, cheese, milk, sardines, soybeans, spinach, and yogurt. Physical activity, avoidance of smoking, and reduction of caffeine and alcohol use will also benefit bone health.

Exercise

Incorporating regular physical activity into daily routines is recommended to help prevent coronary heart disease, hypertension, obesity, and diabetes. In addition, physical activity has been associated with improvements in self-esteem as noted in self-efficacy, self-acceptance, self-concept, and physical competence. Recommended types (aerobic or anaerobic) and levels of exercise are those which are necessary to maintain physical fitness. Chapter 15 discusses exercise in depth.

In counseling the young adult, focusing on the long-term benefits of exercise will be less effective than emphasizing the shorter-term effects of feeling good, improving appearance, and increasing self-esteem. The young adult also needs to be counseled about the potential risks of injury from overvigorous exercise. Young adults have attained their maximum physical and motor functioning and can sustain an overuse injury from trying to push themselves to further limits. The type of activities usually engaged in for regular exercise are running, fast walking, cycling, and swimming, each of which lends itself to the potential for injury. Counseling moderation in distance, intensity, and speed is an appropriate health promotion strategy.

Skin Cancer Prevention

The use of sunscreen should be recommended for any activities that take place outdoors. Sunscreen helps prevent the most common forms of skin cancer, wrinkling, and painful sunburns. Most people do not use enough sunscreen. For complete coverage, an adult needs to apply approximately one ounce of lotion initially, and reapply as sunscreen is sweated, rubbed, or washed off. It should be reapplied hourly while swimming. Even though the day may be cloudy, up to 80 percent of ultraviolet radiation penetrates cloud cover. Other protective recommendations include avoiding being in the sun between 10 AM and 4 PM, wearing tightly woven clothing with long sleeves and pants, wearing a broad-brimmed hat and sunglasses, and staying in the shade whenever possible.

Sunscreen may not be effective in preventing **melanoma,** a malignant skin lesion which develops from repeated exposure to the sun. Melanoma is the cause of approximately 10 percent of skin cancers, but the leading cause of death from skin disease (Berger, 2004). Box 11-9 describes skin lesion characteristics of a potential melanoma.

Rest

Many young adults do not get enough sleep. Causative factors include work schedules, erratic hours, and stress. Young adults may be less senior in their work environments and subject to being placed on a schedule that includes evening or night shifts or both. Or they may be working more than one job in order to make ends meet or to obtain a higher education. In addition, young adults may stay up later socializing or be awakened during the night by small children in the family. Health promotion involves recognizing sleep deprivation and encouraging rest during the day.

BOX 11-9 Malignant Melanomas

A Asymmetry: One half does not match the other half.

B Border irregularity: The edges are ragged, notched, or blurred.

C Color: The pigmentation is not uniform and may have shades of tan, brown, and black.

D Diameter: It is larger than 6 millimeters or has a sudden or continuing increase in size.

Nursing Alert

Sunscreen and UV Protection

For the greatest protection from ultraviolet-type sun rays, recommend a sunscreen with an SPF (Sun Protection Factor) of 15 or higher that contains titanium dioxide, zinc oxide, or avobenzone. A bottle or tube of sunscreen has no expiration date and does not have to be replaced annually. Although it does remain effective over time, any sunscreen that has a foul smell should be discarded.

In addition to contributing to sleep deprivation, stress and anxiety can affect the overall health of young adults. Stress stimulates the fight-or-flight response of the body. Cardiovascular responses are seen in preparation for the violent muscular activity for which the body is being prepared. The sympathetic stimulation of the adrenal glands releases epinephrine into the bloodstream to decrease digestive processes and shunt blood from the internal organs to the skeletal muscle. This epinephrine also increases the clotting tendency of blood. At the same time, there is a release of adrenocorticotropic hormone, which causes the release of fatty acids in the blood, interferes with the action of insulin to increase blood sugar, and suppresses the immune system. The combination of these factors explains the problems which accompany prolonged stress—hypertension, blood clots, and decreased immune system response. One health promotion strategy for stress reduction is meditation. **Meditation** is the intentional focusing of attention on a singular activity, thought, or object such as one's own breathing, a visual image, a religious symbol, or a phrase repeated silently to oneself. The physiologic changes that occur during meditation include reductions in heart rate and blood pressure, decreased breathing rates with lowered oxygen consumption, and an increase in alpha brain waves (Roth & Creaser, 1997). **Alpha brain waves** are rhythmical waves associated with a quiet, resting state in the brain and body (Guyton & Hall, 2006). These body responses are the opposite of those generated by the fight-or-flight response initiated by stress. Studies of individuals who practice meditation have shown that these individuals react differently to stress (Anselmo, 2005). They have a greater anticipatory mental alertness and recover from the psychological and physical effects of stress more rapidly.

Screening

Screening for risk factors or the presence of disease continues to be an important health promotion strategy during young adulthood. The nurse's screening for this age group primarily focuses on substance use, sexually transmitted infections, and malignancies. When risk factors are present, screening for anemia, diabetes, hypercholesterolemia, tuberculosis, and cardiac disease may be needed.

The cost of screening young adults is an issue. More than 13 million young adults lacked health insurance in 2003, an increase of 2.2 million since 2000 (AHANewsNow, 2005). Many of the jobs available to younger workers are low wage or temporary and lack health benefits. Young adults from low-income families are especially likely to lack coverage, with nearly half of 19- to 29-year-olds in households under the poverty level uninsured. About 60 percent of employers who offer health coverage do not cover dependent children after age 18 or 19 unless they are full-time students (AHANewsNow, 2005).

Tobacco, alcohol, marijuana, and cocaine continue to be the primary substances abused by young adults. The nurse should take every opportunity to discuss tobacco-related diseases and recommend cessation of tobacco use when encountered. It may take several times of hearing how tobacco use is a major threat to health to induce users to attempt to stop. Box 11-10 illustrates the National Cancer Institute's recommendation for promoting smoking cessation.

Youthful experimentation with alcohol and other drugs may progress to misuse, abuse, and dependence. Although alcohol users may have occasional episodes of misuse, 15 to 20 percent of drinkers will progress to the abuse category and a smaller percentage will become physiologically dependent. Health promotion strategies should focus on helping individuals who do not have significant problems to take an active role in assessing their substance use and the consequences of continuing their risky behaviors. Changing these behaviors even moderately can have a significant impact on the health of these individuals as well as the health of their families. Using a model similar to the National Cancer Institute's smoking cessation program is helpful. After elucidating a health risk from alcohol use or drug use or both, the nurse should share concerns about the effects of these substances. Educating the individual about the adverse consequences related to use and discussing options for behavioral change help engage the individual in the process. Arranging for follow-up visits and supportive reinforcement of the individual's efforts can help make change more successful. Individuals with serious problems need referral to an addiction specialist.

With over 30 million individuals infected with genital herpes and 1 million infected with HIV, screening for sexually transmitted infections is a key health promotion strategy. Increased personal freedom and the drive to establish meaningful intimate relationships may make young adults vulnerable to sexually transmitted infections. In addition, substance use can promote unsafe sexual behaviors. Information obtained from the sexual history provides direction for health promotion strategies and interventions specifically geared to the individual's personal risk behaviors. The nurse should elicit information regarding the individual's sexual orientation, whether the individual is sexually active in a mutually monogamous relationship or active with multiple partners, whether the individual has recently changed or added partners, and whether the individual has ever had a sexually transmitted infection. If risks are identified, the nurse should provide health education and prevention counseling to help individuals avoid acquiring sexually transmitted infections or to prevent complications and spread of those already acquired. Screening should always be considered for sexually active individuals with multiple sex partners, with a history of sexually transmitted infections, or with a sex partner who has multiple partners or a known sexually transmitted infection.

Screening for malignancies such as breast cancer, cervical cancer, and testicular cancer are important health promotion strategies. Young adult women should be taught breast self-examination (BSE) techniques. From 50 to 90 percent of breast cancer tumors are first detected by self-exam (Giuliano, 2004). These exams are most effective when done one week after the first day of the menstrual period, when the breasts are less dense and less sensitive. Box 11-11 describes BSE techniques. Each of the techniques should be done monthly. Risk factors for breast cancer are listed in Box 11-12.

In the **Papanicolaou (Pap) test,** cells are collected from areas that shed cells and are microscopically examined for early changes which may be related to the development of cancer. Use of the Pap test to screen for cancer in the cervical portion of the uterus has decreased deaths from cervical cancer by 70 percent since the test was developed in the 1940s. Pap smears for cervical cancer should be conducted for all women who are or have been sexually active or who have reached

BOX 11-10 How to Help Clients Stop Smoking

Ask
- Ask about smoking at every visit: "Do you smoke?" "Are you still smoking?"

Advise
- Make a clear statement of advice: "As your nurse, I must advise you to stop smoking now."

Assist
- Set a specific date and provide information about smoking cessation for those interested. For those not interested, refrain from nagging.

Arrange
- Make a follow-up visit within the first two weeks after cessation.

BOX 11-11 Breast Self-Examination (BSE) Techniques

Inspection
- Examine the breasts in front of a mirror, looking for noticeable differences in contour, nipple placement, or dimpling.
- Re-examine with hands on hips, arms raised over the head, and leaning forward.

Palpation in bath or shower
- Using the hand opposite the breast, palpate the entire breast with the flat pads of the first three fingers, using a circular motion.
- Repeat with the other breast.

Palpation lying down
- Raise one arm and tuck it behind the head.
- Using the same technique as in the bath or shower, palpate the breast with the fingers of the opposite hand.
- Repeat with the other breast.

BOX 11-12 Risk Factors for Breast Cancer

- Being female
- Increasing age
- Never having children
- Family history of breast cancer
- Early menarche
- Late menopause
- Higher educational level
- Higher socioeconomic status
- Recent use of estrogen

BOX 11-13 Risk Factors for Cervical Cancer

- Sexually transmitted infections
- First intercourse at an early age
- Multiple sexual partners
- Cigarette smoking
- Low socioeconomic status

described in Box 11-14 and should be performed monthly. Young men should be instructed to look for changes in the testicles. The earliest signs of testicular cancer are pain, swelling, or hardness of the testicle. A painless lump, usually about the size of a pea, may also be cancerous. Risk factors for testicular cancer are listed in Box 11-15.

Psychological Domain

The psychological domain for the young adult includes both cognitive and emotional development. Closely tied to Piaget's theory of cognitive development are both moral and ego development. Kohlberg's and Gilligan's theories of moral development were discussed in the adolescent section of this chapter. Loevinger's ego development theory is considered in this section. There are several psychosocial theories that describe the emotional development of young adults. Along with Erikson's young adult stage of development, observations described by Levinson and Sheehy are discussed.

Cognitive Development

According to Jean Piaget, the cognitive transformation of young adults has progressed to the formal operations

BOX 11-14 Testicular Self-Examination

- Place the index and middle fingers underneath the testicle and the thumb on top.
- Gently roll the testicle between the thumb and fingers.
- Feel for any changes or abnormal lumps.
- Repeat with second testicle.

BOX 11-15 Risk Factors for Testicular Cancer

- Undescended testicle
- Gonadal defect
- Genetic abnormality

age 20. The American Cancer Society recommends screening every one to three years, depending upon results of previous smears. The most important health promotion strategy to prevent cervical cancer is to educate young adult women on risk reduction for sexually transmitted infections. Risk factors for cervical cancer are listed in Box 11-13.

Although testicular cancer has a low incidence rate in the overall population, it is the most commonly occurring cancer in males between age 15 and 35. Young adult men can increase their chances of finding testicular cancer early by performing monthly testicular self-examination (TSE). The best time to perform the exam is after a warm bath or shower when the heat has caused the scrotal skin to relax, making it easier to feel anything unusual on the testicle. TSE techniques are

Testicular Examination in Young Adult Men

Study Problem/Purpose: To describe patterns of testicular self-examination (TSE) in young adult men and to identify factors differentiating men who do and do not practice TSE.

Method: A sample of 191 men 18–35 years of age was given a self-report, 75-item health risk appraisal to identify health-related lifestyle habits.

Findings: Sixty-four percent of 191 participants reported rarely or never performing TSE, and 36 percent practiced TSE monthly or every few months. Men who infrequently performed TSE were more often African American or Hispanic and had less than a college education.

Implications: Both demographic and socioeconomic variables influence whether a young adult man performs TSE. This study supports the need to promote this important cancer-screening activity to all young adult men, especially ethnic minority men.

Wynd, C. (2001). Testicular self-examination in young adult men. *Journal of Nursing Scholarship, 34*(3), 251-255.

reasoning stage with the ability to consider multiple hypothetical possibilities of the consequences of actions (Brainerd, 1978); however, it has been found that some persons may never reach this higher stage of development. Some may use their formal operational abilities in certain aspects of their lives, but use concrete operational thinking in other aspects.

Closely tied to cognitive development are moral and ego development. Jean Piaget emphasized that moral judgment was a developing cognitive process which was stimulated by social relationships. The development of moral judgment was discussed earlier in this chapter.

Ego Development Cognitive and moral development support ego development. Based on the theoretical constructs of Piaget's cognitive developmental theory, Kohlberg's moral development theory, and Sullivan's development of the self system is Jane Loevinger's ego development theory. Ego development refers to the individual's integrative processes and overall orientation to family, friends, and the larger society. Although these stages are defined independently of age, individuals can be characterized through descriptions specific to each stage. The ego development theory represents the individual's movement across the domains of personal relationships, impulse control, moral development, and cognitive style. Table 11-4 summarizes the distinctive features of each stage.

TABLE 11-4 Ego Development: Stages and Individual Behaviors

Impulsive
- Self-centered, concrete thinking
- Self-control viewed as undesirable
- No consideration for intent

Self-protective
- Obedience to rules motivated by self-interest
- Morality governed by pragmatism
- Relationships are manipulative
- Independence is developing

Ritual
- Responses show increased conventionalist tendencies

Conformist
- Beginning recognition of social norms and needs
- Increase in feelings of morality, interpersonal reciprocity
- Concern with material things, conventional behavior, reputation, and status

Self-aware transition
- Growing awareness of relativism in situations
- Able to be self-critical and understanding of motivation
- Freedom from peer pressure

Conscientious
- Interest in differences in individuals, relationships, ideals, achievement, and obligations

Individualistic transition
- Toleration of paradoxical relationships
- Concern for interpersonal relationships
- Growing recognition of emotional interdependence

Autonomous
- Able to cope with inner conflict and conflicts experienced by others
- Concerned with self-fulfillment and individuality of self and others

Integrated
- Able to reconcile conflicting demands and let go of the unattainable

Emotional Development

According to Erik Erikson (1950), the central developmental task of young adulthood is to develop intimacy. Young adults seek to develop intense, lasting relationships with other individuals, thereby increasing their feelings of competency and self-esteem. The developmental task of achieving intimacy is accomplished when an individual can develop an open, supportive relationship with another without fear of losing his or her own individual identity. The capacity to openly share feelings and thoughts, to be empathetic, and to develop mutually dependent emotional ties characterizes an intimate relationship (Sigelman & Rider, 2005). This intimacy may be expressed in a sexual relationship, either heterosexual or homosexual. Without intimate relationships, young adults remain isolated and self-absorbed, often engaging in promiscuous sexual behavior without commitment or psychological security.

Another psychosocial development theory applicable to the young adult stage was developed by Daniel Levinson, who made a biographical, longitudinal study of a group of young men (Levinson, Darrrow, Klein, Levinson, & McKee, 1976). Based on the biographies of the subjects, Levinson proposed a life cycle structure with five eras: Preadulthood, Early Adulthood, Middle Adulthood, Late Adulthood, and Late Late Adulthood. Early Adulthood is divided into four periods. Table 11-5 describes the ages and developmental occurrences Levinson observed. The sequences described male development and may not be descriptive of female development.

One writer who looked at the psychosocial development of adulthood with close attention to the perceptions of both men and women was Gail Sheehy (1974).

Using a similar qualitative research approach of collecting individual biographies, she compared the developmental rhythms of men and women, finding them to be similar, but lacking synchrony. Both genders experience predictable crises in adulthood. Table 11-6 lists these crises for young adults.

Social Domain

Individuals become adults through the process of socialization. The individual learns and adopts norms, values, expectations, and social roles required by the individual's social group. This ongoing process was initiated in infancy and continues throughout adulthood. Changes in role, occupation, family structure, or habitation may necessitate resocialization. For young adults, the major social change is establishing a separate residence from the family of origin and achieving emotional autonomy. (Sigelman & Rider, 2005). Social interaction continues to include the family of origin and may include financial and emotional support; however, there is a restructuring toward a more equal relationship of one adult to another. An individual's transition from adolescence to young adulthood is facilitated by a family that is accepting, empathetic, and supportive.

Heterosexual relationships during this young adult period may result in marriage or cohabitation. The median age at first marriage is 25 years for women and 27 years for men. (U.S. Census Bureau, 2006). The 2005 provisional data show a marriage rate of 7.5 marriages per 1,000 population. The divorce rate for that same period is 3.6 divorces per 1,000 population (Sutton & Munson, 2006). Although the overall marriage failure rate

---

TABLE 11-5 Early Adulthood Periods

Period	Age	Characteristic	Events
Early adult transition	18–23 years	Modification of relationships with family, peers, and other groups Initial exploration and choices in adult world	High school graduation College entry Moving out of family home
Getting into the adult world	Early to late 20s	Exploration and provisional commitment to adult roles and responsibilities	Marriage Occupation choice
Age 30 transition	28–33 years	Modification of provisional life structure	Divorce
Settling down	Early 30s to late 30s	Deeper commitments to occupation, family	Occupational change Long-range plans for specific goals

Adapted from "Periods in the Adult Development of Men: Ages 18–45," by D. J. Levinson et al., 1976, Counseling Psychologist, 6, 21–25.

TABLE 11-6 Crises of Young Adulthood

Period	Age	Characteristic	Events
Pulling up roots	18–20	Separate individual worldview from family worldview Locate self in peer group role, sex role, and worldview	College Military service Travel
The trying twenties	Early to late 20s	Prepare for life work Form capacity for intimacy Construct safe structure for future	Marriage Occupational choice Life pattern choice
Catch 30	Late 20s to early 30s	Outgrow career and personal choices made in the 20s Desire to expand personal and professional life	Divorce/marriage Occupation change Job change Childbirth
Rooting and extending	Early 30s	Increase order, rationality Reduce social life outside family Focus on raising children	Buy home Seek career advancement

Adapted from Passages: Predictable Crises of Adult Life, *by G. Sheehy, 1974, New York: Dutton*

is almost 50 percent, the failure rate for the youngest young adults is even higher. The most important health promotion strategy to help young adults be successful at marriage is to promote communication between the partners. There are many adjustments which must be made in a marriage (emotional, sexual, personal, financial, and social). The degree of marital satisfaction which couples can achieve is dependent upon communication about these tasks during courtship and continued communication following marriage (Sigelman & Rider, 2005).

Marriage has the advantage of recognized social stability where partners share economic resources and property; however, some young adults may decide to live together without marrying. **Cohabitation** as reported by the U.S. Bureau of the Census refers to two unrelated adults of the opposite sex living together without a binding social or institutional contract. In 2000, the U.S. Bureau of the Census recorded over 5 million unmarried cohabitating couples, a 72 percent increase since 1990. Many couples may decide to live together to see if they are compatible for marriage; however, research studies have shown increased levels of physical aggression, lower-quality marriages, and higher rates of divorce after marriage among cohabitating couples. This may be due to a lack of a feeling of permanence. One health promotion strategy for couples contemplating cohabitation would be to review studies and statistics comparing marriage to cohabitation. Enhancing communication between the partners is also important.

The desire for intimacy may also be expressed in a homosexual relationship. There are no definitive statistics on the prevalence of homosexuality. According to advance data from the National Center for Health Statistics (2002), approximately 6 percent of males and 11 percent of females have had same-sex contact in their lifetimes. When asked, "Do you think of yourself as heterosexual, homosexual, bisexual, or something else?" 90 percent of men 18–44 years of age responded that they think of themselves as heterosexual, 2.3 percent of men answered homosexual, 1.8 percent bisexual, 3.9 percent "something else," and 1.8 percent did not answer the question. Societal attitudes of hostility, hatred, and isolation have created psychosocial difficulties for homosexual adolescents and young adults, leading to secrecy in relationships, a lack of opportunity for open socialization, and limited communication with healthy role models. Rejection or harassment by family, peers, or society has led to isolation, substance abuse, domestic violence, depression, and suicide. Health promotion strategies include finding ways to increase the comfort and confidence with which homosexual individuals can interact with health care providers. Recognition of heterosexual bias (seeing the human experience in strictly heterosexual context), homophobia (the irrational fear or hatred of homosexuality), stereotyping, stigmatizing, and social prejudice against homosexuals is essential to a healthy life for heterosexuals as well as homosexuals (see Figure 11-2.)

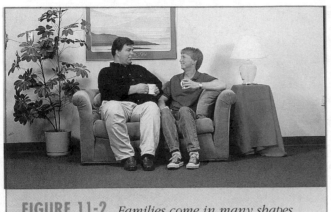

FIGURE 11-2 *Families come in many shapes and configurations.*

Intimate partner violence is a serious social problem affecting heterosexual and homosexual young adults. **Intimate partner violence** is a pattern of assault or coercion to force a partner to comply with the other partner's wishes. Abuse occurs across all cultures, all religions, and all socioeconomic groups; however, young women and those below the poverty line are disproportionately affected. Each year, nearly 5.3 million intimate partner victimizations occur among women age 18 and older, resulting in nearly 2 million injuries and 1,300 deaths (U.S. Department of Justice, 2003). Women experience over 10 times as many incidents of violence by an intimate partner as do men, accounting for 85 to 90 percent of partner abuse. Men are more likely to have been victimized by an acquaintance or a stranger rather than an intimate partner. Abusive relationships intensify during pregnancy, and violence escalates. Women assaulted during pregnancy are more likely to suffer miscarriage or deliver premature, low birth weight infants. Intimate partner violence occurs in both heterosexual and homosexual relationships. Violence within gay and lesbian relationships may go unreported for fear of harassment or ridicule.

Nearly 25 percent of women have been raped, physically assaulted, or both by an intimate partner at some point in their lives (CDC, 2003). For those who had an acute battering incident requiring treatment, most reported that they were battered by their boyfriends or ex-boyfriends. Women reported being punched, kicked, and slapped, being hit with tools such as a hammer, nail gun, and crowbar, and being hit with household items such as pots, pans, dishes, a beer can, and a lamp. Jumping from a moving car, being choked, and being burned with a cigarette caused other reported injuries. Knives and guns were also reported as weapons of injury.

Women with a history of intimate partner violence report 60 percent higher rates of all health problems than do women with no history of abuse (Campbell et al., 2002). Adolescents involved with an abusive partner report increased levels of depressed mood, substance use, antisocial behavior, and, in females, suicidal behavior (Roberts, Klein, & Fisher, 2003). Children who witness intimate partner violence are at greater risk of developing psychiatric disorders, developmental problems, school failure, violence against others, and low self-esteem.

The most important health promotion strategy to stop or prevent intimate partner violence is educating health care professionals to ask about and recognize signs of abusive relationships. Each encounter with an individual enables the health care provider to assess the type of relationship in which the individual is involved. Box 11-16 lists indications of chronic or acute abuse. Individuals tend to seek help several times before being able to leave an abusive situation. Support systems which include health care providers, social services, law enforcement, and emergency shelters need to be in place. Intervening in a timely manner may prevent severe injury, even death. An abused individual returning to the same environment will be abused again.

Political Domain

The young adult no longer is restricted by the minimum age requirements for adult activities. In fact, the young adult, through the ability to vote in local, state, and national elections as well as the opportunity to seek local, state, and national elected office, can be instrumental in determining which laws are passed and which are not. Young adults should be encouraged to be knowledgeable and to actively participate in the political system. They can seek out causes or political candidates that can make a difference in society and should be encouraged to devote time, energy, and effort to effect positive social change.

BOX 11-16 Indications of Intimate Partner Violence

Physical indications
- Bruises on the face, head, breasts, abdomen, or genitals
- Bruises in various stages of healing
- Bite marks
- Repeatedly seeking medical attention for chronic, stress-related disorders

Subtle indications
- Delay seeking prenatal care
- Frequent missed appointments
- Unlikely explanations for bruising
- Overpossessive partner who does not allow the client to respond
- Belittling or oversolicitous partner

Adapted from "Battered," by V. F. Parker, 1995, RN, 58(1), 26–29.

Research Note

Screening for Domestic Violence in Pregnant Women

Study Problem/Purpose: To examine the correlates of violence during pregnancy.

Method: A total of 197 pregnant women 14 to 41, recruited from an inner-city clinic, were assessed for interaction techniques used during conflict, anxiety, depression, perceived stress, social support, negative interactions with the baby's father, and domestic violence. The sample was 49 percent African American, 45 percent Latina, and 6 percent White. Sixty-five percent were unmarried, and 59.6 percent were living with the baby's father. Median annual income was $10,000–$20,000 with 49.4 percent less than $10,000.

Findings: Seventeen percent experienced some form of violence within the last year and 13.3 percent experienced violence from their partner, with 4.8 percent of violence commencing with the pregnancy. Those reporting violence were significantly younger and with lower incomes. African American women reported more verbal aggression than did Latinas. More frequent violence was associated with less support and more negative interactions with the baby's father, rather than associated with cultural subgroup.

Implication: This study supports the need to screen pregnant women for domestic violence in medical settings and indicates that screening for psychosocial variables such as negative interactions may also help detect whether violence is occurring.

Sagrestano, L., et al. (2004). Demographic, psychological, and relationship factors in domestic violence during pregnancy in a sample of low-income women of color. *Psychology of Women Quarterly, 28,* 309-322.

BOX 11-17 Occupational Hazards

Biological
Bloodborne pathogens
Infectious bacteria,
    mold, and fungi
Contagious viruses
Sanitation

Respiratory
Indoor air quality
Asbestos
Tobacco smoke

Chemical
Toxic substances
Lead
Machine fluids
Pesticides

Physical
Confined space
Radiation
Nonergonomic
    workstations
Repetitive strain
High noise levels

Safety
Falls
Machinery-related
    accidents
Fire and explosions

Psychological
Stress
Harassment
Workplace violence

only. Some occupations, such as in microelectronics, food production, teaching, office work, hospitals, banks, and domestic work are predominantly female, exposing women to certain health disorders such as back injuries, repetitive strain injuries, reproductive hazards, and stress. Women are paid workers outside the home and unpaid workers at home, working an average of one to three hours per day longer than a man in the same society. Health problems arising from this situation include stress, chronic fatigue, and premature aging. Women also are more often victims of sexual harassment and discrimination in the workplace. The health care professional must be aware of occupational health hazards and potential gender differences in order to provide health promotion strategies for young adults.

Environmental Domain

Accidents, especially motor vehicle accidents, are the primary cause of death among young adults. Firearms, poisoning, sports injury, drowning, and burns also contribute to accidental injuries in young adults. Table 11-3 on page 231 presents accident prevention strategies applicable to the young adult population.

At least one-third of a young adult's time is spent on the job. Providing a thorough knowledge of the hazards associated with the individual's profession or occupation is the primary health promotion strategy. Box 11-17 illustrates common occupational hazards.

Working conditions and environment are sources of hazards for both men and women; however, the safety and health standards and exposure limits are based on research with male populations and laboratory tests

Sexual Domain

Young adults have accomplished the developmental task of establishing their sexual identity. They know if they are heterosexual, homosexual, or somewhere along the continuum. They may have selected a life partner and be establishing their own homes and careers. The major health promotion strategy in this domain is to help the young adult establish a healthy sexuality.

An assessment of sexuality should be included in the overall health assessment. Problems in sexual relationships for young adults frequently involve poor communication between partners. Facilitating communication between partners, teaching about sexuality, clarifying erroneous information, and providing frank, comprehensive information are health promotion strategies to encourage sexual health.

Young adulthood is the time when many couples decide to raise a family. The tremendous economic, social, and emotional adjustments which accompany parenting responsibilities may affect a couple's sexual desire and responsiveness. Parents may have less time and energy for promoting the marital relationship. Facilitating communication and encouraging couples to make time to be alone is an appropriate sexual health promotion strategy.

A common health problem affecting sexuality as well as the overall quality of life is premenstrual syndrome. **Premenstrual syndrome (PMS)** is the cyclic recurrence of distressing physical, psychological, and/or behavioral changes related to the menstrual cycle. These changes may affect normal activities, relationships, or both. Eighty percent of women report some degree of PMS, with 10 percent having severe symptoms that significantly interfere with daily activities for one to two weeks each month (Dowd, 2005). Symptoms range from changes in mood, thinking, and eating behaviors to bloating, weight gain, headache, and breast tenderness. Researchers have investigated hormonal, nutritional, psychological, biochemical, and metabolic causes with no definitive answers found. Once diagnosis is made, PMS can be treated or controlled. Box 11-18 lists some of the treatments that have been successful.

Spiritual Domain

By the time adolescents reach young adulthood, they have established their own identity and are establishing an intimate relationship with another. This may be a time when they make a conscious commitment toward their religious beliefs. They may struggle and question during the effort to test, learn, and make a decision about their commitment. As they continue to mature, they reexamine their purpose and focus in life. This provides the opportunity to confirm their values, morals, and religious foundation. An appropriate health promotion strategy is to encourage young adult participation in support, learning, fellowship, and spiritual-growth groups. Young adults also take on the responsibility for nurturing the spiritual development of their children. Providing a religious foundation that teaches the value of kindness, goodness, and faithfulness is a parental responsibility. Parents who do not have an active, faithful spiritual life will not be able to impart these values to their children.

SUMMARY

Health promotion in adolescents and young adults focuses on creating healthy lifestyle patterns. Individuals in the adolescent and young adult age groups are primarily healthy; therefore, the majority of health problems addressed in this chapter were potential problems.

Significant physical development, relational change, and emotional turmoil characterize the adolescent period. The potential hazards of adolescence transcend race, gender, and ethnicity; however, adolescents are pliable, adaptable, and responsive to challenge. Their ability to recover from periods of problem behaviors and emotional disorders enables them to mature into responsible and functional young adults. The opportunity to intervene and prevent lifelong health problems is greater and more effective in this age group than in any other. This chapter discussed a wide range of health promotion and preventive care interventions for adolescents organized through biological, psychological, social, environmental, sexual, and spiritual domains.

Young adulthood is a period of stabilization in which the individual makes career and relationship decisions that will be the framework for the rest of her or his life. Young adults develop a balance between autonomy and attachment, separateness and connectedness. Intimacy is expressed in sexual relationships and the choice of a life partner. Health concerns are similar to those of the adolescent as well as those of the middle-aged adult. Lifestyle decisions made during adolescence and young adulthood will determine the quality of life in later years. Health promotion strategies were viewed through biological, psychological, social, political, environmental, sexual, and spiritual domains.

BOX 11-18 Treatment of Premenstrual Syndrome (PMS)

Changing diet
- Decreasing salt, caffeine, refined sugar, and fat
- Restricting alcohol and tobacco use

Changing activity
- Increasing anaerobic exercise such as walking, jogging, or swimming

Supplements
- Daily multivitamin tablet
- Evening primrose oil

Medication
- Oral contraceptives
- Diuretics

Counseling and support groups

Key Concepts

1. Education about the process and normal variations of attaining physical maturity is a key adolescent health promotion strategy. Additional health promotion for adolescents and young adults in the biological domain includes strategies related to nutrition, activity/exercise, and rest.

Objectives/Goals: Through participation in discussion of this case study, participants will have the opportunity to:
1. Discuss the relationship between diet, exercise, and constipation.
2. Discuss the relationship between diet, exercise, and overweight.
3. Relate body image to maintenance of self-concept.

Health Promotion Concern, History and Physical, Present Health Status, Past Health Status, Family History, and Social History

Lisa Flores is a 19-year-old Mexican American college student. She comes to the Student Health Center at the college complaining of abdominal pain. Her health in the past has been good with only minor illnesses such as colds and flu. She has no chronic illnesses, and her immunizations are all up-to-date. Her family history is positive for hypertension (maternal grandmother), coronary artery disease (paternal grandfather), and diabetes mellitus type 2 (paternal aunt). Lisa is single and is a freshman in college studying anthropology. She is currently living in a dormitory on campus and eats either in the cafeteria or at local fast-food vendors. She notes that she has gained 10 pounds since coming to college. She has one sister, 22 years old, and one brother, 15 years old. Both parents are living and well without chronic disease. She does not smoke, drink alcohol, or use street drugs. She uses no over-the-counter medications other than an occasional acetaminophen for headache.

Review of Pertinent Domains
Biological Domain

Physical exam: Reveals a well-developed, well-nourished young adult female, 64 inches tall, weighing 154 pounds for a BMI of 26.4. No abnormal findings were found except for slight tenderness in the left lower quadrant of her abdomen and hard feces in the rectum on digital examination.

Gastrointestinal: Reports that she used to have a soft, formed bowel movement daily, but since coming to college has hard, dry bowel movements every 3–4 days. Her last bowel movement was two days ago. She does not use laxatives or enemas.

Genitourinary: No frequency, burning, urgency on urination. No vaginal itching, burning, or discharge. Her menstrual periods are approximately every 28 days, lasting 5–6 days, with no dysmenorrhea. Her last menstrual period was two weeks ago, and she is not sexually active.

24-Hour Diet Recall: Lisa skipped breakfast except for four ounces of orange juice from cafeteria. She had a 12-ounce regular cola at midmorning, pepperoni pizza and a 10-ounce glass of water for lunch, a 12-ounce regular cola midafternoon, chicken-flavored ramen noodles for dinner, and a late-evening snack of potato chips and half a candy bar.

Diagnostic testing: Complete blood count (CBC) and urinalysis (UA) were in normal range.

Psychological Domain

Cognitive: Lisa has been making above-average grades in school. She appears to lack information about lifestyle changes that establish and promote consistent bowel habits. She also is unaware of the components of a balanced low-fat diet, daily exercise, and her body's daily calorie needs.

Emotional: Lisa is concerned about her body image since gaining extra weight. She says she feels stressed with studying and school activities.

Social Domain

Lisa has been declining invitations to go out socially because she feels unattractive. She stays in her dorm room most days.

Environmental Domain

Before starting college life, Lisa engaged in step aerobics three times weekly, but says she does not have time anymore because she must study so much.

Questions for discussion:
1. What is missing from Lisa's diet? How can daily bowel elimination be promoted? Are there any complications from chronic constipation?
2. What is the "Freshman Fifteen"? What should Lisa do to avoid becoming overweight?
3. What can be done to promote her self-concept?

2. Screening for actual or potential health problems in adolescents and young adults is vital for promoting the quality and quantity of life. Adolescent screening includes hypertension, dental disease, substance use, and sexually transmitted infections. Young adult screening focuses on substance use, sexually transmitted infections, and malignancies.

3. Promoting health in the psychological domain requires understanding of normal cognitive and emotional development. Theoretical frameworks developed by Jean Piaget, Erik Erikson, Lawrence Kohlberg, Carol Gilligan, Daniel Levinson, Gail Sheehy, and Jane Loevinger provide a foundation for determining appropriate health promotion strategies for adolescents and young adults. Depression and potential suicide are adolescent health problems that need careful attention and intervention. Developing the ability to make an intimate relationship during young adulthood is central to emotional security throughout life.

4. Health promotion in the social domain examines relationships with family and peers as well as intimate relationships. Health problems of abuse and intimate partner violence need significant attention for adolescents and young adults.

5. Conservative political forces are attempting to prohibit adolescent access to confidential health care. Reduced access, especially for contraception and sexually transmitted infection treatment, will have a far-reaching negative impact on adolescent health.

6. Accidents, especially motor vehicle accidents, are the leading cause of death for adolescents and young adults. Health promotion focuses on strategies that reduce or prevent accidents in these age groups.

7. The adolescent and young adult mature from a child to an individual capable of reproduction. Sexual health focuses on assisting individuals to develop a comprehensive, accurate knowledge of their own and others' sexuality with relationships based on caring and responsibility between individuals.

8. Adolescents are capable of assuming responsibility for their own spiritual development. Young adults must assume responsibility for the spiritual development of their children.

Learning Activities

1. Describe environmental safety promotion strategies for adolescents and young adults.

2. Observe television news broadcasts for at least three evenings and list the types of crimes reportedly committed by adolescents or young adults or both and compare these crimes with those committed by adults. Document your conclusions. With your class-mates, discuss violence prevention measures for adolescents and young adults.

3. Design a presentation on skin cancer prevention for adolescents and young adults.

True/False Questions

1. T or F Puberty is dependent upon the complex interaction between the hypothalamus, anterior pituitary, gonads, and the muscles and skeleton.

2. T or F Anorexia nervosa and bulimia nervosa are two terms that refer to the same eating disorder.

3. T or F Statistics show that less than 25 percent of adolescents engage in sexual activity.

4. T or F Suicide is a leading cause of death in young adult males.

Multiple Choice Questions

1. Environmental hazards for nurses in the workplace include:
   a. Ergonomics
   b. Dementia
   c. Masculo skeletal injury
   d. Autonomy

1. Breast development in male adolescents is called:
   a. gynecomastia.
   b. male puberty.
   c. menarche.
   d. thelarche.

2. The most accurate blood pressure reading for an adolescent will be obtained using a cuff that:
   a. is four inches wide or greater.
   b. fits the space between the axilla and the antecubital fossa.
   c. extends beyond the antecubital fossa.
   d. is no more than two inches wide.

3. The high rate of motor vehicle accidents in adolescence is related to adolescents':
   a. poor muscle development and motor coordination.
   b. short attention span.
   c. risk taking and experimentation.
   d. inability to pass driver education classes.

4. The type of rhythmic brain waves noted during a meditation session are:
   a. alpha waves.
   b. beta waves.
   c. gamma waves.
   d. delta waves.

5. Precancerous changes in the cells of the cervix are most likely to be caused by:
   a. a high-fat diet.
   b. vigorous exercise.
   c. a sexually transmitted infection.
   d. douching.

Websites

http://www.cdc.gov Centers for Disease Control and Prevention: Offers information related to physical activity and health from a report by the Surgeon General to the Centers for Disease Control and prevention, Division of the National Center for Chronic Disease Prevention and Health Promotion.

http://groups.ucanr.org University of California Agriculture and Natural Resources: Has a nine-lesson educational intervention that uses computer technology to assist adolescents from low-income communities with diet assessment and "guided" goal setting for making healthy lifestyle choices. It is designed to be delivered by middle school teachers for skill building, social support, and goal attainment.

http://www.epi.umn.edu Division of Epidemiology and Community Health: Discusses the Center for Youth Health Promotion (CYHP) at the University of Minnesota that was designed to disseminate to schools and communities innovative youth health promotion programs and materials created by the Division of Epidemiology of the School of Public Health.

http://www.girlshealth.gov Girls Health.gov Website: Developed by the Department of Health and Human Services' Office of Women's Health to respond to adolescent girls' health concerns. Site focuses on friends and family relationships, trust, sexuality, violence and abuse, peer pressure, and self-esteem. The site is intended to motivate girls to choose healthy behaviors without the tediousness of a "you should do this" message.

http://www.mentalhealth.samhsa.gov Substance Abuse and Mental Health Services Administration with the United States Department of Health and Human Services: Focuses on cultural competence in serving children and adolescents with mental health problems in recognition that all cultures practice traditions that support and value their children and that prepare them for living in their society.

http://www.who.int World Health Organization: Provides information from the World Health Organization on the health, growth, and development of children from birth to 19 years of age throughout the world.

Organizations

Centers for Disease Control and Prevention
National Center for Chronic Disease Prevention and Health Promotion
Division of Nutrition and Physical Activity, MS K-46
4770 Buford Highway, NE
Atlanta, GA 30341-3724
Tel: (888) CDC-4NRG or (888) 232-4674 (toll-free)
http://www.cdc.gov
Major source for health promotion information, statistics, and programs.

The President's Council on Physical Fitness and Sports
Department W
200 Independence Ave., SW
Room 738-H
Washington, D. C. 20201-0004
Tel: (202) 690-9000
http://www.fitness.gov
Source for information on fitness and ways to motivate active lifestyles for better health through President's challenge and program offerings

UCLA/RAND Center for Adolescent Health Promotion
1072 Gayley Avenue
Los Angeles, CA 90024
Tel: (310) 794-3000
Fax: (310) 794-2660
http://www.rand.org
Email: adolescent@rand.org
A model for an academic-community partnership to improve adolescent health. Funded by the Federal Centers for Disease Control and Prevention.

References

AHA News Now. (2005). Report highlights nation's 13 million uninsured young adults. Retrieved May, 5, 2005, from http://www.ahanews.com

American Academy of Child & Adolescent Psychiatry (AACAP). (2002, November). Facts for families: Children of alcoholics. Retrieved December 17, 2006, from http://www.aacap.org/page.ww?name=Children+Of+Alcoholics&section=Facts+for+Families

American Academy of Pediatrics (AAP). (2005). Adolescent pregnancy—current trends and issues: 2005. *Pediatrics, 116*(1), 281–286.

American Lung Association. (2006, April). Smoking and teens fact sheet. Retrieved December 17, 2006, from http://www.lungusa.org/site/pp.asp?c=dvLUK9O0E&b=39871

Anderson, S., Dallal, G., & Must, A. (2003). Relative weight and race influence average age at menarche: Results from two nationally representative surveys of US girls studied 25 years apart. *Pediatrics, 111*(4).

Anselmo, J. (2005). Relaxation: The first step to restore, renew, and self-heal. In B. M. Dossey, L. Keegan, & C. E. Guzzetta (Eds.), *Holistic nursing: A handbook for practice*, (4th ed.), (pp. 523–566). Sudbury, MA: Jones and Bartlett Publishers, Inc.

Berger, T. G. (2004). Skin, hair, & nails. In L. M. Tierney, S. J. McPhee, & M. A. Papadakis (Eds.), *Current medical diagnosis and treatment* (43rd ed., pp. 81–114). Stamford, CT: Appleton & Lange.

Campbell, J., Jones, A., Dienemann, J., Kub J., Schollenberger, J., O'Campo, P., et al. Intimate partner violence and physical health consequences. *Archives of Internal Medicine, 162*(10), 1157–63.

Centers for Disease Control and Prevention (CDC). (2003a). Costs of intimate partner violence against women in the United States. Atlanta, GA: CDC, National Center for Injury Prevention and Control.

Centers for Disease Control and Prevention (CDC). (2003b). National survey of children's health. Retrieved December 17, 2006, from http://www.cdc.gov/nchs/about/major/slaits/nsch.htm

Centers for Disease Control and Prevention (CDC). (2004). Surveillance summaries *MMWR, 53* (No. SS-2).

Dowd, S. (2005). Premenstrual dysphoric disorder: A clinical trial approach to assessment. *Advance for Nurse Practitioners, 13*(2), 57–59.

Elkind, D. (1967). Egocentrism in adolescence. *Child Development*, 38, 1025–1034.

Gilligan, C. (1982). In a different voice: Psychological theory and women's development. Cambridge: Harvard University Press.

Giuliano, A. E. (2004). Breast. In L. M. Tierney, S. J. McPhee, & M. A. Papadakis (Eds.), *Current medical diagnosis and treatment* (43rd ed., pp. 669–693). Stamford, CT: Appleton & Lange.

Guyton, A., & Hall, J. (2006). *Textbook of medical physiology* (11th ed.). Philadelphia: W. B. Saunders.

Hagman, J., & Bechtold, D. (2003). Child and adolescent psychiatric disorders and psychosocial aspects of pediatrics. In W. Hay, A. Hayward, M. Levin, and J. Sondheimer (Eds.), *Current pediatric diagnosis and treatment* (16th ed., pp. 172–214), New York: Lange Medical Books/McGraw-Hill.

Hendricks, M. (2005). Risky business: Drug use, pregnancy, alcohol abuse, reckless driving. *Magazine of the Johns Hopkins Bloomberg School of Public Health Online Edition,* Spring.

Henriksen, L., Feighery, E., Yang, Y., & Fortman, S. (2004). Association of retail tobacco marketing with adolescent smoking. *American Journal of Public Health, 94* (12).

Kaplan, D. & Love-Osborne, K. (2003). Adolescence. In W. Hay, A. Hayward, M. Levin, and J. Sondheimer (Eds.), *Current pediatric diagnosis and treatment* (16th ed., pp. 99–143), New York: Lange Medical Books/McGraw-Hill.

Kochanek, K., Murphy, B., Anderson, R., & Scott, C. (2004). Deaths: Final data for 2002. *National Vital Statistics Reports, 53*(5), 1–116.

Kohlberg, L. (1981). *The philosophy of moral development* (Vol. 1). San Francisco: Harper & Row.

Levinson, D. J., Darrow, C. M., Klein, C. B., Levinson, M. H., & McKee, B. (1976). Periods in the adult development of men: Ages 18–45. *The Counseling Psychologist, 6,* 21–25.

Mandleco, B. (2004). *Growth and development handbook: Newborn through adolescent.* Albany, NY: Delmar Learning.

Martinez-Gonzalez, M., Gual, P., Lahortiga, F., Alonso, Y., de Irala-Estevez, J., & Cervera, S. (2003). Parental factors, mass media influences, and the onset of eating disorders in a prospective population-based cohort. *Pediatrics, 111*(2), 315–321.

McKnight, A., & McKnight, S. (2003). Young novice drivers: Careless or clueless? *Accident Analysis and Prevention, 35*(6), 921–925.

Millstein, S. G., & Igra, V. (1995). Theoretical models of adolescent risk-taking behavior, In J. L. Wallander, & L. J. Siegel (Eds.), *Adolescent health problems: Behavioral perspectives* (pp. 52–71). New York: Guilford Press.

Morelli, J., & Weston, W. (2003) Skin. In W. Hay, A. Hayward, M. Levin, and J. Sondheimer (Eds.), *Current pediatric diagnosis and treatment* (16th ed., pp. 400–419). New York: Lange Medical Books/McGraw-Hill.

National Center for Health Statistics Advance Data 362. (2002). Sexual behavior and selected health measures: Men and women 15–44 years of age, United States: Public Health Service 2003–1250. Retrieved December 19, 2006, from http://www.cdc.gov/nchs/ products/pubs/pubd/ad/ad.htm

National Highway Traffic Safety Administration. (2003). Traffic safety facts: Graduated drivers licensing system. Washington, DC: Author.

New York Committee on Safety and Health. (2005). Young workers. Retrieved December 19, 2006 from http://www.nycosh.org

Rennison, C. M. (2003). Intimate partner violence, 1993–2001. *Crime Date Brief.* Bureau of Justice Statistics. Retrieved December 19, 2006, from http://www.ojp.usdoj.gov/bjs/pub/pdf/ ipv01.pdf

Roberts, T. A., Klein, J. D., & Fisher, S. (2003). Longitudinal effect of intimate partner abuse on high-risk behavior among adolescents. *Archives of Pediatrics & Adolescent Medicine, 157*(9), 875–881.

Rome, E., et al. (2003). Children and adolescents with eating disorders: The state of the art. *Pediatrics, 111*(1), 98–109.

Sagrestano, L., Carroll, D., Rodriguez, A., & Nuwayhid, B. (2004). Demographic, psychological, and relationship factors in domestic violence during pregnancy in a sample of low-income women of color. *Psychology of Women Quarterly, 28,* 309–322.

Sahler, O. J., & Kreipe, R. E. (1991). Psychological development in normal adolescents. In W. R. Hendee (Ed.), *The health of adolescents* (pp. 55–88). San Francisco: Jossey-Bass.

Sheehy, G. (1974). *Passages: Predictable crises of adult life.* New York: Dutton.

Sigel, E. (2003). Eating disorders. In W. Hay, A. Hayward, M. Levin, and J. Sondheimer (Eds.), *Current pediatric diagnosis and treatment* (16th ed., pp. 162–171). New York: Lange Medical Books/McGraw-Hill.

Sigelman, C.K., & Rider, E. A. (2005). *Life-span human development* (5th ed.). Belmont, CA: Wadsworth Publishing Company.

Sutton, P. D., & Munson, M. L. (2006, December). Births, marriages, divorces and deaths: Provisional data for April 2006: *National Vital Statistics Reports, 55*(5). Hyattsville, MD: National Center for Health Statistics.

Urberg, L., Luo, Q., Pilgrim, C., & Degirmencioglu, S. (2003). A two-stage model of peer influence in adolescence substance use: Individual and relationship-specific differences in susceptibility to influence. *Addictive Behaviors, 28*(7), 1243–1256.

U.S. Census Bureau. (2006, September). Estimated median age at first marriage by sex 1890 to the present. *Current population survey, March and annual social and economic supplements, 2005 and earlier.* Retrieved December 18, 2006, from http:// www.census.gov/population/socdemo/hh-fam/ms2.pdf

White, J. (2000). The prevention of eating disorders: a review of the research on risk factors with implications for practice. *Journal of Child and Adolescent Psychiatric Nursing, 13*(2), 76–88.

World Health Organization. (2004). Sexual health—A new focus for WHO. *Progress in Reproductive Health Research, No. 67.* Geneva: World Health Organization.

Wynd, C. (2001). Testicular self-examination in young adult men. *Journal of Nursing Scholarship, 34*(3), 351–255.

Chapter 12

THE MIDDLE-AGED ADULT

Jeanette McNeill, Dr.P.H., AOCN, ANP, RN

KEY TERMS

andropause
chronic illness
climacteric
community-level intervention

menopause
outcomes
perimenopause
risk factor

sandwich generation
sensitivity of a
   screening test

specificity of a
   screening test

OBJECTIVES

Upon completion of this chapter, the reader should be able to:

- Describe the characteristics of middle adulthood that influence health promotion activities.

- Discuss the function of health promotion for the middle adult in terms of improved physiological, psychological, sociological, spiritual, and sexual health.

- Identify environmental factors that influence health outcomes for the middle adult.

- Describe guidelines and prevention recommendations for healthy lifestyles for this age group.

- Propose nursing's role in early detection (secondary prevention) activities based on recommended screening tests for middle adults based on age, gender, and risk status.

INTRODUCTION

The middle adult years from 40 to 65 are usually characterized by relative stability in the job arena and increasing job-related responsibility. Middle adults reflect on their accomplishments and consider the meaning of life. There is an increasing awareness of one's own mortality, as many middle adults cope with their own or another's chronic illnesses and disabilities.

Most in this age group demonstrate a heightened sense of caring both for immediate family and for extended family and community. Members of this age group have been identified as the **sandwich generation**, the middle adult period in which people are "sandwiched" between their children who need nurturance and support and their aging parents, who also need care. As they are parenting teen and young adult children, they are also increasingly called upon to care for their aging parents who are living longer. Health promotion and

health maintenance activities are becoming increasingly critical for middle adults. In this chapter, topics such as general wellness, exercise, identification of personal risk factors, and education regarding prevention and screening are addressed. The role of the nurse in promoting health in the middle-aged adult is presented. Primary prevention and screening (secondary prevention) recommendations specific for this age group are presented. Primary prevention comprises activities taken to prevent illness or injury (e.g., immunizations), while secondary prevention refers to activities to detect illness at its earliest stages when treatment can be most effectively begun and have the most beneficial effect.

IMPORTANCE OF HEALTH PROMOTION IN MIDDLE ADULTHOOD

The years between 40 and 65 are critical ones for health promotion. Actions taken during this life stage will influence health in the older years when functional ability and quality of life are increasingly influenced by health status. Because of the developmental tasks of this age, the middle-aged adult is particularly receptive to the development of health promotion lifestyles. Awareness of the aging process has begun, and middle adults are interested in keeping their health and maintaining functional status.

Current Perspective of Health Promotion in Middle-Aged Adults

Over the past few decades, great strides have been made in overall health for those in the middle adult age group. This age group formerly experienced a high rate of mortality and morbidity from heart disease and stroke, but rates since 1970 have decreased by more than 52 percent for coronary artery disease and 63 percent for stroke (Jemal, Ward, Hao, & Thun, 2005). Changes in the ability to control high blood pressure, coupled with lower mean blood cholesterol levels and reduced rates of cigarette smoking, have largely been responsible for decreases in these mortality rates. Deaths from motor vehicle accidents, the highest death rate from nondisease causes, declined by 41 percent, which is attributed predominantly to seat belt use and reduced rates of driving while intoxicated. Fitness and the move toward healthier nutritional practices, along with better control of blood pressure, has caused a significant change in cardiovascular disease incidence over the past 35 years. These changes are reflected in the objectives for health promotion outlined in *Healthy People 2000* and, more recently, *Healthy People 2010*. A summary of selected objectives specific to the middle adult are listed in Box 12-1. Heart disease, stroke, cancer, and other **chronic illnesses** (a type of disease or disorder that causes limitation of activity for a prolonged period, such as chronic liver disease and cirrhosis) have emerged as leading causes of mortality. These trends are also indicated in the objectives, in the form of increasing the participation of high-risk groups in recommended screening. Screening is discussed in further detail later in the chapter.

Demographics of Middle Adulthood

The 2000 census report indicated that about 62 million people, or 22 percent of the population, were between the ages of 45 and 64. Projections, shown in Figure 12-1, are that this percentage will increase to over 25 percent by 2010, because of the continued influx of baby boomers into middle adulthood, and remain over 20 percent through 2050 (U.S. Census Bureau, 2004).

A corresponding increase in the numbers of persons living with chronic illness is also expected. The number of chronically ill persons, defined by the U.S. Bureau of the Census as an individual with a limitation of activity, has been increasing each year and accounted for about 31 million Americans in 1985 (U.S. Department of Commerce, 2000). Approximately 21 percent of these chronically ill are middle-aged adults. Of interest is the finding that as household income increases, the number of persons classified as disabled or with limited activity decreases. This finding appears to indicate that having a higher income may enable individuals to take preventive actions or acquire better medical care that actually decreases the incidence of disability and chronic illness. Additionally, lower income levels may result from disabilities and chronic illness that influence earning power and employment options. Costs of health care are influencing a shift in emphasis to prevention and early detection by some institutions, employers, and insurers in an attempt to maintain or reduce health care expenditures for the greater numbers of chronically ill middle and older adults.

BOX 12-1   Selected Objectives Related to Middle Adults from *Healthy People 2010*

- Increase the proportion of adults who engage in regular, preferably daily, physical activity of at least 30 minutes per day.
- Increase the proportion of adults who are at a healthy weight, and reduce the proportion who are obese.
- Increase the proportion of adults who consume less than 30 percent of total calories in fat, and increase the proportion of those who consume six daily servings of grain products, with at least three being whole grains.
- Reduce tobacco use in adults and increase smoking cessation attempts by adults.
- Increase the proportion of persons appropriately counseled about health behaviors.
- Increase the proportion of adults who follow key food safety practices.
- Increase the proportion of adults who receive flu vaccine and pneumococcal vaccine.
- Increase the proportion of persons who have a specific source of ongoing care.

Regarding disease-specific objectives:

Cancer
1. Increase the proportion of adults who use at least one method of reducing skin cancer (sunscreen, limiting exposure, etc.).
2. Increase the proportion of adults who have colon cancer screening.

Heart Disease
1. Increase the proportion of persons who are aware of the early warning signs of heart attack and stroke and the importance of accessing rapid emergency care by calling 911.
2. Increase the proportion of adults with high blood pressure whose blood pressure is under control.
3. Reduce the mean cholesterol level in adults.

Diabetes and Chronic Disabling Conditions
1. Increase the proportion of adults with diabetes who are identified, have annual eye and foot examinations, and check their blood glucose.
2. Reduce the proportion of adults with osteoporosis.

Adapted from Healthy People 2010, *retrieved from http://www.healthypeople.gov*

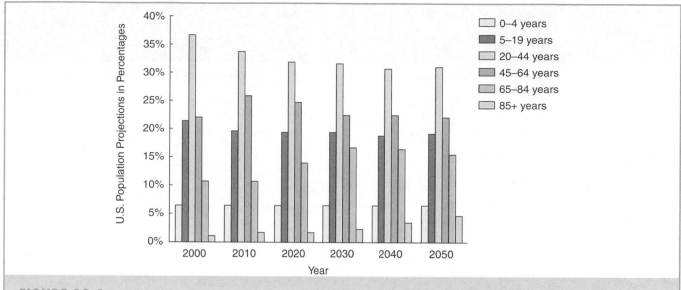

MIDDLE ADULTHOOD: A TIME OF PLANNED CHANGE

Numerous changes in the physical, psychological, social, spiritual, environmental, political, and gender/sexual domains occur during middle adulthood. Some are common to most in this age group. Some are unique to the individual. Many are influenced by lifestyle and health promotion efforts that have occurred during childhood, adolescence, and early adulthood. Many of the health outcomes of middle adulthood can be directly traced to health practices adopted in earlier developmental periods. However, health promotion activities undertaken during this period can still reap benefits and are important to ensuring optimal functioning in late adulthood.

Physical Domain

The middle adult enters the fourth decade usually in good health and in a highly efficient functional state (see Figure 12-2). Although a number of physiological changes occur during this period, most are relatively gradual. General slowing of activity and metabolic rate results in the potential for weight gain and loss of muscle strength and elasticity. These factors predispose to muscle and joint stiffness and a tendency toward respiratory dysfunction. Reproductive changes are the most striking. This period is when perimenopause and menopause occur for women. For men, changes in sexual potency may occur, although reproductive potential for men continues into later years. The occurrence of chronic illnesses, of course, can influence this gradual pace of physical change and can profoundly affect psychosocial development. An estimated 31 million persons of all ages

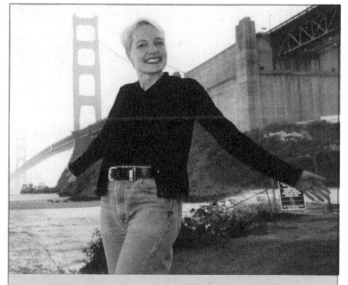

FIGURE 12-2 *Good health and the ability to enjoy physical activity accompany this woman into middle adulthood.*

are affected by chronic illnesses and about 21 percent of these are middle adults (U.S. Department of Commerce, 2000). Table 12-1 depicts important physiological changes by body system.

Female Climacteric

The female **climacteric**, or change of life, occurs gradually over years as ovarian function diminishes resulting in permanent cessation of menses. Perimenopause and menopause are two stages leading to the female climacteric. **Perimenopause** is a time of transition that occurs

TABLE 12-1 Body Changes in Middle Adulthood

Body System	Physiological Change	Implications for Health Promotion
Musculoskeletal	Decreasing bone mass in women Vertebral cartilage hardens Metatarsal spread Loss of muscle mass	Calcium supplementation for women over 40 Safety measures to prevent falls Height decrease may be slowed by hormone replacement therapy Wear properly fitting shoes Maintain physical fitness
Neurological	*Visual changes:* Presbyopia, a gradual decline in ability to focus on close objects Cataract development *Auditory changes:* Presbycusis, progressive hearing loss caused by thickening of capillaries that supply inner ear	Annual eye examinations Avoidance of excessive noise Auditory examination if difficulty
Cardiovascular/ hematologic	Cholesterol and low density lipoprotein (LDL) increases Blood pressure increases Varicosity development	Maintain physical fitness Monitor cholesterol, LDL, triglycerides, BP for changes Maintain regular exercise, use support stockings or socks, avoid dependent position of lower leg
Respiratory	Less elasticity of lung tissue but no loss of functioning unless smoker, respiratory illness	Avoid tobacco use Maintain physical fitness
Integumentary	Loss of elasticity causing sagging and wrinkling Vitiligo and age spots develop May develop skin cancer Callus and corn formation Hair graying and hair loss	Maintain physical fitness and sound nutritional practices Protect skin from sun with sunscreen and cover-ups Participate in skin self-exam Maintain positive body image

gradually over 2 to 15 years as ovarian function gradually diminishes. During perimenopause a woman may experience physical, psychological, and emotional changes related to decreasing levels of estrogen and progesterone.

The premenopausal stage, usually beginning around 40, is characterized by changes in the pattern of menstruation and heightened premenstrual syndrome symptoms. Between the ages of 45 and 55, 95 percent of women actually experience menopause.

The perimenopausal woman may experience hot flashes (flushes), palpitations, loss of muscle strength, increased facial hair, and various gynecological changes associated with decreased amounts of circulating estrogen. Emotional symptoms such as nervousness, irritability, depression, or mood swings may also occur (Carroll, 2005). Although some women might experience adverse

effects of perimenopause and menopause, others experience this passage with a sense of freedom, joy, confidence, and a greater wisdom of life and aging.

Menopause, or the cessation of menses, is considered complete after a year of amenorrhea. Menopause may be induced artifically from surgery such as oophorectomy (the surgical removal of the ovaries) or by other therapies causing sterility such as cancer chemotherapy. In some cases, hormone replacement therapy (HRT) can be helpful in alleviating symptoms. In other cases, such as some malignancies, this therapy may be contraindicated. Concern over the protective effects of estrogen for the skeletal system influences the decisions regarding HRT. Health care providers should discuss cardiovascular, osteoporosis, and cancer risks with women who are considering HRT, whether menopause occurred naturally

TABLE 12-1 Body Changes in Middle Adulthood, *continued*

Body System	Physiological Change	Implications for Health Promotion
Immunological	Slowed cellular repair and regeneration	Maintain physical and emotional well-being to avoid infection and injury
Gastrointestinal	*Dentition:* Periodontal disease, tartar build-up common *Digestive functions:* Slowed GI motility and reduced hydrochloric acid and pepsin production Constipation, also hemorrhoid development Development of lactose intolerance	Preventive and maintenance dental care Balancing diet and fluid needs, avoidance of troublesome foods Regular exercise
Urinary	Gradual decline of glomerular filtration rate Decreased bladder tone Decreased sphincter tone, especially in females Prostate enlargment	Usually causes no dysfunction, may be important in chronic illness or diabetes More frequent urination reduces problems Monitor prostate size for problems with urinary retention, screen for malignancy
Endocrine	Reduced thyroxine due to decreased metabolic rate Reduced pancreatic secretion of insulin	Monitor thyroid function and note signs and symptoms of thyroid disease Screen for non-insulin–dependent diabetes mellitus in high-risk persons or if symptoms occur
Reproductive	*Females:* Diminished ovarian function leading to menopause Risk of breast and other reproductive cancers increases *Males:* Diminished size and firmness of testes Reduced testosterone production Health states may affect erectile function and sex drive	Maintain family planning mechanisms as desired by client Participate in screening procedures and self-exams of breast, vulva Monitor perimenopausal symptoms, manage symptoms, hormone replacement therapy for short-term symptom relief Monitor symptoms, physical and psychological workup for impotence to rule out treatable physical causes

or was surgically induced, so that an informed health promotion decision can be made for each individual woman. In addition to HRT, other considerations for promoting a healthy life during perimenopause and menopause include healthy lifestyle changes, social support, and psychological support.

Male Climacteric

This life change for men occurs at a much more gradual rate than for their female counterparts but begins in midlife. The time may be characterized by many of the same physical and emotional symptoms that women experience. Because many of the resulting symptoms parallel those of women during menopause, this time in a man's life has been termed the male climacteric, or **andropause,** reflective of the diminished levels of the androgen hormone, testosterone, in men. Loss of body hair, gradual weight gain, decreased strength, mood swings, irritability, decreased libido, and memory lapses may occur. Sexual function may begin to decline after 55 years of age, but changes are gradual. For instance, the midlife male may notice he needs more stimulation to achieve an erection, needs more time between erections, and experiences a reduced force of ejaculation (Coray, 2005). Impotence during this period of life should always be completely assessed for physiological causes, such as diabetes, other chronic illness or treatment, and adverse effects of medications, particularly antihypertensives, as well as psychological causes. As with women, considerations for promoting a healthy life for men during this stage of life include healthy lifestyle changes along with social and psychological support.

Psychological Domain

The dynamics of middle age are characterized by psychological changes as depicted in Table 12-2. According to Erikson's theory of human development, individuals in this stage of life are faced with the tasks of achieving generativity, or the passing on of their wisdom and experience to those in succeeding generations. The negative outcome of this stage is self-absorption. When middle life is a continued progression of increasing social influence and economic success, the task of generativity is more likely to be achieved and the adult's self-concept and perception of fulfillment are enhanced. On the other hand, some may view this period as a time when opportunities become more limited or when the chance for achieving success or economic stability is reduced. Some may view midlife as a beginning of changes in health status and loss of earning power and influence in society.

Depression

Depression has been associated with all age groups. Surveys conducted in the 1980s and 1990s showed the younger adult population to be at highest risk for depression, but an escalation of depression has recently been identified with middle-aged adults. Analysis of data from the 2001–2002 National Epidemiologic Survey of Alcoholism and Related Conditions (NESARC), the largest survey ever mounted on the prevalence of psychiatric disorders among U.S. adults, concluded that the highest lifetime risk for depression was among middle-aged adults age 45 to 64 (Neuropsychiatry Reviews, 2005). According to this survey, middle age, female gender, Native American race, low income, and separation, divorce, or widowhood increase the likelihood of current or lifetime major depressive disorder (Neuropsychiatry Reviews, 2005; U.S. Office of the Surgeon General, 2005). Major depressive disorder (MDD), the most common type of major depression in adults, is characterized by one or more episodes that include the following symptoms: depressed mood, loss of interest or pleasure in activities, significant weight loss or gain, sleep disturbance, psychomotor agitation or retardation, fatigue, feelings of worthlessness, loss of concentration, and recurrent thoughts of death or suicide (U.S. Office of the Surgeon General, 2005). Minor depression, with fewer symptoms and less impairment, is not yet recognized as an official disorder, yet its occurrence can have negative consequences on health and well-being. Other findings from the NESARC report are as follows:

1. Asian, Hispanic, and Black race/ethnicity have lower risk.

2. Women are twice as likely as men to experience MDD.

3. Women are somewhat more likely to receive treatment.

4. There is a lag time of about three years between onset and treatment.

5. Of all persons who experienced MDD, age 18 and older, nearly one-half wanted to die, one-third considered suicide, and 9 percent reported a suicide attempt.

TABLE 12-2 Psychosocial Factors in Middle Adulthood

Psychosocial Factors	Health Promotion Implications
Family relationships Spouses Children Aging parents Extended family	Social support can be a motivating factor for health promotion. Stress in family relationships can cause physical and emotional consequences; health promotion activities, particularly exercise, can be an outlet for stress. Demands of caregiving must be balanced with middle adults' own needs.
Career Career changes Retraining/education Responsibility for others	Advise middle adults about the importance of balance in life between work and leisure activities. The perceived need to retrain to increase job security can be a real source of stress. The perceived success as a mentor can be an important source of emotional satisfaction and contribute to self-esteem.
Hobbies and use of leisure time	Hobbies and recreational activities provide balance with work and career. Counsel regarding the safety implications of recreational activities is important. Include assessment for alcohol and recreational drug use by middle-aged clients.
Values clarification **Facing one's mortality** **Midlife crisis** **Planning for retirement**	Assist the middle adult in examining values, mortality issues, evidence of experiencing midlife crisis, and vulnerability to depression. Assess for signs of depression and counsel regarding resources available. Counsel regarding the importance of having a living will, advance directives, or both.

6. Among those with current MDD, 14 percent also have an alcohol use disorder, 5 percent have a drug use disorder, and 26 percent have nicotine dependence.

7. More than 37 percent have a personality disorder and more than 36 percent have at least one anxiety disorder. (Columbia University's Mailman School of Public Health, 2005).

Another study examined racial/ethnic differences in significant depressive symptoms among middle-aged women before and after adjustment for socioeconomic, health-related, and psychosocial characteristics (Bromberger, Harlow, Avis, Kravitz, & Cordal, 2004). Using the Center for Epidemiologic Studies Depression [CES-D] Scale, it was found that, contrary to the NESARC report, Hispanic and African American women had the highest odds, and Chinese and Japanese women had the lowest odds for depression. It was noted that the variation was most likely due to health-related and psychosocial factors that are linked to socioeconomic status.

The effect of depression on function and health of 7,000 preretirement adults at peak earnings potential was the focus of another study (Crown, 2005). It was found that persons with depression were more likely to live alone; report chronic conditions (particularly cancer and lung disease), disabilities, or functional limitations; and have fewer economic resources in terms of income or wealth, or greater reliance on government health insurance such as Medicaid, compared with those who were not depressed. It was concluded that compared to non-depressed peers, adults suffering from depression experience an increased burden of health needs caused by the effects from depression.

Undoubtedly, both major and minor depression are associated with significant disability in physical, social, and role functioning during middle adulthood. Screening for depression using such tools as the Beck Depression Inventory or the Center for Epidemiologic Studies Depression Scale (U.S. Preventive Services Task Force, 2002) provides for early detection and treatment to prevent development of the deleterious affects from depression.

Sociological Domain

Many of the changes of middle adulthood have to do with role transitions regarding family responsibilities. As children grow into adulthood, they establish independence from their parents, while the middle adult's aging parents become more dependent. Another prominent area of potential role alteration is that of job- and career-related change. For many in this period, job security and feelings of accomplishment continue, with the middle adult moving into a mentorship role with younger colleagues. However, in times of economic constraints, downsizing, and technological progress, individuals in this age group may find themselves insecure in a career path. They may pursue career change or cross-training

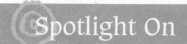

Spotlight On

Grandparent Parenting

The American Association of Retired Persons (AARP) has recognized this growing phenomenon by establishing a hotline for assistance to the group of midlife and older individuals who are primary caregivers for a grandchild (www.aarp.org).

opportunities in order to increase their options. As work is an extremely important part of life for most middle adults, threats to job security result in stress, the effects of which ripple into other aspects of life. Relationships with others are often affected.

One new trend that affects men and women in the middle adult years is the increasing number of grandparents raising grandchildren, due to death, disease, or inability of the parent. This shift in responsibility for child-rearing may occur for the usual reasons but has been shown to be increasingly due to situations involving death of the parent due to violence, substance use, or AIDS.

Another trend caused by rising divorce and remarriage rates is that middle adults are merging with or raising second families or both. Women over 40 years of age are comprising a small but significant group of obstetrical clients whose age has classified them as advanced maternal age. Risks of fetal abnormality, particularly genetic deficits, are thought to increase significantly with age. For women in this age group, special counseling and monitoring are needed in the event of planned or unplanned pregnancy. The trend toward childbearing and childrearing in the 40s and beyond is particularly true for men, whose fertility does not diminish in midlife but may continue into older adulthood.

Environmental Domain

The environment is a crucial factor in health status and health promotion. Many characteristics of the environment contribute to or detract from health, such as air and water pollution, noise, toxic substance exposure, high-stress work situations, economic constraints, and the like. Tobacco use is the single greatest cause of chronic illness, death, and disability in the United States (Fiandt, 2005). Although there has been a decline in cigarette smoking in the United States to a current level of about 25 percent of the population, certain subgroups continue to smoke and use chewing tobacco. Prevalence of tobacco use is inversely related to education and socioeconomic status. See Chapter 17 for further information regarding tobacco and other substance use.

Mortality and morbidity are significantly increased for smokers. Death and disease from tobacco use are seen primarily in the middle and later adult years because of the lag time for the manifestation of harmful effects on the respiratory and cardiovascular systems. Many conditions, including cancer (particularly of the respiratory tract), cardiovascular disease, gastric ulcer, postmenopausal osteoporosis, and low birth weight in offspring of pregnant smokers, are firmly associated with smoking (U.S. Preventive Services Task Force, 2005). Each of these conditions is potentially seen in the middle adult. Further, secondhand smoke has been documented to have important health consequences such as chronic lung disease, coronary artery disease in spouses of smokers, and asthma and respiratory infections in children of smokers.

Another important aspect of the environment is the microenvironment consisting of the relationship of humans to certain bacterial or viral organisms. Some communicable diseases have become increasingly significant threats to health due to world travel and increased population concentrations in urban areas. Emergence of resistant strains of organisms compounds the treatment and eradication of some diseases such as influenza. Screening for communicable disease is an important function in promoting health, yet economics or policy changes in some areas of the United States and the world can have profound effects on adequate detection of communicable disease.

Sexual/Gender Domain

Despite the physiological changes that occur in middle adulthood, the individual in this age group usually continues to be sexually active and may engage in high-risk sexual practices that could result in the risk for sexually transmitted diseases and Acquired Immunodeficiency Syndrome (AIDS). For this reason, individuals seeking treatment for sexually transmitted diseases (STDs) should also be screened for HIV status using the enzyme immunoassay and confirmed if positive with the western blot. Also in need of HIV screening would be individuals who are past or present injection drug users, persons who exchange sex for money or drugs, sexual partners of HIV-infected persons, injection drug users, or bisexual men, and those who received transfusions between 1978 and 1985 (U.S. Preventive Services Task Force, 2005).

Screening for sexually transmitted diseases such as chlamydia, gonorrhea, and syphilis should be performed on all sexually active women at high risk, which would include those with a history of previous STDs, those with new or multiple sex partners (more than two in six months), or those who indicate inconsistent use of safe sex practices. A pelvic examination with an endocervical specimen culture for the selected infections should be performed. Pregnant women should also be screened.

Some conditions, such as anemia, are particularly significant in the middle adult years. This is particularly true for females and for members of certain cultural groups, including Blacks or African Americans and those of Mediterranean descent. All menstruating females should receive a determination of hemoglobin and hematocrit levels and more extensive testing if indicated (U.S. Preventive Services Task Force, 2005). Middle-aged males and postmenopausal females need to receive a nutritional assessment and diet analysis as discussed in Chapter 14.

Spiritual Domain

Spiritual health is the integration of each person's mind, body, and soul or inner spirit to form a harmonious whole. Additionally, beliefs of the individual that subscribe to organized religious faiths are important in health maintenance and health promotion. At times, religious beliefs and practices may be contrary to "scientific medicine." The middle adult and older adult may differ from the child or young adult in their willingness to diversify into prevailing cultural or spiritual norms, preferring instead to retain their individual spiritual or cultural practices. Members of various groups hold certain religious beliefs that may preclude medical practices, such as the use of blood transfusions in a member of the Jehovah's Witness group. Many middle adults find that spirituality becomes even more important in their lives during this period.

CULTURALLY COMPETENT CARE

Health promotion attitudes and behavior are influenced by culture. Cultural considerations were discussed in more depth in Chapter 6, but implications for middle adults will be briefly discussed here as well. Developing cultural competence to effectively work within the cultural context of a community is crucial to nursing interaction with the multicultural populations that are characteristic of health care settings. In consideration of the general developmental tasks of this age group, concern with family issues and work issues within the context of the culture of the client are important. Does the individual value the well-being of the family or the individual more highly? Are there practices that are dictated by the cultural or ethnic group, such as the avoidance of certain activities, that middle adults will feel they must adhere to despite health advice to the contrary? For example, a 55-year-old Asian woman may be advised and taught to perform breast self-examination as part of her screening behavior for breast cancer. For some Asian subgroups, touching oneself, even for a health-related purpose, is considered inappropriate. An important variable in health promotion activities and education regarding health promotion with multicultural groups is language. Health professionals need to obtain or consider developing materials in the target language to ensure relevance to the culture and beliefs. The avoidance of stereotyping and generalizing regarding an individual member of an ethnic group is essential to comprehensive assessment and culturally sensitive intervention (Barry & Wanat, 2005; Office of Minority Health, 2000).

GUIDELINES FOR HEALTH PROMOTION AND SCREENING

Within the past few years, national initiatives have taken place for the purpose of highlighting the health promotion needs of the United States. *Healthy People 2010* was the second of these and represents the results of intense national study. Objectives for the desired health outcomes and health services needed for each population group were outlined. Reduced morbidity, or the effects of disease, from identified chronic illnesses is expected to result from selected preventive and screening activities. The selected objectives that relate to the middle adult were presented in Table 12-1. For example, decreasing cholesterol levels, reducing the incidence of obesity, and increasing the participation in regular exercise are expected to decrease the occurrence of cardiovascular diseases and hypertension.

There are many publications helpful in planning health promotion and screening activities for middle adults. The U.S. Preventive Services Task Force *Guide to Clinical Preventive Services*, which was first published in 1996, assists clinicians in planning evidence-based preventive and screening services, such as tests, and counseling in risk reduction. There are many publications helpful in planning health promotion and screening activities for middle-aged adults. The U.S. Preventive Services Task Force, *Guide to Clinical Preventive Services,* which was first published in 1996, assists clinicians in planning preventive and screening services, such as tests and counseling in risk reduction. Now in its third edition, the guide continues to support the following actions by clinicians in every client encounter (U.S. Preventive Services Task Force, 2005).

- Assess the client's personal health practices.

- Foster shared decision making between clinician and client.

- Use diagnostic and screening services selectively.

- Provide preventive services at every opportunity, particularly for those with limited access to health care.

Additionally, the Task Force suggests support of **community-level interventions** (activities that occur at the community level to promote health or reduce illness or injury, such as fluoridation of the water supply), rather than just individual efforts for certain health problems, when these have been shown to be effective.

The *Guide to Preventive Services* helps the nurse and other health care providers use a scientific basis for screening and for counseling regarding risk modifica-

tion. Table 12-3 provides suggested health promotion actions from these sources that specifically apply to risks in middle adults.

STRATEGIES FOR ACHIEVING LIFESTYLES THAT PROMOTE HEALTH

Middle-aged adults are becoming increasingly conscious of health and health promotion issues. Whether they are caregivers for their aging chronically ill parents, affected by health problems or deaths of family members and friends, or experiencing personal health problem, awareness of the aging process is occurring. Individuals in this age group are usually interested in maintaining health and functional status at optimal levels. Many persons have engaged in certain risk behaviors during their younger years. **Risk factors,** or characteristics associated with increased likelihood of disease or injury, for one condition contribute to the occurrence of other conditions; for example, smokers at risk for lung cancer are also at risk for chronic pulmonary disease. For the middle adult age group, injury, substance abuse, and individual and family violence are important sources of health problems. Middle adults continue to engage in risk behaviors such as tobacco and alcohol use, unprotected sexual activity, lack of seat belt use, and poor nutrition. Primary prevention activities are important because healthier lifestyle changes begun in this period will have positive influences on functional ability in later years

Exercise and Nutrition

The balance between nutrition and exercise to promote health, maintain cardiovascular fitness, and prevent obesity has been well documented (U.S. Preventive Services Task Force, 2005). Nutrition is a key element in a healthy lifestyle and is further discussed in Chapter 14. The companion component is exercise, which is further discussed in Chapter 15. A sedentary lifestyle is common in the United Status. A national survey revealed that over 50 percent of Americans engaged in either little or irregular physical activity (Centers for Disease Control and Prevention, 2004). Sedentary lifestyle and concomitant obesity have been linked to cardiovascular disease, cancer, diabetes, and other chronic illnesses. Figure 12-3 illustrates the dramatic increase in overweight and obesity reported in the United States between 1995 and 2005. Older persons and women are at greater risk for being physically inactive (Fiandt, 2005).

There are documented benefits of a regular exercise program for reducing the risks not only of cardiovascular disease and cancer but also of non-insulin–dependent diabetes mellitus, osteoporosis, and mental health disorders. Cardiovascular disease risk could be reduced significantly even in sedentary persons by initiating an exercise program. Immune system benefit from a regular exercise program has also been suggested.

TABLE 12-3 Risk Assessment for the Middle-Aged Adult

Related Domain	Risk Assessment	Health Promotion Action
Physical	Nutrition	Assess nutrition status and diet. Daily intake should include 25 g of fiber; 30 percent of total calories from fat; 5–6 servings of vegetables and fruits; 6–11 servings of whole grains, breads, and pasta; limited consumption (2–3 servings) of red meat, poultry, eggs, and dairy products.
Physical	Exercise	Encourage 30 minutes of consistent exercise such as brisk walking or swimming five times per week with attention to safety measures and general health maintenance.
Physical Psychological	Tobacco avoidance	Consistently assess regarding tobacco use and interest in cessation, and, if applicable, provide tobacco cessation counseling on a regular basis. Advise the use of pharmacological as well as behavioral interventions for smoking cessation.
Physical Environmental Psychological	Accident prevention	Counseling regarding safety for parents of children, for adolescents, and for adults should be provided. Assess individuals for high risk regarding alcohol and substance use.
Physical	Immunizations	Counsel regarding obtaining and maintaining immunizations, including boosters for tetanus and diphtheria. The primary series should be completed for those who have not completed it. Hepatitis B and influenza immunizations should be obtained, as well as pneumococcal vaccination for persons over 65 years of age or those over 50 living in institutional settings.
Physical Psychological Sociological	Addictive behavior	Assess signs and symptoms of substance use. Advise as to the adverse health consequences associated with alcohol and drug use. Monitor through follow-up for problems with alcohol and drug use.
Psychological Sociological Spiritual Physical	Mental health	Assess for positive development and successful passage through the middle years. Screen for depression or counsel regarding stress management, strategies for stress reduction, and resources for assistance with psychosocial issues.
Sociological Environmental	Workplace exposures and injury	Assess for workplace risk factors for injury and exposures to substances, e.g., carcinogens such as benzene, excessive noise.
Physical Environmental	Dental care	Advise regular annual dental care with daily flossing and brushing with fluoridated toothpaste.
Sexual/Gender Sociological	Sexuality and family planning	Provide counseling about risk factors for HIV and other STDs and measures to reduce risk. Provide information regarding safe sex practice. Specifically counsel individuals identified to be injection drug users regarding HIV and STD risk and refer to appropriate treatment facilities. Offer testing to individuals at risk for specific STDs. Immunize for Hepatitis B. Provide periodic counseling about effective contraceptive methods.

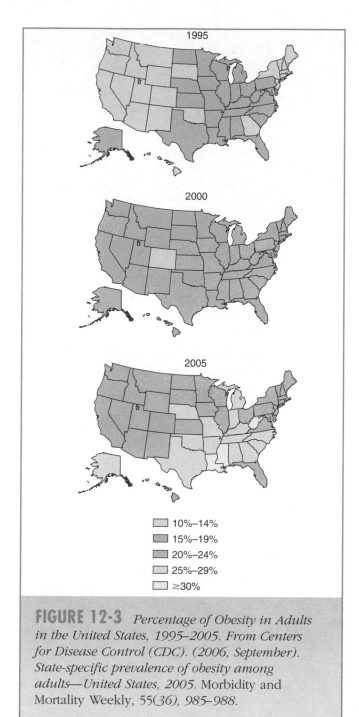

1995

2000

2005

- ☐ 10%–14%
- ☐ 15%–19%
- ☐ 20%–24%
- ☐ 25%–29%
- ☐ ≥30%

FIGURE 12-3 *Percentage of Obesity in Adults in the United States, 1995–2005. From Centers for Disease Control (CDC). (2006, September). State-specific prevalence of obesity among adults—United States, 2005. Morbidity and Mortality Weekly, 55(36), 985–988.*

Beginning an exercise program, particularly for those who are obese and have known cardiovascular disease or hypertension or both, should be approached cautiously and only after a thorough assessment. Additionally, nurses need to advise those who exercise to use warm-up and stretching activities prior to vigorous workouts, to avoid overexercising to the point of exhaustion or pain, and to take basic safety precautions to avoid injury.

Tobacco Avoidance

There are several documented benefits of smoking cessation in the middle adult years. These include immediate cardiovascular reduction in workload, respiratory function improvement with decreased risk of infection, and long-term pulmonary function stabilization and reduction in respiratory cancer risk. Nurses should be knowledgeable about methods that are most effective in helping smokers quit. Health care providers can assist the tobacco user to at least contemplate quitting. If the smoker is already trying to quit, the provider can guide and support this individual in multiple ways to maintain nonsmoking status (Tingen, Andrews, Waller, & Daniel, 2004). Although more study is needed in this area, research supports the effectiveness of a combination of gradually tapering nicotine replacement and behavioral approaches to address the psychological addiction. Chapter 17 provides further discussion on smoking cessation.

The Agency for Health Care Policy and Research has developed guidelines for nurses to assist clients in successful cessation approaches (*Helping smokers quit*, 2005). Support and reinforcement for the smoker must be based on behavioral change principles; long-term follow-up and counseling regarding relapse are essential to successful smoking cessation.

Immunizations

Middle adults should be counseled to keep their immunizations up-to-date. The tetanus-diphtheria-toxoid series should be completed in adults who were not immunized during childhood with the primary series. In adults of any age, regular boosters should be obtained at a recommended interval of every 10 years, barring serious injury during the interval necessitating an additional booster (Weber, 2005). The series of hepatitis B vaccine should be provided to all young adults and any other adults at high risk for infection, including those who are sexually active, are substance abusers, or require blood transfusions or clotting factor concentrates, health care personnel, and those who travel to areas high in endemic disease.

Annual influenza vaccination is recommended for members of high-risk groups, such as chronically ill persons, health care workers, teachers, and young adults in community living arrangements such as dormitories (Weber, 2005). Family members of individuals in these risk groups should also be immunized for influenza

Considering the physiological changes that occur in middle adulthood, exercise functions to maintain bone strength, combat osteoporosis, increase circulation to the periphery, and bolster cardiovascular stamina. The benefits of exercise in lowering the risk of cardiovascular disease and osteoporosis are well established. There is also evidence that exercise decreases the risk of colon cancer as well. Recent studies show that regular moderate exercise can reduce the risk of developing colon cancer by almost 50 percent (Colorectal Cancer Screening, n.d.).

Despite demonstrated benefits, however, it is important to weigh the risks of exercise for certain individuals.

annually. Nurses should obtain immunization histories on all clients seen in health care settings and inform them of needed boosters of primary immunizations. It is also the nurse's responsibility to be aware of community services providing free or low-cost immunizations to indigent or uninsured clients.

Sleep

Difficulty in falling asleep and staying asleep, known as insomnia, is a commonly occurring problem that can have significant consequences. A recent report noted that 40 million to 70 million Americans are estimated to be affected by insomnia (Buscemi et al., 2005). Not only does insomnia cause daytime drowsiness, it may impair quality of life in other ways, including the following:

- Increased health care utilization
- Increased risk of depression
- Poor memory
- Reduced concentration
- Poor work performance
- Perceived or real risk of failure at work (Buscemi et al., 2005)

Transient insomnia is temporary, lasting only a few days and resulting from a variety of causes such as minor illness; different sleeping environment; medications for cold, flu, depression, hypertension, and the like; travel or jet lag; physical or emotional stress, and so on. Addressing the cause is key to overcoming transient insomnia. Insomnia becomes chronic when it occurs at least three nights a week for a month or longer (WebMed, n.d.).

It is important to balance rest and sleep with activity to promote overall health. Some individuals begin to experience changes in patterns and requirements for sleep during the middle adult years. Although the number of hours of sleep recommended for adults, between six and eight hours per night, remains unchanged during the middle years, individuals vary in the amount of sleep that helps them to feel rested and enables them to maintain their desired level of activity. The changes that may occur include more frequent waking at night, less deep sleep, and increased influence of other factors on sleep quantity and quality (Reimer, 2005).

Middle-aged adults should always be queried about their sleep habits and about their satisfaction with their sleep pattern. The nurse can suggest a variety of cognitive and behavioral interventions such as relaxation tapes, relaxing baths, massage, increased exercise, and decreased caffeine and heavy food intake, particularly in the evening. Reliance on medication or alcohol to promote sleep should be avoided.

Dental Health

Dental caries and periodontal disease are problems for many Americans. The National Center for Chronic Dis-

ease Prevention and Health Promotion (2004) has identified the following in regard to dental health in adults:

1. The baby boomer generation, born between 1946 and 1964, will be the first in which the majority will maintain their natural teeth over their entire lifetime, a fact attributed to water fluoridation and fluoride toothpastes.

2. Within the past 20 years, the percent age of adults missing all their natural teeth has declined from over 30 percent to 20 percent for those age 55 to 64 and from 2 percent to 0.4 percent for those adults between 18 and 34 years of age.

3. Most adults show signs of gum disease, with severe gum disease affecting approximately 14 percent of adults age 45 to 54.

4. About 30 percent of poor adults (18 years and older) have at least one untreated decayed tooth compared to 11 percent of non-poor adults.

5. Oral health problems account for more than 164 million hours of work lost each year for employed adults.

6. Over 60 percent of adults report visiting a dentist in the past 12 months. Adults with incomes at or above the poverty level are twice as likely as those with lower incomes to report a visit to a dentist in the past 12 months.

Dental conditions can result in great economic cost and human suffering. Although fluoridating the water supply and increased usage of fluoridated toothpaste have been effective in decreasing the incidence of cavities, problems persist. However, many population groups, particularly those in underserved and low socioeconomic areas, lack information regarding ways to maintain oral health and prevent dental problems (U.S. Preventive Services Task Force, 2005). Nurses can encourage regular dental care and refer low-income clients to available dental services. Regular dental care will also accomplish the goal of routine oral screening, which is important for those at high risk for oral cancer, including smokers, smokeless tobacco users, and heavy alcohol users.

Occupational Safety

Occupational issues are important to the middle-aged adult. Work roles remain a primary concern in this age group. Nurses in both primary care settings and occupational health settings share the responsibility for promoting health and safety. The U.S. Bureau of Labor Statistics reported that there were nearly 6,000 work-related deaths and over 4 million nonfatal illnesses and injuries in private industries during 2004. Nearly 60 percent of the deaths reported were of workers age 25 to 64 (U.S. Bureau of Labor Statistics, 2004).

Primary care providers are in an essential position to assess the effect of the work environment on the middle-aged adult. Some important areas to assess are: (1) work-related potential for stress and violence, (2) risk for back injuries due to personal or occupational history, and (3) exposure to environmental carcinogens. Implications for nurses regarding occupational health are to ask clients about their work, related stresses, and potential for injury. Occupational exposure to carcinogens is an area of concern that nurses should assess in all clients. Nurses in occupational health settings will be particularly concerned with these issues.

NURSING ROLE IN HEALTH PROMOTION AND EARLY DETECTION

Pender's Health Promotion Model (2006) has served as a guide for practice and for research into the complex processes, biological and psychosocial, that determine individual health behavior. This model is further discussed in Chapter 3. It will be applied here as it explains and gives direction to nursing actions to assist clients with their health promotion efforts.

The model applies across the life span and effectively guides practice with the middle adult. Important variables include individual characteristics and experience, behavior-specific cognitions and affect, and outcomes. Each of these variables is discussed in the following sections. Table 12-4 depicts these variables within the context of the domains that frame human existence—psychosocial, biological, environmental, and cultural.

- Individual characteristics and experience: Prior related behavior and personal biological, psychological, and sociocultural factors make up these individual characteristics. For example, the middle adult who has abused alcohol (prior behavior that has caused biological changes) also may have had distinct enabling factors, such as a family pattern of alcoholism (psychological and sociocultural), interacting with the biological factors to perpetuate this dan-

gerous health behavior. Health promotion efforts, to be successful, must include consideration and intervention targeted at each of these areas.

- Behavior-specific cognitions and affect: Perceived benefits and barriers to action, perceived self-efficacy, and activity-related affect are cognitive responses to the known health threat and recommended preventive behavior. These are affected by the individual's characteristics and experiences as well as other interpersonal influences such as family, peers, role models, and situational influences.

- **Outcomes**, or the results of nursing intervention with clients, consist of observable health-promoting behavior that is influenced by other competing demands and level of commitment to a plan of action.

Educating About Risk Reduction and Health-Promoting Activities

Communicating about risk status and risk reduction is a vital role for health care providers, with particular importance for the middle adult. An important component of health promotion is educating the client regarding risk and health-promoting activities for risk modification. The health risks faced by some middle adults are related to lifestyle and behavior. These risks can be very significant. High-risk behaviors tend to be interrelated, for example, alcohol use with unsafe sexual practices, drug use with poor nutrition, lack of exercise with high-fat, low-fiber intake. Sharing risk assessment and risk reduction recommendations with clients gives them control.

Variable	Specific Risk Factor	Health Promotion Activity	Expected Outcome
Individual characteristics	Alcohol abuse	Assist client in identifying need for health promotion. Explore options such as substance abuse programs or support group for help with alcohol abuse. Include client and family members if possible.	Patient attains sobriety. Family members obtain assistance with coping.
Behavior	Excessive caloric intake, obesity	Assist client in identifying need for health promotion. Explore options such as nutritional counseling, local support group, exercise programs. Assist client to adopt new nutritional habits, develop a food diary, and begin an exercise program. Include family members if possible.	Client exhibits healthy meal planning and caloric intake appropriate for body size and activity. Exercise program is maintained as tolerated.
Outcomes	Lack of commitment to exercise program	Explore incentives to increase commitment to an exercise program. Assist in developing an exercise log. Include family members if possible.	Client maintains regular program, develops a relationship with an exercise buddy to maintain schedule. Client reduces weight gradually to within 10 percent of ideal body weight (IBW).

The developmental tasks at this stage influence middle adults to desire control over their lives and the lives of those for whom they feel responsible. The middle adult often perceives a heavy burden of commitment to others, such as aging dependent parents, dependent children, or both. These factors may heighten the client's receptivity to recommendations that will result in decreased risk of illness. Giving individualized feedback regarding risk, rather than routine information about risks, will be more likely to result in behavioral change and adherence to recommendations.

Counseling adults must be based on theories of adult learning which propose that the adult is motivated to learn information and skills that will enhance independence and problem solving, that can be immediately applied to the life situation, and that are congruent with the individual's life experience and role demands (Bastable, 2003). It is also vital to provide opportunities to practice newly acquired skills immediately, such as doing diabetic foot care, monitoring one's blood pressure, or taking cholesterol-lowering medications.

Nurses should advise all individuals in the middle adult years to adopt essential health habits. These include

Nursing Alert

Tips for Teaching the Adult Learner

1. *Make it relate* to the adult's life situation.
2. *Make it fit* the adult's life experience.
3. *Make it work* as the adult carries out old roles, or takes on new roles.

getting regular exercise, reducing the fat and increasing the fiber in the diet, avoiding tobacco and other substance use, and taking measures to prevent accidents. Other health promotion and screening activities should be targeted to groups at risk for a certain disease or injury. This means that certain individuals are more likely to develop the disease or injury or dysfunction than others because of certain characteristics these persons possess. Nurses should be alert for those characteristics which may be unique to the person, such as a person who injects IV drugs. Or risk factors can derive from the environment of the person, such as a plant worker who is exposed to asbestos. For many conditions, risk factors have been identified. For the first situation, the IV drug user, educational and behavioral interventions to reduce the risk of AIDS and hepatitis need to be instituted. For the second, a job-related situation, broad community-based solutions are needed, such as the safety programs instituted by the Occupational Safety and Health Administration. Thus, a key consideration in prevention and early detection is to target education and screening at the individuals in the population who are at risk.

ASSESSMENT OF THE MIDDLE-AGED ADULT

When deciding on the screening tests to use for middle adults, two questions need to be answered. First, is there a benefit to early detection of the condition to be screened for? Second, are the available screening tests accurate?

It is important to consider whether early detection leads to intervention to prevent or delay worsening of the condition. This issue causes one to consider whether treatment for the disease is effective, and if there is any benefit to early detection versus waiting until symptoms arise. This is a particularly important issue for the middle adult because if early treatment can produce a more favorable long-term outcome, it would be important to institute it since the expected life span for men and women has lengthened. An example of this situation is prostate cancer, where "watchful waiting" is sometimes advocated when early prostate cancer is found in older men (Gray, 2005). On the other hand, if detection does not affect the effectiveness of treatment, as in the typical case of lung cancer, the cost of screening will outweigh its benefit.

When considering the accuracy of screening tests, key issues of sensitivity and specificity are involved. The **sensitivity of a screening test** is the ability of the test to correctly give a positive result when the person has the condition. The **specificity of a screening test** refers to the accuracy of the test in correctly giving a negative result when the person being screened does not have the disease (U.S. Preventive Service Task Force, 2005). If a test has low sensitivity, persons with the disease will be missed by the screening procedure. The false-negative results may delay treatment and allow the disease to progress undetected. When a test has low specificity, false positives result and persons who do not have the disease will have to undergo further testing to determine that they are disease free. This problem has been identified with fecal occult blood testing for colon cancer. False-positive results can occur unless the individual pays strict attention to the dietary and medication guidelines for the test (for example, no red meat, cruciferous vegetables, aspirin, nonsteroidal antiinflammatory drugs for

72 hours before the beginning of stool collection and throughout the period needed to collect three stool samples). A positive test will necessitate follow-up with colonoscopy at a significant monetary cost and anxiety for the individual being screened. The cost of false-positives is a problem to the already economically challenged health care system.

There is agreement that for certain acute and chronic illnesses periodic evaluation of all clients based on certain age and gender characteristics is justified. These conditions include hypertension; hyperlipidemia; smoking behavior; colon, breast, and cervical cancer; and alcoholism (U.S. Preventive Services Task Force, 2005). Screening for obesity, because of its relationship to both cardiovascular and cancer incidence, is also recommended. The U.S. Preventive Services Task Force has evaluated evidence about screening practices in primary care (U.S. Preventive Services Task Force, 2005). Tables 12-5 and 12-6 represent a compilation of the screening recommendations for middle adult men and women from the Task Force document. The recommendations of the American Cancer Society (2004) have also been added for some cancer sites.

Health Promotion Measures for Major Deviations from Health

Persons with chronic illnesses, notably diabetes mellitus, cardiovascular diseases such as angina pectoris and hypertension, and renal and pulmonary disease and cancer, have special needs in regard to health promotion. Although they may be maintained on medications, special regimens, or procedures and live with the threat of disease recurrence or exacerbation, these individuals need health promotion and health maintenance activities as do other population groups. Formerly the diagnosis of some diseases such as cancer precluded attention being given to health promotion. These persons may not have been counseled to maintain a more ideal body weight, quit smoking, get regular exercise, maintain sexual function at a level desired by themselves and their partners, or pursue fulfilling career or recreational interests. With the increased longevity made possible by scientific advances in treatment for many of these illnesses, the nurse must be diligent in providing encouragement and education to chronically ill persons regarding health promotion and health maintenance. Similarly, those with, or at risk for, functional impairments need to be specifically targeted for health promotion and screening activities.

Vision and Hearing

Increased IOP, family history, older age, diabetes, severe myopia (nearsightedness), and being of African American descent place an individual at increased risk for glaucoma (U.S. Preventive Services Task Force, 2005). Screening for glaucoma varies among professional groups. The American Academy of Ophthalmology recommends screening

TABLE 12-5 Common Screening Tests and Recommended Frequency for Middle-Aged Adult Females

Screening Tests	Age Range	Frequency
BP monitoring	> 21 years	Every one–two years
Blood cholesterol	45–65	Annually
Height and weight measurement	All ages	At health checkup
Assessment of smoking status, interest in cessation if smoker	All ages Mothers	At health checkup At every visit
Mammography	> 40	Annually
Clinical breast exam	> 40	Annually
Self breast exam	> 20	Every month
Fecal occult blood (FOB), sigmoidoscopy, or colonoscopy	> 50	FOB annually, sigmoidoscopy every 5 years, and colonoscopy every 10 years
Papanicolaou smear	> 18 or sexually active > 65	Every three years if normal May D/C if normal
History, assess use of tobacco, alcohol, other substances	All ages Pregnant women	At health checkup At every visit

Although it lacks scientific support, breast self-exam continues to be a recommended practice by the American Cancer Society.
Adapted from Guide to Clinical Preventive Services, *by U.S. Preventive Services Task Force, 2005.*

TABLE 12-6 Common Screening Tests and Recommended Frequency for Middle-Aged Adult Males

Screening Test	Population Group	Frequency
Blood pressure measurement	21 years	Every one–two years
Blood cholesterol, fasting or nonfasting	> 35–65	Annually
Height and weight	All ages	At health checkup
Assessment of smoking status, interest in cessation if smoker	All ages Fathers	At health check-up Every visit
Fecal occult blood (FOB), sigmoidoscopy, or colonoscopy	> 50	FOB annually, sigmoidoscopy every 5 years, and colonoscopy every 10 years
Digital rectal exam	> 50	
Prostate specific antigen	50–70	Dependent upon personal preference and risk profile in consultation with health care provider
History, questionnaires (CAGE or AUDIT) for alcohol or substance use	All ages	At health check-up

Adapted from Guide to Clinical Preventive Services, *U.S. Preventive Services Task Force, 2005.*

for glaucoma as part of the comprehensive adult medical eye evaluation starting at the age of 20; the Department of Veterans Affairs recommends screening for every veteran over the age of 40 (with frequency depending on age, ethnicity, and family history); and the American Optometric Association recommends annual eye examinations for people at risk for glaucoma. Nonetheless, the U.S. Preventive Services Task Force (2005) concluded that there is insufficient evidence to recommend for or against screening adults not at risk for glaucoma.

Hearing screening should be performed on adults over age 65 as well as on those with exposure to excessive occupational noise, or all middle adults who indicate difficulty with hearing upon questioning.

Diabetes Mellitus

In the United States, diabetes mellitus type 2 is prevalent in approximately 10 percent of adults age 40–59 (National Diabetes Statistics, 2005). There are some population subgroups among adults that have a higher prevalence of diabetes than others. Those include: obese men and women over 40 years of age; members of racial or ethnic groups such as Native Americans, Mexican Americans, and African Americans; and those with a family history of diabetes. Other major risk categories are those adults with hyperglycemia (elevated blood glucose) and hyperlipidemia (elevated low-density cholesterol and total cholesterol). Although the U.S. Preventive Services Task Force (USPSTF, February, 2003) concludes that the evidence is insufficient to recommend for or against routinely screening asymptomatic adults for diabetes mellitus type 2, it does recommend screening adults who have hypertension or hyperlipidemia.

Cancer

Regarding endometrial cancer, high-risk post-menopausal women include Caucasians, those over 50 years of age who are obese, and those with abnormal bleeding. Women over 50 years of age should have a regular pelvic exam for early detection of other gynecological cancers, including ovarian and cervical. High-risk groups for cervical cancer include women with diethylstilbestrol exposure, multiple sexual partners (two or more), AIDS, and human papillomavirus (HPV). The USPSTF strongly recommends screening for cervical cancer in women who have been sexually active and have a cervix (U.S. Preventive Services Task Force, 2003).

Persons who should be screened for head, neck, and oral cancers include past or current tobacco users, frequent alcohol users, and all with suspicious oral lesions. An oral examination as well as a physical assessment of the lymph system should be performed. Those with a history of upper body (head and neck) radiation in childhood should be screened for thyroid cancer with a physical examination and, specifically, palpation of the thyroid (U.S. Preventive Services Task Force, 2005; ACS, 2004).

Osteoporosis

The USPSTF (2002) has identified low body weight of less than 70 kilograms (154 pounds) as the best predictor for the development of osteoporosis. Low body weight, no current use of estrogen therapy, and age (55 and older) are part of the three-item Osteoporosis Risk Assessment Instrument identifying those at risk for osteoporosis and in need of further assessment of bone density. The USPSTF has confirmed that there is less evidence to support the use of other individual risk factors, such as smoking, weight loss, family history, decreased physical activity, alcohol or caffeine use, or low calcium and vitamin D intake, as a basis for identifying high-risk women younger than 65. The USPSTF makes no recommendation for or against routine osteoporosis screening in postmenopausal women who are younger than 60 or in women age 60 to 64 who are not identified as being at risk.

SUMMARY

This chapter has provided an overview of the physiological and psychosocial changes occurring in the middle adult years and their health promotion implications. Recommendations for health promotion activities were presented, as well as specific discussion of recommendations for the special group of chronically ill persons. Finally, screening recommendations were discussed for those conditions for which there is agreement regarding recommended screening procedures and intervals. Screening recommendations for individuals at higher than average risk for certain conditions were presented.

CASE STUDY Laura Jensen: Promoting Health in the Middle-Aged Adult

Objectives/Goals Through participation in discussion of this case study, participants will have the opportunity to:

1. Identify factors affecting exercise in middle-aged adults.
2. Describe interventions to facilitate exercise in middle-aged adults.

Health Promotion Concern, History and Physical, Present Health Status, Past Health Status, Family History, and Social History

Laura Jensen is a 52-year-old female of German descent who is employed in marketing for a successful advertising firm in a Midwest city. She is divorced, with two children ages 20 and 23 who no longer live at home. She is completing a bachelor's degree in business, and her goal is to be chief executive officer of the advertising firm where she is currently employed. She works 12–14 hours a day. She does not cook for herself and has gained 30 pounds in the past two years.

Review of Pertinent Domains

Biological Domain

Physical exam: Reveals a 5'5" female weighing 155 pounds.

Cardiovascular: Laura has a history of hypertension managed with Captopril 25 mg twice daily.

Gastrointestinal: She rarely eats dinner, but tries to eat vegetables twice a week, fruit daily, and snacks often throughout the day just to "keep from getting hungry." Her favorite snack items are granola bars, crackers and cheese, and an occasional cookie.

Psychological Domain

Laura is an intelligent woman completing a bachelor's degree in business. She is an independent and highly motivated person who sets goals and accomplishes them.

Social Domain

Laura has several friends living in the same apartment building. She rarely socializes due to the time spent on her job.

Environmental Domain

Laura lives in a high-rise apartment located adjacent to a public park. Her employing agency offers discounted memberships to the fitness center located in the same building as the agency.

Questions for Discussion

1. What is Laura's Body Mass Index and how is this interpreted? (Refer to Chapter 14 for calculation and interpretation.)
2. What are goals or outcomes that can guide Laura in promoting her health status?
3. Develop a health promotion plan to help Laura in achieving her goals for health promotion.

Key Concepts

1. The middle adult period is characterized by the physiologic changes that accompany menopause and the male climacteric, increasing family and work-related commitments, and beginning concerns regarding retirement and health issues, all of which influence many individuals to adopt more healthy lifestyles.

2. Health promotion activities, even if only recently begun in the middle adult years, reap benefits in older years when functional status and quality of life are greatly influenced by health status.

3. Environmental influences that affect health include air and water pollution, tobacco use and second-hand smoke, work-related exposure and stress, and economic pressures.

4. Prevention recommendations for the middle adult include: engaging in a planned exercise program; consuming a nutritionally sound diet that is high in fiber and low in fat; keeping immunizations up-to-date, including flu vaccination; obtaining restful sleep as appropriate to the individual; maintaining dental health; and taking measures to ensure safety at home, in recreational activities, and at work.

5. Nurses are vitally important in assessing risk for middle adults based on their age, gender, past and current medical history, occupational history, and lifestyle factors and in recommending screening practices specific to the identified risk status and congruent with guidelines established by various national bodies.

Learning Activities

1. Develop a plan to implement a health screening for a group of adults in your community to address the *Healthy People 2010* disease-specific objectives for middle-aged adults. Identify the target population, resources, screening measures to be offered, and health promotion recommendations related to these objectives.

2. Use Table 12-3, Risk Assessment for the Middle-Aged Adult, to perform a health risk assessment on a consenting middle-aged adult relative, friend, or colleague. Develop a health promotion plan addressing your findings.

True/False Questions

1. T or F Health promotion activities are very beneficial, even if they are begun later in life.

2. T or F Spiritual concerns tend to increase as middle adults age.

3. T or F Middle adulthood is a stable period with minimal role transitioning regarding family responsibilities.

4. T or F The percentage of middle adults in the total U.S. population is expected to gradually decrease in the next 25 years.

Multiple Choice Questions

1. Which of the following accurately represents the change in morbidity and mortality rate for coronary artery disease since 1970?
   a. The rate has decreased by 20 percent.
   b. The rate has decreased by 40 percent.
   c. The rate has increased by 20 percent.
   d. The rate has increased by 40 percent.

2. Which one of the following objectives from *Healthy People 2010* is most pertinent for the middle-aged adult?
   a. Decrease the number of injuries from accidents.
   b. Decrease the proportion who have dental caries.
   c. Reduce past-month use of illicit substances.
   d. Reduce tobacco use and increase smoking cessation attempts.

3. Health promotion actions for risk management in middle age would include counseling regarding:
   a. Immunizations, including tetanus and diphtheria, only if continually employed
   b. Risk factors for HIV and other STDs as well as practicing safe sex
   c. The influence of peers on risk-taking activities
   d. The need for less sleep as one ages

4. In regard to accuracy of screening tests for health promotion, which one of the following is the ability of the test to correctly give a positive result when the person has the condition being tested?
   a. Sensibility of a screening test
   b. Sensitivity of a screening test
   c. Significance of a screening test
   d. Specificity of a screening test

Websites

http://www.seekwellness.com Offers practical advice for staying healthy via nutrition, exercise, self-care, humor, play, relationships, and adding meaning and purpose to your life.

http://preventdisease.com Offers Health Headlines, with the latest news in prevention and health matters, including weekly wellness facts on diverse health topics that contribute to a happy life during middle age.

http://www.4women.gov Offers information on health issues important to women of diverse populations throughout the lifespan. Education, outreach, and policy development are highlights.

http://www.aarp.org Organization for mature adults 50 and above in the United States. AARP provides information on health, long-term care, economic security, independent living, consumer affairs, and more.

http://www.healthypeople.gov Government organization that promotes a national health promotion and disease prevention initiative with goals to increase the quality and years of healthy life for all people.

References

American Cancer Society (ACS). (2004). *Cancer facts and figures, 2004*. Atlanta, GA: American Cancer Society.

Barr, D. A., & Wanat, S. F. (2005). Listening to patients: Cultural and linguistic barriers to health care access. *Family Medicine, 37*(3), 199–204.

Bastable, S. (2003). *The nurse as educator: Principles of teaching and learning* (4th ed.). Boston: Jones & Bartlett.

Bromberger, J. T., Harlow, S., Avis, N., Kravitz, H. M., & Cordal, A. (2004). Racial/ethnic differences in the prevalence of depressive symptoms among middle-aged women: The study of women's health across the nation (SWAN). *American Journal of Public Health, 94*(8), 1378–1385.

Buscemi, M., Vandermeer, B., Friesen, C., Bialy, L., Tubman, M., Ospina, M., et al. (2005). Manifestations and management of chronic insomnia in adults. *Evidence Report/Technology Assessment, Number 125*. Retrieved April 11, 2006, from http://www.ahrq.gov/clinic/epcsums/insomnsum.htm

Carroll, R. (2005). Anatomy and physiology review: The reproductive systems. In J. M. Black and J. H. Hawks (Eds.), *Medical-surgical nursing: Clinical management for positive outcomes* (4th ed.). St. Louis: Elsevier-Saunders.

Centers for Disease Control (CDC). (2006, September). State-specific prevalence of obesity among adults—United States, 2005. *Morbididty and Mortality Weekly, 55*(36), 985–988.

Colorectal cancer screening (n.d.). Retrieved March 23, 2006, from http://www.dukehealth.org/HealthLibrary/articles/colorectal_cancer_screening

Columbia University's Mailman School of Public Health. (October 27, 2005). *Largest survey on depression suggests higher prevalence in U.S.* Retrieved April 11, 2006, from http://www.brightsurf.com/

Crown, E. (November 17, 2005). Middle-age depression raises disability risk. *Observer Online: News for the Northwestern University Community*. Retrieved April 11, 2006, from http://www.north-western.edu/observer/issues/2005/11/16/depression.html

Fiandt, K. (2005). Health promotion in middle-aged adults. In J. M. Black and J. H. Hawks (Eds.), *Medical-surgical nursing: Clinical management for positive outcomes* (4th ed.). St. Louis: Elsevier-Saunders.

Gray, M. (2005). Management of men with reproductive disorders. In J. M. Black and J. H. Hawks (Eds.), *Medical-surgical nursing: Clinical management for positive outcomes* (4th ed.). St. Louis: Elsevier-Saunders.

Helping smokers quit: A guide for nurses. (March 2005). Agency for Healthcare Research and Quality. Retrieved March 23, 2006, from http://www.ahrq.gov/about/nursing/hlpsmksqt.htm

Jemal, A., Ward, E., Hao, Y., & Thun, M. (2005). Trends in the leading causes of death in the United States, 1970–2002. *Journal of the American Medical Association, 294*(10), 1255–1259.

National Diabetes Statistics. (2005). *Total prevalence of diabetes among people aged 20 years or older, United States, 2005.* Retrieved April 11, 2006, from http://www.diabetes.niddk.nih .gov/dm/pubs/statistics/index.htm

Neuropsychiatry Reviews. (December 2005). *National survey sharpens picture of major depression among U.S. adults,* 6(10). Retrieved April 11, 2006, from http://www.neuropsychiatryreviews.com/ dec05/surveydepression.html

Office of Minority Health, U.S. Department of Health and Human Services. (2000). *Assuring cultural competence in health care: Recommendations for national standards and an outcomes-focused research agenda.* Retrieved September 25, 2004, from http://www.omhrc.gov/clas/culturalla.htm

Pender, N. J., Murdaugh, C. L., & Parsons, M. A. (2006). *Health promotion in nursing practice* (5th ed.). Upper Saddle River, NJ: Pearson Prentice Hall.

Reimer, M. (2005). Clients with sleep and rest disorders and fatigue. In J. M. Black and J. H. Hawks (Eds.), *Medical-surgical nursing: Clinical management for positive outcomes* (4th ed.). St. Louis: Elsevier-Saunders.

Tingen, M. S., Andrews, J. O., Waller, J. L., & Daniel, S. D. (2004, October). A multicomponent intervention targeting utilization of the Treating Tobacco Use and Dependence guideline in the primary care setting. *Southern Online Journal of Nursing Research,* 5(5), 1–23.

U.S. Bureau of Labor Statistics. (December 2004). *Overview of BLS statistics on worker safety and health.* Retrieved March 24, 2006, from http://www.bls.gov/

U.S. Census Bureau. (2004). *U.S. interim projections by age, sex, race, and Hispanic origin.* Retrieved March 30, 2006, from http://www.census.gov/ipc/www/usinterimproj/

U.S. Department of Health and Human Services. (2000). *Healthy people 2010.* Retrieved September 25, 2004, from http://www .healthypeople.gov

U.S. Department of Commerce, Bureau of the Census. (2000). *Statistical abstracts of the United States.* Washington, DC: Author.

U.S. Office of the Surgeon General. (2005). *Depression in older adults.* Retrieved April 11, 2006, from http://www.surgeongeneral. gov/library/mentalhealth/chapter5/sec3.html

U.S. Preventive Services Task Force (USPSTF). (2005). *Guide to clinical preventive services.* Retrieved March 23, 2006, from http://www.ahrq.gov/clinic/pocketgd/gcps2d.htm

U.S. Preventive Services Task Force (USPSTF). (February 2003). *Screening for diabetes mellitus, adult type 2.* Retrieved April 11, 2006, from http://www.ahrq.gov/clinic/cps3dix.htm

U.S. Preventive Services Task Force (USPSTF). (January 2003). *Screening for cervical cancer.* Retrieved April 11, 2006, from http://www.ahrq.gov/clinic/cps3dix.htm

U.S. Preventive Services Task Force (USPSTF). (September 2002). *Osteoporosis screening.* Retrieved April 11, 2006, from http://www .ahrq.gov/clinic/cps3dix.htm

U.S. Preventive Services Task Force (USPSTF). (May 2002). Screening for depression: Recommendations and rationale. *Annals of Internal Medicine, 136*(10): 760–764.

Weber, C. (2005). Perspectives on infectious disorders. In J. M. Black and J. H. Hawks (Eds.), *Medical-surgical nursing: Clinical management for positive outcomes* (4th ed.). St. Louis: Elsevier-Saunders.

WebMed. (n.d.). *Sleep disorders: Insomnia.* Retrieved April 11, 2006, from http://www.webmd.com/content/article/104/ 107649.htm

Chapter 13

THE OLDER ADULT

Shannon M. Dowdall, MSN, RN

Karyn Taplay, MSN, RNC

Alma Flores-Vela, MSN, RN

Janice A. Maville, EdD, MSN, RN

KEY TERMS

ageism	centenarian	empowerment	heterogeneity
assisted living facility (ALF)	dementia	eustress	polypharmacy
atrophy	dysomnia	geriatrics	spiritual well-being
baby boomers	elder abuse	gerontology	

OBJECTIVES

Upon completion of this chapter, the reader should be able to:

- Identify nursing responsibilities in promoting the health of older adults.

- Explore demographic trends related to aging.

- Examine developmental theories with respect to aging.

- List health promotion tips for expected physiological changes of aging.

- Identify strategies within the biological domain (nutrition, fitness and exercise, sleep, and sex) to promote health in older adults.

- Relate effects from the socioeconomic domain to the health of older adults.

- Describe issues from the psychological domain (stress, depression, and elder abuse) that contribute to the health of older people.

- Consider the influence of spirituality in promoting health of older adults.

- Identify environmental influences that contribute to the health of older adults.

- Discuss future research trends that may influence the health of older adults.

- Identify health promotion resources for this age group.

INTRODUCTION

As the new millennium progresses, it is impossible to ignore the fact that there are an unprecedented number of people in society age 65 and over. Increased life span is the direct result of advances in science, technology, and medicine. Unfortunately, living longer does not always mean living healthier. As mentioned earlier, health problems in the later years of life often are a result of unhealthy or harmful behaviors and events in adolescence and adulthood. Additionally, many seniors address and manage age-related conditions and chronic illnesses commonly identified in the middle adult years.

Geriatrics is a specialized branch of medicine that focuses on the diagnosis and treatment of diseases affecting the elderly. In contrast, the study of the elderly and the aging process is called **gerontology.** Gerontology, which is studied by a variety of disciplines including nursing, encompasses the concepts of health and wellness. As such, gerontology is concerned with the biological, psychological, socioeconomic, and environmental threats and challenges influencing older people. The collective consequences of these influences form important issues for the individual, the community, and society at large.

Growing older is not necessarily a downward spiral. It is often viewed positively as a new beginning or an achievement of the time when freedom and recreation can be enjoyed. Successful healthy aging depends on the individual's ability to cope with the effects of aging, to manage chronic illness, and to confront new threats using personal capabilities and as many existing resources as possible.

The concept of health promotion embodies the attributes of self-care and **empowerment.** These attributes become highly important in older persons regardless of their health status. To become facilitators of health promotion of older adults, nurses must become more knowledgeable about the issues and needs that affect the health and well-being of older adults.

This chapter is based on a gerontological perspective. It addresses demographic characteristics and developmental theories. Nursing responsibilities are discussed as related to health promotion and aging among the various domains (developmental, biological, socioeconomic, psychological, and environmental).

DEMOGRAPHIC CHARACTERISTICS OF OLDER ADULTS

Older adults represent a special segment of the population. Looking at demographics for this age group is helpful in developing a general profile. It must be noted, however, that although a general profile is helpful in forming an understanding of the uniqueness of older adults, recognition of the vast differences among individual members of this group is equally important.

Who Are the Older Adults?

Age identity for older adults has shifted from focusing solely on chronological age to include objective, subjective, and functional perspectives. In other words, an individual's birth date, personal perceptions of age and aging, and ability to function physiologically, psychologically, socially, and economically influence whether that person is considered an older adult. From these perspectives, terms such as *feel-age, cognitive age, stereotype age, comparative age,* and *self-perceived age* have been identified by gerontologists (Kaufman & Elder, 2002). For legal purposes, such as obtaining Social Security benefits and Medicare, age 65 is recognized as the minimal age for entering the elderly population age group.

The marked increase in the numbers of older people, particularly those over 85, will drive many changes in the near future and beyond. From the perspective of a professional health care provider, it is important to remember the **heterogeneity** of the population we call "elderly." Because of the important differences encountered in the various age groups—65 to 74 years (young old), 75 to 84 years (old), and 85 or older (frail old)—each group should be considered a separate entity with a corresponding collection of unique data that should include culture, geographic location, and socioeconomic status as well as mental and physical health.

Because the age range of this group is so large, it is easy to see how variations exist. The lifestyles, health, and behaviors of a 65-year-old person can vary significantly from those of a 90-year-old. It is important, however, to avoid stereotyping elderly people, as many in the old and frail-old categories can be healthier and more productive than those in the younger age ranges.

Regarding gender and marital status, there are more elderly women than elderly men and more elderly widowed women than elderly widowed men. When assessing an elderly client it is important to include an assessment of marital status. Being a widow or a widower frequently has a significant impact on all other aspects of life. Table 13-1 demonstrates that the trend of women outliving men is not expected to change in the future.

Additionally, Table 13-2 summarizes significant demographic characteristics related to the elderly. These demographics are important considerations in planning and implementing health promotion programs for the geriatric population.

Population Trends

In 1776 America celebrated its first Independence Day. A baby born that year could anticipate living to the "ripe old age" of 35. During the next 125 years, or by 1900, the average life span expectancy had only increased to 47 years of age. By the 1990s, however, with scientific advances, medical breakthroughs, and increased focus on healthy living, people could expect to live about 76 years. Life expectancy has increased rapidly in recent years, and a continued, albeit slower, increase is expected. What does this increase in life expectancy mean? It means there are more seniors than ever before.

In 1900 only 4 percent of the population was over the age of 65. By contrast, in 1996 the percentage of the total population of the United States of people age 65 and over was 13. This rising number of senior citizens is only expected to increase as the first of the **"baby boomers"**—the large post–World War II generation—reach 65. It is projected that by 2030 the percentage of persons over 65 will increase to 20 (Centers for Disease Control and Prevention, 2003).

This expected, dramatic increase in the older segment of the population obligates the health care industry to handle tremendous change. The $1 trillion annual expenditure for health care in America currently accounts for 34 million seniors. With the expected increase in seniors, the Department of Health and Human Services estimates that most older persons will have at least one

TABLE 13-1 Projections of Life Expectancy, 1999–2100

Year	Total Population		White		Black		American Indian		Asian		Hispanic Origin	
	Male	Female	Male	Female	Male	Female	Male	Female	Male	Female	Male	Female
1999	74.0	79.7	74.7	80.1	68.3	75.1	72.8	82.0	80.8	86.5	77.1	83.7
2025	76.5	82.6	76.9	82.6	72.4	79.3	77.2	85.3	81.5	86.8	79.0	85.1
2050	79.5	84.9	79.5	84.8	76.6	82.7	80.3	87.3	83.2	88.1	81.4	86.8
2100	85.0	89.3	84.8	89.0	83.9	88.4	85.6	90.6	86.6	90.7	85.8	90.1

Census Bureau terms:
"American Indian" includes American Indian, Eskimo, and Aleut
"Asian" includes Asian and Pacific Islander
"Hispanic Origin" may be of any race (e.g., "Black-Hispanic," "White-Hispanic"; see Chapter 6).

Adapted from Methodology and Assumptions for the Population Projections of the United States: 1999 to 2100, by F. Hollmann, T. J. Mulder, and J. E. Kallan, January 2000, Washington, DC: Bureau of the Census, U.S. Department of Commerce.

TABLE 13-2 Summary of Current Elderly (55 and Over) Population Characteristics

Population size and composition	Total age 55 and over: 59.6 million 26.6 million men and 33.0 million women Ratio of 81 men to 100 women
Married and living with spouse	Age 55–64: 75% men and 63% women Age 65–84: 74% men and 45% women Age 85 and over: 58% men and 12% women
Education **High school graduate**	Age 55–64: 84% Age 64–84: 71% Age 85 and above: 58%
Bachelor's degree	31% of men and 22% of women
Below poverty level	Total age 55 and over: 5.8 million or 9.8% Age 55–64: 8.4% men and 10.3% women Age 65 and over: 10.3% men and 12.4% women

Adapted from The Older Population in the United States: March 2002, by D. Smith, 2003, U.S. Census Bureau Current Population Reports, P20-546, Washington, DC: U.S. Census Bureau.

chronic condition and many will have multiple conditions (Smith, 2003). It is likely that if nothing changes there will be a significant boost in America's health care expenditures. Modifying the focus of health care from curing or caring for the sick to providing comprehensive health promotion and disease prevention strategies is therefore imperative. Several governmental agencies have joined forces to develop the Health Aging Project. This is the first step to examining ways to promote healthy behavior and lifestyle choices in the elderly population.

The dramatic rise in the population of seniors is not confined to the United States. The world's population of older people, in both developing and developed countries, increased 159 million or over 60 percent in the 10-year period between 1990 and 1999 (see Figure 13-1). The world's older population is expected to triple by the year 2050 (see Figure 13-2). The rapid increase in the numbers of older people worldwide reinforces the concept that improving health in all nations requires long-term commitment and participation of all involved in their health and well-being.

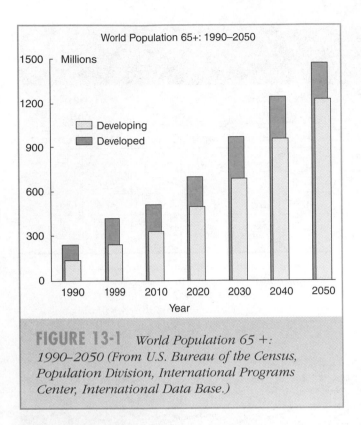

FIGURE 13-1 *World Population 65 +: 1990–2050 (From U.S. Bureau of the Census, Population Division, International Programs Center, International Data Base.)*

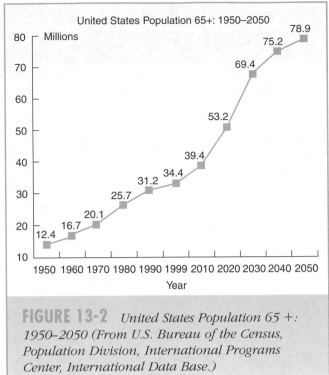

FIGURE 13-2 *United States Population 65 +: 1950–2050 (From U.S. Bureau of the Census, Population Division, International Programs Center, International Data Base.)*

DEVELOPMENTAL DOMAIN

It has been said that some people grow old gracefully, others gratefully, and then there are those who grow old grudgingly. The older adult is subject to significant developmental age-related transitions that affect health. Having knowledge about developmental tasks and theories of how we age physically and mentally will increase the ability of nurses to intervene appropriately to promote a high level of wellness and successful aging.

Developmental Tasks of Aging

To better understand the elderly, several psychosocial theories of aging have been formulated to provide insight into the developmental tasks of the older adult. The psychologist Erik Erikson identified eight stages that cover the life span from infancy to old age. The final stage, which focuses on the older adult, is ego integrity versus despair. Each stage includes specific tasks or challenges that people need to progress through. Successful completion of these tasks or challenges is thought to assist in the successful progression into the next stage. Older people who are able to look back on their lives with a sense of pride and accomplishment are those who enter the final stage of development with satisfaction and contentment. They are symbolic of Erikson's integrity stage. Unfortunately, this is not the case for everyone. It is interesting to note that elderly people who exhibit happiness with their younger phase of life will usually have the same experience with the older phase of life.

As these people age, they accept life and their role in the world. In doing so, they are better able to handle the concerns that come with aging, including the fear of death.

Erikson's theory, although it covers the life span, offers little differentiation in the older adult stage, integrity versus despair. With the elderly population increasing in number and living even longer, greater detail is needed to adequately explore this developmental stage.

Robert Peck enhanced Erikson's old-age stage by adding three specific tasks for the elderly, which influence the outcome of ego integrity versus ego despair (Peck, 1968).

1. Ego differentiation versus role preoccupation: to find satisfaction with oneself instead of satisfaction through parental or occupational roles.

2. Body transcendence versus body preoccupation: to enjoy life instead of being consumed by age-related physical changes.

3. Ego transcendence versus ego preoccupation: to reflect positively on times past rather than obsessing about the limited time remaining.

Additionally, Havighurst (1972) delineated six developmental tasks for the older adult. These tasks relate to adjustments needed for physical, social, and environmental effects of aging.

Table 13-3 demonstrates that psychosocial theories of aging, when used in combination, provide a clear, comprehensive perspective on the developmental tasks of the older adult. Although individuals adapt to the aging

TABLE 13-3 Erikson, Peck, and Havighurst: Developmental Tasks of Aging

Erikson	Peck	Havighurst
Ego integrity versus despair	1. Ego differentiation versus role preoccupation 2. Body transcendence versus body preoccupation 3. Ego transcendence versus ego preoccupation	1. Adjusting to decreasing physical strength and health 2. Adjusting to retirement and reduced income 3. Adjusting to the death of a spouse 4. Establishing an explicit association with one's age group 5. Adapting to social roles in a flexible way 6. Establishing satisfactory physical living arrangements

process in different ways, these psychosocial theories of aging provide a predictable pathway with which to plot progression through various developmental stages or tasks.

Theories Related to Aging

It is predictable that we all age with time. Less predictable is how we respond physically and mentally to aging. Why and how we age have always been of interest to researchers. There was a surge in the creation of developmental theories in the late 1960s and early 1970s that remain pertinent today in understanding human development. These various theories attempt to explain how adults respond differently to the aging process. These can be categorized as of biological, sociological, psychological, and evolving theories of aging as depicted in Table 13-4 on page 272. These theories should be kept in mind when reading about the health promotion domains for the older adult that follow.

BIOLOGICAL DOMAIN

Aging is not a disease. It's a natural process that begins the minute a person is born. The nursing profession has valuable sources of information and research that help with understanding this progression. Providing quality nursing care for clients 65 years or older requires genuine attention to the complex issues that accompany this population. Physiological changes of aging occur in every body system, so it is imperative to understand these changes and how they may impact nursing care. Table 13-5 on page 274 outlines each body system and highlights some of the expected age-related changes. Nursing considerations and health promotion tips are also delineated in this table and are categorized by the age-related changes.

Physical Assessment

Evaluation of a client's health status requires a systematic approach to the collection of information. Having a solid understanding of age-related physiological changes will aid in an accurate evaluation and assessment of the older adult. Comprehensive assessments that address possible functional and mental impairments in older clients are valuable in assuring improved health care outcomes and directing the focus of health promotion (See Figure 13-3). Box 13-1 on page 273 outlines the aspects that should be included in a comprehensive

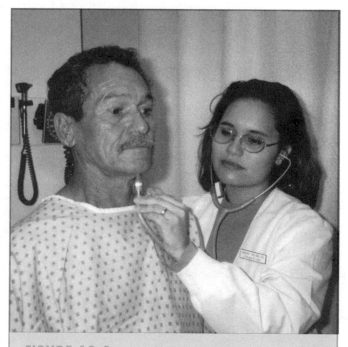

FIGURE 13-3 *Comprehensive assessments are important for promoting health in the older adult.*

TABLE 13-4 Theories of Aging

Category	Selected Theory	Description
Biological	The Genetic Theory	We are programmed to age by a predetermined biological clock.
	The "Wear and Tear" Theory	The body and its cells are damaged by overuse and abuse. Wear and tear is not confined to our organs, however; it also takes place on the cellular level.
	The Neuroendocrine Theory	Hormones are vital for repairing and regulating our bodily functions, and when aging causes a drop in hormone production, it causes a decline in our body's ability to repair and regulate itself as well.
	The Free Radical Theory	Free-radical damage begins at birth and continues until we die. In our youth its effects are relatively minor since the body has extensive repair and replacement mechanisms that in healthy young people function to keep cells and organs in working order. With age, however, the accumulated effects of free-radical damage begin to take their toll.
	Cross-Linkage Theory	A chemical reaction that binds molecules attaches itself to a strand of DNA and damages it. Natural defense mechanisms are inadequate to repair the damage.
Sociological	Disengagement Theory	Older people desire to cut back or to stop working, which provides a mutual benefit to society because younger people are ready and willing to assume these roles.
	Activity Theory	This theory reflects the idea that older people can remain psychologically and socially fit if they remain physically active.
	Continuity Theory	A person's characteristics and coping strategies are in place long before old age occurs. How people age depends on how they adjust to changes throughout their life.
Psychological	Human Needs Theory	Uses Maslow's Hierarchy of Basic Needs. For example, safety and security needs must be met before self-actualization can occur.
Evolving	Evolutionary Theory	Evolutionary theories of aging and longevity try to explain the remarkable differences in observed aging rates and longevity records across different biological species.

Adapted from: American Academy of Anti-Aging Medicine (n.d). Theories on aging: Retrieved June 2, 2006, from www .woldhealth.net/p/90,4863.html; R. Birklow & M. H. Beers (Eds.). (2000). Theories of aging. Merck Manual of Geriatrics. Whitehouse Station, NJ: Merck Research Laboratories; L. A. Gavrilov & N. S. Gavrilov. (2002). Evolutionary theories of aging and longevity. Scientific World Journal, 2 339–356. Retrieved August 6, 2005, from http://longevity-science.org/; and J. L. Powell, (2005). Social theory and aging. Lanham, MD: Rowman and Littlefield Publishers, Inc.

Ask Yourself

Centenarians

Can you picture yourself celebrating your 100th birthday? Where would you be? Who would be with you? Are you interested in living into triple digits?

assessment in order to ensure a holistic approach to nursing the elderly client.

It is entirely possible that a child born today may expect to live to age 100 or older. It's incredible to think of 60 or 70 as middle age. Since 1900, life expectancy has increased by 30 years, and, according to the Census Bureau (Smith, 2003), there are more than 52,000 **centenarians** alive today. That is three times the number of people who were over the age of 100 in 1980.

A comprehensive assessment for the elderly should include all of the following in order to provide holistic care:

Complete medical history	Socioeconomic status	Sleeping pattern	Dental health
Immunizations	Activities of daily living	disturbances	Depression screen
Vision screen	Advance directives	Hearing screen	Nutritional status
Mental status	Sexual assessment	Medications (prescription,	Social support systems
Elimination patterns	Comprehensive physical exam	OTCs, vitamins, herbs)	Risk for falls

People should think of the years remaining in their healthy life span as an open bank account. Each time they exercise, eat nutritious foods, control stress, keep their weight in the normal range, keep regular appointments with their health care provider, and make room for additional types of health-promoting behavior, they are making a sizable deposit into their healthy life span bank account. These deposits accrue benefits, just as money collects interest. These benefits will become increasingly valuable as the years go by. Increased longevity makes attention to health promotion and disease prevention strategies for older adults even more important.

Nutrition

The food consumed each day has a profound and sustained impact on overall health, aging processes, and longevity. Even though good nutrition is so important, it often becomes a progressively lower priority for seniors as they attempt to cope with the demands of daily life. Older people who now live alone sometimes pay little attention to meals or have no interest in cooking for themselves. Inadequate nutrition among the elderly is not uncommon. Nutritional deficits can result from lack of intake of sources of protein, vitamins, and minerals. These nutritional deficits can result in malnutrition. Unfortunately, it is very common for the signs and symptoms of malnutrition to mislead health care professionals. Weight loss, lightheadedness, disorientation, lethargy, and loss of appetite are often misdiagnosed as illness.

A survey completed for the Nutrition Screening Initiative, targeted at improving the nutritional health status of older Americans, showed that while 85 percent of seniors surveyed believe that nutrition is important for their health and well-being, few act on these beliefs (AAFP, 2000). Furthermore, many older adults frequently skip at least one meal a day. Sound nutrition is important in good health for people of all ages. In response to the prevailing lack of nutritional knowledge, the National Council on the Aging has joined forces with other organizations to promote the Nutrition Screening Initiative. The campaign was initiated to increase aware-

ness not only in the older population but also in the health care community.

Nurses encounter a complex challenge when encouraging older adults to eat well and pay serious attention to sound nutrition. There is no simple solution. As a matter of fact, the aging process itself becomes part of the problem. As many people age, they begin to lose lean body mass, which contributes to a decreased appetite. Consequently, interest in food tends to diminish and caloric intake decreases quickly, leading to nutritional deficiencies. This results in eating less which quickly leads to deficiencies. Nutrient requirements do not decline as we age and in some cases may actually increase with age. Other barriers to eating well include a decline in the sense of smell and drying of the oral mucosa. Both of these age-related changes directly affect a person's ability to taste and enjoy food.

In addition, financial concerns play a large role in the nutritional status of the elderly. After people retire, their reduced incomes often force them to make reductions in their monthly expenditures. This possibly leads to a cut in their food budget. Nearly 11 percent of people 65 and over are below the average poverty level for their age group. Lack of funds may lead older people to avoid perishable food items like fresh fruits, vegetables, and meat because of higher cost and possible waste. Also, they may avoid cooking or baking nutritious and cheaper foods like stews and casseroles because recipes for these foods usually yield large quantities.

There are many community-based and national programs to assist the elderly with regard to nutrition. Meals on Wheels and food banks are the primary examples of these programs. These programs provide good nutritional support for the elderly and provide an opportunity to socialize. For those who qualify, food stamps are also available. A one-person household can receive up to $155 a month, depending on individual income and living arrangements (Food Stamp Services, 2007).

Proper nutrition in later years can help lessen the effects of diseases prevalent among older Americans, or improve the quality of life for people who have such diseases. This includes osteoporosis, obesity, high blood pressure, heart disease, certain cancers, gastrointestinal

TABLE 13-5 Nursing Considerations and Health Promotion Tips for Age-Related Physical Changes

System	Age-Related Changes	Nursing Considerations	Health Promotion Tips
Integument	Dry and scaly, decreased elasticity, increased wrinkles and thinning, decreased perspiration. Spotty pigmentation from sun exposure.	Prone to skin breakdown. Alteration in thermoregularity. Lifelong exposure to sun increases risk for skin cancer.	Use a moisturizer. Drink plenty of water (skin becomes dry when dehydrated). Encourage the use of sunscreen. Decrease temperature on hot water heater to 120 degrees F.
Eyes	Decreased visual acuity. Reduced adaptation to darkness and sensitivity to glare. Increased dryness.	May need corrective lenses. Caution should be exercised while driving. Vulnerable to infection.	Encourage annual eye exams and use of prescription sunglasses. Review driving tips for older adults (see Box 13-2).
Ears	Up to 30% of older persons have significant hearing loss.	Hearing loss may lead to social isolation.	Encourage routine hearing exams. Encourage use of hearing aids.
Nose	Decreased sensitivity to odors.	Potential safety hazard. May not be able to detect smoke or harmful odors.	Install smoke and carbon monoxide detectors strategically throughout the home.
Mouth	Drying of oral mucosa. Absence of teeth or ill-fitting dentures. Decreased sense of taste.	Changes can lead to difficulty chewing or pain that can lead to malnutrition.	Have a dental exam every six months. Ensure that dentures fit properly.
Respiratory	Reduced overall efficiency of ventilatory exchange.	Increased susceptibility to infection.	Encourage the client not to smoke. If client smokes, provide support and strategies to quit.
Cardiovascular	Thickening of the wall of the left ventricle. Decreased cardiac output.	May have a decreased response to stress and a higher incidence of arrythmias.	Warning signs for heart attack may present differently in women than in men (i.e., women may have indigestion or pressure in the chest). Have cholesterol levels checked yearly, exercise regularly, eat a low-fat diet.
Gastrointestinal	Decreased salivary secretions, reduced motility.	Swallowing may become difficult. Increased incidence of constipation. Increased incidence of prostate cancer and colon cancer.	Encourage drinking liquids with meals. Increase daily intake of water and fiber. Encourage elderly to have a yearly physical that includes a rectal exam.
Genitourinary	Reduced renal mass. Decreased renal blood flow and functioning.	Drug dosages and administration may need to be altered due to excretion changes.	Encourage Kegel exercises. Encourage adequate fluid intake.

System	Physical Change	Implications	Recommendations
Reproductive	Women: decreased vaginal wall elasticity and vaginal wall thinning. Reduced lubrication during arousal state. Men: erectile dysfunction.	Potential for discomfort during intercourse. Potential for sexual dysfunction. Increased risk for sexually transmitted diseases.	Use a barrier method of contraception if there are multiple partners. Add a water-based lubricant to increase comfort during intercourse.
Musculoskeletal	Decreased muscle mass and strength. Bone demineralization. Decreased rate of autonomic reflexes.	Potential for injury related to decreased ROM and joint motion. May need to alter environment to ensure safety and decrease risks.	Encourage use of multivitamin with calcium or a calcium supplement. Exercise regularly.
Neurological	Decreased ability to respond to multiple stimuli. Insomnia.	Potential for injury. Potential alteration in pain response. Possible cognitive and memory changes.	Encourage elderly to implement recommendations for improving home safety.

From H. M. Seidel, J. W. Ball, J. E. Dains, & G. W. Benedict. (2006). Mosby's guide to physical examination (6th ed.). St. Louis: Mosby; and M. J. Goolsby & L. Grubbs. (2006). Advanced assessment: Interpreting findings and formulating differential diagnoses. Philadelphia: F. A. Davis Company.

problems, and chronic malnutrition. A good diet in later years helps both in reducing the risk of these diseases and in managing their signs and symptoms. Proper nutrition contributes to a higher quality of life and enables older people to maintain their independence by continuing to perform basic daily activities. Poor nutrition, on the other hand, can prolong recovery from illness and lead to a poorer quality of life. Therefore it is imperative that nurses incorporate a nutritional analysis as an integral part of the assessment of the elderly adult. After such an assessment (perhaps a three-day dietary log or journal), the nurse can identify the food groups being neglected and advise clients accordingly.

Fitness and Exercise

The world is a dramatically different place for those people who are now 65 or older. Changes in the ways people live and work today may have been impossible to comprehend during the childhood of today's seniors. Scientific knowledge of the advantages of good nutrition and regular exercise is growing by leaps and bounds. Many elderly people are not aware of these advantages, and nurses can be readily accessible to increase their clients' knowledge base. Research has revealed that only 47 percent of Americans age 50 to 79 exercise regularly (American Association of Retired Persons [AARP], 2002).

Nurses have an obligation to promote the benefits of exercise and its potential to extend quantity of life and improve quality of life. Additionally, nurses may have an even stronger influence through example, with their own physically active lifestyles.

The human body has remarkable capacity to repair itself, and habitual exercise and excellent nutrition enable it to perform even more efficiently. This is especially true for the lungs, heart, veins, arteries, and capillaries, as well as for the musculoskeletal system. Physical activity during midlife corresponds with maintenance of high physical function during early old age, and loss of physical function could be delayed by being physically active (Hillsdon, Brunner, Guralnik, & Marmot, 2005). Recent studies indicate the importance of physical exercise in the elderly to slow down physical degeneration and improve quality of life (Brach, Fitzgerald, Newman, Kelsey et al., 2003). In the absence of exercise, fat displaces muscle and the muscles begin to **atrophy** (become smaller and weaker). Many people, especially those who are older, feel that they are "out of shape" and have absolutely no hope of regaining their physical endurance. Health care professionals know this is not true. It is never too late to begin exercising, and one is never too old to benefit from physical activity.

Research indicates that the ideal combination of exercise combines weight training for strength; aerobics for strength and endurance; and calisthenics (stretching, moving, bending, twisting) for increased flexibility and balance. There is evidence that exercise may minimize and in some cases reverse the syndrome of physical frailty in the elderly and that the elderly can benefit significantly from exercise. Clients who are not in prime physical condition should start off slowly and develop a plan of exercise with health care providers devising their individual exercise programs. Exercising for just five minutes a day is a good starting point.

The WALC model is an example of an evidence-based nursing intervention that was created to enhance exercise self-efficacy in older adults. A study using this model found that using a walking program (Walk), paying attention to physical and psychological effects (Address sensations), gaining knowledge about exercise (Learn), and having exercise role models (Cues) helped older adults to begin and stay with an exercise program (Resnick, 2002).

Exercise intensity for aerobic conditioning is measured by heart rate. People who aren't used to exercise should begin by using 60 percent of their maximum heartbeat and ultimately move up to 80 percent, or what their practitioner recommends. Aerobic exercise not only strengthens bone and muscles, it also helps prevent osteoporosis. If a client's favorite exercise is not aerobics, suggest walking, swimming, or Tai Chi, or advise the client to go dancing. Dancing is often a perfect solution for those who habitually avoid exercise. A regular schedule of dancing 30 to 40 minutes two to three times a week can slow the heart rate, reduce blood pressure, improve cholesterol levels, and strengthen the cardiovascular system (National Institute on Aging, 2004). Benefits include decreased blood pressure and improved function of all major organs. Sustained aerobic exercise can help control type 2 diabetes mellitus because it aids in the metabolism of sucrose.

Sleep

Complaints of sleep disturbances rank high among problems reported by the elderly. In a study by Sukying, Bhokakul, and Udomsubpayakul (2003), insomnia was found in 46.3 percent of an elderly population. Even though older adults spend an increased amount of time in bed, they may have disruptive sleep patterns from a variety of causes that affect the quality of sleep.

Alterations in sleep may be referred to as **dysomnia.** The elderly suffer from these various disturbances as a result of age-related and external influences. Anxiety and psychological factors, including **dementia,** depression, and sensory impairments, have been shown to affect quality and quantity of sleep. Other impacts may include daytime boredom and a lack of social demands. Physiologic reasons such as pain, sleep apnea, periodic limb movements, pathology, altered circadian rhythm, and effects of medication, caffeine, and alcohol also have a strong influence on the elderly and sleep (Miller, 2004).

Commonly reported sleep disturbances include trouble getting to sleep, trouble staying asleep, and early morning awakenings. A combination of physiological, medical, psychiatric, psychosocial, and pharmacologic factors have been found to play a role in sleep disturbances reported in the elderly. Factors associated with sleep problems in the elderly include poor self-rated health, depression, pain, and polypharmacy (Giron et al., 2002). Health conditions more commonly found along with sleep disturbance include arthritis, incident angina pectoris, myocardial infarction or CHF, respiratory symptoms, and depression. Depression was the most important predictive factor associated with the presence of sleep disturbances (Quan, et al., 2005).

Older adults take longer to fall asleep, awaken more easily and more often, and spend more time in the drowsiness stage rather than in deeper sleep referred to as Rapid Eye Movement sleep (Miller, 2004). Disruptions are characterized by a decrease in the amount and amplitude of delta sleep compared to younger persons; in simple terms they spend more time in bed but not sleeping (Miller, 2004). Sleep problems in the elderly may also be explained by their frequent naps during the daytime.

Measures to promote healthier sleep habits should include but are not limited to the following recommendations:

1. Reassure the elderly that alterations in sleep patterns are normal.

2. Establish a bedtime ritual.

3. Avoid food, beverages, and medication that contain caffeine late in the day.

4. Avoid smoking cigarettes, or reduce evening smoking.

5. Avoid alcohol late in the day.

6. Drink milk or chamomile tea, and eat a light snack prior to bedtime.

7. Utilize relaxation methods.

8. Maintain a daily wake-sleep schedule.

9. Perform daily exercise.

10. Sleep in a low-stimulus, dark, cool environment (adapted from Miller, 2004).

Sleep patterns are an integral segment of any health assessment. Dysomnia may provide insight into a biological problem or one of an emotional nature that may not otherwise be detected.

Sex

Sex and sexuality are a basic human need. For unknown reasons, however, this aspect of health promotion and health functioning is often overlooked in the elderly population. Sexuality is vital in a complete assessment of the elderly client. Dysfunction in other areas of the physical domain may disrupt sex and sexuality in the elderly.

Sexuality in the elderly should encompass aspects of intimacy, love, warmth, sharing, and touching as depicted in Figure 13-4. These activities are meaningful for the well-being of the elderly (Nagaratnam & Gayagay, 2002).

Many elderly complain of a less than ideal sex life as well as touch deprivation. This may be a result of physiologic changes of aging. Some of these age-related changes, seen in Table 13-5, include decreased circulation to genitalia, decreased reflex impulses, decreased hormone levels, and alterations in the intactness of genitalia. Therefore it is imperative to incorporate a sexual assessment when doing a comprehensive holistic assessment of an elderly client. If a client is dissatisfied with his or her sexual performance, it may be due to medication or some other variable which the nurse may be able to identify.

Many clients are willing to discuss issues of sex and sexuality with a health care provider but may be less willing if they sense fear or embarrassment from the health care provider.

Viagra, followed by Cialis and Levitra, become the "wonder drugs" of the 1990s, creating a media flourish and, more importantly, allowing topics such as erectile

dysfunction and impotence to become part of mainstream conversation. Drugs such as these may help provide an erection or sustain an erection for those elderly men who were unable to in the past. They have provided success and increased sexual satisfaction for a majority of the affected general population. It is essential, however, that health care providers understand the benefits, side effects, and contraindications of these drugs (Mayo Clinic, 2006). They may be wonder drugs to some, but they may react with many seniors' medications and cause side effects such as headache, runny nose, upset stomach, and diarrhea.

In addition, health professionals must not neglect an awareness of alternative sexual orientations. Homosexuals comprise approximately 10 percent of the population and so also make up 10 percent of the elderly population. Many gay and lesbian seniors take a low profile as they were not able to "come out" in the past. These seniors have families and health concerns common to many others in society. A study by Chamberland (2003) found that aging lesbians suffer social invisibility, which is a major obstacle to the adaptation of residential services to their needs. Families are defined by those within that individual family unit, and therefore it is essential that nurses prevent themselves from passing their own judgment upon their clients.

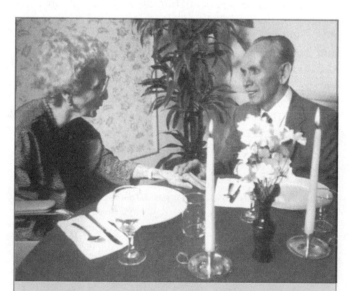

FIGURE 13-4 *Older adults still experience the need for companionship and intimacy.*

Human immunodeficiency virus (HIV) and Acquired Immunodeficiency Syndrome (AIDS) in the elderly are an underestimated and unappreciated reality in the new millennium. HIV/AIDS is not exclusively a disease of youth, and it is commonly underreported in the elderly population. Diagnosing HIV/AIDS in older individuals is also complicated because the symptoms—night sweats, chronic fatigue, weight loss, dementia, and swollen lymph nodes—mimic the natural aging process (Anderson, 2005). In addition, the elderly are at a higher risk for contracting HIV/AIDS because they generally have a more compromised immune system. According to the Centers for Disease Control and Prevention, between 2000 and 2003, an estimated 78,118 persons age 55 to 64 were living with HIV/AIDS. The number of cases in the 65 and over population was estimated to be 21,239 (CDC, n.d.). Fourteen percent of all new AIDS cases are now in people older than 50 years (Janssen, 2005). HIV/AIDS must be considered a differential diagnosis with illness in the elderly, and proper support and education must be provided to prevent the associated depression and isolation. Most importantly, nurses have an obligation to teach safe sex practices regardless of age, lifestyle, or marital status as they would in any other adult population.

SOCIOECONOMIC DOMAIN

A person's socioeconomic level may affect all other domains pertaining to health promotion. A lower economic status is often related to a lower level of education and less ability to afford health care expenses. Awareness of a client's socioeconomic status may change a nurse's focus of health promotion interventions.

Poverty

In spite of significant gains in research, the chronic problem of poverty among the elderly remains a daunting challenge. Understanding that there are differences in poverty characteristics among ethnicities, genders, and geographic locations increases the opportunities for nurses to assist impoverished older Americans. Statistics from the Administration on Aging (2004a) show that the number of people in poverty age 65 and older rose to 3.6 million in 2003. Another million of the elderly were classified as "near poor." In regard to ethnicity, statistics show that one of every 12 elderly Whites, or 8.8 percent, was poor in 2002, compared to 23.7 percent of elderly African Americans, 14.3 percent of elderly Asians, and 19.5 percent of elderly Hispanics. Older persons living in the central cities of the southern United States had the highest poverty rates (11.9 percent). Elderly living in central cities had higher than average poverty rates (13.1 percent) compared to those living in more rural areas (11.0 percent).

In regard to gender, older women had a higher poverty rate (12.5 percent) than did older men (7.3 percent) in 2003. Older persons living alone were much more likely to be poor (18.6 percent) than were older persons living with families (5.8 percent). The highest poverty rate (40.8 percent) was experienced by older Hispanic women who lived alone.

Poverty creates a disparity that can severely diminish access to health care and health promotion education. It is important that nurses recognize that impoverished elderly, as a sub-group of older Americans, have unique strengths as well as challenges in achieving optimal health.

Health promotion programs, including screenings and disease prevention, must be directed at all economic levels without bias and with sensitivity to culture.

Education

Educational levels are increasing in the older population. Between 1970 and 2000, the percentage of those who had graduated from high school rose from 38 to 70. In 1995, almost 15 percent had achieved a bachelor's degree or higher (Federal Interagency Forum on Age-Related Statistics, 2000). What is known is that people with higher levels of education tend to have a higher functional status and to engage in healthy productive behaviors later in life. Low income, less-educated, elderly are less likely to enjoy good health, and they have a higher incidence of smoking, obesity, and sedentary lifestyle. This same population is less likely to have health insurance and less likely to seek preventive care.

Providing affordable or free screening opportunities such as mammograms, blood draws, and diabetic risk profiles allows for early diagnosis and prevention of complications in an otherwise underserviced population. In addition health care providers must consider that living at a poverty level may make compliance with treatment an impossibility. A simple example of this is the diabetic client who may not have electricity to operate a refrigerator to cool his insulin. With education levels of the elderly rising, such problems may be decreasing, but they remain valid concerns for health care providers. This is why it is essential for nurses to include socioeconomic status and barriers to health care or health maintenance when assessing the older adult.

Health Care Expenditures

The majority of people 65 and older have at least one chronic health condition. In 2002, over 12.7 million persons age 65 and older were discharged from short-stay hospitals. This rate is more than three times the comparable rate for persons age 45 to 64. Similarly, length of hospital stay and number of office visits with doctors per year is significantly higher among those 65 and older than for those age 45 to 64. In 2002, older consumers averaged $3,741 in out-of-pocket health care expenditures, an increase of 45 percent since 1992 (AoA, 2004a).

Chronic health conditions, hospital stays, and work absences lead to increases in health care expenditures. This leads to personal financial loss and a drain on the Medicare system. Prevention costs less than treatment. Therefore, the prevention of complications from chronic disease and the prevention of new disease states can lessen the financial burden. It is imperative for nurses to encourage annual exams, wellness screening, and healthy lifestyles in the elderly client.

PSYCHOLOGICAL DOMAIN

Influences within the psychological domain include depression, stress and coping, and issues of abuse. Each of these has a great impact on learning and maintaining healthy behaviors.

Depression

Depression can occur during any stage of life, but the changes that occur to older people may increase their risk for depression. Some common changes that occur in the elderly population include the loss of loved ones, coping with physical and mental changes, illness, and social isolation. Accurately assessing and treating depression in the elderly is a challenge. It is estimated that nearly 6 million of the 35 million Americans over the age of 65 suffer from depression, but only a fraction of these are accurately diagnosed and treated (Shear, Roose, Lenze, & Alexopoulos, 2005). Reasons for the lack of identification and treatment in late life include: atypical symptoms, body system symptoms, apathetic affect, misrepresentation of the problem, **ageism** among health professionals, and stigma among older adults (Tanner, 2005). It is important to screen for and treat depression in the elderly to prevent self-neglect and positively affect quality of life (Tanner, 2005). The Geriatric Depression Scale consisting of 12 to 15 items has been the most widely used to assess for depression among the elderly (Holroyd & Clayton, 2002). A short form of this screening tool in English and in Spanish as well as the original translated Latin American Spanish version are available at *www.stanford.edu/~yesavrage*.

Stress

Stress is a fact of life for each developmental stage. The elderly, however, have some unique factors that may add to stress and influence coping—specifically, the individual's meaning of life, and his or her collection of life experiences, timing, and anticipation of life events, particularly the death of friends and family. Reactions and coping styles may also be influenced by financial resources, social support, social status, spirituality, and connection with organized religion (Miller, 2004). Stress is viewed as having potential for both positive and negative influences on human behavior. **Eustress** refers to the positive stress that mobilizes us to action. Health teaching and screening are examples of this eustress which motivates healthier behavior. In addition, there are many negative stressors that accompany the aging process.

When assessing the elderly client for stress level and stressors, it is imperative to offer creative and individualized stress-reduction techniques. Activities that can reduce stress include but are not limited to the following:

- Physical activity (swimming, dancing)
- Socializing
- Owning a pet
- Listening to music
- Volunteering
- Talking on the phone
- Reading
- Making crafts
- Participating in an organized religion

Figure 13-5 depicts a quiet moment in a chapel, which may reduce stress.

Elder Abuse

Elder abuse is any knowing, intended, or careless act that causes harm or serious risk of harm to an older person, whether it is physical, mental, emotional, or financial. The term is quite broad and encompasses many different types of mistreatment. No one knows exactly how many elders are victims of abuse, but evidence suggests that many thousands have been harmed. Conservative estimates for the United States put the number of elders who have been injured, exploited, or otherwise mistreated at about 1 million to 2 million (National Center on Elder Abuse, 2005). This number is conservative as recent research suggests that only one in 14 domestic elder abuse incidents comes to the attention of the authorities (National Center on Elder Abuse, 2005).

Identification of potential victims and abusers may result as knowledge is gained and as society becomes more aware of the growing problem of elder abuse. Table 13-6 on page 281 highlights specific signs of elder abuse. It is imperative that health care professionals be able to detect signs of elder abuse and take appropriate and immediate actions.

The physically and psychologically debilitated of any age are especially vulnerable to abuse. The responsibility for and the physical and psychological burdens

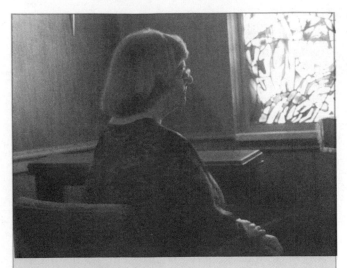

FIGURE 13-5 *Spirituality can help older adults reduce stress.*

Research Note

Understanding Elder Abuse

Study Problem/Purpose: To pilot test a 25-item questionnaire to measure the perception of elder abuse within the population of employees of the long-term care facility where the elderly person resided or in the resident's family members listed as having power of attorney.

Methods: The non-random convenience sample included 49 participants. The questionnaire was mailed to the resident's designated power of attorney or distributed in the employee's paycheck. The participants were encouraged not to sign the questionnaire and to return it upon completion in a self-addressed stamped envelope. Data were analyzed to evaluate the reliability of the questionnaire as a valid instrument.

Findings: The data revealed that the questionnaire on elder abuse was an efficient tool and should be considered an acceptable new instrument. It was suggested that this questionnaire be repeated in numerous populations for reliability comparison.

Implications: Although elder abuse has always existed in our society, defining, understanding, and correcting the problem are difficult. Elder abuse is thought to be significantly underreported; therefore, it is imperative that health care workers and the general population gain a better understanding of elder abuse so that they can better identify it and intervene. This instrument could serve to more clearly identify abuse.

Kottwitz, D., & Bowling, S. (2003). A pilot study of the elder abuse questionnaire. *Kansas Nurse, 78*(7), 4-6.

of caring for any chronically ill person can become unbearable. Perhaps even more important than identification of abuse is to take a more proactive stance aimed at preventing its development in the first place. Health care professionals, for example, can teach families and caregivers helpful techniques to relieve the stresses that often accompany caring for those with multiple needs.

Understanding the physical, cognitive, social, and economic problems that elderly people face can help focus teaching on promoting their health and alleviating their abuse. The study described in the accompanying Research Note was designed to improve understanding and awareness of the prevalent and increasing problem of elder abuse.

SPIRITUAL DOMAIN

Spirituality is often overlooked as an important dimension for health and well-being. To truly promote health in the holistic sense, facilitating health of the mind and the body is incomplete without facilitating the health of the human spirit. Many people look upon spirituality or religion as a resource for coping or stress reduction. There is considerable research linking prayer and/or belief in a higher power with increased health and healing (National Interfaith Coalition on Aging [NICA], 2004).

The National Interfaith Coalition on Aging suggests that relationships and friendships can encourage the deepening of spiritual life in the contexts of congregation and community. Close personal ties across the life span may help people find meaning and purpose in their lives and may enable the elderly to maintain independence and cope with change and loss (NICA, 2004). Having had a lifetime of experiences upon which to reflect, the older adult has the opportunity to harmoniously connect personal beliefs, faith, and hope with life. This becomes very important in progressing successfully through Erikson's final stage of development, ego integrity versus despair.

Many elderly use a variety of spiritual sources to cope with the stressors of everyday life and respond to illness, the death of loved ones, and anticipation of their own death. Spiritual groups or associations within organized

TABLE 13-6 Recognizing Abuse of Older Adults

Signs and symptoms of maltreatment of older adults include, but are not limited to, the following.

Physical abuse
- Unexplained injuries
- Frequent visits to the emergency department for treatment of traumatic injuries
- Untreated injuries in various stages of healing
- Broken eyeglasses/frames
- Loss of patches of hair, pulling of hair
- Signs of being restrained, including rope marks
- Laboratory findings of medication overdose or underutilization of prescribed drugs
- Elder's report of being hit, slapped, kicked, or mistreated
- Elder's refusal to disrobe for bath; trying to hide injuries
- Caregiver's refusal to allow visitors to see an elder alone

Sexual abuse
- Bruising around the breasts or genitalia
- Unexplained venereal disease or genital infections
- Unexplained vaginal or anal bleeding; torn, stained, or bloody underclothing
- Elder's report of being sexually assaulted or raped

Emotional/psychological abuse
- Emotionally upset or agitated; paranoid
- Extremely withdrawn and noncommunicative or nonresponsive; depressed
- Unusual behavior usually attributed to dementia (e.g., sucking, biting, rocking)
- Elder's report of being verbally or emotionally mistreated

Psychological neglect
- Dehydration or malnutrition
- Untreated health problems
- Poor personal hygiene
- Hazardous or unsafe living environment (e.g., improper wiring, no heat, or no running water)

- Unsanitary living environment (e.g., dirt, fleas, lice on person, soiled bedding, fecal/urine smell, inadequate clothing)
- Social isolation
- Low self-esteem
- Elder's report of being mistreated

Financial or material exploitation
- Sudden changes in bank account or banking
- Unauthorized withdrawal of the elder's funds
- Abrupt changes in a will or other financial documents
- Substandard care or living though adequate financial resources are available
- Elder's signature being forged for financial transactions
- Sudden appearance of previously uninvolved relatives claiming rights to an elder's affairs and possessions
- Purchase of services or supplies that are not indicated
- Elder's report of financial exploitation

Self-neglect
- Dehydration or malnutrition
- Untreated health problems
- Poor personal hygiene
- Hazardous or unsafe living environment (e.g., improper wiring, no heat, or no running water, animal/insect infestation, no functioning toilet, fecal/urine smell)
- Unsanitary living environment (e.g., dirt, fleas, lice on person, soiled bedding, fecal/urine smell)
- Inadequate or inappropriate clothing
- Social isolation
- Lack of the necessary health aids (e.g., eyeglasses, hearing aids, dentures)
- Grossly inadequate housing or homelessness

Adapted from National Center on Elder Abuse (2005, June). 15 Questions & Answers About Elder Abuse. Retrieved August 6, 2005, from http://www.elderabusecenter.org/; and National Center on Elder Abuse (2005). Types of elder abuse in domestic settings. Elder Abuse Information Series No. 1. Retrieved August 1, 2005, from http://www.elderabusecenter.org/default.cfm?p=statistics.cfm

religions may provide an excellent arena for socialization. Additionally, many organized religions offer wellness or health promotion programs such as weight reduction programs. They offer social and emotional support essential to coping and provide incentive to participate in healthy group activities.

To guide nurses in identifying spiritual needs, the North American Nursing Diagnoses Association identi-

fied two diagnoses related to spirituality: (1) spiritual distress and (2) potential for enhanced **spiritual well-being.** If an elderly client seems distressed, or is not a part of a spiritual group, or does not see himself or herself as spiritual, the potential for enhanced spiritual well-being could be explored. A nurse should identify personal bias in this area, as well as the client's culture, before beginning any intervention.

CULTURAL DOMAIN

Incorporating cultural considerations is imperative in providing individualized and holistic nursing care for all clients. Population trends and ethnicity related to older adults presented earlier in this chapter highlight a corresponding increase in diversity. In 2002 approximately 17 percent of persons greater than 65 years of age were members of minorities; by 2030 the older minority population is expected to increase by 217 percent (Administration on Aging [AoA], 2004b).

The increase in elder minorities is accompanied by challenges that create opportunities for health promotion. These challenges are based on the knowledge that the older population at risk for chronic conditions will become more diverse; that disparities exist among ethnicities regarding access to health care; that and literacy, language, and communication problems affect comprehension and adherence to health teaching (Ihara, 2004).

Considering the client's culture helps the nurse to understand the client's values, attitudes, and behaviors, which also helps to eliminate stereotyping and biases that would undermine health promotion efforts. Miller (2004) has suggested that nurses perform a cultural self-assessment to gain insight into their own feelings regarding culture and older clients. Nurses who can focus on their own cultural identity and on how that identity influences their attitude toward older adults from diverse cultures and health practices enhance their ability to provide culturally competent care, as discussed in Chapter 6.

ENVIRONMENTAL DOMAIN

Many environmental factors may contribute to, or hinder an elderly client from, initiating or maintaining a healthy lifestyle. Knowing your client's activities is important to planning health promotion for their safe enjoyment. The health promotion focus for this environmental domain will include safety on the road, safety at home, safety in the use of medications, and safety related to health care services and facilities.

Safety in Driving

Access to friends, families, employment, shopping, personal care, cultural enrichment, and religious expression depends on one's ability to move from one location to another. A high level of mobility means easy access to choice and opportunity, which can lead to self-fulfillment and enrichment. Low levels of mobility often mean isolation, depression, and social impoverishment.

The rapid growth of our aging population presents special transportation challenges. When people with diminishing capabilities continue to drive, this creates increased safety risks for all members of society. Yet,

older Americans have grown up in a culture that depends on the ability to drive, and the loss of this option may present a major life crisis.

As the U.S. population ages, more older drivers will be on the road. It is estimated that there will be over 40 million licensed drivers over the age of 65 by the year 2020 (Dellinger, Langlois, & Li, 2002). The National Highway Traffic Safety Administration (2003) reported that older drivers account for 12 percent of all traffic fatalities and 12 percent of vehicle occupant fatalities. Statistics show that over 80 percent of traffic fatalities involving older drivers occur during the daytime and over 70 percent occur on weekdays (NHTSA, 2003).

Many national and international organizations have developed suggestions to help compensate for the aging effects on driving. Everyone ages differently, so some people are perfectly capable of continuing to drive in their 70s, 80s, and even beyond. Many older adults, however, are at higher risk for road accidents due to loss of hearing acuity, loss of visual acuity, chronic diseases, physical impairment, and medications. When working with elderly clients, it is imperative to assess whether or not they drive. Box 13-2 suggests driving tips for the eld-

BOX 13-2 Driving Tips for Older Adults

1. Limit driving to daytime hours if seeing or driving at night is a problem.
2. Turn the head frequently to compensate for diminished peripheral vision.
3. Add a larger rear-view mirror.
4. Limit distractions.
5. Keep fit. Physical activity is needed to keep a person strong and flexible for quick reactions that are needed for driving.
6. Avoid driving for a few days after the start of new medication. Side effects of medication can worsen after a couple of days.
7. If medication causes sleepiness or disorientation, DON'T DRIVE.
8. Attend a driver refresher course for the elderly.

erly that can help accommodate for age-related physical changes. These driving tips can increase the confidence of the driver, make driving less stressful, and make the roads safer for everyone.

Safety at Home

A majority of older Americans are active members of their families and communities and relish the independence of living in their own homes. In many cases, the home where they live is the place where they raised their children and enjoyed the happiest years of their lives. Millions of other seniors, however, are at risk of losing their independence, including 4 million Americans age 85 and older. Many of these people live alone and have no immediate family nearby to give them assistance.

The Centers for Disease Control and Prevention (2006) has stated that falls in the home are the leading cause of fatal and nonfatal injuries to people 65 and older. It is predicted that 30 percent of people 65 or older will fall each year. In fact, statistics suggest that falls led to emergency room visits for an estimated 1.8 million Americans age 65 or older in 2000 (CDC, 2006). Box 13-3 lists important recommendations to keep in mind when teaching the elderly, their caregivers, and their families about home safety.

One way to reduce falls in the home is by modifying homes in order to eliminate or abate common hazards for frail persons. Using a relatively new concept known as universal design, AARP (n.d.) advocates for a home that is architecturally designed to allow people to stay in it at any age. As the nation grows older at a record pace, this

Spotlight On

Facts About Falls, Hip Fractures, and Older Adults

Falls account for 90 percent of the more than 352,000 hip fractures in the United States each year. It is estimated that by 2050, there will be 1,800 hip fractures daily and 650,000 hip fractures yearly.

Hip fractures occur two to three times more in women than men. One of every seven White, post-menopausal women will have a hip fracture. Taller women, 5'8" or more, have twice the risk of those under 5'2". Almost half of all women who reach age 90 have suffered a hip fracture.

Twenty-five percent of those with hip fracture have a full recovery, and 24 percent of those over the age of 50 will die within 12 months due to complications. Approximately 220,000 total hip replacements were performed in the United States in 2003. Increased risk factors of an adverse outcome of the surgery include advanced age, male gender, black race, existing health problems, and a low income.

Adapted from "Falls and Hip Fractures," American Academy of Orthopedic Surgeons n.d., retrieved May 9, 2006, from orthoinfo.aaos.org and D'Angelo, K. D. (2003). *News release: New analysis indicates age, gender, race, income, and coexisting medical conditions affect rates and outcomes of primary and revision total hip replacements.* American Academy of Orthopedic Surgeons, February 2, 2003.

BOX 13-3   Nursing Teaching Tips: Safety in the Home

Ensure that fire detectors and carbon monoxide detectors are in working condition.
Clear front and back walkways of clutter, snow, and ice.
Ensure that all entrances inside and out are well maintained.
Keep flashlights or battery-operated lights handy throughout the house.
Get to know the neighbors if not already acquainted.
Consider placing a phone in the bedroom and bathroom.
Remove scatter rugs.

When using the stairs:
Provide enough lighting to see steps clearly, and keep them free from clutter.

Cover stairs with a nonslip surface such as tightly woven carpet.
Install sturdy handrails on both sides of the stairs.

In the kitchen:
Avoid climbing and reaching to high shelves.
Use a stable step stool with handrails, if climbing is necessary.
Arrange storage at counter level.
Clean spills as soon as they happen.
Don't wax floors.

In the bathroom:
Keep a night light on.
Use rugs with nonskid backing.
Install handrails in the bathtub and toilet areas.

will be an increasingly important feature. The house has step-free front and garage entrances. It features nonslip tile, extra-wide doorways and showers, and a barrier-free design. Although people often refer to the "safety of home," the home poses many opportunities for injury. Therefore it is essential for nurses to promote safety in the home.

A monitoring device can be a helpful safety feature for older adults who live alone. These devices are transmitters that can be worn hanging around the neck or wrist and can even be worn while bathing in a tub or shower. They are connected remotely via telephone service to a 24-hour monitoring center that will know the wearer is in trouble with in seconds of pushing a button on the transmitter. Many transmitters have an open voice channel for communication with the elderly person.

Medications and the Elderly

The geriatric population consumes approximately 25 percent of all medications produced. Approximately 70 percent of over-the-counter medications are used by people over the age of 65. The use of multiple medications is called **polypharmacy.** Some elderly people take as many as 15 different medications a day. The risk of drug interaction directly corresponds with the number of drugs being taken. As an example, an elderly person taking five medications has a 50 percent chance of a

---

BOX 13-4 Polypharmacy Risk Assessment Questions

- Do you take five or more prescription medications?
- Do you take dietary supplements, vitamins, or over-the-counter medications?
- Do you take homeopathic or herbal remedies?
- Do you get your prescription filled at more than one pharmacy?
- Is more than one doctor prescribing your medications?
- Do you take your medications more than once a day?
- Do you have trouble opening your medication bottles?
- Do you have poor eyesight or hearing?
- Do you live alone?
- Do you have a hard time remembering to take your medications?

Adapted from Peterson, E. A. (2003). Are you at risk for polypharmacy? Health Alliance Plan. Retrieved August 6, 2005, from http://www.hap.org/info/formulary/polypharmacy_risk.php

---

drug interaction, and when the number increases to eight medications there is a 100 percent chance of a drug interaction (Thompson, 2005). Box 13-4 lists ten risk questions, any one of which can lead to polypharmacy. It is essential to improve problem-solving abilities in the clinical setting by understanding an elderly client's medications, including herbal and other nonprescription drugs. Teach elderly clients about their medications, when to take them, how to take them, what the medication is expected to do, and potential side effects. Box 13-5 offers additional guidelines to teach the elderly about their medications. Additionally, nurses will want to teach elderly clients to keep a current medication list with them at all times. Keeping an accurate medication record provides many benefits for the elderly client. It provides a quick, easy reference when meeting with the health care worker. It is easier than carrying all of the medication bottles. It may prevent the possibility of duplicate or contraindicated prescriptions from being ordered. Most importantly, a medication record empowers the elderly client by involving him in his own care. Table 13-7 provides a sample medication record.

Safety and Assisted Living Facilities

An **assisted living facility (ALF)** is designed to provide a special combination of personalized care, supportive services, and health-related services for care of the elderly. There are thousands of ALFs in communities across the United States with such names as residential care facility, community-based retirement facility, personal care facility, adult living facility, adult foster care, adult homes, congregate care, supportive care, enhanced care, and elder care facility. Although the types of services and levels of care vary, most facilities provide assistance with bathing, dressing, grooming, personal hygiene, ambulating, and monitoring of medications and dietary intake. Additionally, meals, transportation, laundry, and housekeeping are usually provided; however, the amount of health care provided varies widely among facilities.

With no common definition, operations of ALFs range from residential retirement homes to nursing homes. Each state has a different set of regulations governing its ALFs, and most, but not all, require some type of licensure, certification, or both. Although nursing homes must operate under strict federal regulation, inconsistency in regulating ALFs has created issues of safety for residents. Having adequate and qualified staff to provide care and to supervise residents is one major area of concern. Some ALFs accept those who are severely ill and who require skilled personnel to prevent development of pressure sores and complications associated with feeding and elimination. Those ALFs that do not accept severely ill clients must still have adequate personnel to supervise residents who, for example, might have wandering tendencies that could result in tragedy.

The following guidelines are helpful for all who take medications and are especially important for older individuals.

1. Know the names of all medications, what they are for, and when to take them.
2. Keep a current medication list with you at all times (sample list, see Table 13-7).
3. Wear a medical alert bracelet for allergies or a chronic health condition.
4. Follow the exact instructions provided by your doctor or nurse practitioner.
5. Never stop taking a medication on your own. Contact your doctor or nurse practitioner first.
6. Have prescriptions filled in advance to prevent running out.
7. Choose over-the-counter (OTC) medications that have only the ingredients that you need.
8. Use OTC medication as directed on the label.
9. Keep medications out of the reach of small children.
10. Take only your own medications. Never take medications that have been prescribed for someone else and never offer your medications to another person.

TABLE 13-7 Sample Current Medication List for Elderly Clients

Note: Include all prescription medications, over-the-counter medications, vitamins, minerals, and herbal remedies. Important: Have all medications reviewed annually by your primary physician.

Name of Client _____ Allergies _____

Medication Name	Dosage	Dosage Schedule	Prescribing Doctor	Purpose	Side Effects (if any)
Example: Lasix	20 mg (one tab) twice per day	Take one tab at 8:00 AM & one at 2:00 PM	Dr. Brown	Hypertension	Dizziness, blurred vision, urinary frequency, low blood pressure

The following common criteria have been suggested for state law that would preclude a person's admission to assisted living facilities (Downey, 2004):

- Is a threat to self or others
- Has a contagious or an infectious disease
- Requires care beyond the facilities' skill
- Requires physical or chemical restraints or both
- Requires 24-hour nursing or other care
- Is bedridden
- Requires specialized long-term care
- Has stage III/or IV pressure sores or both
- Requires more than minimal assistance in moving to a safe area during an emergency
- Is less than 18 years old
- Requires help with tube feeding

Choosing a quality care facility that is also safe and affordable is an important decision for older persons and their family members. Location or setting, cost, types and extent of services, condition of the other residents, the reputation of the managing company, and the rights of residents are all important considerations. Before making a decision, it is important to visit several facilities, talk to the staff, talk to residents, ask to have a meal at mealtime, and check for reviews or comments on the Internet.

In an effort to enhance the safety of older persons living in ALFs, the Joint Commission on Accreditation of Healthcare Organizations (JCAHO) has delineated goals and actions to achieve the goals. This information is presented in Table 13-8.

Goals for health promotion of older individuals are based on risk assessment. Table 13-9 provides selected risks for older adults arranged according to related domains. Suggested health promotion actions are provided as a guide.

TABLE 13-8 The 2007 Assisted Living National Patient Safety Goals

Goal	Action
Improve accuracy of patient identification.	• Use at least two resident identifiers when providing care treatment or services. • Prior to the start of any invasive procedure, conduct a final verification process to confirm the correct patient, procedure, site, and availability of appropriate documents. This verification process uses active—not passive—communication techniques.
Improve effectiveness of communication among caregivers.	• For verbal or telephone orders or for telephonic reporting of critical test results, verify the complete order or test result by having the person receiving the order or test result "read back" the complete order or test result. • Standardize a list of abbreviations, acronyms, and symbols that are to be used throughout the organization. • Implement a standardized approach to "hand off" communications, including an opportunity to ask and respond to questions.
Reduce risk of health care–associated infections.	• Comply with current U.S. Centers for Disease Control and Prevention (CDC) hand hygiene guidelines. • Manage as sentinel events all identified cases of unanticipated death or major permanent loss of function associated with health care–associated infection.
Accurately and completely reconcile medications across the continuum of care.	• There is a process for comparing the resident's current medications with those ordered for the resident while under the care of the organization. • A complete list of the patient's medications is communicated to the next provider of service when a patient is referred or transferred to another setting, service, practitioner, or level of care within or outside the organization. The complete list is provided to the patient upon discharge.
Reduce the risk of resident harm resulting from falls.	• Implement a fall reduction program and evaluate the effectiveness of the program.
Reduce the risk of influenza and pneumococcal disease in institutionalized older adults.	• Develop and implement a protocol for administration and documentation of the flu vaccine. • Develop and implement a protocol for administration and documentation of the pneumococcus vaccine. • Develop and implement a protocol to identify new cases of influenza and to manage an outbreak.

Adapted from "Joint Commission Announces 2006 National Patient Safety Goals for Assisted Living Facilities," Joint Commission on Accreditation of Healthcare Organizations (JCAHO), 2005, retrieved March 27, 2007, from http://www.jointcommission.org .NewsRoom/NewsReleases/nr_npsg_al.htm

TABLE 13-9 Risk Assessment for the Older Adult

Related Domain	Risk Assessment	Health Promotion Action
Physical	Nutrition	Recommend a daily caloric intake of 1,600–2,000 for females and 2,000–2,800 for males depending upon activity, health status, and metabolism. Consume extra vitamin B12 and vitamin D in fortified foods. Daily intake should include 25 g of fiber, < 30 percent of total calories from fat, 5–6 servings of vegetables and fruits, 6–11 servings of whole grains, breads, and pasta, limited consumption (2–3 servings) of red meat, poultry, eggs, and dairy products.
Physical	Exercise	Advise to stretch every day. Engage in consistent exercise, such as walking or swimming, 30 minutes each time for three to five times per week. Pay special attention to safety measures and general health maintenance.
Physical Psychological	Tobacco avoidance	Assess use of tobacco, interest in cessation, and, if applicable, provide tobacco cessation counseling on a regular basis. Advise the use of pharmacological as well as behavioral interventions for smoking cessation.
Physical Environmental Psychological	Injury prevention	Counseling regarding safety in the home and while driving. Assess individuals for high risk regarding alcohol and substance use. Evaluate all medications for adverse interactions. Assess for abuse.
Physical	Immunizations	Counseling and intervention regarding the obtaining and maintenance of immunizations, including boosters for tetanus and diphtheria. The primary series should be completed for those who have not completed it. Hepatitis and influenza immunizations should be obtained.
Psychological Sociological Spiritual Physical	Stress and mental health issues	Assess for risk factors for depression or other mental health problems, including suicidal ideation. Counsel regarding prevention or management of depression or both. Discuss preferences on limits of medical interventions and other advance planning needs.
Physical	Oral and skin care	Advise regular annual dental care and daily care of teeth, dentures, or dental appliances. Report any signs of gum disease. Report any changes in skin condition or appearances of lesions.
Sexual/Gender Sociological	Sexuality	Provide counseling about risk factors for HIV and other sexually transmitted infections and about measures to reduce risk.

SUMMARY

Individual development through the different stages of the life cycle requires both individual initiative and an enabling environment. An emphasis on wellness is an integral part of many health promotion programs for all age groups. Health promotion programs throughout the nation provide a necessary community link with resources and support for acute and chronic disease, and they reassure the elderly with regard to expected age-related changes.

Throughout the nation wellness programs are in keeping with the agenda of *Healthy People 2010*. The *Healthy People 2010* goals are to increase the years of healthy life and to reduce health disparities among Americans. These goals are consistent with the goals nurses have for health promotion in the elderly.

The 21st century brings a challenging vision for the health of the aging population. Persons age 65 and older constitute the fastest-growing population worldwide. This unprecedented societal trend places a heavy demand on professionals throughout the health care field. Health care professionals need to become knowledgeable about the developmental tasks and physical changes specific to this age group. Additionally, health care providers must be well informed about programs and resources that exist for health promotion in this population. Older adults should be given every opportunity to age in good health. Healthier aging will contribute to a healthier society.

CASE STUDY Beatrice Hernandez: Activity Intolerance, Sleep Pattern Disturbance, and Depression

Objectives/Goals: Through participation in discussion of this case study, participants will have the opportunity to:

1. Discuss factors contributing to activity intolerance, sleep pattern disturbance, and depression in an elderly female client.
2. Identify health risks related to biological, psychological, cultural, and spiritual domains.
3. Explore health promotion interventions in increasing exercise and sleep in an elderly female client.

Health Promotion Concern, History and Physical, Present Health Status, Past Health Status, Family History, and Social History

Ms. Hernandez, an 83-year-old female Hispanic and a retired department store clerk, arrives at the rural health clinic requesting to have her blood pressure checked. Her past medical history is significant for mild hypertension, which is being controlled by Bumex 0.5 mg every day. She admits to taking up to six regular-strength aspirin per day for arthritic pain. Ms. Hernandez complains that she is very tired and has no energy. She says she has difficulty walking out to the end of her driveway to get her mail and has been unable to sleep well for the past three months, getting between four and five hours of sleep most nights. She admits to drinking at least two cups of chamomile tea every evening before bedtime, but says that she still cannot sleep. She lights a candle by her bed every night and prays for sleep to come. She has not seen a health care provider in the last 12 months.

Review of Pertinent Domains:

Biological Domain

Physical exam: Reveals a female, 5 feet 2 inches tall, 135 pounds, with a blood pressure of 165/95, pulse 85. Heberden's nodules of arthritis are observed on fingers of both hands. Skin is dry and lacks elasticity. There are numerous purple lesions over her arms which she says happen with the slightest bump. Eyes have a sunken appearance and her affect is dull.

Gastrointestinal: Ms. Hernandez admits to snacking because she is too tired to cook. She recalls breakfast as a bowl of instant oatmeal and coffee; dinner yesterday was an apple and four cookies; lunch yesterday was a cold meat sandwich and a glass of tea.

Integumentary: Easily bruises.

Cardiovascular: No chest pain or discomfort.

Musculoskeletal: States that arthritis in fingers and knees is sometimes painful.

Neurological: Balance intact, no gait disturbances.

Psychological Domain

Cognitive: Completed high school, is coherent, and is fluent in English and Spanish.

Emotional: Ms. Hernandez reports that she often feels depressed and is currently taking no medication for this. She drinks two cups of chamomile tea every night. She frequently eats only one or two times a day and averages five hours of sleep at night.

Social Domain

Ms. Hernandez has two sons in their mid-50s and has been divorced for 30 years. Her parents died in their mid-50s of unknown causes. Ms. Hernandez has three brothers, two of whom have undergone open heart surgery.

Environmental Domain

Ms. Hernandez states that her sons have taken away her car as she was having difficulty operating the controls due to arthritis in her hands and knees. Although one son takes her shopping for groceries every Saturday, she reports feeling very lonely.

Cultural/Spiritual Domain

Herbal remedies: Ms. Hernandez has had problems sleeping before, and she has obtained relief by drinking chamomile tea.

continued

Questions for Discussion

1. List all the possible factors that may contribute to Ms. Hernandez's sleeplessness, activity intolerance, and depression.
2. What health risk factors does she have that are unrelated to her complaints?
3. What risks are specifically related to her cultural and spiritual practices?
4. What measures could be taken to help relieve sleeplessness, increase activity, decrease depression, and promote the general health of an elderly person such as Ms. Hernandez?

Key Concepts

1. As facilitators of health promotion, nurses must be aware of issues and needs of older adults in order to empower them in self-care, personal health, and well-being.

2. The elderly population is the fastest-growing population worldwide. By the year 2050 there will be more elderly than children.

3. The psychosocial theories of development as perceived by Erikson, Peck, and Havighurst along with theories of aging provide a comprehensive view of the developmental tasks of older adults. These theories can be a helpful guide to understanding how individuals adapt to physical, psychosocial, and environmental effects on aging.

4. Each body system goes through age-related changes. Special nursing consideration needs to be taken and health promotion tips offered to clients going through these changes.

5. There are many physical, psychological, and environmental challenges to consider when encouraging an older adult to eat a well-balanced diet. Exercise, such as swimming, dancing, and walking, is proven to stop or slow some of the physical changes of aging. There are many simple ideas that can be taught to the elderly that will assist in improving their quality of sleep. Because sex and sexuality are important to the health of the elderly, a sexual assessment should be included in your comprehensive assessment, and teaching should include information on safe sex.

6. Low economic status and low level of education are two socioeconomic influences on health-promoting behaviors in the elderly that affect accessibility to and availability of health resources.

7. For many elderly, the stresses of living are compounded by physical, psychological, social, economic, and environmental changes. Incidences of stress among the elderly and elder abuse are occurring frequently; research in this area is ongoing.

8. Spiritual well-being is important for many elderly to achieve or maintain harmony as they progress through the later stages of life.

9. The rapid growth of our aging population presents special environmental challenges. There is a disproportional number of accidents involving the elderly compared to the time they spend driving. Many accidents can be the result of age-related physical changes; therefore, it is imperative to teach driving safety tips.

10. There is a multitude of wellness programs and health promotion resources available for the elderly within their communities, across the nation, and on the Internet.

11. Health care workers must be knowledgeable in properly identifying and assessing elder abuse and in understanding the warning signs of elder abuse.

12. Assisted living facilities provide a special combination of personalized care for the elderly. These facilities exist throughout the nation, and many different levels of care are provided.

Learning Activities

1. List five of the possible physiologic changes of aging. Suggest creative nursing tips to teach your elderly clients about these changes.

2. Develop a pamphlet for healthy sleep patterns for the elderly.

3. List three signs of elder abuse.

4. Give three examples of simple ways the elderly can make their homes safer.

5. Select an older adult, such as a grandparent or neighbor. Ask the person to list or show the medications being taken. Utilize the suggested medication table.

True/False Questions

1. T or F There are more elderly men than elderly women.

2. T or F Each day, there are approximately 6,000 Americans celebrating their 65th birthday.

3. T or F Depression is the most important predictive factor associated with the presence of sleep disturbances.

4. T or F Elder abuse is a legal term referring to physical harm to an older person.

5. T or F Operations of assisted living facilities could range from a residential retirement home to a nursing home for the severely ill.

Multiple Choice Questions

1. In 2002, the percentage of minority persons greater than 65 years of age in the United States was approximately:
   a. 8 percent
   b. 17 percent
   c. 26 percent
   d. 37 percent

2. Which of the following is Erikson's developmental stage for the older adult?
   a. Body transcendence versus body preoccupation
   b. Ego integrity versus despair
   c. Ego differentiation versus role preoccupation
   d. Establishing an explicit association with one's own age group

3. Which one of the following theories is based on the concept that humans are programmed to age by a predetermined biological clock?
   a. Free radical theory
   b. Genetic theory
   c. Human needs theory
   d. Neuroendocrine theory

4. Which of the following is most responsible for fatal and nonfatal injuries to people age 65 and older?
   a. Auto accidents
   b. Cigarette smoking
   c. Falls
   d. Polypharmacy

Websites

http://www.redhatsociety.com Source to generate connections with women over 50 who want to find some support, camaraderie, and comedy relief associated with the responsibilities of middle and older adulthood.

http://www.stanford.edu Site for the Geriatric Depression Scale and various interpretations.

http://www.aoa.dhhs.gov Offers a wealth of information related to health and aging resources for minorities and diverse populations. Also includes a guidebook for providers of service to elderly clients to promote culturally competent care for the elderly and their families.

Organizations

American Association of Retired Persons (AARP)
601 E Street, NW
Washington, DC 20049
Tel: (800) 424-3410
http://www.aarp.org
The American Association of Retired Persons is dedicated to promoting the health and welfare of Americans over the age of 50.

Fifty Plus Fitness Association
Box 20230
Stanford, CA 94309
Tel: (650) 323-6160
http://50plus.org
Promotes activity and fitness for better health of the body and mind. Offers a newsletter, books, and videos as well as sponsoring activity events for mid-life and older adults.

Administration on Aging, Dept. of Health & Human Services
One Massachusetts Ave.
Washington, DC 20201
http://www.aoa.gov
Tel: (202) 619-0724
Provides access to information, resources, and issues related to aging.

National Institute on Aging
Building 31, Room 5C27
31 Center Drive, MSC 2292
Bethesda, MD 20892
Tel: (301) 496-1752
http://www.nia.nih.gov/
Leads the federal effort on aging research. Provides links to health and research information.

Sexuality Information and Education Council of the United States
130 West 42nd Street, Suite 350
New York, NY 10036-7802

Tel: (212) 819-9770

http://www.siecus.org

Serves as the national voice for sexuality education, sexual health, and sexual rights. Provides information to the public to promote sexuality education for all ages.

United States Census Bureau

4700 Silver Hill Road

Washington, DC 20233

Tel: (301) 763-2378

http://www.census.gov

Provides statistics on the United States population.

Office of Disease Prevention and Health Promotion

U.S. Department of Health and Human Services

200 Independence Avenue, SW, Room 738G

Washington, DC 20201

Tel: (202) 401-6295

http://www.osophs.dhhs.gov

Works to strengthen the disease prevention and health promotion priorities of the U.S. Department of Health and Human Serprices.

References

Administration on Aging (AoA) (2004a). *Statistics. A profile of older Americans 2004*. Retrieved July 31, 2005, from http://www.aoa.gov/prof/Statistics/profile/2004/10.asp

Administration on Aging (AoA) (2004b). *The elderly nutrition program*. Retrieved August 6, 2005, from http://www.aoa.gov/Press/Fact/alpha/fact_elderly_nutrition.asp

American Academy of Anti-Aging Medicine (n.d.). Theories on Aging: Retrieved June 2, 2006, from www.worldhealth.net/p/90,4863.html

American Association of Retired Persons. (AARP). (n.d.). *Understanding universal design*. Retrieved January 2, 2006, from http://www.aarp.org/life/homedesign/Articles/a2004-03-23-whatis_univdesign.html

American Association of Retired Persons. (2002, May). *Exercise, attitudes and behaviors: A survey of midlife and older adults.* Retrieved July 29, 2005, from http://www.aarp.org/research/health/healthquality/aresearch-import-65a.html

Anderson, M. (2005, May 24). *HIV/AIDS and the elderly*. Retrieved July 31, 2005, from http://www.finalcall.com/artman/publish/article_2010.shtml

Birklow, R., & Beers, M. H. (Eds.). (2000). Theories of aging. *Merck manual of geriatrics*. Whitehouse Station, NJ: Merck Research Laboratories.

Brach, J. S., Fitzgerald, S., Newman, A. B., Kelsey, S., Kuller, L., VanSwearingen, J. M., & Kriska, A. M. (2003). Physical activity and functional status in community dwelling older women: A 14-year prospective study. *Archives of Internal Medicine 163*(21), 2565–2571.

Centers for Disease Control and Prevention. (n.d.). Cases of HIV infection and AIDS in the United States, 2003. In *HIV/AIDS Surveillance Report* (Vol. 15). Retrieved July 30, 2005, from http://www.cdc.gov/hiv/stats/2003SurveillanceReport.htm

Centers for Disease Control and Prevention. (2003, February 14). Public health and aging United States and worldwide. *Morbidity and Mortality Weekly Report, 52*(06), 101–106.

Centers for Disease Control and Prevention. (2006). Falls among older adults. *National Center for Injury Prevention and Control.* Retrieved January 2, 2006, from http://www.cdc.gov/ncipe/factsheets/adultfalls.htm

Chamberland, L. (2003). Elderly women, invisible lesbians. *Canadian Journal of Community Mental Health, 22* (2), 85–103.

D'Angelo, K. (2003). *News release: New analysis indicates age, gender, race, income, and coexisting medical conditions affect rates and outcomes of primary and revision total hip replacements.* American Academy of Orthopedic Surgeons, February 2, 2003.

Dellinger, A. M., Langlois, J. A., & Li, G. (2002). Fatal crashes among older drivers: Decomposition of rates into contributing factors. *American Journal of Epidemiology, 155*(3), 234–241.

Downey, J. (2004). *Increased safety in assisted living*. Retrieved July 8, 2005, from http://www.rkmc.com/Increased_Safety_in_Assisted_Living.htm

Food Stamp Services. (January 4, 2007). *Applicants & recipients.* Retrieved March 21, 2007, from http://www.fns.usda.gov/fsp/applicant_recipients/default.htm

Gavrilov, L. A., & Gavrilov, N. S. (2002). Evolutionary theories of aging and longevity. *Scientific World Journal, 2*; 339–356. Retrieved August 6, 2005, from http://www.longevity-science.org/

Giron, M. S. T., Forsell, Y., Bernsten, C., Thorslund, M., Winblad, B., & Fastbom, J. (2002). Sleep problems in a very old population. *The Journals of Gerontology Series A: Biological Sciences and Medical Sciences, 5*, 236–240.

Havighurst, R. J. (1972). *Developmental tasks and education* (3rd ed.). New York: David McKay.

Hillsdon, M. M., Brunner, E. J., Guralnik, J. M., & Marmot, M. G. (2005). Prospective study of physical activity and physical function in early old age. *American Journal of Preventive Medicine, 28*(3), 245–250.

Holroyd, A., & Clayton, A. (March 25, 2002). *Measuring depression in the elderly: Which scale is best?* Retrieved July 25, 2005, from http://www.medscape.com/viewarticle/430554

Ihara, E. (February 2004). Cultural competence in health care. *Issue briefs on challenges for the 21st century: Chronic and disabling conditions.* Center on an Aging Society. Retrieved May 15, 2006, from http://www.ihcrp.georgetown.edu/agingsociety

Janssen, R. S. (2005). *HIV/AIDS in persons 50 years of age and older.* Testimony presented on May 12, 2005, at the Special Committee on Aging, U.S. Senate. Retrieved May 10, 2006, from www.hhs.gov/asl/testify/t050512a.html

Joint Commission on Accreditation of Healthcare Organization (JCAHO). (2005). *2007 national patient safety goals for assisted living facilities.* March 27, 2007, from http://www.jointcommission.org/NewsRoom/NewsReleases/nr_npsg_al.htm

Kaufman, G., & Elder, G. H. (2002). Revisiting age identity: A research note. *Journal of Aging Studies, 16*, 169–176.

Kottwitz, D. & Bowling, S. (2003). A pilot study of the elder abuse questionnaire. *Kansas Norse, 78*(7), 4–6.

Mayo Clinic. (2006). *Erectile dysfunction: Viagra and other oral medications.* Retrieved May 10, 2006, from http://www.mayoclinic.com/health/erectile-dysfunction

Miller, C. (2004). *Nursing for wellness in older adults: Theory and practice.* Philadelphia: Williams and Williams.

Nagaratnam, N., & Gayagay, G. (2002). Hypersexuality in nursing care facilities. A descriptive study. *Archives of Gerontology and Geriatrics, 35*(3), 195–203.

National Center on Elder Abuse. (2005). *15 questions & answers about elder abuse.* Retrieved August 6, 2005, from http://www.elderabusecenter.org/

National Center on Elder Abuse. (2005). Types of elder abuse in domestic settings. *Elder Abuse Information Series No.1.* Retrieved

August 1, 2005, from http://www.elderabusecenter.org/default .cfm?p=statistics.cfm

National Highway Traffic Safety Administration (NHTSA). (2003). *Traffic Safety Facts 2002: Older Population.* Retrieved December 28, 2006, from http://www-nrd.dot.gov/pdf/nrd-30/NCSA/ TSF2002/2002oldfacts.pdf

National Interfaith Coalition on Aging (NICA) (2004). *Faith communities and aging: No longer silent.* Retrieved August 6, 2005, from http://www.asaging.org/media/pressrelease.cfm?idz77

National Institute on Aging. (May, 2004). *Health information.* Retrieved July 29, 2005, from http://www.niapublications.org/ engagepages/exercise.asp

Perk, R. (1968). Psychological developments in the second half of life. In B. Neugarten (Ed.), *Middle age and aging* (pp. 88–92). Chicago: University of Chicago.

Peterson, E. A. (2003). *Are you at risk for polypharmacy?* Health Alliance Plan. Retrieved August 6, 2005, from http://www.hap .org/info/formulary/polypharmacy_risk.php

Powell, J. L. (2005). *Social theory and aging.* Lanham, MD: Rowman and Littlefield Publishers, Inc.

Quan, S. F., Katz, R., Olson, J., Bonekat, W., Enright, P. L., Young, T., & Newman, A. (2005). Factors associated with incidence and persistence of symptoms of disturbed sleep in an elderly cohort: The cardiovascular health study. *Southern Society for Clinical Investigation, 329* (4), 163–172.

Resnick, B. (2002). Testing the effects of the WALC intervention on exercise adherence in older adults. *Journal of Gerontological Nursing, 28*(6), 40–49.

Seidel, H. M., Ball, J. W, Dains, J. E, & Benedict, G. W. (2006). *Mosby's guide to physical examination (6th ed.).* St Louis: Mosby.

Shear, K., Roose, S. P., Lenze, E., & Alexopoulos, G. S. (August 2005). Depression in the elderly: The unique features related to diagnosis and treatment. *CNS Spectrums, 10*(18), 33–42.

Smith, D. (2003). *The older population in the United States: March 2002.* U.S. Census Bureau Current Population Reports, P20-546. Washington, DC: U.S. Census Bureau.

Sukying, C., Bhokakul, V., & Udomsubpayakul, U. (2003). An epidemiological study on insomnia in an elderly Thai population. *Journal of the Medical Association of Thailand, 86*(4), 316–324.

Tanner, E. K. (2005). Recognizing late-life depression: Why is this important to nurses in the home setting? *Geriatric Nursing, 26*(3), 145–149.

Thompson, D. (2005). *Exercise and nutrition: The true fountains of youth.* Healthfinder. Retrieved May 15, 2006, from http://www .healthfinder.gov

WebMD. (n.d.). *Erectile dysfunction: Alternative treatments.* Retrieved May 10, 2006, from http://www.webmd.com/content/ article/94/102933.htm

SECTION IV

HEALTH PROMOTION STRATEGIES AND INTERVENTIONS

CHAPTER 14
Embracing Proper Nutrition

CHAPTER 15
Engaging in Physical Fitness

CHAPTER 16
Controlling Weight

CHAPTER 17
Avoiding Tobacco, Alcohol, and Substance Abuse

CHAPTER 18
Enhancing Holistic Care

Chapter 14

EMBRACING PROPER NUTRITION

Carolina G. Huerta, EdD, MSN, RN
Esperanza R. Briones, PhD, RD, LD

KEY TERMS

anorexia nervosa	Dietary Reference	exchange system	nutrients
basal metabolic rate	Intakes (DRIs)	Food Guide Pyramid	nutrition
bulimia	ESADDI	MyPyramid	phytochemicals
Dietary Guidelines	essential nutrients	nonessential nutrients	RDA

OBJECTIVES

Upon completion of this chapter, the reader should be able to:

- Recognize those nutrients that are essential to maintaining health.
- Identify the major goals of *Healthy People 2010*.
- Describe how the biological, psychological, sociocultural, spiritual, and environmental domains influence eating behaviors.
- Develop an awareness of how nutritional excesses and deficits affect health promotion.
- List dietary strategies that promote a healthful diet.
- Utilize the food guide pyramid in planning a healthy diet.
- Recognize how the exchange system can be utilized as a tool for menu planning.
- Recognize how the nursing process may be utilized in developing a nutritionally balanced health promotion plan.

INTRODUCTION

Obesity among the U.S. population has become a significant social as well as health problem. Obesity rates have increased throughout this decade, and obesity is partly to blame for soaring health care costs. Spending on obesity-related illnesses has increased tenfold in the United States since 1987 and now accounts for 12 percent of the national health budget (Gardner, 2005). Yet, as is evident by the growing number of health food stores, nutritional supplements, and vitamins, it is obvious that the public continues to be obsessed with con-

trolling weight, dieting, and knowing what foods actually promote good health, to little or no avail.

It is understood that everyone wants to have a healthy, long, and productive life and delay the onset of chronic diseases. It is also apparent that eating patterns and knowledge of a balanced diet are essential to maintaining the quality of life, especially when entering the senior years. What is not as well understood or accepted is the ease with which diet-related health problems, due to excess, lack, or inappropriate amounts of the essential nutrients, can be alleviated.

Among nursing and health care professionals, there is an awareness that nutrition plays a major role in disease prevention and health promotion. Nurses, thus, are an important asset to clients who are intent on achieving a nutritionally balanced diet in addition to their other health promotion goals. The previous chapters have addressed the conceptual foundations of health promotion and described various factors that are related and that impact individual health promotion throughout the life cycle. This chapter presents the concepts of nutrition and nutrition's role in maintaining health. General nutritional guidelines will be emphasized as well as the role of the nursing process and health promotion model in meeting nutritional needs.

IMPORTANCE OF NUTRITION IN HEALTH PROMOTION

Nutrition is the study of food substances essential for health. Nutrition is also the study of how the body uses these substances to promote and support growth and maintain health throughout the life cycle. It includes the study of digestion, absorption, transportation, metabolism, and storage of nutrients, as well as excretion of waste products.

Foods contain **nutrients** that our bodies can use for the maintenance of body functions throughout life. Nutrients may be essential or nonessential. A variety of health problems can occur when persons lack **essential nutrients** or consume excessive or inappropriate nutrients. A nutrient is considered essential when the body requires it for growth or maintenance but it is not manufactured in sufficient amounts to meet the body's needs. It must be supplied by foods in our diet. Nutrients that the body can make are considered **nonessential.**

The nutrients are classified into six categories. They are water, carbohydrates, lipids, proteins, vitamins, and minerals. Only carbohydrates, lipids, and proteins provide energy. Vitamins and minerals do not provide energy but are essential nutrients, required in very small amounts for specific metabolic function, health promotion, and disease prevention. Table 14-1 provides a list of the most well-known vitamins and mineral supplements and their health promotion implications.

Spotlight On

Dietary Reference Intakes (DRIs)

The DRIs focus on the role of certain nutrients in reducing the risk for chronic diseases and are a set of four reference values: Estimated Average Requirements (EARs), Recommended Dietary Allowances (RDAs), Adequate Intakes (AIs), and Tolerable Upper Intake Levels (ULs). The development of DRIs expands on the periodic reports called Recommended Dietary Allowances, which focus on preventing deficiency diseases and which have been published since 1941 by the National Academy of Sciences (National Academies Press, 2004). DRIs have been established for vitamins, minerals, carbohydrates, fats, and proteins and for water and electrolytes. As with the RDAs, DRIs are intended for maintaining a healthy population.

TABLE 14-1 Vitamins, Mineral Supplements, and Health Promotion Implications

Vitamins and Minerals	Dietary Use	Health Promotion Implications
Beta carotene	Antioxidant nutrient that neutralizes harmful substances called free radicals, resulting from body cells' normal metabolism.	Damage from free radicals may contribute to cardiovascular disease and cancer. Some studies have found that beta carotene increases risk of lung cancer in smokers.
Folic acid	Found to prevent spinal cord birth defects during pregnancy.	The Food and Drug Administration has mandated that all breads, cereals, pasta, and grain products be fortified with folic acid. Intake is kept below 1 mg to prevent risk of masking a vitamin B_{12} deficiency that may occur in the elderly.
Vitamin C (ascorbic acid)	Essential for formation of collagen and fibrous tissue, teeth, bone, cartilage, connective tissue, skin, and capillary walls.	Studies have found that people who have high vitamin C intakes have lower cardiovascular disease and cancer. The National Institutes of Health (NIH) Study has proposed raising the RDA from 60 to 200 mg. This recommendation is achieved with five servings of fruits and vegetables.
Vitamin D and calcium	Vitamin D and calcium work together. Vitamin D helps in absorbing dietary calcium and depositing it in the bones. Studies show that people who supplement their diets with Vitamin D and calcium experience slower bone loss and reduced number of fractures.	NIH scientists have recommended increasing the RDA of calcium from 800 mg to 1500 mg for those over the age of 65. This is equivalent to five eight-ounce glasses of milk per day. Age affects the ability to use vitamin D and calcium. Supplements may be appropriate for those who do not get enough of this vitamin and mineral in their foods, or who live in cloudy areas or rarely go outside.

(continued on next page)

Vitamins and Minerals	Dietary Use	Health Promotion Implications
Vitamin E	Fat-soluble antioxidant that protects against cardiovascular disease. Thought to prevent or slow progression of atherosclerosis. Also thought to prevent or slow progression of side effects associated with psychotropic drugs. Acts as an antihemolysis and is essential for reproduction and muscle development.	Vitamin E may affect prostaglandins that regulate a variety of body processes. More evidence of its efficacy and safety is needed prior to recommending vitamin E to the general population.
Selenium	Antioxidant thought to prevent cancer and cardiovascular disease.	More research is needed on this trace mineral. Taking excessive amounts of selenium may cause hair and nail loss.
Vitamin A	Necessary for vision, healthy epithelial tissue, proper bone growth, and energy regulation.	Dietary deficiencies may produce night blindness or impaired dim-light vision. Long-term intake of large amounts of vitamin A may lead to bone abnormalities.
Vitamin B complex (thiamine, riboflavin, B_6, B_{12}, folic acid, niacin, pantothenic acid, biotin)	Function as oxidative coenzymes by joining with enzymes to activate them. Group of vitamins essential for carbohydrate, fat, and protein metabolism and for nerve conduction; also participates in the synthesis of fatty acids; B_{12} is essential for normal red blood cell formation.	Deficiencies in B complex vitamins may cause peripheral neuropathy. Increased risk of deficiency found among those who smoke, miss meals, drink excessive alcohol, lose weight, or consume excessive sugars. Deficiencies may cause dermatitis, oral lesions, and anemias; Folic acid has been found to prevent spinal cord birth defects during pregnancy.
Vitamin K	Active role in blood clotting. Recently has been identified as needed for regulation of serum calcium levels.	Use may affect action of prescribed anticoagulants. Instructions regarding vitamin K intake should be provided to those taking warfarin.

From Nutrition and Diet Therapy, *by C. Lutz and K. Przytulski, 2006, Philadelphia: F. A. Davis; and* Nursing for Wellness in Older Adults: Theory and Practice *(4th ed.), by C. A. Miller, 2004, Philadelphia: Lippincott Williams & Wilkins.*

Water is a major part of every tissue of our bodies. It functions as the fluid in which substances are dissolved, broken down, and reformed for use by our bodies. Tables 14-2 (on pages 298–301) and 14-3 (on pages 300–303) list the nutrients, their functions, food sources, and deficiency and toxicity symptoms as well as the recommended dietary allowance (RDA) for each nutrient and/or the estimated safe and adequate daily dietary intake **(ESADDI). RDA** is the daily dietary intake that is sufficient to meet the nutrient requirements of 97 to 98 percent of all healthy individuals in the specific life-stage and gender groups. ESADDI provides a range of recommended intake for some nutrients, since not enough information is available to set a specific RDA.

Dietary Reference Intakes (DRIs) have also been established as bases for the amount of dietary intake that is sufficient to meet the nutritional requirements of the body. DRIs are four reference values that include the estimated average requirements, recommended dietary allowances, adequate intake levels (AI), and tolerable upper intake levels (UL). RDAs and DRIs may both be used as goals for individual dietary intake (Institute of Medicine of the National Academies, 2004).

Healthy People Goals and Nutritional Health

The goal of health promotion is to improve the overall health of all individuals. The United States has been actively pursuing this goal for almost three decades. National objectives related to health and health promotion have been established and serve as the basis for development of state and community health promotion plans (USDHHS, 2005b). *Healthy People* is a national health initiative under the jurisdiction of the U.S. Department of Health and Human Services (USDHHS) that identifies the most significant preventable threats to health and focuses efforts toward eliminating them. The *Healthy People* process began in 1979, and at the start of each decade the program sets goals for improving the nation's health during the following 10 years. One of the major accomplishments of *Healthy People 2000* included surpassing the target for reducing deaths from coronary heart disease and cancer. The nation also made progress toward the goal of reducing health disparities for more than one-half of the special population identified to be at increased risk.

An important development for the next decade is the publication of *Healthy People 2010: Understanding and Improving Health and Objectives for Improving Health* (USDHHS, 2000). As the third generation of 10-year goals for the nation, it builds on initiatives pursued over the past two decades. Central to *Healthy People 2010* are its two broad goals, which challenge the nation to (1) increase quality and years of healthy life and (2) eliminate health disparities. Like its predecessors, *Healthy People 2010* is the product of an extensive cooperative national process involving both the public and private sectors, including the Healthy People Consortium, which, by the end of the 20th century, had grown to include some 350 national organizations and 250 state public health, mental health, substance abuse, and environmental agencies. *Healthy People 2010* includes for the first time a set of 10 Leading Health Indicators (LHIs). These reflect major public health priorities in the United States at the beginning of the 21st century. The 10 LHIs are physical activity, overweight and obesity, tobacco use, substance abuse, responsible sexual behavior, mental health, injury and violence, environmental quality, immunization, and access to health care. Box 14-1 provides a description of *Healthy People 2010* Nutrition and Overweight Objectives. Box 14-2 provides a listing of *Healthy People 2010* focus areas.

BOX 14-1   *Healthy People 2010* Nutrition and Overweight Objectives

- Increase the proportion of adults who are at a healthy weight.
- Reduce the proportion of adults who are obese.
- Reduce the proportion of children and adolescents who are overweight or obese.
- Reduce growth retardation among low-income children under age 5.
- Increase the proportion of persons age 2 and older who consume at least two daily servings of fruit.
- Increase the proportion of persons age 2 and older who consume at least three daily servings of vegetables, with at least one-third being dark green or orange vegetables.
- Increase the proportion of persons age 2 and older who consume at least six daily servings of grain products, with at least three being whole grains.
- Increase the proportion of persons age 2 and older who consume less than 10 percent of kcalories from saturated fat.
- Increase the proportion of persons age 2 and older who consume no more than 30 percent of kcalories from total fat.
- Increase the proportion of persons age 2 and older who consume 2400 mg or less of sodium.
- Increase the proportion of persons age 2 and older who meet dietary recommendations for calcium.
- Reduce iron deficiency among young children, females of childbearing age, and pregnant females.
- Reduce anemia among low-income pregnant females in their third trimester.
- Increase the proportion of children and adolescents age 6 to 19 whose intake of meals and snacks at school contributes to good overall dietary quality.
- Increase the proportion of schools that teach all essential nutrition education topics in one course.
- Increase the proportion of work sites that offer nutrition or weight management classes or counseling.
- Increase the proportion of primary care providers who provide nutrition assessment when appropriate and who formulate a diet plan for those who need intervention.
- Increase the proportion of physician office visits made by patients with a diagnosis of cardiovascular disease, diabetes, or hyperlipidemia that include counseling or education related to diet and nutrition.
- Increase food security among U.S. households and in so doing reduce hunger.

Note: "*Nutrition and Overweight*" *is one of 28 focus areas, each with numerous objectives.*
From: Healthy People 2010, *www.healthypeople.gov.*

BOX 14-2 *Healthy People 2010* Focus Areas

- Access to quality health services
- Injury and violence prevention
- Arthritis, osteoporosis, and chronic back conditions
- Maternal, infant, and child health
- Cancer
- Medical product safety
- Chronic kidney disease
- Mental health and mental disorders
- Diabetes
- Nutrition and overweight
- Disability and secondary conditions
- Occupational safety and health
- Educational and community-based programs
- Oral health

- Environmental health
- Physical activity and fitness
- Family planning
- Public health infrastructure
- Food safety
- Respiratory distress
- Health communication
- Sexually transmitted diseases
- Heart disease and stroke
- Substance abuse
- HIV
- Tobacco use
- Immunization and infectious diseases
- Vision and hearing

From Healthy People 2010, *Department of Health and Human Services, 2000,*
http://www.healthypeople.gov/documents/tableofcontents.htm#Volume2.

TABLE 14-2 Energy Nutrients and Vitamins: Their Functions and Food Sources

Nutrients	Functions	Food Sources
Water	Body fluids—blood, saliva, digestive juices, urine	Water, beverages, foods
Energy nutrients **Carbohydrates: (glucose)**	Provides energy; protein sparing	Cereals, fruits, vegetables, milk
Lipid (fat) (essential lipid: linoleic acid)	Provides essential fatty acids and energy; absorbs and transports fat-soluble vitamins (A, D, E, and K); protects vital body tissues; insulates body	Fats and oils, meats, fish, nuts, some seeds, dairy products
Protein (essential amino acids: histidine, isoleucine, leucine, lysine, methionine, phenylalanine, threonine, tryptophan, valine)	Growth and repair of tissues; maintains fluid and acid-base balances; provides energy	Meats, fish, dairy products, eggs, nuts, legumes, cereals
Vitamins **Fat-Soluble** A	Affects vision; health of skin; growth of hair, nails, bones, and glands; prevents infections	Dairy products; liver; green, yellow, and orange fruits and vegetables; dairy products
D	Calcium and phosphorus absorption; bone mineralization	Dairy products, egg yolks, fatty fish

DOMAINS INFLUENCING EATING BEHAVIOR

Good health depends on many factors such as adequate diet, family health history, level of physical activity, and other lifestyle behaviors. Adequate nutritional status not only is important in maintaining structural integrity but also adds to our quality of life. Our food choices as well as food-related activities are usually associated with pleasurable events, social and cultural interactions, and caring and comfort (Miller, 2004). Although healthy eating can be simple, eating behaviors can be influenced by multiple factors. These multiple factors can be categorized in terms of the biological, psychological, sociocultural, spiritual, and environmental domains that have been previously identified as influencing health promotion. Technology has also affected eating behavior as well as food preparation.

Biological Domain

Energy requirements affect eating behavior. Infants, children, and adolescents, for example, require a high caloric intake that should contain adequate amounts of the recommended nutrients. Older adults, too, have special nutritional needs. Evidence indicates that older adults require an increased intake of several nutrients because of diminished absorption and utilization of nutrients. In addition, food interactions with multiple medications must be considered and adjustments made. Medications can affect food consumption through adverse effects such as anorexia, constipation, and chewing discomfort (Miller, 2004). If caloric intake is inadequate to meet energy needs, fatigue, listlessness, and apathy can result. If the body's energy requirements are not met, growth retardation may occur in children.

Deficiency	Toxicity	RDA***
Dehydration: thirst, loss of appetite, nausea, headache, lightheaded, fatigue, low blood pressure, low pulse, shock	Water intoxication: loss of appetite, edema, loss of conciousness, increased blood pressure	Adults 19-30 years: 3.7 liters for men and 2.7 liters for women; 30+ monitored individually; Infants: 1.5 ml per kilocalorie ingested
Protein store breakdown, fat breakdown, ketosis, fatigue, nausea, lack of appetite	None	45–65% of kilocalories consumed
Increased hunger, inadequate minerals, vitamins, and fatty acids	Increased cardiovascular risk, obesity, diabetes	Children: 25-40% of kilocalories ingested Adults: 20-35% of kilocalories ingested
Lack of energy, poor wound healing, thinning hair, marasmus, kwashiorkor, muscle wasting, mental retardation, albumin, deficiency, edema, lower immunity levels	None	Men: 56 g Women: 46 g Lactating women: 71 g
Night blindness, xerophthalmia, poor growth, dry skin	Fetal malformations, hair loss, skin changes, bone pain	*Females* 800 RE (4000 IU)* *Males* 1000 RE (5000 IU) 5–10 ug (200–400 IU)
Rickets, osteomalacia	Growth retardation, kidney damage, calcium deposits in soft tissue	

TABLE 14-2 Energy Nutrients and Vitamins: Their Functions and Food Sources, *continued*

Nutrients	Functions	Food Sources
E	Antioxidant—prevents cell damage	Vegetable oils, nuts, seeds, whole grains
K	Blood clotting	Green vegetables
Water-Soluble C	Antioxidant—prevents cell damage; causes collagen formation; affects health of teeth and gums	Citrus fruits, green peppers, broccoli, cantaloupe, kiwi fruit, cabbage, strawberries
B complex Thiamine (B$_1$)	Muscle nerve function; coenzyme for energy metabolism	Whole grains and enriched cereals, pork, legumes, seeds, nuts
Riboflavin (B$_2$)	Coenzyme for energy metabolism	Whole grains and enriched cereal products, eggs, meats, fish, green leafy vegetables
Niacin	Coenzyme for energy metabolism	Meats, fish, nuts, whole grains, eggs
Pyridoxine (B$_6$)	Metabolism of amino acids and protein, neurotransmitter synthesis	Whole grains, most high-protein foods, spinach, broccoli
Folic acid (folacin)	Aids metabolism of DNA and RNA (genetic material); red blood cell maturation	Green leafy vegetables, nuts, legumes, grain products
B$_{12}$	Folate metabolism, nerve function	Foods of animal origin; microorganisms in fermented foods
Pantothenic acid	Coenzyme for energy metabolism	Most foods of plant and animal origin
Biotin	Coenzyme for energy metabolism	Most foods of plant and animal origin

*Retinol Equivalents
**Tocopherol Equivalents

***RDAs and DRIs (Specifically AIs) may both be used as goals for individual intake (Institute of Medicine of the National Academies, 2004).

TABLE 14-3 Minerals: Their Functions and Food Sources

Nutrients	Functions	Food Sources
Macrominerals Calcium	Forms bones and teeth; blood clotting, nerve function, muscle contraction	Dairy products, dark green vegetables, fortified orange juice
Phosphorus	Forms bones and teeth; part of some coenzymes; major ion of intracellular fluid	Dairy products, meats, processed foods, soft drinks
Magnesium	Nerve and muscle function; part of some coenzymes, bone strength	Green vegetables, whole grain cereals, nuts, chocolate, legumes

Deficiency	Toxicity	RDA***
Red blood cell destruction, nerve destruction	None; no supplements with anticoagulant drugs	*Females* 8 mg or-TE** *Males* 10 mg or-TE
Hemorrhage	Anemia, jaundice	*Females:* 65 mg *Males:* 70 mg
Scurvy, poor wound healing, pinpoint hemorrhages, bleeding gums	> 2 g can cause diarrhea, kidney stone formation	60 mg
Beriberi, poor coordination, edema, weakness	None	*Females:* 1.1 mg *Males:* 1.5 mg
Ariboflavinois, cheilosis, glossitis, seborrheic dermatitis, pellagra	None	*Females:* 1.3 mg *Males:* 1.7 mg
Pellagra, dermatitis, diarrhea, dementia	Vasodilation, liver damage	*Females:* 15 mg NE *Males:* 19 mg NE
Headache, anemia, convulsions, nausea	Nerve destruction > 2 g/day	*Females:* 1.6 mg *Males:* 2.0 mg
Megaloblastic anemia, poor growth, birth defects	None	*Females:* 180 mg *Males:* 200 mg
Megaloblastic anemia, poor nerve function	None	2.0 mg
Fatigue, headache, nausea	None	4–7 mg
Dermatitis, anemia	None	30–100 mg

Deficiency	Toxicity	RDA* or ESADDI
Osteoporosis	May cause kidney stones in susceptible people	800 mg (age > 24 yrs) 1200 mg (age 11–24 yrs)
None	Hampers bone health in people with kidney failure	800 mg (age > 24 yrs) 1200 mg (age 11–24 yrs)
Weakness, muscle pain, poor heart function	Weakness in people with kidney failure	*Females:* 280 mg *Males:* 350 mg

TABLE 14-3 Minerals: Their Functions and Food Sources, *continued*

Nutrients	Functions	Food Sources
Sulfur	Part of amino acids and vitamins, drug detoxification	Protein foods
Sodium	Nerve and muscle function and body fluid balance	Salt (sodium chloride), soy sauce, processed foods, cheese, chips
Potassium	Nerve and muscle function and body fluid balance	Dairy products, fruits and vegetables (especially bananas), whole grains, legumes, meats
Chloride	Nerve and muscle function, body fluid balance; forms hydrochloric acid in the stomach	Salt, soy sauce, salted foods, cheese, processed foods
Microminerals (Trace minerals) Iron	Transports oxygen (in hemoglobin in blood)	Meats, legumes, cereals, eggs
Zinc	Coenzyme; heals wounds; affects taste, sexual development	Whole grains, seafood, tea, meats, greens
Iodine	Part of thyroid hormones	Seafood, iodized salt, dairy products, some breads
Selenium	Part of antioxidant system, glutathione peroxidase; acts with vitamin E	Seafood, whole grains, meats
Fluoride	Affects tooth and bone structure	Fluoridated drinking water, seafood, tea, seaweed
Copper	Coenzyme	Cocoa, seafood, nuts, legumes, liver
Chromium	Glucose and energy metabolism	Brewer's yeast, seafood, meat, liver
Manganese	Coenzyme	Whole grains, fruits, nuts, vegetables
Molybdenum	Coenzyme	Cereals, legumes, some vegetables

*RDAs and DRIs (specifically AIs) may both be used as goals for individual intake (Institute of Medicine of the National Academies, 2004).

Biological changes can also affect the eating behaviors of people in all age groups. This is especially true as a person gets older. Changes that occur as a result of aging include diminished taste and smell acuity, which, as might be suspected, contribute to a decreased enjoyment of food. Other changes that occur as a result of aging may contribute to nutritional deficiencies. Energy requirements depend on age and body size. Older individuals experience a decrease in energy requirements with a subsequent reduction in lean body mass (Pender, Murdaugh, & Parsons, 2006). Other changes include a decrease in the body's basal metabolic rate and composition. **Basal metabolic rate** is the rate at which the body uses energy to support its involuntary activities that are necessary to life, such as breathing and digestion. The biological domain is quite important when considering nutrition and its implications for health promotion. The ease with which our bodies burn energy determines whether we will gain or lose weight. Adjustment in caloric intake is essential to maintaining a healthy weight. Other biological factors that influence our energy requirements include gastrointestinal motility and caloric absorption. If there is a decreased gastrointestinal motility, constipation may result. A high intake

Deficiency	Toxicity	RDA* or ESADDI
None	None	None
Muscle cramps	Hypertension in susceptible individuals, hypercalciuria	500 mg
Irregular heartbeat, appetite loss, muscle cramps	Slow heart rate	2000 mg
Convulsions in infants	Hypertension in susceptible people, when combined with sodium	700 mg
Low blood hemoglobin levels	Seen in people with hemochromatosis	*Females:* 15 mg *Males:* 10 mg
Skin rash, loss of taste, hair loss, poor wound healing, poor growth and development	Decreased immune function, diarrhea, cramps	*Females:* 12 mg *Males:* 15 mg
Goiter, poor growth in infancy	Inhibits thyroid function	150 mg
Muscle pain and weakness	Nausea, vomiting, hair loss, weakness	55–70 mg
Increased risk of dental caries	Mottling of teeth during development, bone pain	1.5–4 mg
Anemia, poor growth	Vomiting, nervous system disorders	1.5–3 mg
High blood glucose	None	50–200 mg
None	None	2–5 mg
None	None	75–250 mg

of high-fiber foods, such as fruits, vegetables, and whole wheat grains, and an increase in fluids increase motility. Likewise, a decrease in hydrochloric acid may result in decreased absorption of some nutrients such as iron, calcium, and vitamin B_{12}.

Psychological Domain

In American society, the media bombard us with images of what constitutes the ideal body image. We are led to believe that the average person is eternally young and slim, and, of course, beautiful. The supermodels with their waiflike appearance and ultraslim bodies encourage an anorexic, unhealthy weight and look. Our goal, it seems, should be to lose weight and eat as if we are on a perpetual weight-reduction diet. Many of the programs on television and radio, as well as all of the literature available to our communities, stress dieting as the ultimate goal. Television programs, advertisements, magazines, newspapers, and movies are proponents of this ultraslim body that is presumed to bring fame, success and happiness. Unfortunately, young people are especially susceptible to these messages and are more likely to alter their eating behaviors to maintain slim bodies.

Researchers have reported that as much as 1 percent of the adolescent female population has anorexia. That means that one out of every 100 females between the ages of 10 and 20 is starving herself, sometimes to death. No reliable figures for younger children and older adults exist, but cases are not very common (ANRED, 2005). Many people such as models, actresses, ballet dancers, figure skaters, and gymnasts, whose professions require slim bodies, have long-standing histories of anorexia nervosa or bulimia.

Food is also linked with personal emotional experiences. Many of our memories may be closely associated with foods. Food is a source of both comfort and pleasure. Eating certain foods can have the ability to stimulate the release of certain substances, called opioids, that produce a sense of calm and euphoria in the human body. Some foods such as those that contain chocolate have been found to produce these effects and thus may be overconsumed.

Sociocultural, Religious, and Spiritual Domains

The United States is considered the melting pot of the world since its people come from many different cultural and ethnic backgrounds. The different types of foods found in this country reflect the intermingling of cultures. It is not unusual to walk or drive on a main street and see restaurants offering foods, even fast foods, from different ethnic origins. Some of these ethnic foods featured in restaurants include Mexican tacos, Chinese egg rolls, Italian lasagna and pizzas, Greek gyros, and French croissants. The choices are endless and usually only restricted by what the consumers can afford.

Ethnic, religious and spiritual, and cultural backgrounds influence eating behaviors as do a person's parents' beliefs and knowledge about what constitutes a healthy diet. The consequence of this is that the foods people eat may be totally different from the foods recommended by different scientific organizations and dietary associations. Many food habits are culturally based. One example of foods that are firmly intertwined with culture is the inclusion of tortillas and beans as a staple in the diet

of the Mexican American. These foods in combination, fortunately, provide sufficient nutritional benefits. Neither corn nor beans alone supply the essential amino acids to maintain optimum health. Combined, they provide a complete protein. Culturally based dietary customs are usually not a source of concern in health promotion. The primary concern, however, is whether the foods usually eaten are nutritious and do not aggravate any underlying health conditions. For example, some of the foods like tamales (lard and corn dough filled with a variety of meats or fruit or both) and menudo (tripe) enjoyed by Mexican Americans are loaded with saturated fats and may not be suitable eating choices for those who are overweight or who have diabetes or high levels of blood cholesterol.

A limited income may also influence food choices and food purchases. If nutrient intake is inadequate due to financial limitations, the nutritional status of the individual may be affected. This may be especially true in older adults who may have age-related changes in nutritional needs (Miller, 2004). Also, in certain parts of the world, some foods may not be available to or accessible by the general population. In some countries, people may have a narrower choice of food selection. In many countries, some of the staples that make up sound nutritional choices may be simply unattainable.

Although religious and spiritual beliefs are not necessarily synonymous, it is important to note that these may play a part in a person's eating behaviors. Some individuals belonging to a particular religious sect, for example, may have certain food restrictions. Others may follow food regimens that are based on spiritual beliefs. Seventh-Day Adventists, for example, have guidelines about what their congregational members can eat. Orthodox Jews require that some foods be consumed only in certain combinations. Spiritual beliefs can also guide food preferences. Followers of the Indian Ayurvedic principles, for instance, focus on a holistic approach that involves the entire body, including spiritual fulfillment. According to Ayurveda, all foods have their own heating or cooling energy and a postdigestive effect. Food combinations are also of great importance in Ayurveda. If two or more foods have different energies, tastes, and postdigestive effects, they can overload the stomach and inhibit enzymes, resulting in toxin production. If these same foods are eaten separately, they may stimulate digestion and help to burn energy. Poor food combinations can result in indigestion, fermentation, and putrefaction, and, if eaten on a regular basis, can lead to toxemia and disease (Lad, 2003). Geographical location as well as whether an individual lives in the city or the country also influence what foods are consumed.

Environmental Domain

The American food environment is changing toward healthier eating behavior. Currently there are thousands of low-fat products sold in grocery stores, and these foods continue to increase. New mandatory food labels on all packaged foods contain useful and accurate information to assist individuals and families in making healthy food choices.

Convenience foods make up a large percentage of the American diet (Wardlaw, 2000). However, the nutrient quality of many fast foods is questionable. Such foods are usually high in fat, salt, and refined carbohydrates and low in dietary fiber and important nutrients. With the increased awareness of a healthful diet, fast-food restaurants are now providing lower-fat food choices for consumers. Ease of preparation also plays an important role in food selection. Quick preparation techniques appeal to families who have busy schedules.

Technical Domain

The food environment has changed throughout the world as a result of revolutionary technology that affects food production, food preparation, safety, and composition. Food engineering has resulted in bigger, more attractive, and better-tasting crops. It has also been used to develop the type of nutrition needed by livestock so that these animals are bigger and produce better-tasting and more tender meats. Technology has also changed the landscape of food preparation. Foods can be prepared faster, for example, in convection ovens and can be made to taste and look like the foods that previously took hours to cook, broil, or brown. These foods are now more visually appealing when prepared that way and may be more likely to be eaten than when prepared in a microwave or conventional oven.

Technology has also been used to protect foods and make them safer for consumption. For example, synthetic cysteine, used to condition dough and to produce meat flavors, is used instead of natural cysteine derived from hair or feathers. Technology can also be used as a diagnostic tool to determine the level of nutrients needed by certain age groups. Levels of antioxidants in tissues, for example, can be scanned in minutes, revealing information about the current state of health and a person's health future (Adams, 2005).

NUTRITIONAL EXCESSES, DEFICITS, FADS, AND HEALTH PROMOTION

Nutritional excesses as well as nutritional deficits can affect the health of individuals young and old. These nutritional states known commonly as overnutrition, or obesity, and undernutrition, or anorexia, are quite prevalent in the United States and the world today. Popular nutritional fads capitalize on our need to be thin, beautiful, and active. Many nutritional fads exist and influence our consumption, whether the fad is to eliminate excess weight or provide for optimal energy. All nursing professionals who are involved in client teaching should be aware of the impact of nutritional excesses and deficits and nutritional fads on health promotion and health-promoting client behaviors.

Overnutrition

Although hunger still exists in the United States, a more significant problem is overnutrition rather than undernutrition. Of the leading causes of death in the United States, several are associated with dietary excesses and with excessive alcohol consumption (CDC, 2003). It has been noted that an increase in chronic diseases is associated with an excessive intake of certain nutrients such as saturated fats, cholesterol, sodium, and sugars. Government agencies, voluntary health associations, and scientific associations have made dietary recommendations to address the problem of increases in diet-related diseases such as heart disease, hypertension, cancer, diabetes, osteoporosis, and obesity. There is consensus among these agencies that dietary guidelines are essential for the maintenance of good general health. Recommendations from these groups have been issued as national goals. There is agreement that obesity is of national concern and that the intake of total fat, saturated fat, cholesterol, and sodium should be reduced, starting at about 2 years of age. Further recommendations include avoidance of excessive caloric intake and increased intake of dietary fiber, complex carbohydrates, fruits, and vegetables. These goals are the basis of health promotion efforts for chronic disease prevention.

Undernutrition

It may seem that overnutrition and obesity are the primary problems facing U.S. citizens; however, there are many people in the United States that are going hungry today. Some reasons for the incidence of undernourishment in our population may include poverty, ignorance of what constitutes a healthy diet, and eating disorders such as anorexia nervosa and bulimia.

Anorexia Nervosa

Anorexia nervosa may be defined as the relentless pursuit of thinness or a prolonged refusal to eat or maintain normal body weight for age or height. This condition is seen primarily in adolescent girls although it has also been found (infrequently) to occur in males, young children, and the elderly (ANRED, 2005). The disorder is thought to originate from emotional or stress-related conflicts such as anger, irritation, body-image disturbance, and fear of losing control. Anorexia nervosa often includes depression, irritability, withdrawal, and peculiar behaviors such as compulsive or strange eating habits (ANRED, 2005). The goals of treatment are to help the client achieve emotional as well as physical health.

Bulimia

Bulimia is an eating disorder that is also referred to as the diet-binge-purge disorder (ANRED, 2005). A food-gorging binge is followed by a period where the individual feels out of control and purges the food. These episodes usually involve the uncontrolled, rapid ingestion of large quantities of food and usually begin in adolescence or early adult life. The typical bulimic is female and college-aged or in her early twenties (Keltner, Schwecke, & Bostrom, 2003). Research suggests that about 4 percent, or four out of 100, college-age women have bulimia. Anorexics can also develop bulimia. In fact, 50 percent of people who have been anorexic develop bulimia or bulimic patterns. Because people with bulimia are secretive, it is difficult to know how many older people are affected. Bulimia is rarely seen in children (ANRED, 2005). The goal of treatment in bulimia is similar to that of anorexia. The client is helped to focus on resolving psychological issues that may have precipitated the eating disorder and to progress to a state of physical health.

Nutritional Fads

Nutritional fads and myths abound in today's media and literature. These fads and nutritional myths can be costly in terms of money and in terms of impact on a person's health. There are thousands of health claims associated with what we eat (University of Iowa Health Center, 2005). These health claims or myths are frequently taken as truth. For example, there are claims that certain foods such as grapefruits can burn fat and that foods like garlic prevent heart disease. Although these claims are quite popular, the truth is that many of these claims have not proven to be clinically significant (Almada, 2001). Individuals are always looking for the quick results approach. Normally what is proposed to be the wonder solution for making us lean or more energetic is a very ordinary, everyday item that will neither kill us nor make us better (Loeschorn, 2002). On a daily basis, every magazine and newspaper on the newsstand propose a new magical diet plan, food, or nutrient that can make us thinner, younger, healthier, and probably more beautiful. The truth is that certain foods are good for us and that a balanced diet and activity plan are essential to maintaining health. A variety of nutritious foods can replace fad diets and supplements. See Chapter 16 for more information on different fad diets and issues surrounding weight control.

Fad diets have been around for decades. These diets have included drinks that increase physical endurance, vitamins and herbs that improve physical stamina, and protein and amino acids that supposedly build muscle and improve the immune response. The latest and hottest nutritional fads today include a wide variety of energy drinks. These drinks are used as nutritional supplements and usually contain high concentrations of carbohydrates and amino acids and some caffeine. These substances have not proven to have any noticeable effect on performance (Bonci, 2002). In fact, because there is little or no regulatory control on these products, they can pose a potential health risk and in some cases may be fatal.

DIETARY STRATEGIES TO PROMOTE A HEALTHFUL DIET

A healthful diet consists of the essential nutrients and calories needed to prevent nutritional deficiencies and excesses. Nurses are increasingly responsible for determining appropriate strategies to assist clients to select healthy diet choices. These strategies should ensure that the diet selected provides the right balance of carbohydrate, fat, protein, vitamins, and minerals. Such a diet is not difficult to achieve since there is a large variety of foods that are available and enjoyable. The following sections will describe dietary guidelines that are necessary in promoting wellness and healthful eating.

Dietary Guidelines for Americans 2005

Dietary Guidelines for Americans is published jointly every five years by the U.S. Department of Health and Human Services (USDHHS) and the U.S. Department of Agriculture (USDA). The **Dietary Guidelines** provide authoritative, science-based advice for people 2 years and older on how to promote health and reduce the risk for major chronic diseases through diet and physical activity (USDHHS, 2005). The purposes of the *Guidelines* are to summarize and synthesize knowledge regarding individual nutrients and food components and to make recommendations for a pattern of eating that can be adopted by the public. Key recommendations are grouped into nine interrelated focus areas (see Table 14-4). These recommendations are based on the preponderance of scientific evidence for lowering the risk of chronic disease and promoting health by eating fewer calories, being more active, and making wise food choices.

Nutrient needs should be met primarily through the consumption of foods. Foods that provide an array of essential nutrients have a beneficial effect on individual health. Fortified foods and dietary supplements may be

TABLE 14-4 *Dietary Guidelines for Americans* Focus Areas and Selected Recommendations

Focus Area	Recommendations
Adequate nutrients within calorie needs	Consume a variety of nutrient dense foods. Limit fats, sugars, salt, and alcohol.
Weight management	Balance calories consumed with calories expended. Make small decreases in food and beverage calories and increase physical activity.
Physical activity	Engage in regular physical activity and reduce sedentary activities. Engage in at least 30 minutes of moderate-intensity activity most days of the week. Include cardiovascular conditioning, stretching exercises for flexibility, and resistance exercises for muscle strength.
Food groups to encourage	Consume a sufficient amount of fruits and vegetables. Consume three or more ounces of whole grain products per day. Consume three cups per day of fat-free or low-fat milk or equivalent milk products.
Fats	Consume less than 10 percent of calories from saturated fatty acids and less than 300 mg of cholesterol. Keep total fat intake between 20 and 35 percent of calories. Limit intake of fats and oils high in saturated or trans fatty acids or both.
Carbohydrates	Choose fiber-rich fruits, grains, and vegetables often. Practice good oral hygiene to prevent dental caries caused by sugar- and starch-containing foods.
Sodium and potassium	Consume less than 2,300 mg of sodium per day. Consume potassium-rich foods, such as fruits and vegetables.
Alcoholic beverages	Consume no more than one drink per day for women and two for men. Avoid alcohol when engaging in activities that require attention.
Food safety	Clean hands, food contact surfaces, and fruits and vegetables. Meat and poultry should be washed or rinsed. Cook foods to a safe temperature. Chill perishable foods. Avoid raw (unpasteurized) milk or any products made with it. Avoid raw eggs and foods that contain raw eggs.

Adapted from Dietary Guidelines for Americans, *2005, Washington, DC: US. Department of Health and Human Services, http://www.health.gov/dietaryguidelines.*

useful sources of one or more nutrients that otherwise might be consumed in less than recommended amounts. Dietary supplements, while recommended in some cases, cannot replace a healthful diet.

One example of an eating plan that is based on the premises of the *Dietary Guidelines* is the DASH (Dietary Approaches to Stop Hypertension) Eating Plan. This plan is designed to assist adults in making healthy lifestyle choices that include foods that speed the rate of sodium excretion and help in avoiding high blood pressure

(Schultz, 2003). DASH recommendations include foods low in total fat, saturated fat, and cholesterol, and foods such as fruits, vegetables, and low-fat dairy products. The diet is constructed across a range of calorie levels to meet the needs of the various age and gender groups. The DASH diet recommends that people make healthy changes in their lifestyle to avoid developing high blood pressure and its complications (Schultz, 2003).

In describing the *Dietary Guidelines* it is essential to understand how culture affects individual dietary plans.

Research Note

Improvement of Weight and Fat-Free Mass with Oral Nutritional Supplementation

Study Problem/Purpose: To examine the effects of oral nutritional supplements (OS) on body weight, body composition, nutritional status, and cognition in elderly clients with Alzheimer's disease. Nutritional deficiencies in the elderly who have a cognition problem occur frequently.

Methods: This was a prospective, randomized, controlled study conducted in geriatric wards and day care centers in France. Ninety-one Alzheimer's disease subjects age 65 and older at risk of undernutrition as evaluated by the Mini Nutritional Assessment were included in this study. After randomization, 46 clients received three months of OS. The other 45 received the usual care without OS. Weight, body composition, cognitive function, activities of daily living, eating behavior, and dietary intakes were evaluated at the beginning of the study and at three months and six months.

Findings: Between the first evaluation and three months, energy and protein intakes significantly improved in the group receiving OS, resulting in a significant increase in weight and fat-free mass. No significant changes were found for dependence, cognition function, or biological markers. The six-month benefit of OS was maintained in the intervention group even after discontinuation of the OS at three months.

Implications: The results indicate that even three months of OS improves body weight. OS is practical and effective, and regular courses of OS may help to maintain the fat-free mass and improve the nutritional status of clients.

Lauque, S., et al. (2004). Improvement of weight and fat-free mass with oral nutritional supplementation in patients with Alzheimer's disease at risk for malnutrition: A prospective randomized study. *Journal of the American Geriatrics Society, 52*(10), 1702-1707.

It is important to incorporate the food preferences of different racial/ethnic groups, vegetarians, and other groups when planning diets and developing educational programs and materials. Cultural sensitivity in relation to types of foods eaten and meaning of foods for ethnic populations is essential when counseling people about dietary and nutritional needs.

MyPyramid

MyPyramid replaced the Food Guide Pyramid introduced in 1992 by the U.S. Department of Health and Human Services and the U.S. Department of Agriculture (USDA, 2005). The **Food Guide Pyramid** was designed to help in following the *Dietary Guidelines for Americans* by providing a guide to the amounts and kinds of foods that we should eat daily to maintain health and to reduce risks of developing diet-related diseases. The guiding principles for MyPyramid are the same. These principles focus on overall health, provide up-to-date research, and focus on an individual's total dietary needs. The main goals of MyPyramid are to: (1) improve its effectiveness in motivating consumers to make healthier food choices, and (2) ensure that the USDHHS/USDA food guidance system reflects the latest nutritional science. MyPyramid incorporates recommendations from the 2005 *Dietary Guidelines for Americans* and makes Americans aware of the vital health benefits of simple and modest improvements in nutrition, physical activity, and lifestyle behavior (see Figure 14-1). In contrast to the previous Food Guide Pyramid, MyPyramid's approach to nutrition is not "one size fits all." Instead, it demonstrates an individualized, personalized recommendation about daily food intake. A personalized recommendation on the kinds and amounts of food to be eaten to gain weight, lose weight, or maintain weight can be found at MyPyramid.gov. This new food pyramid encourages gradual nutritional improvements and suggests that each individual can benefit from taking small steps to improve diet and lifestyle patterns each day.

MyPyramid is a very comprehensive guide for achieving nutritional health. Much thought was given to providing a pictorial depiction of the food guidelines. Physical activity as well as dietary planning are emphasized and are represented by the steps found on the pyramid graphic. Variety of the food groups is symbolized by the six color bands representing the five food groups and oils. Foods from all six groups are needed each day for good health. Moderation is one of the key messages of MyPyramid. Moderation is represented by the narrowing of each food group from top to bottom. The wider base stands for foods with little or no solid fats, added sugars, or caloric sweeteners. These should be selected more often to get the most nutrition from calories consumed. Proportionality is also shown by the different widths of the "good group" bands. The width suggests how much food a person should choose from each group. Caution should be taken, however; the widths are just a general guide and not exact proportions.

The website MyPyramid.gov contains interactive activities that make it easy for individuals to key in their age, gender, and physical activity level so that a personalized recommendation can be made. The site also provides motivational tools and educational resources for

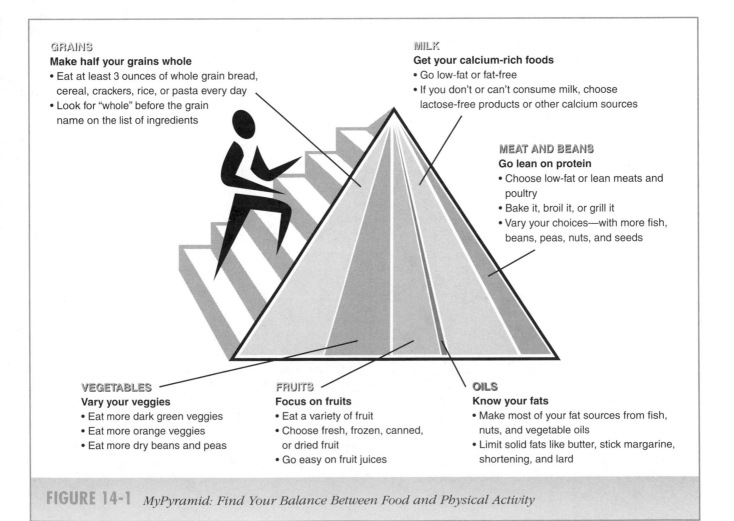

GRAINS
Make half your grains whole
- Eat at least 3 ounces of whole grain bread, cereal, crackers, rice, or pasta every day
- Look for "whole" before the grain name on the list of ingredients

MILK
Get your calcium-rich foods
- Go low-fat or fat-free
- If you don't or can't consume milk, choose lactose-free products or other calcium sources

MEAT AND BEANS
Go lean on protein
- Choose low-fat or lean meats and poultry
- Bake it, broil it, or grill it
- Vary your choices—with more fish, beans, peas, nuts, and seeds

VEGETABLES
Vary your veggies
- Eat more dark green veggies
- Eat more orange veggies
- Eat more dry beans and peas

FRUITS
Focus on fruits
- Eat a variety of fruit
- Choose fresh, frozen, canned, or dried fruit
- Go easy on fruit juices

OILS
Know your fats
- Make most of your fat sources from fish, nuts, and vegetable oils
- Limit solid fats like butter, stick margarine, shortening, and lard

FIGURE 14-1 *MyPyramid: Find Your Balance Between Food and Physical Activity*

consumers. Individuals can find general food guidance and suggestions for making smart choices from each food group. A tracker is included so that an individual can receive more detailed information on diet quality and physical activity status by comparing a day's worth of foods eaten to the current nutritional recommendation.

Because the previous "one size fits all" approach is no longer appropriate, it is difficult to determine the number of daily servings needed according to food groups in relation to gender, physical activity, and age. Instead, personalized and individualized food group information is provided, including daily amounts in commonly used measures like cups and ounces. Examples and everyday tips are also included. Downloadable suggestions on all of the food groups and required physical activity are also available.

The Exchange System: A Menu Planning Tool

The **exchange system** is another valuable tool for quickly estimating the energy, protein, carbohydrate, and fat content of a meal. It was developed by the American Dietetic Association and the American Diabetes

Association (American Diabetes Association, 2005). It is a system for classifying foods into numerous lists based on their macronutrient composition and for establishing serving sizes so that one serving of each food on a list contains the same amount of carbohydrate, protein, fat, and energy (calories). By using the exchange system, people may plan daily menus without having to look up the nutrient values of numerous foods.

The meal planning exchange lists have been expanded to include a greater variety of commonly consumed foods, carbohydrate counts for each food portion, portion weights in ounces, reduced-fat and fat-free foods, and vegetarian alternatives as well as fast foods. The revised exchange system remains the same in many ways, but new food groups have been added, thus allowing more flexibility in choosing foods (American Diabetes Association, 2005).

Exchange lists are designed so that when the proper serving size is used, each food on a list provides about the same amount of carbohydrate, protein, fat, and energy. This equality allows the exchange of foods on each list. Thus an individual is able to choose favorite foods from each list while controlling the amount and kind of carbohydrates consumed throughout the day. Since the exchange lists encourage variety while helping to control calories and grams of carbohydrates, protein, and fats, these lists have been adapted to meet the needs of weight reduction programs and medical nutrition therapy planning. See Chapter 16 for other weight control strategies.

Food Labels

Food labels are the best way for consumers to see how individual foods fit their own nutritional needs. In 1993, the Food and Drug Administration made it easier to figure out serving sizes by improving the nutrition labels that appear on food packages. An example of a label for processed foods is shown in Figure 14-2.

The nutrition facts panel lists the quantities of energy (calories), fat, and specific other nutrients in a serving: total food energy, food energy from fat, total fat, saturated fat, cholesterol, sodium, total carbohydrates, dietary fiber, sugars, protein, vitamin A, vitamin C, calcium, and iron. The information on the label is not based on the entire contents of the package. It is calculated for a typical portion, or serving, of that food.

Paying attention to serving sizes can help an individual make informed choices about what to eat. However, labels are not available in a restaurant. About a third of all meals are eaten at restaurants today, and many entrees can contain up to a day's worth of servings from several food groups. Although the cooking method or the serving size in a restaurant cannot always be controlled, a person can always request a take-home container if there is too much food on the plate. This will reduce the serving size of a meal and, perhaps, allow for continued enjoyment of the food at a later time.

Nutrition Facts

Serving Size 1/2 cup (114g)
Servings Per Container 4

Amount Per Serving

Calories 90	Calories from Fat 30

	% Daily Value
Total Fat 3g	5%
Saturated Fat 0g	0%
Cholesterol 0mg	0%
Sodium 300mg	13%
Total Carbohydrate 13g	4%
Dietary Fiber 3g	12%
Sugars 3g	
Protein 3g	

Vitamin A	80%	•	Vitamin C	60%
Calcium	4%	•	Iron	4%

• Percent Daily Values are based on a 2,000 calorie diet. Your daily values may be higher or lower depending on your calorie needs:

		Calories	2,000	2,500
Total Fat	Less than		65g	80g
Sat Fat	Less than		20g	25g
Cholesterol	Less than		300mg	300mg
Sodium	Less than		2,400mg	2,400mg
Total Carbohydrate			300g	375g
Fiber			25g	30g

Calories per gram:
Fat 9 • Carbohydrate 4 • Protein 4

FIGURE 14-2 *Sample Food Label*

The Five a Day Program

The Five a Day program is the first government and private industry partnership intended to improve our health. This is a collaborative effort of the National Cancer Institute, DHHS, and the Produce for Better Health Foundation, a nonprofit consumer education foundation (National Cancer Institute, 2000; CDC, 2006). The purpose of the program is to increase our consumption of fruits and vegetables to at least five servings a day. By doing so, goals of the *Dietary Guidelines for Americans, Healthy People 2010*, and other dietary recommendations may be achieved.

By focusing on fruits and vegetables, the Five a Day guide becomes an easy way to decrease the intake of fats since fruits and vegetables are naturally low in fat. There are a variety of chemical compounds present naturally in foods that include some of the well-known vitamins and other components of food. They include carotenoids such as beta-carotene, vitamins C and E, selenium, dietary fiber, and other substances such as dithiolthiones, isothiocyanates, indoles, phenols, and phytoestrogens. These are known as **phytochemicals**, which are bioactive compounds of plant origin that can provide protection against heart disease, arthritis, and some types of cancer (Phytochemicals, 2006). With five servings of fruits and vegetables each day, increased consumption of these phytochemicals will also occur.

The National Cancer Institute has spent a lot of effort researching the anticancer constituents of plant foods. Those foods and herbs found to possess anticancer activity include garlic, soybean, ginger, and cruciferous vegetables (brocooli, cabbage, and Brussels sprouts) (Warner, 2002). Other plant foods are currently being evaluated to determine their safety, efficacy, and applicability for preventing and treating cancer.

Nutritional Issues and Health Promotion Strategies

Although nutritional health is an important health promotion focus area, little attention has been paid to nutritional issues despite the cultural and biological importance of food and eating, and the deleterious effects of malnutrition and overnutrition (Perry & McLaren, 2004). Adequate nutritional status is dependent on a whole array of contributing factors and issues that can impact nutritional outcomes. These may include such factors as amount and type of dietary intake, quality of life issues, economic concerns, emotional issues, poor eating behaviors, structural defects, and underlying diseases and conditions. Poor nutritional status and substantial dietary inadequacy may result from poor self-esteem; for example, anorexia is typically seen in adolescent girls and is considered to be related to self-esteem issues.

Depression may also play a part in poor eating habits. The elderly, for example, frequently experience malnutrition that can be attributed to depression, lack of

social support, or eating-related disabilities. The effects of mood and social support are well recognized, and intervention in these areas might achieve improvements in nutritional health and quality of life. Several conditions such as menopause and inherited factors have also been noted to impact nutritional status. See Box 14-3 for a listing of some factors that can impact nutritional health.

BOX 14-3 Selected Factors Impacting Nutritional Health

Age-Related Changes and Conditions
  Calcium deficit in menopause
  Anorexia, bulimia in adolescence
  Malnutrition in the elderly
Hereditary Conditions
  Diabetes
  Cardiovascular disease
  Hypercholesterolemia/lipidemia
Disease Conditions
  Cancer
  Diabetes
  Obesity
  Heart disease
  HIV
Lifestyle Behaviors
  Overindulgence
  Alcoholism
  Smoking
  Eating patterns/cultural eating habits
  Workaholic behavior

THE NURSING PROCESS IN PROMOTING NUTRITIONAL HEALTH

The role of the nurse in promoting a nutritionally balanced health promotion plan cannot be overemphasized. As described in Chapter 4, the nurse utilizes the nursing process in identifying the health needs of clients and determines an appropriate plan for addressing the identified needs. Likewise, the nurse involved in the care of a client carefully assesses the client's nutritional health and devises a plan to ensure optimal nutritional health. The following nursing process steps are useful in promoting a client's nutritional health: assessment, diagnosis, planning, implementation, and evaluation.

Assessment

Assessment is the key step in determining a client's nutritional health needs. This very important step is quite complex and involves the initial recognition of those factors that might affect nutrition and lifestyle. Each of the domains previously described as influencing eating behaviors should be identified and considered in this phase of the nursing process. Assessment of the biological domain, for example, demonstrates the importance of gender and age in determining nutritional requirements. The body's actual energy requirements as well as the body's ability to absorb nutrients are also essential assessment considerations. The psychological domain assessment may reveal emotional issues that are affecting a person's appetite. The way that a person interacts with others as well as her or his interpersonal relationships can reveal much about eating habits and should not be overlooked. A client's sociocultural and religious beliefs related to foods, as well as the impact of the environment, are important areas to be assessed when determining nutritional health. Table 14-5 identifies specific domain areas to be assessed when utilizing the nursing process to determine a nutritionally balanced health promotion plan.

Refer to Chapter 16 for a sample assessment form that can be used in the nutritional screening of adults and children.

Nursing Diagnosis

The next step in the nursing process is identification of the nursing diagnosis or diagnoses. Nursing diagnoses are based on the thorough analysis of data obtained through the nursing assessment. According to NANDA (2007), there are a number of nutrition-related nursing diagnoses that could be applicable in a client situation. These can usually be classified as:

- Imbalanced nutrition: Less than body requirements

- Imbalanced nutrition: More than body requirements

- Risk for imbalanced nutrition: More than body requirements.

Selection of the actual nursing diagnosis will rest on what is causing the alteration or risk for alteration of the nutrition status. That is, the nursing diagnosis is always stated as in the following examples, to indicate the cause for the alteration:

- Imbalanced nutrition: Less than body requirements related to anorexia

- Imbalanced nutrition: More than body requirements related to excessive intake and sedentary activity (NANDA, 2007).

There are a number of nutrition-related nursing diagnoses and, for the most part, these can be classified according to the domains covered in this chapter. For example, an alteration in nutrition may be related to the biological domain in that it is caused by a physiological problem such as painful ulcers, or it could be related to the environmental domain if the cause of the nutritional alteration is related to a change in diet. The psychological domain can also have a major influence in nutritional alterations.

Planning

Following determination of the appropriate nursing diagnoses, the next step of the nursing process is to develop a plan of care. The planning phase includes a careful identification by both the client and the nurse of the goals, outcomes, or both that will assist both the client and the nurse in resolveing the problems identified. The goals identified are mutually established and should be measurable and, above all, realistic. For example, it is not enough to state that the client will recognize reasons for weight loss. Realistic and measurable objectives may include goals or outcomes such as follows: The client will identify five factors that contribute to weight loss; or, the client will identify four situations that lead to a decreased appetite. The planning phase is extremely important since this sets the stage for implementation of those measures that will promote the client's health.

The planning phase arises from the nursing diagnoses and must be congruent with them. That is, if a

TABLE 14-5 Assessment of Domains Influencing Nutritional Health

Domain	Specific Assessments
Biological	Client's age, weight, and height Weight changes Problems or conditions affecting nutritional status Caloric intake, number of meals, servings per day Oral health Allergies Alcohol, caffeine, and sugar consumption daily Physical activities and exercise Client 24-hour diet recall Laboratory values indicative of nutritional problems: e.g., hemoglobin, hematocrit, lymphocytes, red blood cells, globulins, blood urea nitrogen, fasting blood sugar, and electrolytes (Jaffe & McVan, 1997)
Psychological	Family issues affecting nutrition Interpersonal relationships Emotional disorders Aversion to specific foods
Sociocultural	Lifestyle Ethnic food preferences Meal preparation by whom? Regular meals eaten at home or out Number of snacks per day and type
Spiritual/Religious	Feelings regarding certain foods Foods related to religious or spiritual events (e.g., Lent, Passover) Religious food prohibitions Meaning of foods
Environmental	Eats alone or with others Lives alone Salt readily available Other condiments used in food preparation Comfort foods, favorite snacks
Technological	Client's age Educational status Economic status Computer literacy Availability of technology Comfort level with technology

diagnosis is Imbalanced nutrition: Less than body requirements related to decreased appetite due to anorexia nervosa, the nursing plan should focus on those measures that address the cause of the decreased appetite such as, perhaps, low self-esteem and poor interpersonal relationships. Additionally, the plan could address the need for consultation with a nutritionist and the need for an increase in the client's knowledge base relative to nutritional information. Refer to Chapter 16 for further information on planning care for a client with nutritional alterations.

Implementation

Though the previous phase of the nursing process established goals or outcomes or both related to nutritional health and identified a plan of action to achieve these goals, the implementation phase actually attempts to put the identified plan into action. The implementation phase is the most dynamic aspect of the nursing process since it determines which interventions relative to the nutritional goals are appropriate and which are not. This constant evaluation of interventions can subsequently lead to a modification of the plan and perhaps even a reassessment of the client situation and the identification of new nursing diagnoses.

While the implementation phase is the most dynamic, it is also the most difficult phase since it will involve considerable effort in motivating clients to make changes and perhaps even adopt a healthier lifestyle that will lead to a positive nutritional status. The domains previously identified as influencing nutritional health can be utilized in determining which interventions are necessary to achieve the client goals. For example, interventions directed toward the biological domain are useful and can include a monitoring of the client's weight, a continued assessment of dietary status, and identification of any abnormal lab values that are influenced by nutritional status. Likewise, interventions directed to the sociocultural domain may include dietary counseling for both the client and the family members affected by needed dietary changes. The environmental domain is also a major consideration when implementing a nutritional plan that might require lifestyle changes. Table 14-6 identifies some specific nutrition-related interventions according to domain areas.

Later chapters also provide useful information on implementation of interventions for promoting nutritional health.

Health Promotion Model and Nutritional Status

Pender's revised Health Promotion Model (HPM) is also a useful tool that can be utilized to determine and implement actions that direct behaviors that enhance health (Pender, Murdaugh, & Parsons, 2006). As described in Chapter 3, the HPM focuses on motivation for health behaviors, identifies interactions among cognitive, behavioral, and environmental factors that influence health behaviors, and does not use fear or threats to effect change. Thus, according to this model, interventions implemented to achieve nutritional health will not be effective if the client is threatened with dire outcomes such as obesity-related consequences or even death. Rather, the nurse works with the client in determining which required client actions and behaviors have positive personal value and assists in identifying the motivational significance for successfully achieving these changes. An assessment of the client's perceived self-efficacy or ability to carry out the required actions and identification of competencies required in achieving goals is essential in establishing a health-promoting plan for the individual. For example, if the nurse is establishing a plan for Larry, an extremely obese individual weighing 100 pounds over the weight limit, it is important to determine whether he believes that a 100-pound

TABLE 14-6 Nutrition-Related Nursing Interventions Categorized by Domain Areas

Domain	Interventions
Biological	Monitor client's weight. Assess client's dietary intake. Modify dietary intake if necessary. Identify abnormal laboratory values and report. Monitor energy levels and expenditure. Encourage moderate levels of physical exercise.
Psychological	Encourage client to evaluate meaning of foods and situations where too much or too little food is eaten. Refer client for psychological counseling if needed.
Sociocultural	Refer client for dietary counseling by licensed nutritionist. Provide information on dietary guidelines, low-fat foods, exchange system as needed. Include cultural or ethnic-specific food choices or both in meal planning. Include individual who cooks for the client in the dietary counseling and exchange of nutrition-related information.
Spiritual/Religious	Incorporate specific spiritual or religious beliefs in menu planning.
Environmental	Encourage and support needed lifestyle changes. Include client's lifestyle in planning of menus. Provide client education regarding the needed environmental changes that will positively influence nutritional health.

weight loss is achievable. Larry's physical abilities, cognitive and individual characteristics, and external influences must be considered in establishing a realistic nutritional health-promoting plan. The biological, psychological, sociocultural, spiritual, and environmental domains previously described as influencing eating and nutritional behaviors are also essential components to be considered in utilizing the HPM in achieving adequate nutritional status in all clients.

Evaluation

The evaluation phase of the nursing process focuses on goals that were established initially in the planning phase. Any unforeseeable changes that have caused the plan to be unworkable must be evaluated and the plan must be modified. A nursing plan, for example, that includes teaching the client about the need to eat two five-ounce servings from the meat group daily must be based on an awareness of the client's food preferences. If the nurse is unaware that the client is a strict vegetarian, the plan must be evaluated and then modified to include foods that are acceptable as meat substitutes. All client preferences, behaviors, and attitudes must be noted when thoroughly evaluating the client's progress in achieving the goals set out in the nursing process plan. Table 14-7 provides an example of a nursing process plan that focuses on a client's nutritional status. A Case Study for an individual at risk for malnutrition is included at the end of this chapter.

SUMMARY

Nutrition is essential for health promotion. The role of nutrition in health promotion is to maintain health through the consumption of an adequate diet containing the essential nutrients and calories to prevent nutritional deficiencies. There are several tools that can guide us toward healthful eating. These are: *Dietary Guidelines for Americans*, MyPyramid, exchange system, food labels, and the Five a Day Program. By utilizing these tools, nurses can plan a balanced diet that contains a variety of foods that supply nutrients essential to life, health, maintenance, and prevention of diet-related chronic diseases.

TABLE 14-7 Nursing Process for a Slightly Below-Weight Adolescent

Assessment: A medium-framed 18-year-old active female; weight = 108 lbs; height = 5'6"; average caloric intake = 1,600; ideal body weight = 120 pounds

Nursing Diagnosis(es)	Goals/Outcomes	Interventions
Imbalanced nutrition: Less than body requirements related to stressful adolescent relationships evidenced by loss of appetite.	Will consume a daily balanced diet as determined by activity level and metabolic needs.	Establish client goals. Consult dietitian on the appropriate dietary intake.
	Will gain two pounds per month until ideal weight is achieved.	Provide diet high in complex carbohydrates and fiber and low in sugar, fats, and salt. Weigh monthly.
	Will verbalize stress-provoking situations.	Encourage client to verbalize stress-provoking situations. Provide support.
Deficient knowledge related to inadequate understanding of what constitutes a well-balanced diet.	Will verbalize foods needed for a well-balanced diet.	Inform client on five food groups, food pyramid, diet guidelines, and the importance of well-balanced diets. Reinforce the information both in writing and orally.
	Will recognize possible causes of dietary inadequacy.	Have client list possible causes of her poor appetite. Work with client in developing plan that includes food preferences. Discuss need for moderate exercise as way to promote health and to stabilize weight.

Objectives/Goals: Through participation in discussion of this case study, participants will have the opportunity to:

1. Discuss factors that impact nutritional status in the elderly.
2. Discuss the relationship between these impacting factors and the risk for malnutrition in the elderly client.

Health Promotion Concern, History and Physical, Present Health Status, Past Health Status, Family History, and Social History

Monica Avery is a black, 72-year-old widowed female who lives alone in her own home although she does have a housekeeper who cleans her house and buys and prepares food for her twice a week. On the other days, Monica is responsible for preparing her own meals. Her two children live more than 100 miles away and can only visit every two to three months. Her past medical history includes a broken left hip, which occurred four months ago and required surgery. She is on several medications for her hypertension and cardiovascular insufficiency, takes oral hypoglycemic agents for her type 2 diabetes mellitus, and takes multiple vitamins and fiber supplements. Monica has always engaged in physical activity until recently when she fell and broke her leg. Her family history is positive for diabetes on both sides of her family, and both her father and mother died of a massive heart attack in their early 60s. Her mother also had a positive history for depression.

Monica is visited once a week by a home health nurse who notices that Monica has been losing weight gradually since her dismissal from the hospital. She appears to have lost interest in eating and exercises infrequently. Her primary mode of entertainment is watching soap operas on television.

Review of Pertinent Domains

Biological Domain

Physical exam reveals an underweight individual who is 62 inches tall and weighs 105 pounds. She has kyphosis, which is evidence of osteoporosis in her back and shoulders. She has full range of motion in her right leg but not in her left leg or arms. Gastrointestinal: Reports no problems in this area. She has regular bowel movements. The fiber supplement helps in regulating her bowel movements. Her dietary pattern consists of eating three meals only when the housekeeper cooks. Usually she eats one egg and two slices of bread for dinner and supper when she is alone. Occasionally she will eat a sandwich with lean ham and a slice of processed cheese. She will eat a banana or fruit when offered. She drinks black caffeinated coffee without sugar, two to four cups a day.

Genitourinary: Nonremarkable. Urinates frequently with no discomfort. Urine is clear, straw colored, with no foul odor.

Diagnostic testing: Glucose readings have been slightly below normal for the last two months.

Psychological Domain

Psychologically she appears to be slightly depressed. Monica states that she has felt very "down" since she broke her hip.

Social Domain

Cognitively she is alert and oriented. She is able to verbalize her understanding of her current physical condition. She gets along well with her children and other family members. Monica enjoys visiting with family and friends. She was a member of a church club but has not been able to participate recently due to her physical condition.

Environmental Domain

Because she lives alone, Monica does not interact with anyone on a regular basis. She does see her housekeeper twice a week and has a pleasant relationship with her. Monica needs information on the importance of a balanced diet and moderate exercise. She needs to know what foods she should include in her diet and what foods to avoid. She also needs information on health care activities and resources in her community.

Questions for Discussion

1. What foods should Monica include in her diet?
2. What are some lifestyle modifications for Monica in relation to food choices?
3. Which of Monica's medicines can affect her appetite?
4. What community resources might be helpful to Monica?

Key Concepts

1. The essential nutrients to maintain health are water, carbohydrates, protein, lipids, vitamins, and minerals.

2. *Healthy People 2010*, a document by the U.S. Public Health Service, provides health promotion and disease prevention objectives for Americans that include a reduction in the incidence of heart disease, cancer, overweight, and growth retardation, an improvement of nutritional health, and the delivery of nutrition services to be achieved by the year 2010.

3. The biological, psychological, sociocultural, environmental, and technological domains can influence eating behavior and can also affect caloric and nutrient intake of an individual.

4. Nutritional excesses such as obesity and deficits such as anorexia or bulimia significantly affect the nutritional status of all Americans.

5. Eating a variety of foods such as grain products, vegetables, fruits, lean meats, and fish will ensure provision of essential nutrients for health maintenance and prevention of diet-related chronic diseases.

6. Following MyPyramid guidelines daily is the key to a healthy diet.

7. The food exchange list is a valuable guide that can be used in menu planning.

8. Paying attention to food labels can help an individual choose foods lower in fat so as not to exceed the recommended intake.

9. The nursing process and Pender's HPM can be effectively used to plan strategies that will improve a client's nutritional status.

Learning Activities

1. Record all the foods you eat and all the beverages you drink in one typical 24-hour period. Include items such as amount of sugar or cream in coffee, sugar in iced tea, and so forth.

2. Record the number of servings you obtained from each food group. Estimate the amount of your intake (use ounce for meat serving; cup for vegetables, potatoes, beverages; small, medium, large for fruits).

3. How does your diet compare to the MyPyramid recommendations? Which food groups are underrepresented in your diet?

4. If you did not follow MyPyramid guidelines for each food group, list the reasons why.

5. List six strategies you can use to improve your diet.

True/False Questions

1. T or F Biological changes can change the eating behaviors of people.

2. T or F Approximately 50 percent of anorexics develop bulimia.

3. T or F Weight is not a contributing factor in development of type 2 diabetes.

Multiple Choice Questions

1. Which of the following nutrients has been found to prevent spinal cord birth defects during pregnancy?
   a. Beta carotene
   b. Folic acid
   c. Vitamin C
   d. Selenium

2. Vitamin D is necessary because it does which of the following?
   a. Affects vision
   b. Affects gums and teeth
   c. Helps in the absorption of calcium and phosphorus
   d. Protects vital body tissue

3. Anorexia nervosa primarily affects which of the following?
   a. Adolescent girls
   b. Mature males
   c. Elderly females
   d. Young children

4. Which of the following is the typical bulimic individual?
   a. Child in elementary school
   b. College-educated female
   c. Male in his early 40s
   d. Senior citizen

Websites

http://www.aedweb.org Academy for Eating Disorders. The Academy for Eating Disorders is an international transdisciplinary professional organization that promotes excellence in research, treatment, and prevention of eating disorders. The AED provides education, training, and a forum for collaboration and professional dialogue.

http://www.wpic.pitt.edu Western Psychiatric Institute and Clinic (WPIC). This organization has been a national leader in the diagnosis, management, and treatment of mental health and addictive disorders.

http://www.fns.usda.gov Food and Nutrition Service Assistance Program (FNS). This program provides children and low-income people access to food, a healthful diet, and nutrition education.

Organizations

American Dietetic Association
120 South Riverside Plaza, Suite 2000
Chicago, Illinois 60606
Tel: (800) 877-1600
http://www.eatright.org

The nation's largest organization of food and nutrition professionals, ADA serves the public by promoting optimal nutrition, health, and well-being.

American Obesity Association
1250 24th Street NW, Suite 300
Washington, DC 20037
Tel: (202) 766-7711
Fax: (202) 776-7712
http://www.obesity.org

Offers the most comprehensive site on obesity and overweight on the Internet.

National Association of Anorexia Nervosa and Associated Disorders
P.O. Box 7,
Highland Park, Illinois 60035

Tel: (847) 831-3438
http://www.anad.org

The oldest eating disorder organization in the nation. This organization assists individuals and their families to find resources and provides referrals to professionals.

National Cancer Institute
6116 Executive Boulevard, Room 3036A
Bethesda, MD 20892-8322
Tel: (800) 422-6237
http://www.cancer.gov

The National Cancer Institute website provides a comprehensive site for information on cancer, including latest cancer-related news, research, and cancer statistics.

The North American Association for the Study of Obesity (NASSO)
8630 Fenton Street, Suite 918
Silver Springs, Maryland 20910
Tel: (301) 563-6526
Fax: (301) 563-6595
http://www.naaso.org

The leading scientific society dedicated to the study of obesity. Since 1982 NAASO has been committed to encouraging research on the causes and treatment of obesity and to keeping the medical community and public informed of new advances.

References

Adams, M. (2005). *The pharmanex biophotonic scanner revolution.* Retrieved April 6, 2006, from http://www.truthpublishing.com/bluelaser.html

Almada, A. (2001). Garlic and heart disease. *Nutrition Science News*, September 2001. Retrieved December 1, 2005, from http://www.newhope.com

American Diabetes Association. (2005). *Meal planning exchange lists.* Retrieved October 15, 2005, from http://www.diabetes.org

ANRED. (2005). *Anorexia nervosa and related eating disorders.* Retrieved November 23, 2005, from http://www.anred.com

Bonci, L. (2002). Energy drinks: Help, harm or hype? *Sports Science Exchange 84*, 15(1). Retrieved January 18, 2006, from http://www.mtnrnr.com

Centers for Distance Control and Prevention (CDC). (2003). *National center for health statistics report.* Volume 54(1). http://www.cdc.gov/nchs/

Centers for Disease Control and Prevention (CDC). (2006). *Five a day program.* Department of Health and Human Services. Retrieved April 20, 2006, from http://www.cdc.gov

De Castro, J. M. (2002). Age-related changes in the social, psychological and temporal influences on food intake in free living, healthy, adult humans. *Journal of Gerontology: Medical Sciences, 57*(A), M368–M377.

Gardner, A. (2005). Obesity sends costs soaring. *Health on the Net Foundation.* Retrieved April 27, 2006, from http://www.hon.ch/News

Institute of Medicine of the National Academies. (2004). *Dietary reference intakes.* Retrieved April 27, 2006, from http://www.iom.edu.

Jaffe, M. S., & McVan, B. F. (1997). *Davis laboratory and diagnostic test handbook.* Philadelphia: F. A. Davis.

Keltner, N. L., Schwecke, L. H., & Bostrom, C. E. (2003). *Psychiatric nursing* (4th ed.). St. Louis: Mosby.

Lad, V. (2003). Food combining. In Usha & V. Lad, *Ayurvedic cooking for self-healing.* Albuquerque, NM: The Ayurvedic Institute.

Lauque, S., Amaud-Battandier, F., Gillette, S., Plaze, J., Andrieu, S., Cantet, C., & Vellas, B. (2004). Improvement of weight and fat-free mass with oral nutritional supplementation in patients with Alzheimer's disease at risk for malnutrition: A prospective randomized study. *Journal of the American Geriatrics Society, 52*(10), 1702–1707.

Loeschorn, J. (2002). Be wary of nutrition fads: They promise fantastic results, but can they deliver? *John Loeschorn's Running Lifestyle.* Retrieved May 2006 from http://www.mtnrnr.com/healthfads.htm

Lutz, C., & Przytulski, K. (2006). *Nutrition and diet therapy.* Philadelphia: F. A. Davis.

Miller, C. A. (2004). *Nursing for wellness in older adults: Theory and practice* (4th ed.). Philadelphia: Lippincott Williams & Wilkins.

NANDA. (2007). *Nursing diagnoses: Definitions and classification 2007–2008.* Philadelphia: NANDA International.

National Academies Press. (2004). *Dietary reference intakes for water, potassium, sodium, chloride, and sulfate.* Retrieved April 27, 2006, from http://www.nap.edu

Pender, N. J., Murdaugh, C. L., & Parsons, M. A. (2006). *Health promotion in nursing practice* (5th ed.). Upper Saddle River, NJ: Pearson Prentice Hall.

Perry, L., & McLaren, S. (2004). An exploration of nutrition and eating disabilities in relation to quality of life at 6 months post-stroke. *Health and Social Care in the Community, 12*(4), 288–297.

Phytochemicals. (2006). Retrieved April 6, 2006, from http://www
.phytochemicals.info

Schultz, M. (2003). Dietary approaches to stop hypertension. *Super-market Guru*. July 19, Retrieved April 28, 2006 from http://www
.supermarketguru.com

University of Iowa Health Center. (2005). *Nutrition fads and myths*. Retrieved April 20, 2006, from http://www.uihealthcare.com

U.S. Department of Agriculture (USDA), Center for Nutrition Policy and Promotion. (2005). *MyPyramid: Steps to a healthier you*. Retrieved April 25, 2006, from http://www.mypyramid.gov

U.S. Department of Health and Human Services (USDHHS). (2000). *Healthy people 2010: Understanding and improving health and objectives for improving health*. Washington, DC: U.S. Government Printing Office.

U.S. Department of Health and Human Services (USDHHS), U.S. Department of Agriculture. (2005a). *Dietary guidelines for Americans*. Washington, DC: U.S. Government Printing Office. http://www.healthierus.gov/dietaryguidelines/

U.S. Department of Health and Human Services (USDHHS), Office of Disease Prevention and Health Promotion. (2005b). *Healthy People 2010*. Retrieved May 2, 2006, from http://www
.healthypeople.gov

Wardlaw, G. M. (2000). *Perspectives in nutrition* (4th ed.). Boston: WCB McGraw-Hill.

Warner, J. (2002). *Broccoli pill prevents breast cancer*. WebMD Medical News. Retrieved April 6, 2006, from http://www.WebMD.com

Bibliography

Bascetta, C. (2005). *Childhood obesity* [electronic resource]. Washington, DC: U.S. Government Accountability Office.

Caballero, B. (2003). *Encyclopedia of food sciences and nutrition* (2nd ed.). Boston: Academic Press.

Cupp, J., & Tracy, T. S. (2003). Dietary supplements [electronic resource]. In M. J. Cupp (Ed.), *Toxicology and clinical pharmacology*. Humana Press.

Ford, J. (2006). *Diseases and disabilities caused by weight problems: The overloaded body*. Philadelphia: Mason Crest.

Grodner, M., Long, S., & De Young, S. (2004). *Foundations and clinical applications of nutrition, a nursing approach* (3rd ed.). St. Louis: Mosby.

Katz, S. (Ed.). (2003). *Encyclopedia of food and culture*. New York: Charles Scribner's Sons.

Lucas, A. (2004). *Demystifying anorexia nervosa: An optimistic guide to understanding and healing* [electronic resource]. New York: Oxford University Press.

Chapter 15

ENGAGING IN PHYSICAL FITNESS

Carolina G. Huerta, EdD, MSN, RN
Sue G. Mottinger, PhD

KEY TERMS

ballistic stretching
body composition
body mass index (BMI)
cardiovascular fitness
cooldown
flexibility
heart rate reserve

intensity
maximum heart rate
muscular endurance
muscular strength
overload principle
performance-related
  fitness

physical fitness
plantar fasciitis
principle of
  progression
principle of specificity
rate of perceived
  exertion

RICE
sprain
static stretching
strain
target heart rate
warm-up

OBJECTIVES

Upon completion of this chapter, the reader should be able to:

- Explain why exercise is important in health promotion.
- Define physical fitness, including health-related fitness and motor-performance fitness.
- Assess the various components of health-related fitness.
- Identify the general principles of fitness training.
- Plan a fitness program using the FITT Model.
- Understand the principles and concepts of cardiovascular fitness.
- Describe the essential elements of training.
- Identify frequent problems related to exercise.
- Describe the RICE concept for injury treatment.
- Identify myths and fallacies about exercise.
- Describe how the health promotion model is useful in developing a fitness program.
- Recognize how the nursing process may be utilized in developing a physical fitness plan.
- Identity practical tips for increasing physical activity.

INTRODUCTION

"Be All That You Can Be" is a popular slogan that applies to all individuals. The slogan may be interpreted in terms of applying the best effort to develop in all aspects of life and then applying talents and capabilities to achieve desired goals. To achieve these goals, a person must be as healthy as possible. The healthier one is, the more completely one achieves personal potential. This chapter is about achieving goals and being "all that you can be"—a healthy and physically fit individual.

Many Americans today are emphasizing **physical fitness,** which is the ability to be physically active on a regular basis. People are more aware of the role of fitness in achieving a healthy lifestyle and are inundated from many sources such as TV, magazines, books, and even the Internet about how to include some form of exercise in their busy schedules.

Each day more and more people are choosing to take responsibility for their own well-being by becoming physically active through health-promoting behaviors. Unfortunately, the majority of people are not. For example, despite the proven benefits of physical activity, more than 50 percent of American adults do not get enough exercise to achieve health benefits. Twenty-five percent of adults are not active at all in their leisure time. It is a fact that activity decreases with age. Physical activity is less common among women than men and among those with lower income and educational level (U.S. Department of Health and Human Services, Centers for Disease Control and Prevention [CDC], 2005). Statistics further indicate that Blacks and Hispanics engage in less physical activity than non-Hispanic Whites.

Chapter 14 presented the concepts of nutrition and nutrition's role in maintaining health. This chapter will focus on the importance of physical fitness in health promotion. The relationship between physical fitness and health, benefits of exercise, development of a fitness program, and the role of the nurse in promoting health through physical fitness will be emphasized.

EXERCISE AND HEALTH PROMOTION

It is not unusual for a client to ask a health care professional "Why should I exercise?" While the immediate response might be "Because it is good for you," most people are not necessarily interested in finding out what is good for them. Rather, they are interested in engaging in those activities that feel good. An ideal response to this question is that physical activity or exercise is fun, feels good, and is in fact beneficial. All three of these general reasons are true and people who agree and respond to this rationale have made a commitment to fitness and are actively pursuing their commitment.

In *Healthy People 2010* (U.S. Department of Health and Human Services, 2005) a major goal is to improve physical fitness and the healthy life span of people through physical activity. The benefits of a fitness program that involves cardiovascular and strength-developing exercises, then, are physiological as well as psychological, such as improvement in one's self-perception. In fact, a health-promoting fitness program may have multiple benefits that can be categorized according to the domains listed in Chapters 4 and 14. As previously indicated, physical exercise has multiple physiological benefits and psychological benefits. The sociocultural domain may also be influenced by physical activity in that a physically fit individual is more likely to exude confidence and engage in social activities, making that person a well-rounded individual.

The Surgeon General's Call to Action to Prevent and Decrease Overweight and Obesity (U.S. Department of Health and Human Services, 2001) recommends that American adults accumulate at least 30 minutes per day of moderate physical activity most days of the week. The

recommendation for children is 60 minutes per day most days of the week. More exercise may be needed to prevent weight gain, to lose weight, or to maintain weight loss. To promote health, cardiovascular endurance activities should be included, and these should be supplemented with strength-developing exercises at least twice per week. *Healthy People 2010* also focuses on the benefits of physical activity and the acquisition of physical fitness. In fact, *Healthy People 2010* includes two overarching goals: to "increase quality and years of healthy life" and "eliminate health disparities" (USDHHS, 2005). In keeping with these goals, *Healthy People 2010* emphasizes physical activity and fitness.

The development of modern technology such as cellular telephones, computers, riding lawn mowers, even automatic garage door openers provides numerous opportunities for individuals to develop chronic conditions attributed to lack of physical activity. Being physically fit can help to reduce these chronic conditions such as heart disease, diabetes, osteoporosis, hypertension, low-back pain, and obesity.

Members of the health professions can make a difference, both a personal difference and a difference in others. Health care professionals have an opportunity to counsel adults and young people about physical activity as well as other healthful behaviors such as nutrition and stress management. Client education is an integral part of nursing practice. It is a primary focus for nurses regardless of the setting. Nurses can certainly influence, though not control, a client's health promotion outlook through education (Craven & Hirnle, 2003).

PHYSICAL FITNESS

The term "physical fitness" means different things to different people. To some people fitness may mean having a good figure or physique. To a runner, fitness may mean the ability to run a 10K, a common racing distance of 10.2 miles, in a given amount of time. To a teenager, it may mean the ability to perform at a high, sustained

Ask Yourself

Skill Performance or Health Benefit?

Why would an athlete who is striving for maximum performance to achieve a performance goal train differently than the individual who is seeking a change in lifestyle to improve and maintain a healthy lifestyle?

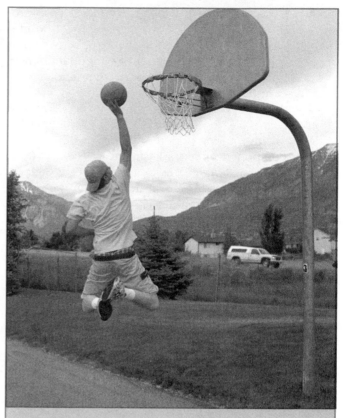

FIGURE 15-1 *Physical fitness means many things to many people. What does it mean to you?*

athletic level. A college student may deem fitness to be looking good and being free of stress. All these descriptions can apply to a definition of fitness (See Figure 15-1).

Because physical fitness is defined in numerous ways and may include attributes that contribute to skill or athletic performance versus health-related components, a distinction is made between performance-related fitness and health-related fitness. As indicated in Box 15-1, health-related fitness pertains to the health and well-being of the individual and is necessary to maintain a healthy lifestyle. It includes the components of cardiovascular fitness, strength and muscular endurance, flexibility of the lower back and hip region, and body composition (Teach PE.com, 2005).

Performance-related fitness (PRF) components are associated more with performance than good health. Both are necessary in determining the physical fitness of an individual. For example, to compete in selected sporting activities, one must have a high level of health-related fitness plus performance-related fitness. PRF components include agility, reaction time, power, coordination, balance, and speed and, most often, also includes the health-related components (Teachnet.ie, 2005). The health-related components have significance for everyone, not just for the athletically inclined. Although health-related fitness and performance-related fitness often overlap, it is the goal of the individual that determines which component of fitness to pursue.

COMPONENTS OF HEALTH-RELATED FITNESS

Health is often based upon a continuum with the extreme ends consisting of positive and negative poles (refer to Chapters 2 and 3 for a review of the health-illness continuum). Health is no longer considered merely absence from disease but a capacity to enjoy life and meet challenges. In addition to the ability to function physically, cognitively, and socially, the concept of health is related to the environment, socioeconomic level, race, and geographic location (Edelman & Mandle, 2006). The health-related components contribute to the overall well-being of the individual without any specific skill-related or motor-performance expertise. The four components of health-related fitness—cardiovascular fitness, muscular strength/endurance, flexibility, and body composition—are described in the following sections.

Cardiovascular Fitness

Cardiovascular fitness is synonymous with cardiorespiratory fitness, aerobic fitness, or cardiorespiratory endurance. All are terms that commonly refer to the circulatory system and respiratory system and how effectively and efficiently they function to transport oxygenated

BOX 15-1	Health- and Performance-Related Fitness
Health-Related Fitness	**Performance-Related Fitness**
cardiovascular strength	strength, power, agility
muscular strength	balance, coordination
muscular endurance	speed, reaction time
flexibility	
body composition	

blood to working muscles for an extended period of time. The function of these two systems must be efficient to allow the body to perform more effectively during physical activity. Perhaps the most important benefit of cardiovascular fitness is that it is a deterrent to chronic heart disease (CHD).

To develop cardiovascular fitness, large muscle groups must work together in the form of contractions during a relatively long period of time while the cardiovascular components make adjustments to the activity as necessary. For example, the more efficient the heart, lungs, and blood vessels are in transporting the air we breathe to the contracting muscle fibers, the easier it is to walk, run, swim, study, and concentrate for longer periods of time. Activities conducive to developing cardiovascular fitness include walking, running, swimming, stair stepping, rowing, cycling, step aerobics, low-impact aerobics, hiking, cross-country skiing, in-line skating, cross-country ski simulator, and rowing machines. All are commonly labeled aerobic activities.

Muscular Strength and Endurance

Muscular strength is the ability to exert force with a muscle against resistance, under maximal conditions in a single effort. For example, being able to lift an object or client without undue stress or suffering sprain, strain, or muscular difficulties requires a certain amount of muscular strength. Muscular strength such as strength of the abdominal muscles helps to maintain proper posture and prevents lower-back problems.

Muscular endurance refers to the ability of a muscle or group of muscles to perform or sustain a muscle contraction over an extended period of time. When a person has good muscular endurance, he or she has the ability to carry something over a long period of time as well as repeat a movement without becoming tired. It is recommended that individuals incorporate some form of resistance training, such as weight lifting, in their fitness programs to promote muscular strength and endurance. Furthermore, resistance training helps maintain or develop muscle mass and bone strength.

Females typically have lower levels of upper body strength than of lower body strength. Therefore, in general, females should engage in a program of regular, upper body strength development.

Flexibility

Flexibility is the ability of a joint or group of joints to move freely through a range of motion (ROM). The ROM for a joint may be restricted by the shape of bones and cartilage of the joint, and the muscles, tendons, ligaments, and fascia that cross the joint. On a continuum, an extreme lack of flexibility would be the knee of a person with arthritis and on the extreme other end would be the individual with knees that hyperextend.

Ask Yourself

Changing Lifestyle Behaviors

Linda is a 38-year-old female 5.4" tall and weighing 126 lbs. She is employed as an executive with a large technology company and is feeling stressed at having to perform her duties at work and also handle her home responsibilities. She is always complaining of being fatigued and weak. She has never played any sports and feels too inept to start a physical fitness and exercise program sponsored by her employer. As the nurse at the company where Linda works, what would you recommend to Linda that would promote a change in her health status?

Body Composition

Body composition refers to the relative amount of fat in the body compared to fat-free weight such as muscle, bone, and other elements in the body. In terms of health-related fitness, an excessive amount of fat or being overweight is unhealthy because it requires more energy for movement, may reflect a diet high in saturated fat, and places numerous demands on the cardiovascular system.

A major health problem in the United States is people who are overweight. Statistics indicate that 61 percent of adults in the United States are overweight or obese and that 13 percent of children aged 6 to 11 years and 14 percent of adolescents age 12 to 19 are overweight. These statistics show that overweight and obesity have tripled in the American population over the last two decades and that overweight and obesity cut across all ages and racial and ethnic groups as well as both genders (U.S. Department of Health and Human Services [USDHHS], 2001). Many of the leading causes of death can be linked to obesity. For example, cardiovascular disease, stroke, and even cancer may be associated with obesity. As a result of this close link, there is obviously economic cost associated with obesity. In 2000, for example, the United States incurred $117 billion in economic costs that were associated with obesity (USDHHS, 2001).

ASSESSING HEALTH-RELATED FITNESS

Although it is wise to start a fitness program early in life, a person is never too old or too sedentary to begin. The key is realizing that success is gradual and that the present state of fitness or lack of fitness did not occur overnight. A common question a nurse receives is "Where do I begin?" The appropriate response is determined after conducting an individual fitness assessment.

One of the first things to be assessed is the client's desire and/or reasons for wanting to become fit. Is it to feel better, look better, join a group, or play on the company's softball team? Fitness requires effort and the fuel for effort is motivation. Determining the reason and goal is essential.

As difficult as it may sound, a person cannot sit and become fit. Before recommending that a client engage in exercise, it is important to know as much about the person as possible. A fitness program should start with an inventory of the individual that includes the current level of fitness and medical history. Prevailing factors such as age, previous medical conditions, pregnancy, and present medication may necessitate a physical examination. People are often unaware of preexisting conditions that might pose a risk when participating in new or vigorous physical activity programs. A sample of preliminary questions that may be answered by a yes or no can be a starting point for a pre-exercise program inventory.

Cardiovascular Fitness

Prior to beginning a cardiovascular or aerobic fitness program, the present condition of the individual must be assessed. The level of cardiovascular fitness is determined by the maximal amount of oxygen the human body is able to use per minute of physical activity. The greater the oxygen consumption, the more efficient the cardiovascular system. Tests for levels of cardiovascular fitness may incude maximal or submaximal measures.

Submaximal tests do not require the individual to "gut it out" or push to the limit of exercise tolerance. These tests are a good alternative to the maximal oxygen consumption laboratory tests. By performing these activities periodically, individuals can assess how well they are doing on the road to a healthier lifestyle.

Muscular Strength

Several methods can be used to measure muscular strength, or the ability to exert force against resistance,

under maximal conditions in a single effort. The most common way to measure muscular strength is by using a one maximum repetition (1-RM) to determine how much weight one can lift in a single effort. How much weight to use initially for testing purposes must be safely estimated by trial and error. Caution must be exercised for the beginning individual since injury from maximum lifting may occur. It is recommended that inexperienced individuals estimate maximal strength by using a 6-RM—the amount of weight lifted six times and no more and no less.

Muscular Endurance

Muscular endurance allows the individual to repeat a movement over a period of time without getting tired. When muscles become fatigued they do not relax after each contraction, and the potential for injury increases. Prior to assessing muscular endurance, a person should perform a 5- to 10-minute warm-up using large-muscle groups such as in walking and calisthenics.

A muscular endurance assessment may be done by having the individual lift a certain amount of weight for as long as possible. An example is the bicep curl—lifting a weight toward the chest using the arm flexors—counting the number of completed times the weight is lifted and returned to the starting position.

Assessing Flexibility

Flexibility in an individual can vary throughout the body depending on the specific body part. To develop and maintain flexibility and ROM one must continually do flexibility exercises. Stretching exercises are best for improving flexibility and can be performed in two ways: **ballistic stretching** (repeated bouncing) and **static stretching** (slow and deliberate). Caution should be used when performing ballistic stretches since these are prone to cause injury or soreness. Static stretching is preferred, is considered safer, and involves using a slow and gradual lengthening of the muscle. An example is sitting on the floor with one leg extended and the other bent at a 45-degree angle and slowly moving forward toward the wall, bending at the waist, and extending the hands in a forward position.

Testing for flexibility may involve the sit-and-reach test. The sit-and-reach test as well as other versions provide essentially the same information: the ability to sit on the floor and bend forward at the waist. Good flexibility in the joints can help prevent injuries through all stages of life. Activities that lengthen the muscles such as swimming or a basic stretching program are excellent ways to increase flexibility.

Assessing Body Composition

There are several methods for assessing body composition, including height-weight tables, body mass indexes, and laboratory methods such as bioelectrical impedance, BOD POD, and underwater weighing. In laboratory settings, hydrostatic weighing (underwater) is often done rather than skinfold measurement, although hydrostatic weighing is more time-consuming.

Hydrostatic weighing involves applying Archimedes' principle to determine the body's density. The person is weighed outside water, then submerged and weighed again accounting for air in the lungs. The density is determined which in turn allows for the total body fat to be calculated.

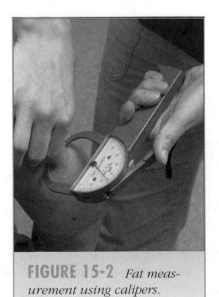

FIGURE 15-2 *Fat measurement using calipers.*

Skinfold calipers (see Figure 15-2) used by a trained person can give a good estimate of body fat. Although body fat is located throughout the body around organs, muscles, and under the skin, measuring thickness of skinfolds at certain multiple locations provides a good estimate of total body fatness. However, skinfold measurements are not accurate with the obese.

Body mass index (BMI) is a convenient tool and is relatively easy to calculate (see Box 15-2). It is used to relate height and weight to determine whether the individual is considered overweight or obese. Caution is required when using BMI as well as height-weight tables in that BMI cannot distinguish how much weight fat contributes to the total weight of the individual. The National Institutes of Health have set more stringent BMI guidelines for men and women. A value of 25 to 29.9 is considered overweight and a value of 30 or greater is considered obese.

STARTING A FITNESS TRAINING PROGRAM: MAKING THAT DECISION

Once the decision to improve fitness is made and assessments are completed, regular training or work must begin. Starting and maintaining a fitness program is a conscious choice, one that requires planning, goal setting, and executing the plan. Motivation is one of the key ingredients. A fundamental reason to start a program and continue is simple: fun and enjoyment. If a person does not like the workout, does not think he or she can perform the exercises, is not having fun, and is getting overly sore, or if exercising is becoming a chore, then the individual probably will not continue regardless of the benefits to be reaped.

BOX 15-2 Calculating Body Mass Index

1. Divide your weight in pounds by 2.2 to convert weight to kilograms.
2. Multiply your height in inches by .0254 to convert height to meters.
3. Square your height in meters.
4. Divide weight in kilograms by height in meters squared.
5. Use the Rating Scale for BMI to obtain your BMI rating.

Body Mass Index Rating

Classification	Women	Men
High risk	27.3	27.8
Marginal	24.5–27.2	25.0–27.7
Good fitness	18.0–24.4	19.0–24.9
Low	15.0–17.9	17.9–18.9

A fitness program does not have to be confined to a gym. People do not have to hurt when they train. Clients should be encouraged to exercise with others or make a new friend who has an interest in exercising. It has been noted that individuals who exercise with others are more inclined to continue the exercise regimen.

GENERAL PRINCIPLES OF FITNESS TRAINING

There are three general principles that must be applied in a fitness program to reap the benefits from the effort expended. These include (1) the principle of overload, (2) the principle of specificity, and (3) the principle of progression.

Principle of Overload

For a muscle, including the heart muscle, to get stronger, the **overload principle** must be applied. Overload means the body is being forced to do more than it normally does. An overload stimulus can be applied to any muscle or body part for a specific component of fitness—lifting weights for improving strength, walking for cardiovascular endurance, or stretching to improve flexibility. The body may adapt to the overload or higher level of work, in which case fitness improves, or it may fail to adapt and injury may occur.

Principle of Specificity

The **principle of specificity** applies to all types of training and states that one must overload the body systems or the specific fitness component to achieve a specific outcome. Different methods of exercise place specific demands on the body, and an individual must participate in a specific program to develop each of the four components of fitness. Stretching is specific to flexibility and does not improve cardiovascular endurance. Overload is specific also to each body part. To develop upper body strength, the muscles involved improve only when they are used in the specific way they are trained. A vertical press lift makes it easier to lift heavy objects up to the top shelf of an equipment stand but does not make it easier to carry objects in front of the body. Aerobic exercises concentrate on the cardiovascular system while resistance training is more effective in developing muscular strength. Flexibility exercises are low-energy activities but are the most effective way to develop joint ROM. The overload principle does not imply that spot reducing can be achieved (see Myth 3 later in chapter).

Principle of Progression

Principle of progression implies that gradually the overload stimulus is increased as adaptations to the existing workload occur. As the body adapts to one level of exercise, a new overload must be applied to stimulate improvements in physical fitness. For positive fitness results, the progression principle should not be increased too slowly or too rapidly. Minimum and maximum levels of training are based on the progressive exercise principle.

PLANNING A FITNESS PROGRAM

Questions such as "How often should I exercise?" and "What type of exercise is the best for achieving fitness?" and "How hard should I work?" are often asked of health care professionals. Once again, it is important that the goal for fitness of the individual be clearly established. Does the client want to achieve overall fitness such as a change in cardiovascular endurance, muscular strength and endurance, flexibility, and body composition or concentrate on one or a combination of the various components? Remember that the greater the number of large muscles involved in an exercise regime, such as a cardiovascular program, the greater the return on additional health-related benefits.

Physiological variables impact a person's decision to become physically fit. Behavioral and psychological variables also influence the decision to be physically active. Maintenance of physical fitness and regular physical activity are dependent on sources of personal and social motivation within a person's day-to-day environment (Pender, Murdaugh, & Parsons, 2006). Part of the planning procedure to enlist a person in a physical fitness program is to determine variables impacting exercise ability and to determine the frequency, intensity, time involved, and type of training (FITT) to incorporate into the fitness program.

Frequently, when planning an exercise or fitness program, variables such as culture or lack of personal motivation are not taken into account. These variables are quite obvious and yet health promotion planners may not be aware of their impact on the decision to exercise. For example, people may be motivated to exercise to music if the type of music is relevant to their age group, lifestyle, or culture. An older American may adhere to an exercise plan using music referred to as "Golden Oldies" while younger adults may prefer rap music.

Research has found that exercise programs that take into account culture create personal interest and increased adherence. One study conducted by researchers from the University of California–San Francisco School of Nursing found that 96 percent of the participants completed a 12-week Tai Chi exercise program for older Chinese women at risk for coronary heart disease. The researchers attributed the success of the program to the fact that it was culturally in tune with the exercise group (American Heart Association, 2005a). Incorporating culture into exercise routines may prove beneficial in other ethnic populations. For example, use of salsa music in an exercise regimen has been found to spark the interest of Cuban Americans as well as other Hispanic groups (Sankofa, 2006). Box 15-3 identifies factors that impact a person's decision to participate in exercise.

Frequency (F)

Frequency is how many times per week a person is physically active or participating in an exercise program. The Surgeon General recommends that a person exercise most days of the week (USDHHS, WHS 2001). The more often a person exercises during the week, the greater the caloric expenditure. A good practice is to establish a pattern for training such as exercising at the same time each day. Clients should be encouraged to write the times on their calendar; that is, plan time in their schedule that suits them.

Intensity (I)

Intensity describes how hard a person must work to improve physical fitness. The intensity of exercise is determined by the maximum heart rate of the individual. In the beginning stages of a fitness program, the intensity should be kept low. High intensity can often lead to soreness, injury, and frustration.

Time (T)

Time indicates how long the individual should work during an exercise session and how often a person should work out during a given time in a week. It is recommended that workout sessions be from 20 to 60 minutes each and that a time pattern for training be set, such as the same time on a specified day (American Academy of Family Physicians, 2005).

Type of Training (T)

The last element of the FITT model is the type of training a person plans to do for each fitness component. For cardiovascular fitness, the training should be some type

BOX 15-3	Factors Impacting the Decision to Exercise

- Age
- Boring exercises
- Culture
- Depression
- Fatigue
- Finances
- Insufficient time
- Lack of motivation
- Lack of self-confidence
- Personal health problems

of aerobic exercise such as walking, running, swimming, hiking, and so on. Weight lifting for muscular strength and endurance may include working with free weights such as barbells and dumbbells, weight machines, or some other type of weight resistance. Flexibility training should involve some type of stretching. To make a change in body composition necessitates a combination of aerobic exercise, weight resistance, flexibility, and good daily nutrition.

PRINCIPLES AND CONCEPTS OF CARDIOVASCULAR FITNESS

Prior to undertaking an aerobic or a cardiovascular fitness program, an individual must first understand the concepts of resting, target, and recovery heart rates and rate of perceived exertion. Each of these components is integral for determining the intensity of the workout and is discussed next.

Resting Heart Rate

Resting heart rate can be an initial indicator of a person's fitness level. An active lifestyle tends to produce a lower resting heart rate while a sedentary lifestyle is associated with a higher resting heart rate.

The resting heart rate is best determined by counting the pulse either at the carotid artery or the radial artery for one minute upon awakening in the morning. For best results, several resting heart rates should be taken and then the average should be determined. When taking the carotid pulse, care should be taken to use only two fingers, the index and middle fingers, to press lightly at the carotid artery, and to count the pulse. Be sure that the thumb is not used since it has a beat of its own. The radial pulse is taken at the radial artery on an upturned wrist below the heel of the hand, as per usual. The two-finger method previously described should be used to take the pulse. Some people have a difficult time taking the radial pulse when at rest and when exercising.

Target Heart Rate

The **target heart rate** is the level or zone one should attain during aerobic activity to receive any training benefit. During exercise the heart rate increases and immediately after exercise the heart rate gradually decreases. The better the cardiovascular condition of the individual, the quicker the recovery time for the heart rate to return to its resting rate. The age and heart rate of the individual determine the intensity at which the client should exercise, especially for cardiovascular endurance. The intensity of the workout uses the **heart rate reserve,** which is the difference between the resting heart rate and the maximum heart rate. The **maximum heart rate** is the fastest rate the heart can attain under maximal exercise conditions and still receive benefit. The target heart rate zone is from 60 to 80 percent of the maximum heart rate. Staying within this range when exercising is ideal (American Heart Association, 2005b).

To calculate a target heart rate zone (THR), the maximum heart rate (MHR) and the heart rate reserve (HRR) must first be determined. To calculate the MHR the person's age is subtracted from the constant 220. The HRR is then calculated by subtracting the resting heart rate from the MHR. For example, a 30-year-old with a resting pulse of 65 beats per minute would have a 190 MHR (220 – 30 years). The same individual would have an HRR of 125 (190 – 65). The THR zone can then be calculated as either a minimal target heart rate (50 percent heart work intensity) or a maximal target heart rate (85 percent heart work intensity). To determine the minimal target heart rate, 50 percent of the HRR is added to the resting heart rate. To calculate MHR, 85 percent of the HRR is added to the resting heart rate. The 30-year-old with a resting pulse of 65 would thus have a minimal target heart rate of 127 beats per minute (50 percent of 125 HRR plus 65) and a maximal target heart rate of 171 (85 percent of 125 HRR plus 65).

It is recommended that the intensity of training be from 50 to 85 percent of the HRR or 60 to 90 percent of the MHR for developing and maintaining cardiovascular fitness, muscular strength and endurance, and body composition (Pierson, 2005).

Frequency and time are important components for increasing the body's response to cardiovascular fitness. Beyond the recommended frequency and time, exercise does not benefit the individual and injury may result. The guidelines previously discussed should be achieved gradually over several months.

Once people become experienced exercisers, they perceive or have a feeling for the amount of intensity or exertion that they are achieving (their **rate of perceived exertion**). Perceived exertion calls upon individuals to be "in tune" with their bodies physiologically and psychologically during exercise. Essentially they are using their sensory information to predict their working capacity.

Ask Yourself

Intensity

You are engaged in a walking program. How fast should you walk? How do you know you are within your target zone? Can you carry on a normal conversation with your exercise partner or are you gasping for breath?

Nursing Alert

Reaching Client Fitness Goals

A well-rounded fitness program should include cardiovascular work, resistance training, and flexibility exercises, all incorporated with a sound nutritional plan. Reaching a client's fitness goals will require a multidisciplinary approach that includes a professional nurse, trainer, and nutritionist.

Exertion ranges from very, very light to very, very hard, with very light, somewhat hard, hard, and very hard categories in between. If you are walking on a treadmill for 20 to 30 minutes, for example, you might perceive your workout to be between mildly hard and somewhat hard. However, if you struggled to complete the 30 minutes on the treadmill, you might judge your workout to be extremely hard. It is recommended that you try to maintain your workout somewhere between *somewhat hard* to *hard*.

In the FITT model, frequency and intensity are directly related. The less intense the workout, the longer an individual must work to achieve the same benefit as if the workout were more intense and the duration shorter. When starting a program one can accomplish his or her goals by working at the minimum threshold target or submaximally for a longer period of time. Gradual progression is an important key to remaining motivated and enjoying a fitness program.

A BALANCED FITNESS PROGRAM

A well-balanced fitness program includes achieving and maintaining good body composition, which includes the relative amount of fat in the body compared to fat-free weight such as muscle, bone, and other elements. Rather than be consumed with weight-measuring scales, a different set of scales can be used—one focused on energy consumption. This set of scales depends on one's energy expended versus energy consumed. A balanced fitness program includes both physical activity and change in food consumption. To change or decrease weight, lower food intake must be accompanied by more energy output, such as exercise. Moderate exercise burns 240–420 calories per hour (Murray & Zentner, 2001). There are numerous activities that can be incorporated into a fitness program that is designed to achieve the client's specific goal.

Result Expectations

How soon can results be expected from a fitness program? To experience change such as feeling or seeing results, one has to not only actively engage in physical activity but continue in physical activity as well. Immediate results are unrealistic for people just beginning an exercise program. Clients should be reminded that results take time and that they should not be discouraged if their results from the fitness program are slow. All changes toward a healthy behavior take time.

During the initial two weeks of an organized physical activity program, people express that they feel better and experience a sense of accomplishment. The actual physiological improvements usually take 6 to 12 weeks. The key is progression: not to do too much, too soon, and not to expect too much, too soon. Caution should be taken when recommending the type of activity and prescribing an exercise program for the novice exerciser. People new to exercise should be told to start slow, stay with it, and have fun. A good suggestion is to tell clients to keep their fitness goals on the refrigerator or some other prominent location.

IMPLEMENTATION OF FITNESS PROGRAM: ESSENTIAL ELEMENTS OF TRAINING

Once the assessments are complete, and the goal and plan are determined, it is time to begin the actual program. Clients should be encouraged to dress comfortably favoring clothing such as loose shorts and T-shirt, socks, and appropriate shoes. Although image may be important, comfort when exercising is more important than looks.

Athletic shoes for the specific types of exercise are important, and certainly an abundance of sport shoes are manufactured. The essential characteristics of the appropriate training shoe are proper support and cushion, the fit, and shoe performance specific to the activity such as running, walking, aerobics, or cross-training.

The essential elements of a training program include the warm-up, workout, and cool-down. The **warm-up,** which consists of stretching and mild exercise to gradually increase the heart rate, circulation, and body temperature, occurs prior to the actual workout and should be gradual. An increase in body temperature is essential for a better workout. For some people, stretching is done after the initial 10 to 15 minutes of slow walking or jogging or some other large muscle activity. For others, stretching may be done prior to and at the conclusion of the exercise session.

The actual cardiovascular workout should be from 20 to 30 minutes, depending upon the initial assessment, present physical condition, and fitness component. It may take a period of time to reach the initial minimum 20 minutes of involvement, depending on the condition of the client. Benefits such as a sense of accomplishment and feeling better can be immediate. It is the starting of a program, or taking the first step, that often requires the most determination.

The **cooldown** or warm down is gradual and should be the last 5 to 10 minutes of the completed workout. Slow jogging or walking (cardiovascular workout) followed by static stretching helps the body to readjust to a resting phase without abruptly coming to a halt. The heart rate should be monitored during the actual workout and after completing the workout. This provides immediate feedback for intensity purposes such as staying within the THR zone. After completing the workout and cooldown, the quickness with which the heart rate returns to a resting phase is an indicator of the condition of the client.

FREQUENT PROBLEMS RELATED TO EXERCISE

It can be discouraging when an individual begins an exercise program only to become injured because of doing too much too soon or because of an improper exercise technique. Understanding potential dangers as well as "listening" to the body through different aches and pains can prevent many of the injuries that often occur. Several frequent injuries may occur and there are ways to prevent and treat each. Environmental conditions including warm or cold weather and pollution also affect exercise.

Side Stitch

The exact cause of the sharp pain that occurs in the side during exercise or in the shoulders or upper back is unknown. Some experts suggest that it relates to a lack of blood flow to the respiratory muscles during exercise. Usually it occurs with novice exercisers, particularly in the beginning stages, and with experienced exercisers when higher intensities than usual occur. The remedies are to slow down, breathe deeply and slowly, or stop altogether, if it persists. When exercising, particular attention should be given to breathing in a slow rhythmic pattern. This is a reminder to warm up prior to exercising.

Muscle Soreness

Exercising when not accustomed to exercise tends to produce muscle soreness. Usually the soreness subsides gradually and disappears within several days. This soreness is different from the burn felt when doing extreme and heavy workouts or total fatigue. Lactic acid is a byproduct of heavy exercise and can cause pain that is different from the usual soreness. Careful and deliberate warm-ups plus exercising within the THR zone should help in preventing extreme muscle soreness. Remember to apply the principle of progression.

Strains and Sprains

Strains, which are injuries to muscles, and **sprains,** injuries to ligaments, can occur during exercise. Without a proper warm-up and cooldown, and with overloading body parts, strains most often occur in the quadriceps, hamstring muscles, and back (from improper lifting techniques). **Plantar fasciitis**, or arch pain most often occurs in walkers and runners. Shin splints, which occur in the front and sides of the tibia, can be extremely painful.

Warm Weather Conditions

Whether the individual is a beginner or already an experienced exerciser, extreme caution must be taken when exercising in hot, humid weather. Prolonged exposure to extreme heat as well as high humidity can result in heat cramps, heat exhaustion, or heatstroke. To exercise in heat one must gradually acclimatize to the environment and then take certain precautions.

The time of day to exercise is important, and the hottest parts of the day should be avoided at all times. Exercising either in early morning or late afternoon or in an air-conditioned facility is recommended. The type of clothing is important and should be adjusted to accommodate the heat. A change in the intensity and duration of time during workouts helps to accommodate the environment.

When exercising it is essential to replace fluids lost through evaporation by drinking large quantities of fluids whether thirsty or not. The average daily fluid intake for an adult is 1,300 milliliters. An additional 1,000 milliliters of water are obtained from foods such as fruits and vegetables, which are 80 to 90 percent water (Craven & Hirnle, 2003). A good precaution is to weigh yourself prior to exercising and again after and replenish the weight loss with fluids, preferably water.

Exercising in Cold Weather

Conserving heat becomes a major concern when exercising in cold weather. Additional problems occur when cold weather is accompanied by wind or wet conditions, or both creating a wind-chill factor. Dress in thin layers that can be altered as the body temperature rises.

Pollution Problems

Exercising in polluted conditions or smoggy weather warrants the same caution as exercising during extreme weather conditions. Avoid exercising outdoors particularly in urban areas where pollutants such as carbon monoxide, ozone, and others adversely impact the body. Like heat, pollution levels are often at their highest during midafternoon.

The nurse involved in promoting health through exercise should stress to all clients that they must learn to self-monitor their bodies during exercise. Fatigue and discomfort that accompany training are often foretelling an injury. Progressive pain during and after exercising is alerting that something is wrong and the client should slow down and rest.

RICE CONCEPT FOR INJURY TREATMENT

Minor injuries are not uncommon to anyone who exercises. The **RICE** method is a good modality to use with muscle sprains or strains or other minor discomforts. The first onset of pain or injury indicates an immediate

reduction from the exercise routine; therefore, *rest* the body for a day or more, depending on the extent of the injury. Immediately after injury apply *ice* to decrease pain and promote vasoconstriction. It is widely accepted that ice packs should be applied to the injured area for no longer than 30 minutes at a time for 72 hours after an acute injury. A light covering such as a dry-cloth towel should be applied next to the skin prior to applying the ice pack to prevent possible cold burn to the area.

Compression is vitally important in conjunction with the use of ice to control swelling. The best way to reduce the amount of space available for swelling is to apply an elastic wrap firmly and evenly around the injury. This should be done following the application of ice.

The fourth aspect of the RICE model is *elevation* of the injured part to assist in controlling swelling. In order to provide a decrease in the swelling, the injured part must be elevated above the heart. The greater the degree of elevation above the heart, the more effective the control is for the swelling. It is important to elevate as much as possible during the first 72 hours of the injury. The goal is to return to exercise and use the injured part as soon as possible; thus the treatment must be aggressive.

MYTHS ABOUT EXERCISE

The enthusiasm for fitness and exercise seems to be at an all-time high, yet this enthusiasm is puzzling since less than 25 percent of Americans engage in high levels of physical activity daily. In fact, only one in four engages in any type of physically demanding activity per day (Wellner, 2003). People who do not engage in physical activity often succumb to myths or fallacies about exercise. These myths or fallacies or both are quite difficult to dispel and must be addressed by all health care professionals if fitness and exercise are the national goal. Box 15-4 provides a description of the myths and facts related to exercise and physical activity. These should be shared with all clients who express an interest in physical fitness or who are in dire need of a physical fitness program.

HEALTH BELIEF AND HEALTH PROMOTION MODELS

Changing behavior particularly in promoting health involves choices and decisions. Having the required information such as knowledge about health-related fitness components is insufficient and incomplete for achieving fitness. Daily choices about how to live a life to influence overall health must continually be made. There are several conceptual frameworks that can provide a basis upon which to build a successful fitness program that will be adhered to by nursing's clients. These frameworks indicate that people are more likely to change their health-related behavior when they believe that there are benefits to doing so or that they can, in fact, impact their own health outcomes.

The Health Belief Model, for example, assumes that everyone wants to achieve well-being and that the person's belief that health is attainable is critical in attaining this well-being (Rosenstock, 1990). Additionally, Pender's (1996) Health Promotion Model proposes that health-promoting behavior is related to an individual's perceptions of health and perceived control over health status. The individual's belief that a certain behavior is possible, that there are benefits associated with this behavior, as well as recognition of the perceived barriers

---

BOX 15-4 Myths and Facts About Exercise

Myth 1: Exercise is too hard and time-consuming.
  Fact: An investment of 60 minutes per week divided into bouts of 20 minutes three times per week and working at a minimum of 60 percent of maximum heart rate can yield healthy benefits.

Myth 2: Exercise is not a quick way to lose weight; you have to do so much to lose even one pound of fat.
  Fact: Walking at 60 percent of maximum heart rate, people weighing between 120 and 150 pounds can expend 258 to 318 kcal per hour, respectively. Good nutrition and exercise can lead to loss of about one pound per week (Corbin & Lindsey, 2007).

Myth 3: Passive or no-sweat exercise is effective in losing fat in specific areas of the body and can increase fitness.
  Fact: Passive exercise equipment such as vibrating belts, muscle stimulators or vibrators, rubber "fat" belts, and body fat–suction suits are examples of passive exercise equipment that are ineffective. Exercise involving large muscle groups stimulates the entire body, including fat deposits.

Myth 4: Exercise causes an increase in appetite and, therefore, weight gain.
  Fact: If a weight-lifting program is selected, an increase in fat-free weight occurs and there is a possible weight gain since lean muscle mass weighs more than fat. Fat-free tissue expends more energy than fat tissue. A decrease in appetite occurs with moderate exercise. A balanced nutrition plan combined with exercise is effective in sensible weight reduction.

Myth 5: If I stop exercising all my muscle will turn to fat.
  Fact: Exercise increases fat-free tissue. Inactivity decreases fat-free tissue and increases fat tissue. The positive health benefits gained from exercise are reversed with inactivity.

in achieving the health promotion outcomes, are essential components of this model. The health care professional establishing a physical fitness program should recognize that clients are more likely to change health-related behavior if the current behavior is perceived to be detrimental to their health status. Behavior may also change if the client becomes aware that considerable unpleasantness affecting work, family, and health will occur if there are no changes. In educating clients, it is thus important to recognize that the client must believe that the benefits of the new behavior are achievable and worth the effort.

UTILIZING THE NURSING PROCESS IN DEVELOPING A PHYSICAL FITNESS PLAN

As previously described, the nursing process can be utilized in developing a health promotion plan. The nursing process is an appropriate planning tool for nurses involved in addressing physical activity and fitness needs. Frequently the nurse is the primary health provider working with clients who are experiencing health problems related to obesity, high blood lipid levels, nutritional deficiencies, or all three that will require interventions, possibly including interventions in the area of physical fitness. In determining the interventions that focus on physical fitness and activity, a complete assessment must be done followed by the establishment of the appropriate nursing diagnosis(es). Once this is done, the planning, implementation, and evaluation phases logically follow.

Assessments

The assessment phase is critical to the establishment of a physical fitness plan for any client. The assessment phase explores all of those areas that have a direct bearing on the client's ability, motivation, or both to consistently follow through with the physical activity as designated. The domains described throughout this textbook and found to influence the attainability of physical fitness must be assessed in order to individualize the health promotion plan for each client. For example, some specific assessments that pertain to the biological domain may include identification of medical conditions that affect or may limit physical activity. The client's age, weight, and height as well as body fat composition and current levels of physical activity are also important areas to include in the assessment of the biological domain.

An assessment of the client's mental status and levels of alertness as well as motivation are crucial aspects of the psychological domain that must also be included in a thorough assessment. A person's lifestyle and cultural beliefs related to physical activities might also be included as part of the assessment of the sociocultural domain. Certainly religious beliefs might influence whether a client embarks on a physical fitness plan and when the actual activities will take place. The environmental domain and its influence on physical fitness have been described previously in this chapter and must, of course, be assessed. Table 15-1 identifies the specific assessments to be made, and that may influence the physical fitness plan, according to the domains.

Nursing Diagnosis

Following the thorough assessment of the domains and all areas that might affect the physical activity and fitness plan, the appropriate nursing diagnosis(es) must be identified. For the most part, physical fitness and activity are considered interventions rather than problem areas. Many of the possibly applicable nursing diagnoses do not always directly relate to the area of physical fitness, though there are several that may. For example, there are nursing diagnoses that relate to a person's mental outlook that indirectly influence a person's desire to perform physical activity. Physical impediments, attributes, or both may also indirectly relate to physical activity and fitness nursing diagnoses.

There are some nursing diagnoses that might be appropriate for problems associated with physical fitness and activity. These are usually classified as Activity Intolerance, and Risk for Activity Intolerance (NANDA, 2007). There are also other nursing diagnoses that are specific to problems with mobility that may be a consequence of a poorly implemented physical fitness plan (Impaired Physical Mobility). These diagnoses, however, do not seem to fit in as well with the area of physical fitness and activity as does the diagnosis of Activity Intolerance.

The determination of the nursing diagnosis will always reflect the actual cause for the alteration or impairment or both. For example, the nursing diagnosis may be stated as Risk for Activity Intolerance related to deconditioned status, or Activity Intolerance related to pain or limited mobility (NANDA, 2007). The domains described throughout this textbook are useful in determining the contributing cause of the alteration. Activity Intolerance, for example, may be related to psychological problems such as major depression or poor self-concept. The actual cause of the alteration must be determined and is important in implementing appropriate interventions in the health promotion plan. Table 15-2 includes select nursing diagnoses that may affect physical activity and fitness potential categorized according to domains.

Planning

The planning phase is crucial in establishing a realistic physical fitness plan. This phase determines the proposed course of action that will ultimately lead to the client's success in initiating and maintaining physical fitness. Goals and expected outcomes should be mutually

TABLE 15-1 Assessment of Domains Influencing Physical Fitness

Domain	Specific Assessments
Biological	Client's age, weight, and height Caloric intake, basal metabolic rate Problems or conditions affecting physical activity Medical conditions affecting exercise limitations Medications that might influence energy levels and heartbeat Respiratory conditions such as allergies Blood flow to extremities Heartbeat, respiration, and blood pressure Laboratory values indicative of problems associated with obesity or other diseases such as diabetes mellitus and heart: e.g., cholesterol levels, triglyceride levels, fasting blood sugar, high/low density lipoproteins Body fat composition Current and past level of physical fitness and activity Muscular strength and flexibility
Psychological	Client's desire for fitness Motivation level, mental status, mood Client's self-perception Current stress levels Beliefs regarding benefits of physical fitness
Sociocultural	Lifestyle Self-confidence levels, attitude toward exercise Client's social activities Cultural beliefs regarding physical activities Exercise preferences
Spiritual/Religious	Client's introspection Meaning of exercise and fitness for client Religious prohibition of exercise on certain days
Environmental	Lives alone Work environment conducive to exercise Environmental influences affecting ability to exercise
Technological	Client's technological competence Ability to adapt to new technology

established between the nurse and the client. In addition to being realistic, the goals should be measurable and be based on sound rationale. Realistic and measurable outcomes may include goals such as: The client will engage in physical exercise, such as walking, for 30 minutes three times a week, or The client will progressively increase current level of activity by adding five extra minutes to his or her physical activity routine.

It is important to note that the planning phase arises from the establishment of nursing diagnoses and should be in congruence with them. For example, if the cause of the lack of physical activity or activity intolerance is related to fatigue or another biological condition, then the planning phase should address the cause. Refer to

Chapters 14 and 16 for information on how physical fitness is used as a strategy in planning care for individuals with nutritional and weight control problems.

Implementation

The implementation phase determines which interventions are more likely to resolve problems identified and achieve expected outcomes. It is an always-changing dynamic phase that is one of the most difficult in determining a nursing process plan. Knowledge of the Health Promotion Model is essential for establishing a plan that will lead to positive improvements in physical fitness and activity. Considerable efforts in motivating the

TABLE 15-2 Selected Nursing Diagnoses Related to Physical Activity and Fitness Potential According to Domains

Domain	Nursing Diagnoses
Biological	• Activity Intolerance Related to Generalized Weakness • Risk for Decreased Activity Intolerance Related to Circulatory Problems • Decreased Cardiac Output Related to Altered Heart Contractility • Impaired Physical Mobility Related to Obesity
Psychological	• Ineffective Coping Related to Inadequate Resources • Fatigue Related to Stress • Hopelessness Related to Lost Belief in God
Sociological	• Ineffective Health Maintenance Related to Ineffective Family Coping
Cultural	• Noncompliance Related to Cultural Values • Impaired Physical Mobility Related to Cultural Beliefs Regarding Age-Appropriate Activity
Environmental	• Risk for Disuse Syndrome Related to Prescribed Immobilization • Sedentary Lifestyle Related to Deficient Knowledge
Spiritual/Religious	• Spiritual Distress Related to Social Alienation • Risk for Spiritual Distress Related to Environmental and Natural Disasters
Technological	• Impaired Wheelchair Mobility Related to Impaired Ability to Operate Wheelchair

clients to make these positive changes must be made by the nurse or health care worker involved.

In order to succeed, clients must decide how they want to look and feel, not how they think someone wants them to look and feel. It is important to design an exercise program with a goal to achieve the maximum health benefit at the lowest risk. The program should emphasize regular physical activity and, more than likely, a change in lifestyle.

The various domains described earlier and throughout this text as influencing health promotion can be utilized in determining an appropriate plan necessary to achieve the established goals. For example, interventions related to the psychological domain may include referral for counseling if the client is unable or unwilling to engage in physical fitness due to depression. Interventions that address the environmental domain can, likewise, be determined and may include educating the client on appropriate clothing and gear for strenuous physical activity. Table 15-3 describes some specific physical fitness–related interventions according to the domain areas.

Evaluation

The evaluation phase is ongoing once the actual interventions are implemented. This phase will focus on outcomes and goals and determine if these have been met.

In the event that the various interventions are not working or addressing the identified nursing diagnoses, the evaluation phase leads to a modification of the plan and reevaluation phase. An example of an evaluation and modification of the plan could be one in which the nurse determines that the client must walk vigorously three times a week and is unaware that the client has a painful heel spur on his right foot that prevents him from doing so. The plan must be modified to include other types of exercise that will not cause physical stress on the right foot. Table 15-4 describes a nursing process plan that focuses on establishing a physical fitness program for a client in a deconditioned status. A case study focusing on physical fitness or activity or both is include at the end of this chapter.

GETTING STARTED AND STICKING TO IT

The most difficult aspect of becoming physically fit is getting started. As previously described, a person's motivation level for engaging in a physical fitness program or activity is crucial to success. There are several helpful hints that a nurse and health promotion expert can share with clients that will help them build or maintain motivation. Participation in a fun exercise program will reap many healthful benefits and nurses

TABLE 15-3 Physical Fitness–Related Nursing Interventions Categorized by Domains

Domain	Interventions
Biological	Monitor client's activity levels Identify abnormal lab values and report Determine plan for intensity level of activity Start fitness program gradually according to client ability Determine fitness program using FITT model Educate client on proper activity equipment, including appropriate attire and shoes Specify importance of warm-up and cooldown exercises Set up self-monitoring diary Establish exercise contract
Psychological	Refer to appropriate counseling if stress levels high Set up fitness plan utilizing small attainable goals Refer to kinesiology specialist, if necessary
Sociocultural	Encourage involvement with formal and informal fitness groups Involve significant others in fitness plan Encourage and support needed lifestyle changes
Spiritual/Religious	Encourage client to discuss spiritual/religious needs that may be influential in setting up fitness program Include specific spiritual/religious beliefs in the fitness plan
Environmental	Include environmental conditions affecting activity and fitness plan Counsel client to be cognizant of environmental influences on exercise, e.g., excessively hot or cold temperatures, pollution levels Educate on the appropriate clothing to wear when exercising
Technological	Educate client on new exercise machinery Monitor client's use of exercise equipment

TABLE 15-4 Nursing Process for an Inactive Adult Male

Assessment: A heavy-set, 40-year-old male; weight = 200 lbs.; height = 5'9"; is a smoker who has a sedentary lifestyle. The only daily exercise routine consists of parking his vehicle and climbing a flight of stairs to his office.

Nursing Diagnosis	Goals/Outcomes	Interventions
Risk for activity intolerance, related to deconditioning	Will describe five reasons for participating in progressive physical activity. Increase current activity level as evidenced by participation in a progressive fitness program.	Educate client on the importance of physical activity. Refer to the benefits of exercise according to the identified domain areas. In consultation with exercise expert, determine activity regimen using FITT. Set up attainable goals. Determine what motivates client. Monitor activity level. Increase activity level according to client tolerance. Educate on the appropriate clothes to wear when exercising. Encourage use of self-monitoring diary.

BOX 15-5   Helpful Training Tips

- Take the right step—get out the front door.
- Select activities for the program based upon the four components of fitness.
- Set aside time for exercising. Make it a part of your daily schedule.
- Select the proper equipment for exercising and have it gathered in an accessible place.
- Set your goals and plan of action. Let everyone know; this helps with motivation.
- Locate a friend or group to exercise with. It is more difficult to quit if someone else depends on you.
- Don't overdo. Listen to your body and be gradual in progression.
- Work out in different locations and facilities.
- Keep a record of your physical activities and monitor your progress.
- Reward yourself upon reaching a goal, no matter the size.
- Determine fitness goal, establish a plan incorporating the principles of overload, progression, and specificity, and act on the plan gradually.
- Resistance training should be rhythmical, performed at slow speed through a complete ROM, and with normal unforced breathing.

BOX 15-6   Practical Tips for Increasing Physical Activity

- Choose activities that you like.
- Make exercise fun, not exhausting.
- Join a neighborhood gym.
- Park your car as far away from where you are going as possible.
- Add variety to your routine.
- Find a convenient time and place to exercise.
- Dance to music you enjoy.
- Walk with a friend.
- Make Saturday family biking day.
- Spend an afternoon in a park that has a playground.
- Register for a fun run or walk.
- Share activity time with the family.
- Make walking before dinner or after dinner your family routine.
- If you have a toddler, use the stroller to walk briskly or push your toddler on a swing.
- Go swimming; don't just soak up the sun.
- Work in the yard raking leaves, planting flowers, and trimming trees.

should encourage this behavior. Box 15-5 describes helpful training tips that you can share with your clients. Box 15-6 provides some practical tips for increasing activity.

SUMMARY

Exercise and physical activity are essential to the achievement of health and wellness. Although the public in general recognizes that fitness is important to achieving a healthy lifestyle, far too many people are choosing to remain physically inactive. Physical fitness has been defined in numerous ways and, for the most part, people think of fitness in terms of athletic performance. As a health care worker, the nurse recognizes that there are different types and levels of physical fitness. Physical fitness may be described as health-related

fitness or performance and motor-skill fitness. Not all clients will achieve motor-skill fitness; however, health-related fitness is achievable.

Cardiovascular fitness, muscular strength and endurance, flexibility, and body composition are all components that must be assessed in developing a realistic physical fitness plan. The general principles of overload, specificity, and progression must also be incorporated in a physical fitness plan. Part of the planning process must include a determination of the frequency, intensity, time, and type of training that the individual is capable of. Many feel incapable of performing any type of physical activity because they succumb to myths or fallacies related to exercise. It is the responsibility of the nurse to work through these myths to help dispel them. The Health Belief and Health Promotion Models are conceptual frameworks that can be utilized in building a successful fitness program that will be adhered to by clients.

Objectives/Goals: Through participation in discussion of this case study, participants will have the opportunity to:

1. Describe factors that impact a client's ability to engage in a physical fitness program.
2. Discuss the relationship between these impacting factors and Marguerite's physical fitness status.

Health Promotion Concern, History and Physical, Present Health Status, Past Health Status, Family History, and Social History

Marguerite Brown is a 68-year-old divorced Caucasian female who lives alone in her own home in a retirement park. She is new to the area and is eager to meet people in her community. She is sedentary now because she has osteoarthritis in her knees and slight emphysema. Marguerite is somewhat overweight at 5 feet 4 inches tall and 165 pounds. Her past medical history includes a right knee replacement approximately six years ago. Her right knee is painful at times, but she is able to control the inflammation with nonsteroidal anti-inflammatory medicines. She has been a smoker since she was in her early 20s and is on several medications for her chronic bronchitis and hypertension. She sees her nurse practitioner every 12 months for her checkups or more often if she needs to. Marguerite's family history is negative for any major illnesses. Both of Marguerite's parents lived well into their 80s and did not suffer from anything other than slight hypertension. Marguerite is eager to get involved with the activities enjoyed by her neighbors in the retirement park. Although she recognizes that she is out of shape at this point, she wants to play tennis, join a yoga program, and go dancing like the others.

Review of Pertinent Domains

Biological Domain

Physical exam reveals a well-developed, overweight individual. She has no major structural disabilities that prevent her from exercising. She does smoke a pack of cigarettes a day and as a result she has a chronic cough with lung congestion and some difficulty breathing. She has some mobility problems due to osteoarthritis in her right knee.

Gastrointestinal: Reports no problems in this area. She has regular bowel movements. She loves to eat fruits and vegetables and gets her fiber from them.

Genitourinary: Nonremarkable. Urinates frequently with no discomfort. Urine is clear, straw colored, with no foul odor. She eats a light breakfast and makes lunch and dinner for herself. She loves to bake and enjoys eating what she bakes as dessert. She drinks Coca-Cola with her lunch and dinner and caffeinated coffee with breakfast.

Diagnostic testing: Marguerite's blood tests are normal with the exception of an elevated cholesterol reading.

Psychological Domain

Cognitively she is alert and oriented. Loves to read the latest news and enjoys reading novels regularly. Although she is divorced, she is happy to be able to travel and enjoy her retirement.

Social Domain

Marguerite wants to meet her neighbors. She is very sociable and eager to get involved. She loves to spend time outdoors and used to engage in a physical fitness routine. She enjoys dancing and playing tennis and hopes to find people with similar interests in her retirement community.

Environmental Domain

Marguerite lives alone in a middle-class retirement park. She is able to perform all activities of daily living without assistance. Marguerite's retirement park has a recreation room that has several exercise machines.

Technological Domain

Some of the exercise machines in the park's recreation room are brand new and computerized. Marguerite needs to have someone show her how to use the machines. She is feeling technologically incompetent and has hesitated to go exercise with the rest of her neighbors. Marguerite needs information on how to go about increasing her physical fitness so that she may resume some of the physical activities she enjoys. She also needs information on physical fitness activities and resources in her community.

Questions for Discussion

1. What should Marguerite do initially to improve her physical fitness status?
2. What types of activities can Marguerite engage in when she is alone or at home?
3. Can any of Marguerite's physical problems or medicines affect her ability to do physical activity?

Key Concepts

1. More people are choosing to take responsibility for their own well-being by becoming physically active through health-promoting behaviors.

2. Health-related fitness includes the cardiovascular, muscular strength and endurance, flexibility, and body composition components.

3. Motor-skills–related fitness, which is associated with athletic endeavor, includes power, speed, agility, balance, and reaction time.

4. Cardiovascular fitness requires large muscle groups to work together in the form of contractions during a relatively long period of time while the cardiovascular components of the heart, lungs, and vessels make adjustments to the activity as necessary.

5. Muscular strength is the ability or capacity to exert force against resistance under maximal conditions in a single effort while muscular endurance sustains a muscle contraction over an extended period of time.

6. The general principles of fitness that should be applied to a fitness program include the overload principle, principle of progression, and principle of specificity.

7. For exercise to be effective, the FITT model should be employed: frequency, intensity, time, and type of training.

8. The heart rate reserve is used to determine the intensity of a cardiovascular workout.

9. The essential elements of a training program include the warm-up, workout, and cooldown.

10. Understanding potential danger as well as "listening" to the body through different aches and pains can prevent many injuries that occur during exercise.

11. The RICE method is a good modality to use with muscle strains or sprains or other minor discomforts.

12. People who do not engage in physical activity often believe or adhere to myths and fallacies about exercise.

13. The Health Promotion and Health Belief Models can be influential in helping people make choices and decisions about engaging in health-promoting behaviors.

Learning Activities

1. Calculate your threshold of training and target heart rate zone using the method described in this chapter.

2. Select either yourself or a client, assess the health-related components, and design a walking program as the primary form of exercise for a novice exerciser using the following suggestions. The program

is only a guideline for six weeks and is not engraved in stone. It is progressive in nature and should include the essential elements of training with the FITT model.

   a. Determine your goals and plan your action. For example, begin walking at a comfortable pace (conversation oriented and walking with a friend) for 12 to 15 minutes each session, three times per week with a day of rest in between each session. Distance is less important than the actual time involved in walking. Continue with the following plan.

   b. Week 1: Walk 15 min. each day, 3X/week for a total of 15 min. each day.

   c. Week 2: Increase 3 min. each day, 3X/week for a total of 18 min. each day.

   d. Week 3: Increase 3 min. each day, 3X/week for a total of 21 min. each day.

   e. Week 4: Increase 3 min. each day, 3X/week for a total of 24 min. each day.

   f. Week 5: Increase 3 min. each day, 3X/week for a total of 27 min. each day.

   g. Week 6: Increase 3 min. each day, 3X week for a total of 30 min. each day.

This program does not have to be completed in six weeks. It is merely a guideline for a basic beginning program. Remember, if you cannot carry on a normal conversation, slow down. Use the rate of perceived exertion (RPE) to help indicate the intensity of the workout. Monitor your heart rate based upon your calculations in Learning Activity 1. Record your progression, and reward yourself upon completion of your goals.

3. Incorporate the suggested basic exercises in a warm-up and cooldown routine.

True/False Questions

1. T or F   Health is considered to be the absence of disease.

2. T or F   Statistics indicate that just under half of adults in the United States are overweight or obese.

3. T or F   Behavior and physiological and psychological barriers influence the decision to become physically active.

4. T or F   Feelings of depression negatively influence the desire to exercise.

Multiple Choice Questions

1. The *Surgeon General's Call to Action to Prevent and Decrease Overweight and Obesity* recommends that American adults exercise at least:

a. 15 minutes per day
b. 30 minutes per day
c. 45 minutes per day
d. 60 minutes per day

2. Statistics indicate that in the United States, approximately what percent age of individuals are overweight or obese?
   a. 25 percent
   b. 48 percent
   c. 61 percent
   d. 75 percent

3. Muscular endurance refers to which of the following?
   a. The ability of the muscle to perform or sustain a muscle contraction
   b. The capacity of a muscle to exert force against resistance
   c. The relative amount of fat in the body needed to sustain exercise
   d. The ability of a joint and muscle to move freely

4. Which of the following is a technique used for rehabilitative purposes as well as in clinical settings?
   a. Ballistic stretching
   b. Body mass indexing
   c. Flexibility stretching
   d. Proprioceptive neuromuscular facilitation

5. Which of the following is a general principle of fitness training?
   a. Principle of exercise behavior
   b. Plantar fasciitis principle
   c. Principle of specificity
   d. Strength and sprain principle

6. The target heart rate is which of the following?
   a. Level or zone one should attain during aerobic activity
   b. The same as the resting heart rate
   c. The maximum heart rate reserve
   d. The rate of perceived exertion

Websites

http://www.aap.org American Academy of Pediatrics. Organization dedicated to the welfare of all children.

http://www.50plus.org Fifty-Plus Lifelong Fitness (formerly Fifty-Plus Fitness Association). A nonprofit organization whose mission is to promote an active lifestyle for older people. Publishes a newsletter, distributes books and videos, and sponsors physical activity events for midlife and older adults.

http://www.osophs.dhhs.gov The Office of Disease Prevention and Health Promotion, Office of Public Health and Science, Office of the Secretary, U.S. Department of Health and Human Services. Works to strengthen the disease prevention and health promotion priorities of the department within the collaborative framework of the HHS agencies.

http://www.prevent.org Partnership for Prevention™. A national membership organization dedicated to building evidence of sound disease prevention and health promotion policies and practices and advocating their adoption by public and private sectors.

http://medlineplus.gov Medline Plus. Provides information from the National Library of Medicine and the National Institutes of Health.

http://phpartners.org Partners in Information Access for the Public Health Task Force. A collaboration of U.S. government agencies, public health organizations, and health sciences libraries focusing on health objectives.

http://www.scouting.org To Be Physically Fit. Website emphasizing physical fitness for Cub Scouts, Boy Scouts, venturers, and leaders.

References

American Academy of Family Physicians. (2005). Exercise: A healthy habit to start and keep. Retrieved December 12, 2005, from http://www.familydoctor.org

American Heart Association. (2005a). Culture-specific exercise sparks interest of older women. Retrieved May 10, 2006, from http://www.americanheart.org

American Heart Association. (2005b). Target heart rate. Retrieved December 12, 2005, from http://www.americanheart.org

Corbin, C., & Lindsey, R. (2007). *Fitness for Life (5th ed.)*. Champaign, IL: Human Kinetic Publishers.

Craven, R., & Hirnle, C. (2003). *Fundamentals of nursing: Human health and function* (4th ed.). Philadelphia: Lippincott Williams & Wilkins.

Edelman, C. L., & Mandle, C. L. (2006). *Health promotion throughout the lifespan* (6th ed.) St Louis: Mosby.

Murray, R. B., & Zentner, J. P. (2001). *Health promotion strategies throughout the lifespan* (7th ed.). Upper Saddle River, NJ: Prentice Hall.

NANDA. (2007). *Nursing diagnoses: Definitions and classification 2007–2008*. Philadelphia: NANDA International.

Pender, N. J. (1996). *Health promotion in nursing practice* (3rd ed.). Norwalk, CT: Appleton & Lange.

Pender, N. J., Murdaugh, C. L., & Parsons, M. A. (2006). *Health promotion in nursing practice* (5th ed.). Upper Saddle River, NJ: Pearson Prentice Hall.

Pierson, V. R. (2005). Understanding your target heart rate. Retrieved May 10, 2006, from http://www.primusweb.com

Riebe, D., Blissmer, B., Greene, G., Caldwell, M., Ruggiero, L., Stillwell, K. M., & Nigg, C. R. (2005). Long-term maintenance of exercise and healthy eating behaviors in overweight adults. *Preventive Medicine, 40*(6), 769–778.

Rosenstock, I. M. (1990). The health belief model: Exploring health behaviors through expectancies. In Glanz, K., Lewis, F. M., & Rimer, B. K. (Eds.), *Health behavior and health education: Theory, research, and practice*. San Francisco: Jossey-Bass.

Sankofa, P. (2006). Afro-Cuban dancing with Rene Thompson adds culture to exercise regimen. *Journal of Community News, Business and Arts*. Insight News. Retrieved May 10, 2006, from http://www.insightnews.com

Teachnet.ie. (2005). Retrieved December 12, 2005, from http://www.teachnet.ie/coconnor/componentsoffitness.htm#backtotop

TeachPE.com. (2005). http://www.teachpe.com/cloze/health_related_fitness.htm

U.S. Department of Health and Human Services, Office of Disease Prevention and Health Promotion. (2005). *Healthy People 2010*. Retrieved December 12, 2005, from http://www.healthypeople.gov

U.S. Department of Health and Human Services, Centers for Disease Control and Prevention. (2005). *Nutrition, physical activity, and obesity prevention program: Resource guide for nutrition and physical activity interventions to prevent obesity and other chronic diseases*. Retrieved December 2, 2005, from http://www.cdc.gov

U.S. Department of Health and Human Services. (2001). *The surgeon general's call to action to prevent and decrease overweight and obesity*. Retrieved May 10, 2006, from http://www.surgeongeneral.gov/reportspublications.html#public

Wellner, A. S. (2003). More Americans see fit to sit: Fewer than 25 percent of Americans engage in high levels of physical activity on a regular basis. Retrieved May 11, 2006, from http://findarticles.com

Bibliography

Burbank, P. M., & Riebe, D. (Eds.). (2002). *Promoting exercise and behavior change in older adults*. New York: Springer.

Bushman, B. A. (2005). *Action plan for menopause*. Champaign, IL: Human Kinetics.

Gordon, M. (2002). *Manual of nursing diagnosis: Including all diagnostic categories approved by the North American Nursing Diagnosis Association* (10th ed.). St. Louis: Mosby.

Hong, S., Farag, N. H., Nelseen, R. A., Ziegler, M. G., & Mills, P. J. (2004). Effects of regular exercise on lymphatic subsets and CD62L after psychological vs. physical stress. *Journal of Psychosomatic Research, 56*(3), 363–370.

Jakicic, J. (2002). Relationship of physical activity to eating behaviors and weight loss in women. *Medicine and Science in Sports Exercise, 34*, 1653.

Padden, D. L. (2002). The role of the advanced practice nurse in the promotion of exercise and physical activity. *Topics in Advanced Practice Nursing Journal, 2*, 1.

Wenzel, L., Glanz, K., & Lerman, c. (2002). Stress, coping, and health behavior. In K. Glanz, B. K. Rimer, & F. M. Lewis (eds.), *Health behavior and health education* (3rd ed.). San Francisco: Jossey-Bass.

Chapter 16

CONTROLLING WEIGHT

Linda Eanes, EdD, RN
Carolina G. Huerta, EdD, MSN, RN

KEY TERMS

balance
basal metabolic rate
body image
    disturbances
central obesity
desirable body weight

ideal body weight
negative energy
    balance
obesity
optimal body
    composition

positive energy
    balance
regular physical
    exercise
set-point of weight
    control theory

severe obesity
sleep apnea
weight control
weight cycling

OBJECTIVES

Upon completion of this chapter, the reader should be able to:

- Identify physiological, psychosocial, and economic consequences of obesity.
- Recognize obstacles encountered in weight control.
- Identify theories associated with obesity.
- Describe how the domains fundamental to health promotion influence weight.
- Describe how the biological/physiological domains influence obesity.
- Recognize the role of heredity in obesity.
- Describe environmental domain influences on obesity.
- Identify biological theories that influence weight control.
- Describe how the sociocultural domain influences weight control.
- Recognize how the nursing process may be utilized in developing a weight control health promotion plan.
- Utilize nursing's health promotion model in determining strategies for weight control.
- Explain ways to help promote lifestyle changes and successful weight control.

INTRODUCTION

The United States is a prosperous, highly mechanized, technologically advanced society, but is enjoying this land of plenty and convenience costing people their health and well-being? Sadly, the answer is yes. With economic growth and prosperity, there is a parallel rise in obesity and obesity-related problems. More than half of the U.S. population is considered overweight. Rates of obesity among this population are climbing. Overweight and obesity statistics are found not only in adult populations. It is estimated that the percentage of children and adolescents who are obese has doubled in the last 20 years (Medline Plus Medical Encyclopedia, 2004). Many health care problems can be linked to overweight and obesity. Most experts conclude that many of these problems are a result of individual lifestyle choices. Lack of activity and obesity and their consequences are correlated with increased incidence of cardiovascular diseases, diabetes mellitus, and other general problems that may be life-threatening and could also lead to immobility. Through the use of weight control health-promoting strategies, many of the health care problems that are associated with a sedentary and technologically enhanced lifestyle may be prevented.

The two previous chapters addressed the importance of nutrition and physical fitness in health promotion. This chapter will focus on the physiological, psychosocial, and economic consequences of obesity and will highlight weight control as a strategy for health promotion. The nursing process and health promotion model will also be emphasized.

CONSEQUENCES OF OBESITY

The prevalence of **obesity**, or being above ideal body weight by 20 percent or more, among adults living in the United States is at an all-time high. The National Heart, Lung, and Blood Institute estimates that about 97 million adults in the United States are overweight or obese. Obesity and overweight substantially increase the risk of morbidity from hypertension, dyslipidemia, type 2 diabetes, coronary heart disease, stroke, gallbladder disease, osteoarthritis, sleep apnea and respiratory problems, and endometrial, breast, prostate, and colon cancers. Higher body weights are also associated with increases in all-cause mortality (National Heart, Lung, and Blood Institute, 2000).

Americans are increasingly becoming overweight but the verdict is still out on whether this trend applies to clinically **severe obesity.** Severe obesity refers to being 100 pounds or more (45 kg) over normal body weight (Sturm, 2003). Severe obesity may have different causes than overweight and creates different challenges for the health care system. Severe obesity is not that easy to explain. It is considered a complex disorder that has been linked to biochemical, physiologic, genetic, or inherited influences on weight maintenance. Other domains, such as environmental, cultural, socioeconomic, and psychological, are thought to be contributing factors associated with obesity (Wallace, Schulte, Nakeeb, & Andris, 2001). Box 16-1 describes one way in which obesity has been defined.

A variety of medical problems, including high blood pressure, heart problems, diabetes, sleep apnea, depression, and arthritis, have been associated with being overweight. There are numerous physiological consequences associated with obesity. Cardiovascular problems, for example, are common among obese people. High blood pressure is also associated with obesity, and it can lead to heart problems, kidney failure, and stroke as well. Severely obese people are six times more likely to develop heart disease because the heart in an obese person is required to work harder, which can lead to early development of congestive heart failure. Severely obese people often have elevated cholesterol levels, which can also contribute to heart disease and the hardening of blood vessels. Diabetes, which frequently strikes the obese, is another risk factor for developing coronary heart disease and is 10 times more likely to develop in overweight individuals. Respiratory problems are also a consequence of obesity since the chest wall is heavier to lift than in the normal weight person. Obesity

Ask Yourself

Psychosocial Consequences of Obesity

How many people are not employed because of their appearance? Are obese persons more likely to suffer from some form of discrimination by their employers because they are viewed as less healthy, less intelligent, weak, or lazy? Are obese persons frequently subjected to disapproving looks or comments? Because we equate being slender with power, control, beauty, happiness, goodness, and fitness, are those who are obese viewed as helpless, ugly, unhappy, and lazy?

can aggravate a previously diagnosed condition such as asthma and may also cause **sleep apnea**, a condition that is characterized by recurrent periods of absence of breathing for 10 seconds or longer, occurring at least five times per hour (American Sleep Apnea Association, 2006). Musculoskeletal problems, gastroesophageal reflux, and urinary incontinence can also result from obesity as can hormone imbalances in women (Wallace, Schulte, Nakeeb, & Andris, 2001).

The location of body fat appears to be of particular importance in determining risk factors. **Central obesity** is a pattern of obesity in which a high proportion of body fat is localized around the abdomen and upper body. Central obesity is associated with a higher probability of developing plasma lipid disorders, abnormalities of insulin action (insulin resistance), increased insulin production, polycystic ovary syndrome, and syndrome X (Wikipedia, 2006).

In addition, obesity has important psychosocial and economic consequences. Obesity-related diseases create a huge financial burden to taxpayers as the result of increased health, life, and disability insurance premiums, as well as increased sick leave coverage According to Finkelstein, Fiebelkorn, and Wang (2003), medical costs associated with being overweight or obese accounted for 9.1 percent of the total U.S. medical expenditures in 1998 and may be as high as $78.5 billion in 2003. Approximately half of these costs were paid by the taxpayer through Medicare and Medicaid. As can be seen in Chapter 4, the psychosocial domain also plays a significant role in promoting wellness and preventing disease. The psychosocial impact of obesity, though difficult to measure, can create major obstacles in achieving optimal health. These obstacles will greatly challenge nursing skills in caring for obese clients.

Unfortunately, there is very little information about the psychological impact that obesity may have on persons who are severely obese. Most studies have been limited to severely obese persons seeking treatment and,

BOX 16-1 Obesity Defined

Overweight:

Above ideal body weight by less than 20%

Obesity:

Mild	20% to 40% above ideal body weight
Moderate	40% to 100% above ideal body weight
Morbid	50% to 100% above ideal body weight
Severe	100 lbs. or more above ideal body weight

therefore, may not be representative of the general population. From knowledge of the importance of the concept of person in nursing's metaparadigm, however, it is easy to recognize the importance of self-concept and self-esteem to all people. As may be recalled, Chapter 2 describes Maslow's hierarchy of needs, which includes the need for self-esteem. This need for self-esteem also incorporates the need for approval and feelings of self-worth. It stands to reason, then, that an obese person who is the subject of disapproval by society because of an overweight condition will probably suffer from low self-esteem.

Given the magnitude and seriousness of obesity, nurses should address weight control in promoting the health of their clients. **Weight control** involves the change, acquisition, and maintenance of a desirable body weight, whereas a **desirable body weight** entails achieving a balance between adequate nutrition, proper body fat, and physical activity (Craven & Hirnle, 2007). The key word is **balance.** Balance implies that the total energy intake in the form of nutrient calories does not exceed the body's expenditure of energy. As discussed in Chapter 14, food intake and energy needs are met in a way that reduces the risk of disease and promotes the overall stability between the body and mind.

HEALTH PROMOTION AND WEIGHT CONTROL

Current emphasis has been placed by the U.S. government on health promotion and disease prevention. Since the late 1980s the Public Health Service of the U.S. Department of Health and Human Services (USDHHS) has set forth health promotion objectives in both *Healthy People 2000* and *Healthy People 2010.* Overweight and obesity are two leading health indicators that have been chosen as a focus area among children, adolescents, and adults.

There are several objectives related to overweight and obesity; however, two objectives that are used to measure progress for this leading indicator of health are (1) reduce the proportion of children and adolescents who are overweight or obese and (2) reduce the proportion of adults who are obese (USDHHS, 2000). The USDHHS promotes efforts to maintain a healthy weight and emphasizes the need for regular physical activity. Over time, even a small decrease in calories eaten and a small increase in physical activity can help prevent weight gain and facilitate weight loss.

Although nurses may be viewed as pioneers addressing potential health problems and needs, the future of the profession may hinge on nurses' ability to take an active role in guiding clients to increase self-understanding and to learn new skills that promote the adoption of sound dietary practices and increased physical exercise. Nurses practicing both in a hospital setting and outside have a unique opportunity to implement a variety of preventive interventions to assist clients in gaining control of their weight and promoting their overall health and well-being.

OBSTACLES TO WEIGHT CONTROL

Finding the necessary balance to achieve weight control is difficult for many. No theory fully explains the nature and causes of obesity. Obesity is a complex phenomenon involving the interaction of multiple factors, including genetic susceptibility, diet composition, inactivity, psychological influences, culture, and physiologic mechanisms.

Although some Americans realize that their dietary habits and inactivity are adversely affecting their health, problems resulting from existing behaviors frequently may not be manifested for decades. Adopting sound nutritional habits is a lifestyle choice. Because many of the diseases that affect individuals as they age are related to their food consumption, dietary modifications may decrease overweight- and obesity-related diseases. People who are knowledgeable about the type of health problems they may acquire may be more willing to modify their diets to maximize health (Lutz & Przytulski, 2006). Educating individuals about lifestyle choices may be costly for society but is less costly than treating diseases in the long run.

Our culture and values impact our choices of foods and nutritional patterns. Ethnic identity, nationality, and even educational preparation and religion are factors that influence food choices. Some aspects of culture related to food choices are passed on from birth (Lutz & Przytulski, 2006). Other food patterns and choices are learned and differences may exist among cultures.

Other cultural factors may also be important determinants of eating and physical activity. Within our society, certain groups may place a greater emphasis on patterns of eating and less importance on physical activity and weight control, which may predispose them toward obesity. Attitudes about specific food preferences and physical size may also contribute to obesity.

Ideal body weight refers to what a person should reasonably weigh as compared to height. It results from a balance between adequate nutrition, proper body fat, and physical activity. This definition, as well as definitions for beauty and health, has changed over time. In the 1950s, the Rubenesque, or well-rounded, body was desired. The anorexic look (the thinner, the better) led by Twiggy, an English model, dominated the 1960s. Today, the thinness mania is waning. Looking fit and muscular is more popular. It seems that the most realistic approach, then, is to assist people in achieving a balance between food intake and activity and to encourage them to focus on the total consumption of food rather than individual foods. Thinking of foods as either good or bad is not as important as eating a variety of foods in moderate amounts and including regular physical exercise.

Nevertheless, most Americans are inactive. Although the health benefits of physical exercise are well documented, estimates indicate only 10 to 20 percent of the adult population between the ages of 18 and 65 exercise with the intensity and frequency that would lead to positive health outcomes. Many of today's adults and, alarmingly, children lead a sedentary lifestyle.

If being fit and muscular is considered vogue, then why are so many adults inactive? Interventions that focus on factors that influence physical activity are thought to be more useful in increasing physical activity among populations. An intervention protocol that focuses on self-efficacy, social support, perceived benefits of exercise, and perceived barriers to physical activity may result in behavioral changes (Pender, Murdaugh, & Parsons, 2006). Perhaps many adults believe they were born to be overweight and have no control over their weight. Some may accept weight gain as a normal aging process. Some may lack confidence in their ability to change. Others may think they are too out of shape, are too tired, or do not have time to exercise. The negative consequences associated with exercise, such as exercise taking too much time and causing pain and sore muscles, may be enough to stop some from trying. Also, the results from exercise—lost pounds and inches—are not immediate. Visible results take weeks of consistent effort.

Conceivably, the primary reason many Americans resist change is that they continue to search for a painless, quick fix. There are a number of people claiming to be experts who try to appeal to our desire for immediate results. In fact, dieting and weight control have become big business. Billions of dollars are spent annually in America on weight loss. Indeed, even a quick glance at a typical magazine or book rack will probably reveal an assortment of eye-catching titles like *Weight-Loss: Tips That Work; Lose Fat Faster;* or *Lose Ten Pounds In Ten Days.* Unfortunately, there are no quick and easy fixes. In most cases, these quick fixes actually compound the problems.

As might be surmised by now, the causes of obesity are not usually well understood. Some individuals have a genetic predisposition; others have neurological or hormonal disorders that contribute to obesity. Others may live a very sedentary lifestyle or lack responsibility for their health and well-being. Studies suggest that about

Research Note

Effect of Body Mass Index Recording in Clients' Records

Study Problem/Purpose: To evaluate the effectiveness of body mass index (BMI) tables placed in exam rooms as an intervention to encourage providers to calculate and record BMI scores in clients' medical records. Overweight and obesity have increased dramatically in the United States over the past decade. Provider attention to the issue of obesity has been shown to have a positive effect on weight control.

Methods: Medical record data for 276 adult clients at a federally funded community health center were examined over a period of two years. Prominent, multicolored, laminated BMI tables were posted in the exam rooms of one of the site's three primary health care teams. Data collected included documentation of BMI, documentation of an obesity diagnosis, and inclusion of heights and current weights in medical records. Frequency distributions were calculated and chi-square tests were used to identify associations.

Findings: Clients treated by the intervention team were more likely to have BMI recorded in the medical record. A statistically significant increase in the diagnosis of obesity was observed throughout the health center after the intervention.

Implications: Awareness of BMI encourages providers to focus attention on the issue of obesity. Posting the BMI tables in exam rooms contributed to increased documentation of obesity in clients' medical records.

Lemay, C. A., Cashman, D. B., Savageau, J. A., and Reidy, P. (2004). Effect of a low-cost intervention on recording body mass index in patients' records. *Journal of Nursing Scholarship, 36*(4), 312.

25 to 40 percent of individual differences in body weight and body fat is dependent on genetic factors. Evidence also suggests that some people are more susceptible to either weight gain or weight loss than others. Obesity and overweight are not always the result of lack of adherence to prescribed dietary modifications. Obesity may be related not only to genetic tendencies but also to ethnicity and ethnic disparities (Black & Hawks, 2005). While it is true that genetic tendencies for overweight and obesity are often observed in family units, obesity is more prevalent among certain ethnicities. The reasons for this are not clear, so it is necessary to consider culture in a sensitive manner when developing health promotion approaches.

Childhood and Adolescent Obesity

Unfortunately obesity is not a health promotion problem affecting only adults. Obesity in children is a very serious problem that may cause health and social problems into adulthood (American Obesity Association, 2005). There is a likelihood that obesity beginning in early childhood will persist throughout the lifespan. Teaching healthy behaviors and promoting lifestyle changes in early childhood is important since change always becomes more difficult with age.

It is estimated that about 15.5 percent of adolescents (ages 12 to 19) and 15.3 percent of children (ages 6 to 11) are obese. Childhood obesity has doubled since 1976 and almost tripled in adolescents (American Obesity Association, 2005). This increase in obesity among American youth over the past two decades is dramatic and must be addressed by health care professionals.

Parents may not recognize the consequences of obesity. Being overweight does not mean that the child is well nourished. Obesity can lead to many complications that are similar to those that occur in obese adults. Obesity can increase the risk for hypertension and heart disease. It can also lead to bowing of legs and pain in the hip joint as a result of the excessive weight. Chances of diabetes mellitus, elevated cholesterol, and gallbladder disease also increase (Pediatric Oncall Child Health Care, 2001). Physical activity and appropriate nutrition are essential to preventing obesity. A health promotion approach in children and adolescents should focus on proper nutrition, selection of low-fat foods, increased exercise, and reduction in sedentary activities such as watching television, playing video games, and so forth.

DOMAINS INFLUENCING OBESITY, WEIGHT CONTROL, AND EATING BEHAVIORS

There are a number of theories that may help explain why some people are prone to excessive accumulation of fat and have difficulty achieving weight control. There is no common agreement, however, among experts on what causes overweight and obesity to be prevalent among some individuals. Understanding factors influencing weight control and obtaining knowledge on how some of the health promotion domains influence obesity and weight control may help nurses intervene more appropriately. The biological, environmental, psychological, and social domains are primary focus areas when discussing and identifying intervention strategies to prevent overweight and obesity.

Biological Domain

Are some people born to be fat? There are many biological factors that influence whether an individual becomes obese or remains lean throughout a lifetime. According to the theory of genetics and obesity, genetics influences human body mass and stature. The underlying assumptions of this theory are that people resemble their biological parents and that obesity and fat deposition are largely under genetic control. These assumptions, however, should not be taken to mean that a person will become obese regardless of dietary behaviors. The following are some biological factors influencing whether an individual will become obese.

Theory of Thermogenesis and Weight Control

According to the theory of thermogenesis and weight control, weight control is the result of a balance between caloric intake and energy expenditure. When there is an imbalance, that is, when the calorie (energy) intake exceeds the calories used, the surplus calories are stored as fat (Lutz & Przytulski, 2006). Because adipose tissue is the major energy storage organ, body weight increases as body fat deposits increase. Therefore, obesity results from overeating, a decreased expenditure of energy (inactivity), or a combination of both. Overeating appears to be an important factor in the cause of obesity.

The Five-Hundred Rule states that to lose one pound of body fat per week, a person must eat 500 kilocalories fewer per day than the body expends for seven days. To gain a pound of body fat per week, a person must eat 500 kilocalories more per day for seven days than the body expends. As such, weight control is very influenced by expenditure of energy through activity. Decreased energy expenditure may cause or perpetuate obesity (Lutz & Przytulski, 2006). In order to maintain a balance between caloric intake and energy expenditure, dietary patterns should be adjusted. Energy expenditure is dependent on the **basal metabolic rate**, which is the amount of energy required to carry out involuntary activities at rest (e.g., breathing, body temperature, circulation; Craven & Hirnle, 2007). In other words, if too much food is consumed, a person will gain weight or be in what is referred to as a positive energy balance. **Positive energy balance,** then, occurs when the amount of food consumed exceeds the energy used by the body. Conversely, if a person's energy needs exceed that produced by the food consumed, a **negative energy balance** occurs. For body weight to remain constant, food intake must equal energy needs. Therefore, to lose weight a person must burn more calories each day than the calories consumed.

Theory of Equilibrium Set-Point of Weight Control

Body weight usually remains relatively constant. This point is particularly significant when one considers that the amount of calories required to function varies widely from hour to hour or day to day. Some individuals who are more prone to gain weight are thought to require fewer kilocalories to perform normal body functions than do lean individuals. Some experts believe that it is true that some obese individuals have a slow metabolism. The **set-point of weight control theory** states that all individuals have a unique, stable, adult body weight that is the result of several biological factors. The obese person is thought to have a higher set-point than does the lean individual (Lutz & Przytulski, 2006). The underlying premise of this theory is analogous to setting a thermostat to maintain a constant room temperature. If you set the thermostat at 76 degrees, an air conditioner will turn on or off in order to maintain room temperature at 76 degrees. The thermostat is equivalent to the set-point for body weight, whereas the air conditioner is equivalent to either an increase or decrease in metabolic activity required to maintain this body weight (set-point). Each person has an internal set-point that is established by biological or genetic factors and controlled by the hypothalamus. Because of this set-point, starving or overfeeding will be followed by a rapid return to the original weight. In other words, during times of famine, the body survives by lowering its set-point or energy requirements (basal metabolic rate).

The set-point of weight control theory may help explain excessive weight gain. When a person diets, the basal metabolic rate is lowered. The body does not know a person is dieting to lose weight on purpose. The body interprets extreme calorie deprivation as starving and tries to compensate. After the dieting has ended, the effects of the lowered metabolic rate continue. Many researchers believe that stringent dieting triggers binge eating. Eating after starving may be as natural as gasping for air after being deprived of oxygen.

Weight cycling is losing and regaining weight as seen in yo-yo dieting. Yo-yo dieting is the repeated practice of dieting followed by the return to normal eating patterns or in some cases overeating and then dieting again. This practice is not only counterproductive, but may have potentially harmful effects. Weight cycling appears to alter the set-point for weight control. When the basal metabolic rate is lowered, as with a diet-only approach, the muscle-to-fat ratio is altered. Muscle is lost and fat is gained. The energy required to sustain life is taken from muscle. Thus, the results of dieting may be a loss of muscle mass and a gain in body fat.

Although the results are inconclusive, diets very low in calories (800 calories per day or less) may lead to a protein-sparing effect. It bears mentioning that dieting not only results in loss of body fat. There is always loss of protein during weight loss because lean body mass is more metabolically active and burns more kilocalories than fat tissue (Lutz & Przytulski, 2006, p. 377). The greater the amount of weight loss, the more organ and muscle mass is lost.

The long-term detrimental effects of weight cycling remain undetermined. However, the health risks associated with obesity are known. Therefore nurses should encourage those who have a history of weight cycling to gain control of their weight through lifestyle changes. Nurses can be instrumental in assisting clients with lifelong commitments to better eating and activity patterns.

Theories of Biochemical Influences and Eating Behaviors

Out-of-control eating and obesity may be the consequence of a broken brain or malfunctioning central nervous system. According to theory of biochemical influences and eating behaviors, obesity may occur as a result of a malfunction of the mechanisms within the brain that regulate appetite and satiety (Payne & Hahn, 2000). While the physiology of eating is a poorly understood complex process, the limbic system and the hypothalamus have been identified as the command centers of the brain that control hunger, food intake, and satiety. The hypothalamus, located at the base of the brain, serves as a mediator between the brain and body by regulating the endrocrine system (Guyton & Hall, 2006). The ventromedial hypothalamus has been identified as the satiety center, where electrical stimulation (an action potential) of this area reduces appetite. Innervation, or electrical stimulation, of the ventrolateral hypothalamus increases hunger and appears to initiate feeding behavior. Studies with mice have shown that electrical stimulation of the feeding center evokes eating behavior and destruction of the satiety center leads to hyperphasia and hypothalamic obesity (Ganong, 2005).

Many neuroscientists believe that the problem in the brain leading to obesity is a breakdown in neurotransmitter systems. Within the central nervous system, of which the hypothalamus is a part, cells (neurons) communicate with each other through chemicals called neurotransmitters. Molecules seep out of one cell and excite another cell, triggering electrical signals (action potentials). Norepinephrine (also known as noradrenaline) and serotonin are two neurotransmitters that have been implicated as playing an integral role in appetite, eating behaviors, and satiety. The norepinephrine-containing cells originate in the brainstem and ascend in a netlike manner (like electrical wiring) through the midbrain, the hypothalamus, and throughout the cerebral cortex. The serotonergic system also originates in the brainstem and projects to portions of the hypothalamus, the limbic system, the cerebral cortex, and the spinal cord (Ganong, 2005).

Anorectics (antisuppressing drugs) presented for the treatment of obesity are not intended as a cure for obesity, but rather as an adjunct treatment while an individual makes lifestyle changes in eating and activity behaviors. Anorectics have not been considered a safe alternative to dieting since the fen-phen scare in 1997. Currently, few appetite-suppressing drugs are being prescribed by health care providers. The question of risk versus benefit has come under great scrutiny with these drugs. After the approval in the 1940s and 1950s of a number of amphetamine and amphetamine-like compounds for the treatment of obesity, the U.S. Food and Drug Administration struggled to define the efficacy and safety of these agents. Labeling restrictions on duration of use and warnings about abuse and addiction ultimately have contributed to the reduced use of anorectics. The reduced use of prescribed anorectics continued until the mid- to late 1990s, when the off-label use of fenfluramine plus phentermine (fen-phen) and the approval of dexfenfluramine gave rise to widespread, long-term use of anorectics to treat obesity. The adverse effects that have come to be associated with fenfluramine and dexfenfluramine, leading to their eventual withdrawal from the market, have given pause to regulators, health care providers, clients, and drug companies alike. Very few prescribed diet drugs are currently in use. Two of the most popular are sibutramine (Meridia) and xenical (Orlistat). Xenical works in the intestine where it blocks fats by preventing their absorption or digestion or both. Many physically and socially unpleasant side effects are associated with xenical. These include gastrointestinal distress, oily bowel movements, urgency, and flatulence. The rate of adverse effects is related to how much fat is ingested. If more fats are ingested, there are more adverse effects (Health Facts, 2004). Sibutramine, the latest anorectic to enter the market, is now the focus of a landmark trial that is examining, for the first time, whether drug-induced weight loss reduces the risk for fatal and nonfatal cardiovascular disease (Colman, 2005). Evidence suggests that anorectic drugs increase the likelihood of hypertension, stroke, and other possibly fatal consequences.

Not all theories of biological influences and the development of obesity are widely accepted. According to another theory of biochemical influences and eating behaviors, the hypothalamus does not act alone. It influences and is influenced by other systems. The endocrine system is a group of glands located throughout the body. The hypothalamus communicates with these various glands through substances known as hormones. Hormones are chemical messengers that travel through the bloodstream in order to reach the glands they control. The hypothalamus receives continuous feedback from the organs of the endocrine system, which also produce hormones. It is through this feedback system that the hypothalamus monitors the pituitary (Guyton, 2005). The thyroid has been considered an important gland in the endocrine system contributing to obesity. Thyroid hormones increase metabolic rate and energy expenditure. Conversely, a deficiency of thyroid hormone causes a decrease in metabolic rate. One could conclude that a hypometabolic state produced by deficient quantities of circulating thyroid hormones could cause obesity and that treatment with thyroid hormones would increase the resting metabolic rate and reduce hunger. However, long-term treatment of obesity with thyroid replacement has not proven successful.

Environmental Domain

There are, of course, other factors that influence whether a person will become obese. The environment, for example, plays an indirect—but powerful—influence. This is good news, because nurses may assist individuals with learning how to modify their environment to promote weight control. The environment is thought to be a major determinant of overweight and obesity. Environmental influences are related to food intake and physical activity behaviors. The overabundance of food in the United States plus the aggressive marketing of foods promote high calorie consumption. It seems that the U.S. environment is intent on perpetuating and promoting overweight and obesity while the U.S. government is intent on controlling overconsumption and obesity.

Theories of Environmental Influences

Nature versus nurture has been debated for years. As previously stated, there appears to be some genetic component to the development of obesity, but the environment clearly influences whether someone will become obese. According to cognitive-behavioral theorists, people's early environmental experiences influence behaviors. Eating patterns stem from the home environment. If the home environment encourages overeating, then overeating becomes an ingrained pattern of behavior. In other words, people may be obese because they were taught to eat large meals high in calories and fat.

Moreover, according to cognitive-behavioral theorists, people learn to eat excess amounts of food because of the abundance of foods available to them. In other words, in prosperous environments where foods are plentiful, there is a parallel rise in obesity. Con-

affect eating patterns. Some people tend to eat more when they are sad, upset, depressed, anxious, or stressed. This may create a vicious cycle since overeating may lead to overweight that can then have psychological consequences. These psychological consequences can result in overeating, thus continuing the cycle. Research has shown that psychological factors are in part responsible for obesity and overweight. These psychological factors must be addressed if weight loss is the ultimate goal. In addressing health promotion in overweight clients, the nurse must recognize that a person-centered approach that enables understanding of the psychology behind eating behaviors is essential (Sharman, 2004).

Understanding the psychological consequences of being overweight cannot be minimized. Traditional models of obesity treatment and management have sometimes neglected to include the psychological domain. One important psychological consequence of obesity is **body image disturbance** (Lutz & Przytulski, 2006). Body image disturbance refers to a distorted image that a person has of himself or herself. This distorted image can lead to eating disorders such as anorexia or bulimia (see Chapter 15). Obese clients may also present with poor self-esteem, self-worth, and self-confidence. There are clear obesity-depression links in the literature, but there is no conclusive evidence as to which comes first (Sharman, 2004).

Sociocultural Domain

The sociocultural domain is also integral to a discussion about weight control. Societal expectations include having a lean and trim body. The United States seems, in particular, to be obsessed with leanness. Our society often

versely, in poorly developed environments where foods are less available, the incidence of obesity is far less.

Recognizing that obesity is probably the result of both genetic and environmental forces interacting with each other, nurses should assist clients in modifying their environments to reduce the risk of developing obesity. Perhaps something as simple as pointing out that grocery shopping on an empty stomach may influence the selection of fat-laden, calorie-rich foods is all the information that a client needs to modify this behavior. It is essential that a client also recognizes that unhealthy behaviors that have been learned may be unlearned.

Psychological Domain

The psychological domain influences and is influenced by weight-related lifestyle behaviors. Emotional status is very important to weight control since emotions can

equates attractiveness with thinness, especially in women. Societal expectations may cause those who are overweight or obese to feel unattractive and ashamed. The assumption is that overweight and obese people are gluttonous, lazy, or both. This, of course, is not true (Wellman, 2002). Obese people face prejudice or discrimination at work, at school, while job hunting, and in social situations every day. Feelings of rejection, shame, or depression are common. Obesity has severe psychological consequences in all age groups. Overweight or obese children also encounter prejudice and discrimination in society. Many children are teased or receive negative comments that will be remembered throughout life. Disparagement of obese individuals persists as one of the last socially accepted forms of prejudice (Loke, 2002).

Cultural expectations as well as ethnicity also influence weight control. The foods that we eat and the type of activity that we participate in may also be related to acculturation factors. There may be a lack of pressure to lose weight among certain cultures. There are also sociocultural differences in preferences and attitudes about diet, body weight, and body image. For example, many African American and Latino cultural foods have a high fat content (Bryant & Neff-Smith, 2001; Foreyt, 2003). A health promotion approach to weight control in obese and overweight clients must incorporate culturally based food preferences and reinforce healthy food choices.

ISSUES RELATED TO WEIGHT CONTROL

There are many issues related to weight control. It seems that on a daily basis Americans are bombarded with the latest fad in weight management and control. Fads such as the Sugar Busters, Atkins, Zone, South Beach, Ornish, and Low Glycemic Index diets have been quite prevalent over the last few years. The thinking behind these diets is that some foods are worse than others in impacting weight control. There are diets that limit sugars and sweets (Sugar Busters), are low in carbohydrates (Atkins), include only the right carbohydrates and the right fats (South Beach), are vegetarian and low-fat (Ornish), and banish foods based on their effect on blood levels (Low Glycemic Index), to name a few. People all over the world are turning to trendy exercise routines, a myriad of fad diets, pills or supplements, and even hypnotism to battle obesity. Even restaurants are now offering weight control in the form of food choices that are part of a particular fad diet. Lawsuits pitting people who are obese against fast-food restaurants are not unheard of. Admittedly all these efforts have made an impact, but there are still a number of people who have had little or no success using these methods. Bariatric surgery seems to be the answer for those who are severely obese (100 pounds or more over ideal weight). Bariatric surgery involves reducing in the size of the stomach in order to reduce the amount of food a person consumes. There are several surgical treatment options such as open gas-

tric bypass or gastric banding laparascopic surgery. The surgical method may differ but the same desired result, which is to lose weight, is achieved. A generally accepted statistic is that at least 50 percent of individuals receiving bariatric surgery maintain the weight loss for five years or longer (Stiles, 2003).

Obsession with weight management and control can lead people to accept the latest fad diet or bariatric surgery as the answer to weight loss. Among all the choices of fad diets and surgery, research affirms that fad diets do not work on a long-term basis and that bariatric surgery is only long-term for 50 percent of those undergoing the surgery. Research also reaffirms that weight loss can best be accomplished through a reduction in the number of calories consumed. A reduction in calories must also be coupled with an increase in exercise (Davis & Turner, 2001). Those interested in weight control and maintenance should be advised that there are no quick fixes but rather that small changes in eating behaviors will produce desired results. Eating well and exercising regularly can result in a healthier status. A change in lifestyle as opposed to diet deprivation is the best way to ensure that the pounds will stay off. Eating a variety of foods such as lean proteins, low-fat dairy items, legumes, fruit, vegetables, and whole grains is recommended for controlling or maintaining weight or both. See Box 16-2 for suggestions on maintaining or controlling weight or both.

THE NURSING PROCESS IN WEIGHT CONTROL

Chapter 4 covered the role of the nurse in health promotion and included the use of the nursing process in identifying the health needs of clients and in determining health-promoting strategies. Likewise, the nurse caring for an obese client utilizes the nursing process in

---

BOX 16-2 Weight Control and Maintenance Suggestions

- Eat breakfast daily.
- Eat a low-calorie/low-fat diet.
- Avoid sugar-laden soft drinks.
- Surround yourself with a support system.
- Engage in physical activity.
- Eat a variety of foods from all of the food groups.
- Substitute healthy alternatives for fat-laden favorite foods.
- Avoid fast-food restaurants.
- Don't eat standing up or while watching TV.
- Eat only when you are hungry.
- Measure progress in small increments.
- Maintain a daily food and activity log.

gathering and interpreting data essential to the formulation of a plan that includes weight control strategies. This nursing process focuses primarily on health promotion planning and utilizes the original steps of assessment, diagnosis, planning, implementation, and evaluation.

Assessment

Assessment is the foundation for the nursing process. The purpose of doing an assessment is to develop a baseline of information in order to identify problems or potential problems that a client may have and to plan how to assist a client in making necessary changes to promote health. Understanding what factors may have contributed to an individual's obese state depends on the nurse's effectiveness in obtaining appropriate information. Critical to this process is the ability of the nurse to communicate with a client in such a way that promotes a therapeutic relationship.

As described in Chapter 5, effective communication involves awareness of communication skills and attitudes toward others. This awareness is especially important when dealing with clients who are obese. By developing some insight or self-awareness about negative thoughts or emotions, it may be possible to avoid acting on them. It is only by taking a nonjudgmental approach to clients that nurses are able to build therapeutic relationships. A nonjudgmental approach may best be defined as accepting clients without harsh criticism and encouraging them to express their thoughts and feelings (the individual's point of view).

In performing a nursing assessment, it is critical to understand the difficulties someone may encounter in making needed lifestyle changes. Conceivably, the greatest obstacles to overcome may be related to some commonly held myths about how to achieve an optimal body composition. In fact, it is possible that nurses may also believe some of these same myths. In order to do an accurate assessment and follow through with a health promotion plan, it is essential to be knowledgeable about these commonly held myths. Box 16-3 provides a listing of some commonly held myths.

The first myth listed in Box 16-3 is one of the most difficult to dispel. It is critical that nurses be knowledgeable about the normal aging process and provide appropriate information to clients. If a client states that she has gained weight after hitting 40, it must be remembered that although gaining weight after turning 40 years old may be common, it is not necessarily a normal process. Overeating and inactivity are more likely to account for the excess weight gain. A decline in overall physical and mental health may be more related to lifestyle than a natural process of aging.

In the role of a health promotion educator, the nurse is asked for advice by many people. At some point, clients, primarily female, will approach the nurse for some advice on how to get rid of that special fat called cellulite. Although the news and television media may frequently provide information on "fat busters" and special lotions and treatment that eliminate cellulite, it is important to know that cellulite is not a special kind of fat. The dimpling effect is nothing more than connective tissue surrounding a layer of excess fat beneath the skin. Many advertisers who are in the business of promoting books, diets, or equipment for profit are guilty of misleading the public in that they have given ordinary fat a fancy name. Appealing to a desire to have smooth, tight, and firm thighs, they have attempted to convince the public that this type of fat, cellulite, requires special treatments, such as body wraps, rolling machines, or intense massages. Nurses can educate clients about the best approaches to reducing fat, which include balancing nutrition with physical exercise.

Thinking that dieting is the best way to control weight gain is another one of those myths that is most difficult to dispel. Dieting may lead to a short-term weight loss, but chances are the weight will be regained. Unfortunately, there are no quick fixes or miracle cures. Attempting to shed pounds by dieting pits the dieter against the body's own physiology. Dieting is a negative word that probably should be deleted from our vocabularies. Nurses working with clients who are trying to control their weight must inform them that learning moderation, eating a variety of foods, and including physical exercise will lead to positive results. Nurses may also assist clients by teaching that the best way to lose weight forever is by eating the same healthy foods in reasonable amounts that they will continue to eat after they have lost weight.

One of the best ways to sabotage a weight-control program is to avoid certain foods. This way of thinking

---

BOX 16-3 Common Myths Related to Weight Control

1. It is a normal part of aging for people over 40 to gain weight.
2. Cellulite is a special kind of fat.
3. The best way to gain control of weight is by dieting.
4. Gaining control over weight means avoiding certain foods.
5. The terms low-fat and fat-free mean a product is low in calories.
6. Obese people are weak and lack willpower to resist overeating.
7. Some people were born to be fat.
8. Gaining control of weight requires large amounts of time exercising.
9. Some people are too out of shape to exercise.
10 Everyone can have a perfect body

Low-Fat or Nonfat Foods and Calories

Even though some foods are labeled low-fat or fat-free, they still contain calories. Most low-fat and fat-free foods have excessive amounts of sugars. Weight control, then, involves learning to eat smaller portions of a variety of foods.

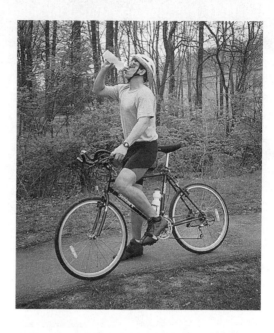

FIGURE 16-1 *Everyone can benefit from exercise.*

automatically sets one up for failure. For example, Jill, proud of her efforts to change her unhealthy eating habits, ordered broiled fish, dry, no oil, a tossed salad without dressing, steamed vegetables with no butter, and no dessert. Although we have increased public awareness about the importance of reducing fat intake, many like Jill have taken this message to an extreme. The food industry has capitalized on our obsession to avoid fats. No-cholesterol, no-fat, or low-fat products sell quite well. Although overloading on fats can cause weight gain and increased risks for health problems, some fat is essential for life. Fat supports the cell walls within the body. Fat enables the body to absorb, circulate, and store fat-soluble vitamins. Fat provides a layer of insulation. It is needed for the production of hormones and surrounds vital organs for protection and support. Avoiding all fats not only is unhealthy but reduces the chances of making a lifelong change in eating behaviors. The key to success is learning to balance intake with energy expenditure. The message of weight control is that it's okay to have a pizza—just not the extra-large one.

Another one of the most common myths is that low-fat and fat-free foods are also low in calories. This is a common mistake. Many believe that because foods are labeled as low-fat or fat-free, this means that people can consume larger amounts. Joe sampled a bite of a low-fat coffeecake and said, "This is great! I bet I could eat the whole thing." He did. Does this sound familiar?

As stated previously, one of the hardest barriers to overcome is the mistaken belief that obese people are weak people who lack the willpower to resist overeating. This broad generalization is unfair, especially when even experts do not have a full understanding about the causes or physiology involved.

Although some people may be genetically susceptible to obesity, modifying lifestyles by balancing food intake with physical activity can help control weight. Exercising may require no more than 20 to 30 minutes, three days a week, to improve health and control weight. Generally, people find the time for the things that are important to them. The myth that some individuals are too out of shape to exercise must also be debunked. The truth is that people should exercise because they are out of shape. If they wait until they are in shape, it will never happen. Exercising will help individuals get into shape. They should make the effort, begin slowly, and gradually build muscle strength and endurance.

The myth that everyone can have a perfect body is also difficult to discount. It is important to remember that human bodies are genetically coded and that for some, even faithful adherence to a healthy lifestyle will not result in a perfectly sculptured body. Therefore, all people should focus on reaching an attainable or reasonable weight. A reasonable weight is one that an individual can maintain over time.

Professional nurses make an assessment that includes many facets of a client's lifestyle. This will include a review of individual dietary habits. Information obtained about overall food consumption patterns can enhance one's understanding regarding the nature of the problem and can serve as a way of making a client aware of individual eating behaviors and serve as the basis for decisions regarding change. A guideline for gathering information on nutritional practices is offered in Table 16-1 and Table 16-2. In addition, a three- or seven-day food diary kept by a client may serve as an assessment tool to evaluate dietary status and related behaviors, as well as a client's thoughts and feelings surrounding eating.

Before a nurse and client may continue to develop the next phases of the nursing process, the degree of

TABLE 16-1 Nutrition Assessment for Adults and Adolescents

Nutritional screening

Height _____ Usual weight _____ Actual weight _____

Has your weight changed in the past six months? _____ yes _____ no

If yes, how much? _____ Describe associated events _____

_____

Have you been on a weight-reduction diet?   _____ yes   _____ no

Have you had any recent change in appetite?   _____ yes   _____ no

Do you have any food allergies?   _____ yes   _____ no

If yes, please list _____

Do you take any medication?   _____ yes   _____ no

If yes, please list prescription _____

If yes, is your appetite affected? How? _____

Nutritional practices

Who plans the meals? _____

Who shops for groceries? _____

Who prepares the meals? _____

How many days a week do you eat? _____

A morning meal? _____

A lunch or mid-day meal? _____

An evening meal? _____

During the evening or night? _____

How many days a week do you have snacks and when do you have them? _____

In mid-morning? _____

In mid-afternoon? _____

In the evening? _____

During the night? _____

Where do you usually eat your meal?

Morning _____ Mid-day _____ Evening _____

How many times a week do you usually eat away from home? _____

Describe mealtime (who is present, when, where, and atmosphere?) _____

Would you say your appetite is good? _____ Fair? _____ Poor? _____

Are you on a special diet? _____ If yes, what kind? _____ Who prescribed? _____

Are there foods you don't eat for other reasons? _____

What foods do you particularly like? _____

Dislike? _____

Do you add salt to the food at the table? _____

Do you use canned or packaged foods? _____

---

obesity must be determined. **Optimal body composition** refers to the proper balance between body fat, muscle mass, and bone. Ideal body weight and optimal body composition are not necessarily one and the same. A person may be within an accepted range of ideal weight, as determined by height, weight, and frame charts, but may have a high body fat composition. The percentage of body fat for the average male should be between 15 and 19 percent and for the average female 18 and 22 percent (Lutz & Przytulski, 2006). The minimum body fat acceptable for good health is 5 percent for males and 12 percent for females. Low body fat may be found in athletes who believe that low body fat is related to athletic performance. Although the body fat percentage is increasing in the United States and Europe, a low body fat percentage is a major health problem (About.com, 2006).

Dietary fat

How many times per week do you eat the following (at any meals or between meals)?

Red meat, fish, and poultry   0 1 2 3 4 5 6 7 > 7

Specify _____

Cheese _____	0 1 2 3 4 5 6 7 > 7 What kind?
Cold cuts	0 1 2 3 4 5 6 7 > 7
Eggs	0 1 2 3 4 5 6 7 > 7
Fat in cooking	0 1 2 3 4 5 6 7 > 7
Milk, dairy products	0 1 2 3 4 5 6 7 > 7
Butter or margarine	0 1 2 3 4 5 6 7 > 7

Complex carbohydrate and fiber

How many times per week do you eat the following?

Fruit	0 1 2 3 4 5 6 7 > 7 (juices, fresh, canned?)
Vegetables	0 1 2 3 4 5 6 7 > 7 (canned, frozen, fresh?)
Bread	0 1 2 3 4 5 6 7 > 7 (whole grain, white?)
Pasta	0 1 2 3 4 5 6 7 > 7
Potatoes	0 1 2 3 4 5 6 7 > 7

Sugar consumption

Do you use sugar in cooking? Do you buy candy, pastries, sweetened cereal?

Do you eat desserts? _____ If yes, how often? _____

Do you use sugar substitutes in packet form or in drinks? _____

Alcohol consumption

How often do you use alcohol? _____

Caffeine

How much coffee, tea, or cola do you drink per day? _____

Water consumption

Do you drink water? _____ How often during the day? _____

How much each time? _____

Economics

Do you receive any supplementary income to purchase food items? _____

Source of nutrition information

School, journals, magazines, friends, family members, health food stores.

While some of the body's composition is genetic, for most of us the percentage of body fat is directly related to poor eating and exercise behaviors as well as to lifestyle. Box 16-4 demonstrates assessment methods for determining body composition.

There are acceptable techniques used to determine ratio of body fat to lean muscle mass. The hydrostatic weighing, bioelectrical impedance, densitometry, and skin-fold measurements are generally accepted and reliable techniques. The drawback with these techniques is that they require special equipment and charts, thus making their use impractical for the general population. Therefore, although a less reliable indicator of body fat percentage, a derivation of the Mahoney Formula may be used to determine ideal body weight (Healthy/Living Radio, 2005). The formula is as follows: for men, take the

TABLE 16-2 Physical Activity Questionnaire for Adults and Adolescents

Please place a check by the statement that most accurately describes you.

_____ I currently do not exercise.

_____ I do not exercise but I am thinking about starting.

_____ I exercise some but not regularly.

_____ I exercise regularly.

If you marked a space indicating that you exercise, what sort of activities do you do? _____

_____

If you currently exercise, how much time per session do you spend? _____

How many days per week do you exercise? _____

Do you exercise alone or with someone else? _____

If you are considering starting an exercise program, what sort of exercises would you enjoy?

_____

Do you feel confident that you can participate in regular exercise? yes _____ no _____

What are some of your concerns about starting a regular exercise program?

_____

What are some of the benefits of regular exercise? _____

_____

What are some of the barriers to exercising? _____

_____

height in inches and multiply by 4, then subtract 128; for women, take the height in inches and multiply by 3.5, then subtract 108. If the skeletal frame is large (wrist size greater than 7 inches for men and 6.5 inches for women), add 10 percent to the total. If the skeletal frame is small (wrist size less than 7 inches for men and 6.5 inches for women), subtract 10 percent of the total. For example, a small-boned woman 5 feet 6 inches tall should weigh 111 pounds.

Although the Mahoney Formula has been used to measure ideal body weight for a number of years, there are other methods that can also be used as easy methods of assessing body composition. One method to calculate ideal body weight is to add five pounds for women and six pounds for men for each inch over five feet of height to a baseline of 100 pounds for women and 106 pounds for men. Adjustments for frame size are made by adding or subtracting 10 percent from the obtained weight. For example, a small-framed woman 5 feet 6 inches tall would ideally weigh 117 pounds (130 pounds minus 13). After the ideal weight is calculated, the current weight divided by the ideal weight multiplied by 100 will provide the percentage of ideal body weight. A percentage of the ideal weight over 110 percent is considered overweight, over 119 percent is considered obese, and over 200 percent is morbidly obese (Dudek, 2006). Anything under 90 percent is considered malnourished. Taking the same example as above, if the woman

weighs 139 pounds, her percentage over ideal body weight is 119 percent. She is considered to be overweight (139 divided by 117 multiplied by 100 equals 118.8 percent).

Although these formulas for determining ideal body weight are limited in the information they provide, they do provide a frame of reference from which to measure outcomes and may also be useful for calculating a baseline daily caloric intake.

The hip-waist circumference ratio and the body mass index (BMI) may be used to determine risks associated with fat and weight distribution (Black & Hawks, 2002). The hip measurement in millimeters (1 millimeter = 1/16th inch) is divided into the waist measurement in millimeters. Less than .90 for men and .80 for women is considered low risk. For example, Sue, a 35-year-old female, measured her hips and waist. She had a hip measurement of 35.5 inches (35.5 × 16 = 584 millimeters) and a waist measurement of 26.5 inches (424 millimeters). Her hip-waist circumference is .73 (424 divided by 584 = .726 or .73). Therefore, she is considered low risk for the development of cardiovascular disease.

Abdominal circumference
Hip circumference

The BMI defines the level of fat composition according to the relationship of weight to height, independent

BOX 16-4 Assessment Methods for Body Composition

Hydrostatic (underwater) weighing

1. Weigh client on land.
2. Seat client on a scale.
3. Have client blow out air in lungs.
4. Submerge client for about five seconds.
5. Record registered weight on the scale.
6. Calculate fat percentage according to formula.

Biolectrical impedence

1. Attach electrodes to client's right hand and right foot.
2. Record results from portable instrument.

Skinfold method

Female	Male

1. Use caliper to measure skinfolds:

   Triceps   Chest
   Iliac crest   Abdomen
   Midthigh   Midthigh
2. Measure each skinfold three times and average.
3. Sum the three skinfolds.
4. Calculate fat percentage according to formula.

of frame size. The BMI is an indicator of optimal weight for health and considers only weight and height. It is an indicator of risk for disease and can be used by health care providers in clinical settings. It ids important to note, however, that the BMI may not be accurate in clients who have much muscle mass, such as weightlifters and body builders. A BMI of 20 to 25 is considered normal for those individuals who do not have large muscles. Anything over 30 is considered obesity and any BMI over 40 is considered morbid obesity (Lutz & Przytulski, 2006).

To determine the BMI, take the weight in kilograms (weight in pounds divided by 2.2 = weight in kilograms) and divide by the height in meters squared (height in inches multiplied by .0254 = height in meters).

$$\frac{Weight\ (kg)}{Height\ (m)^2}$$

For example, Gloria is 5 feet 6 inches tall and weighs 122 pounds. Her BMI is calculatd as follows:

$$\frac{122/2.2}{(66 \times .0254)^2}$$

Gloria's BMI is 19.67. According to this value, is Gloria at risk for early death? The answer is no. She has a good fat percentage and should not be at risk for early death from obesity or obesity-related diseases.

Nursing Diagnosis

As described in Chapter 4, the next step of the nursing process is the determination of a nursing diagnosis. This nursing diagnosis is formulated after objectively analyzing all of the client's data. Since this chapter deals with weight control as a strategy for health promotion, the most likely nursing diagnosis(es) will deal with nutrition, although other nursing diagnoses may also be related to weight control. For example, a person's nursing diagnosis of Situational Low Self-esteem may also relate to the need for control of weight. It should be noted, however, that whether a client is trying to reduce weight or gain weight, the most likely nursing diagnosis related to weight control will be Risk for Imbalanced Nutrition: More than body requirements related to excessive intake and sedentary activity level, or Imbalanced Nutrition: Less than body requirements related to inability to digest food (NANDA, 2007). Remember that nursing diagnosis may deal with actual identified needs or ones that could develop in the future. With that in mind, then, Risk for Imbalanced Nutrition: More (or Less) than Body Requirements might also be a nursing diagnosis to address.

Planning

Once the nursing diagnoses are determined, the plan of care is then formulated and implemented. Some basic knowledge about nutrition and physical exercise is necessary to effectively assist the client in setting reasonable goals and ways to increase the likelihood that the goals may be accomplished. The goals should be stated as realistically as possible and should be accomplished within a designated time frame. For example, to set a goal that states that a significantly obese individual will lose 10 pounds per month may not be realistic. For that reason, the planning stage is of considerable importance and should be determined in collaboration with the client. All goals should be stated in measurable terms in order for them to be evaluated.

Dietary guidelines for reducing chronic disease risk are recommended (see Box 16-5). These recommendations include: (1) reducing fat intake to 20 to 35 percent or less of the total calories consumed daily (saturated fats should not exceed 10 percent of calories and cholesterol should not exceed 300 mg/day); (2) daily intake should include sufficient servings from all five food groups; green and yellow vegetables and citrus fruits; (3) choose fiber-rich fruits and vegetables; (4) select lean cuts of meat and maintain protein intake at a moderate level (0.36 grams of protein per pound of ideal body weight per day). These guidelines may be incorporated in the planning phase for the client.

The most realistic nursing approach for obese clients is to encourage them to: (1) focus on the total daily consumption of food rather than individual foods; (2) avoid thinking of foods as either good or bad; and (3) balance food intake with a variety of foods in a moderate amount.

Eating a variety of foods is particularly important, because varying foods provides a much greater range of nutrients. In addition, eating a variety of foods increases the probability that a change in eating behaviors can be sustained over time. Eating the same foods, as with many diets, is boring.

The total caloric intake should not be less than 1,200 calories per day for women and 1,500 calories per day for men. In addition, to either lose weight or maintain weight, most of the total caloric intake should occur early in the day. In other words, eat a light supper and avoid snacking before going to sleep.

The best way to achieve weight control is through a lifestyle change that includes balancing proper nutrition and physical exercise. The human body is not designed to be sedentary. Sitting for long periods causes fatigue and sluggishness. When less energy is expended than consumed, an imbalance is created, which results in those added pounds. Physical activity burns calories. Regular physical exercise must be included to achieve and maintain a balance between fat and lean.

Although exercising specific areas, such as doing abdominal crunches, will enhance muscle tone, trying to eliminate a flabby midsection cannot be achieved by working that area alone. The body burns calories uniformly. In order to lose excess adipose deposits, the calories burned must exceed those consumed. Therefore, probably the best way to achieve the optimal body composition is to include a combination of aerobic (calorie burning) and isotonic (muscle toning) exercises along with a proper diet (Dudek, 2006).

Nurses should recognize the difficulty most people have in changing long-standing behavioral patterns. Help-

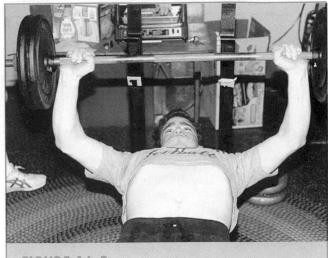

FIGURE 16-2 *Regular physical activity is essential to maintain weight.*

ing clients break goals into smaller, more achievable short-term objectives may increase their confidence that they can make lifestyle changes. Clients should establish reasonable goals to avoid becoming overwhelmed with the tremendous amount of weight they need to lose. Setting a short-term goal for losing one to two pounds instead of focusing on the entire number of pounds to be lost can build confidence that an overall goal can be accomplished.

Implementation

How can nurses motivate clients to change long-standing behavioral patterns? Despite the considerable efforts directed toward motivating individuals to adopt healthy lifestyles, to date there has been little progress. Although researchers have sought to identify factors relevant to an individual's decision to make significant lifestyle changes, most health treatment plans continue to be determined by the nurse. Even though nurses are taught to include the client in formulating a treatment plan and recognize the importance of gaining the client's cooperation for therapies requiring self-care, input from the client's point of view is seldom encouraged. Individuals are viewed as passive recipients of care. They are given directions in the guise of client education, and it is assumed that knowledge will lead to behavioral change.

Health intervention strategies for weight control typically include diet instructions and an exercise program. Generally, limited information is given to the client regarding the positive effects of weight loss and exercise or the risk associated with obesity and inactivity. Feedback about the client's intentions to carry out the prescribed plan is often excluded.

BOX 16-5 Dietary Guidelines for Reducing Chronic Disease Risk

Reduce fat intake to 20 to 35 percent or less of total calories/day.

Include 2 cups of fruit and 1½ cups of vegetables daily.

Consume 3 or more ounces of whole grain products per day.

Select lean meats.

Balance amount eaten with the amount of physical exercise.

Limit alcohol consumption.

Limit amount of salt.

Consume 3 cups per day of fat-free or low-fat dairy products.

Adapted from Dietary Guidelines for Americans, *U.S. Department of Health and Human Services, 2005, Washington, DC: U.S. Government Printing Office.*

Discharge Planning

How many times have you witnessed a nurse reciting a long list of discharge plans as the client is packing to leave the hospital? Usually the importance of social support and individual perceptions regarding the benefits and barriers to adopting a lifestyle change are omitted. How can we expect clients to comply with our treatment plans if they have not been included in devising the plan?

Behavioral Change and Weight Control

Before a person decides to initiate a behavioral change, such as weight control, that person must develop self-awareness. According to Bandura (1986), enduring behavioral patterns are sustained because they are cued and reinforced by aspects of the environment. Interventions for enhancing a person's decision to alter diet and to include physical exercise involve the promotion of the individual's awareness of existing behaviors, feelings, or attitudes that are important. It is the nurse's responsibility to raise client awareness by asking the client to engage in self-observation and self-judgment. Ask the client to list the anticipated gains or losses associated with weight control or to keep a diary recording eating and activity patterns along with associated thoughts and feelings.

Health Promotion Model and Weight Control

Derived from social learning theory, Pender's Health Promotion Model may be an alternate, more effective approach because it explores human behavior in terms of a continuous interaction among cognitive, behavioral, and environmental factors (Pender, Murdaugh, & Parsons, 2006). As described in Chapter 3, the Health Promotion Model may help explain why people adopt health promotion behaviors when there is no perceived threat. In other words, people do not have to wait until they experience a heart attack to make a behavioral change. According to this model, behaviors may be either health-protecting or health-promoting. Health-protecting behaviors are aimed at stabilizing, whereas health-promoting behaviors are directed toward developing an increased level of well-being. Within this model, concepts have been categorized into cognitive-perceptual factors (individual perceptions) and modifying factors (variables affecting the probability of action). For example, Marissa, who has a family history of heart disease, has been primarily sedentary for years. After reading a magazine article about how exercise reduces the risks of heart disease, she joined a fitness center. Even though she initially changed behaviors because of a perceived threat, she continued to attend regular exercise classes because she enjoyed the company of others, felt more energetic, and liked the way she looked.

The importance of knowledge cannot be negated; however, knowledge cannot be considered separate from other factors that have been identified as essential motivational determinants of behavioral change. In conjunction with knowledge, other factors proposed by the Health Promotion Model as directly affecting the likelihood of behavior change are (1) individual characteristics and experiences such as those related to self-esteem, (2) perceived benefits of action, (3) perceived barriers to change, (4) perceived self-efficacy or the confidence in one's ability to make the change, and (5) interpersonal influences such as family, peers, and social support. In addition, situational factors and behavioral factors, such as previous experience with dieting and exercise, indirectly influence behavioral change (Pender, Murdaugh, & Parsons, 2006).

Behavior, Attitude, and Weight Control

Attending to specific behaviors, attitudes, or feelings associated with weight control enables a participant to become aware of the factors that fostered an unhealthy lifestyle. Understanding what conditions lead to certain behaviors allows for the possibility of modifying things to effect change (Sharman, 2004). For example, if pain or discomfort is associated with exercise, ways to reduce or prevent muscle soreness can be discussed. Also, if a person discovers passing a doughnut shop on the way to the office without stopping is impossible, altering the route may reduce the temptation to indulge. However, record keeping should be considered a short-term (one week) intervention strategy. The goal is not to create people who obsess about food and calories, but to increase their awareness about habits, and the conditions that foster those habits, and to get a general idea about total caloric intake. In addition, it is not practical to expect clients to carry calorie counters and diaries around with them forever.

Identifying triggers or cues to behavior is an important step toward change. In order to successfully modify one's habits, environmental changes to support the desired behaviors and to weaken the competing behaviors must be made (Bandura, 1986). Careful scrutiny of current situations may reveal conditions that suppress desired behavior (weight control) and facilitate unwanted behavior (overeating). Sometimes the simplest solution is to modify the environment. For example, if a client finishes all of the food on her plate because that is what she has been taught to do, she can learn either to remove herself or the plate from the dinner table when she is full. Using a smaller plate or serving smaller portions may also modify existing habits.

Another strategy that may be effective in promoting behavioral change is cognitive restructuring, that is, correcting maladaptive thinking. For example, if an individual voices that there is no time to exercise, questioning whether the lack of time is real or artificial, since most people seem to find the time for things that are most important to them, may change that person's thinking process.

Restructuring thoughts about dieting is also important. Many people think that eliminating one meal per day is a logical way to lose weight. For example, Carol stopped eating breakfast, because she figured she could cut approximately 3,500 calories per week, the amount needed to lose a pound. Her problem was she more than made up for this calorie reduction at supper. In addition, she found that she was feeling sluggish most of the day. She did not lose weight. Grazing or eating small amounts throughout the day is a more effective way to lose weight. Not only is this more nutritionally sound, but it also helps control appetite and increases the basal metabolic rate. Just as a car needs fuel to run, so does the human body.

Shaping and Guided Practice Weight Control Techniques

There are no quick and easy fixes. Dieting, appetite suppressants, and surgery do not work for the long term. Shaping and guided practice may be useful techniques. Rather than prescribing a weight reduction diet and a rigorous exercise program, teaching clients to try putting

three-quarters of their usual portions on their plate for the first week and then half of the usual portions thereafter may assist them in altering their eating habits without feeling deprived. In addition, balancing foods to reduce the fat content and increase complex carbohydrates (fruits, vegetables, and grains) and lean proteins is not only nutritionally sound but will help suppress appetite. Moreover, thinking in terms of making a healthy lifestyle change instead of thinking in terms of dieting is more likely to lead to adherence to the suggested behavioral changes. Altering eating habits, with the goal of losing one or two pounds a week, is a more reasonable approach than undertaking more drastic and potentially harmful measures such as fasting, skipping meals, fad diets, appetite suppressants, laxatives and diuretics, binge eating and purging, or surgical removal of fat. Focusing on the attempts to change rather than reaching an ideal body composition may increase the likelihood of success.

The principle of shaping behavior should also be applied to exercise. If a person has been generally inactive, exercising at the recommended intensity and duration to achieve cardiovascular fitness will be overwhelming and will increase the chance of dropping out. Beginning at a relaxed pace (low intensity) for 10 minutes or less and gradually increasing the time and intensity will increase the chance the person will change behavioral patterns. Even taking a relaxed walk to the end of the block and back is beneficial, because it is an increase over a previous activity level and alters existing behavioral patterns. In addition, clients should be encouraged to choose physical activities that they enjoy. They are much more likely to engage in regular exercise if it is fun. Moreover, clients should be encouraged not to weigh themselves daily. Because changes are not readily apparent, weighing daily may reinforce returning to the previous, more comfortable sedentary lifestyle.

Developing a positive support system may be the most important factor influencing behavioral change. Social support refers to the social interactions that are perceived as being available and supportive or that actually provide support. Positive social support can be of an emotional nature, can be advisory or informational, can include provision of resources, can lead to personal introspection, or all of these (Pender, Murdaugh, & Parsons, 2006). Clients should be encouraged to get their social support systems such as families or friends involved in their weight control program.

Evaluation

The last phase of the nursing process is the evaluation phase. It is during this phase that a nurse uses her professional judgment in determining whether the goals determined in the planning phase have been achieved. Any changes that have been observed, whether it is the client's attitudes and behaviors or in actual weight loss or gain, should be duly noted. Some of the questions

TABLE 16-3 Nursing Process for the Sedentary Overweight Client

Assessment: A small-framed, 35-year-old female; weight = 150 lbs., height = 5'6"; does not engage in any exercise; average daily caloric intake = 1,690; ideal body weight = 117 lbs.

Nursing Diagnosis(es)	Goals/Outcomes	Interventions
Activity intolerance related to sedentary lifestyle as evidenced by deconditioned status	Will engage in physical activity by_____(date)	Have client list anticipated barriers to exercise and ways to overcome them. Encourage client to keep a diary to record thoughts and feelings. Examine types of exercise to include in program. Utilize behavioral contracting to encourage some exercise commitment.
Imbalanced nutrition: More than body requirements	Will lose 1–2 lbs/week	Have client keep diary to record types of foods, eating patterns, thoughts, feelings. Reduce caloric intake to 1,400/day. Schedule time for breakfast, lunch, and dinner. Balance meals with various food groups. Reduce serving portions. Limit weighing to 1–2 times/week. Drink 8–10 glasses of water/day.

that come to mind when evaluating the client's progress include the following: Have the goals been attained? Do the goals need to be modified? What types of lifestyle changes have taken place? Is the client watching her nutritional intake? Exercising? Has weight been gained or lost? Does the client seem to have developed self-awareness regarding appropriate nutrition? These questions are only meant as a guide. Naturally the important questions in the evaluation phase will be those that adequately describe the changes that the client has exhibited as a result of focusing on weight control as a means to achieve health promotion. Table 16-3 provides an example of how the nursing process may be used in promoting health in the client requiring weight control. A case study for an individual who has weight control issues is also included at the end of this chapter.

SUMMARY

Obesity and obesity-related problems are of concern to the health care community. There are consequences associated with being overweight. A majority of the problems that clients experience are life-threatening and related to obesity states. Health-promoting strategies that focus on weight control and obesity are important to the professional nurse who will be dealing with clients who are in need of education and support. The professional nurse recognizes the obstacles encountered in weight control and utilizes the nursing process in developing a weight control health promotion plan.

The obese not only suffer the health consequences of their size but also are faced with psychosocial as well as economic consequences. They face public intolerance and have difficulty finding employment. Individuals who have difficulty controlling their weight must also deal with the propaganda in the advertising world that promise miracles. Finally they are often faced with the fact that obesity is generally misunderstood.

There are many theories that address the reasons for obesity. There are theories related to genetics, biological, and environmental influences. Not all theories are widely accepted. For that reason, it is easy to see why individuals in need of weight control strategies receive erroneous or misleading information. It is the nurse's responsibility to assist the client with decision making related to fads, drugs, diets, and exercise. The public looks to the professional nurse for advice on how best to control weight.

The nursing process is appropriate for addressing the health needs of a client and in devising a realistic plan to address these needs. This nursing process utilizes concepts found in the health promotion model to determine appropriate health-promoting strategies for those in need of weight control. Use of the assessment, planning, implementation, and evaluation phases of the nursing process demonstrate an effective method for clients who need assistance in controlling their weight.

Objectives/Goals: Through participation in discussion of this case study, participants will have the opportunity to:

1. Identify appropriate weight ranges for certain individuals.
2. Describe methods that promote weight control in the morbidly obese person.
3. Discuss theories related to weight control and management.

Health Promotion Concern, History and Physical, Present Health Status, Past Health Status, Family History, and Social History

Alma Sandoval is a 28-year-old Mexican American female with a long history of being overweight. She is a pharmaceutical representative with a professional degree and lives with a former college roommate who works for the same pharmaceutical company. Alma is 5′7″ tall and weighs 190 pounds. Alma is quite active in her community and church. She enjoys cooking and entertaining friends on weekends. As part of her job, she is expected to take potential clients to dinner three to four times a week. She sees her nurse practitioner every 12 months for her gynecological checkups or more often if she needs to. Alma's parents are both alive and her family history is negative for any major illnesses. Alma is frustrated with her yo-yo dieting patterns and wants to achieve a normal weight so that she can look better in her clothes. She needs information on what choices she has in terms of managing her weight and what resources are available to her in her community.

Review of Pertinent Domains

Biological Domain

Physical exam reveals an obese young woman with no major health complaints. She has not had any major illnesses and no surgeries but due to her weight she is at risk for diabetes mellitus and hypertension. She denies any problems with alcohol but does enjoy having mixed drinks with her meals and includes alcoholic beverages when she entertains. She exercises only occasionally and her favorite form of exercise is walking. She does not smoke and finds that she experiences an allergic reaction if she is around a lot of smoke.

Gastrointestinal: Reports no problems in this area. She has occasional constipation due to the fact that she likes to eat highly refined foods such as baked goods and any type of breads. She loves to eat and gets very little fiber from her dietary habits.

Genitourinary: Nonremarkable. She reports no problems in this area. She urinates frequently with no discomfort. Urine is clear, straw colored, with no foul odor. Her dietary pattern is varied. She rarely eats breakfast because she is always in a hurry to get to work. She eats lunch and dinner out most of the time. She does not usually frequent any fast-food restaurants since she has an expense account to take her clients to fine dining establishments.

Diagnostic testing: All of Alma's blood tests are normal.

Psychological Domain

Cognitive: Cognitively she is an intelligent individual with a degree in business administration. She is well aware that she is having a problem controlling her weight. She has gained 10 pounds in the last year, which coincides with her employment with her company. Her source of entertainment is watching movies and television. With the exception of feeling "fat," she seems happy most of the time. She and her roommate have a lot in common and get along very well. She recently broke up with her boyfriend, who would occasionally point out that she needed to lose weight.

Social Domain

Alma is very gregarious. She gets along well with her family and enjoys an active social life.

Environmental Domain

Part of Alma's problem is that her job requires that she entertain her clients socially. She usually takes her clients to the best dining establishments. Alma has very little self-control when it comes to food.

Cultural Domain

Alma is a Mexican American and her mealtimes are very important, especially if she is socializing with friends and family. She tends to like high-calorie Mexican fried dishes such as fried stuffed chili peppers and homemade flour tortillas.

Technological Domain

Alma can afford to buy some of the most sophisticated exercise and weight control equipment available. She is very technologically adept at using computerized calorie counters and exercise machines. Using sophisticated equipment does not pose any challenge for Alma.

Questions for Discussion

1. Because of her long history with weight control issues, Alma is very frustrated and wants to know what her ideal weight should be. What information would you give her?

2. Alma wants to know if she would be a good candidate for a gastric bypass. What would you tell her?

3. Alma has not been able to lose more than 30 pounds every time she attempts to diet. She says that she has been able to lose the weight but her weight always fluctuates between 160 and 162 pounds. She wants you to tell her why.

Key Concepts

1. Many common health problems are linked to lifestyle.

2. Weight control health-promoting strategies can alleviate many of the health problems associated with sedentary, hedonistic, and technologically enhanced lifestyles.

3. There are numerous physiological consequences associated with obesity such as diabetes mellitus, hypertension, coronary artery disease, some forms of cancer, and lipid disorders.

4. Obesity has important psychosocial and economic consequences such as discrimination, lowered self-esteem, and poor economic compensation.

5. Inactivity, difficulty with behavioral changes, lack of personal responsibility, and attitudes related to "quick fixes" are major obstacles to achieving weight control.

6. There are a number of theories associated with excessive accumulation of fat and difficulty achieving weight control. These include hereditary, environmental, and biological theories.

7. The nursing process can be utilized in formulating a plan of care for the obese client.

8. Effective communication skills along with recognition of commonly held myths are essential to the performance of an adequate assessment of the client.

9. The degree of a client's obesity can be assessed through several techniques: bioelectrical impedance, hydrostatic weighing, skinfold measurements, hip-waist circumference, and body mass index.

10. Pender's Health Promotion Model can be used effectively in planning approaches to dealing with the client in need of weight control.

11. Self-awareness regarding specific behaviors, attitudes, or feelings associated with weight control issues enables clients to recognize unhealthy lifestyle behaviors.

Learning Activities

1. Perform and record a nutritional and activity assessment on a client.

2. Plan a weight control program for someone who has a history of unsuccessful attempts at dieting.

3. Plan an educational program designed to assist a client in learning the difference between dieting and weight control.

True/False Questions

1. T or F More then half of the U.S. population is overweight.

2. T or F Central obesity refers to accumulation of fat in the thighs.

3. T or F Even a small decrease in calories eaten and a small increase in exercise can help prevent weight gain.

Multiple Choice Questions

1. An overweight female, age 25, wants to lose weight. She has an average frame, is 5 ft. 6 in. tall, and weighs 160 pounds. Using the Mahoney Formula, how much weight should she lose?
   a. 27 pounds
   b. 37 pounds
   c. 47 pounds
   d. 57 pounds

2. Appetite suppressants are based on which of the following theories?
   a. Biological
   b. Environmental
   c. Genetic
   d. Social learning

3. A client would like to lose weight. She asks the nurse which diet is recommended. The nurse's best response would be:
   a. Eating an assortment of foods in moderate amounts is the best way to lose weight.
   b. I lost weight on the grapefruit diet. You may want to consider it.
   c. If you increase your proteins, you will lose weight.
   d. To lose weight you should eliminate all fats from your diet.

4. A male client, age 25, has a BMI of 25. He is concerned that he might be at risk for cardiovascular disease related to obesity. The nurse's best response would be:
   a. Body mass index has no relationship to the risk of developing heart disease.
   b. I think you should discuss your concerns with your doctor.
   c. If you are concerned, you need to reduce your calories and exercise more.
   d. Your BMI of 25 indicates that you are at low risk for the development of heart disease.

5. A client is 30 pounds overweight. You plan on including strategies to help your client lose weight. Of the following, which is your highest priority?
   a. Asking the client how she feels about making a change.
   b. Consulting with a dietician.
   c. Performing a history and physical.
   d. Providing her with a list of foods she should avoid.

6. A male client is 20 pounds overweight. You are to assist him with learning how to balance his nutrition. His total caloric intake is 1,600 calories. Approximately what percentage of his total calories should come from protein?
   a. 20
   b. 30
   c. 40
   d. 50

Websites

http://www.aasmnet.org American Academy of Sleep Medicine. Involved in advancing sleep medicine and improving health.

http://www.sleepapnea.org Comprehensive site that addresses problems associated with sleep apnea and offers practical health information related to this disorder.

Organizations/Agencies

American Sleep Apnea Association
1424 K St. NW
Washington, DC 20005-2410
Tel: (202) 293-3650
http://www.sleepapnea.org

The American Sleep Apnea Association is a non-profit organization dedicated to reducing injury, disability, and death from sleep apnea and to enhancing the well-being of those affected by this common disorder.

American Obesity Association
1250 24th Street, NW
Suite 300
Washington, DC 20037
Tel: (202) 776-7711
http://www.obesity.org

The American Obesity Association was founded to combat a condition that affects more than one-quarter of all adults and one in five children. The association focuses on changing public policy and perceptions about obesity. It is the authoritative source for policy makers, media, professionals, and patients about the obesity epidemic.

International Food Information Council
1100 Connecticut Avenue, NW
Suite 430
Washington, DC 20036
Tel: (202) 296-6540
http://www.ific.org
foodinfo@ific.org

The International Food Information Council communicates science-based information on food safety and nutrition to health and nutrition professionals, educators, journalists, government officials, and others providing information to consumers. IFIC is supported primarily by the broad-based food, beverage, and agricultural industries.

References

About.com. (2006). Body composition basics. *About.com. A part of the New York Times Company*. Retrieved May 19, 2006, from http://sportsmedicine.about.com

American Obesity Association. (2005). *Childhood obesity*. Retrieved May 25, 2006, from http://www.obesity.org

American Sleep Apnea Association. (2006). *Enhancing the lives of those with sleep apnea*. Retrieved May 19, 2006, from http://www.sleepapnea.org

Bandura, A. (1986). *Social foundations of thought and action: A social-cognitive theory*. Englewood Cliffs, NJ: Prentice Hall.

Black, J. M., & Hawks, J. H. (2005). *Medical-surgical nursing: Clinical management for positive outcomes* (7th ed.). St. Louis: Elsevier Saunders.

Bryant, S. A., & Neff-Smith, M. (2001). Risk factors and interventions for obesity in African-American women. *Journal of Multicultural Nursing and Health* (Winter 2001).

Colman, E. (2005). History of medicine: Anorectics on trial; A half century of federal regulation of prescription appetite suppressants. *Annals of Internal Medicine, 143*(5), 380–385.

Craven, R. F., & Hirnle, C. J. (2007). *Fundamentals of nursing: Human health and function* (5th ed.). Philadelphia: Lippincott Williams & Wilkins.

Davis, R. B., & Turner, R. W. (2001). A review of current weight management: Research and recommendations. *Journal of the American Academy of Nurse Practitioners, 13*(1), 15–22.

Dudek, S. G. (2006). *Nutrition essentials for nursing practice* (5th ed.). Philadelphia: Lippincott Williams & Wilkins.

Finkelstein, E. A., Fiebelkorn, I. C., & Wang, G. (2003). National medical spending attributable to overweight and obesity: How much and who's paying? *Health Affairs*, W3, 219–226.

Foreyt, J. P. (2003). Cultural competence in the prevention and treatment of obesity: Latino Americans. *Permanente Journal, 7*(2).

Ganong, W. F. (2005). *Review of medical physiology* (22nd ed.). New York: Lange Medical Books/McGraw-Hill.

Guyton, A. C., & Hall, J. (2006). *Textbook of medical physiology* (11th ed.). Philadelphia: W. B. Saunders.

Health Facts. (2004). Two weight loss drugs: Meridia and Xenical; The pros and cons of each. *29*(2), 3.

Healthy Living Radio. (2005). http://www.cooperaerobics.com/radio

Lemay, C. A., Cashman, S. B., Savageau, J. A., & Reidy, P. A. (2004). Effect of a low-cost intervention on recording body mass index in patients' records. *Journal of Nursing Scholarship, 36*(4), 312.

Loke, K. Y. (2002). Consequences of childhood and adolescent obesity. *Asia Pacific Journal of Clinical Nursing, 11*(3): 5702–5704.

Lutz, C., & Przytulski, K. (2006). *Nutrition and diet therapy*. Philadelphia: F. A. Davis.

Medline Plus Medical Encyclopedia. (2004). Obesity. Retrieved May 19, 2006, from http://www.nlm.nih.gov/medlineplus

NANDA. (2007). *Nursing diagnoses: Definitions and Classification 2007–2008*. Philadelphia: NANDA International.

National Heart, Lung, and Blood Institute, Obesity Education Initiative. (2000). *The practical guide: Identification, evaluation, and treatment of overweight and obesity in adults*. Bethesda, MD: National Institutes of Health. NIH Publication Number 00-4084. Retrieved May 19, 2006, from http://www.nhlbi.nih.gov

Payne, W. A., & Hahn, D. B. (2000). *Understanding your health* (6th ed.). Boston: McGraw-Hill.

Pediatric Oncall Child Health Care. (2001). *Obesity*. Retrieved May 25, 2006, from http://www.pediatriconcall.com

Pender, N. J., Murdaugh, C. L., & Parsons, M. A. (2006). *Health promotion in nursing practice* (5th ed.). NJ: Pearson Prentice Hall.

Sharman, K. (2004). From compliance to concordance: A psychological approach to weight management. *Healthcare Counseling and Psychotherapy Journal, 4*(4).

Stiles, S. (2003). A focus on obesity, part 1. *Permanente Journal, 7*(2). Retrieved May 19, 2006, from http://xnet.kp.org/permanentejournal

Sturm, R. (2003). Increases in clinically severe obesity in the United States, 1986–2000. *Archives of Internal Medicine, 163*(18), 2146–2148.

U.S. Department of Health and Human Services. (2000). *Healthy people 2010*. U.S. Government Printing Office. Retrieved May 15, 2006, from http://www.healthypeople.gov

U.S. Department of Health and Human Services. (2005). *Dietary guidelines for Americans*. Washington, DC: U.S. Government Printing Office.

U.S. Department of Health and Human Services, Centers for Disease Control and Prevention. (2005). Overweight and obesity: Economic consequences. Retrieved May 15, 2006, from http://www.cdc.gov

Wallace, J. R., Schulte, W. J., Nakeeb, A., & Andris, D. A. (2001). Health problems related to severe obesity. *Health Link: Medical College of Wisconsin*. Retrieved May 19, 2006, from http://healthlink.mcw.edu/article/984434798.html

Wellman, N. (2002). Causes and consequences of adult obesity: Health, social and economic impacts in the United States. *Asia Pacific Journal of Clinical Nursing, 11*, 5705–5709.

Wikipedia: The free encyclopedia. (2006). *Central Obesity*. Retrieved September 23, 2005, from http://en.wikipedia.org

Bibliography

American Dietetic Association. (2004). Position of the American Dietetic Association: Dietary guidelines for healthy children ages 2 to 11 years. *Journal of the American Dietetic Association, 104*(4), 660–677.

Bessesen, D. H. (2002). Obesity as a factor. *Nutrition Review, 58*(3), S12–15.

Institute of Medicine. (2002). *Dietary Reference Intakes for energy, carbohydrate, fiber, fat, fatty acids, cholesterol, protein, and amino acids*. Washington, DC: The National Academies Press.

International Food Information Council Foundation (2003). Calories count: Balancing the energy equation. *Food Insight* (March–April): 1, 6.

Chapter 17

AVOIDING TOBACCO, ALCOHOL, AND SUBSTANCE ABUSE

Jane A. Newman, PhD
Debra Otto, DM, RNP

KEY TERMS

addiction
comorbidity
cross tolerance
detoxification
drug abuse
drug misuse

dual diagnosis
environmental tobacco
  smoke (ETS)
half-life
over-the-counter (OTC)
  drugs

polypharmacy
polysubtance abuse
prescription drugs
primary prevention
protective factors
psychotropic drugs

relapse prevention
risk factors
secondary prevention
tertiary prevention
tolerance
triad diagnosis

OBJECTIVES

Upon completion of this chapter, the reader should be able to:

- Describe the impact of substance use, abuse, and addiction on society.

- Differentiate among prescription, nonprescription, and psychotropic drugs.

- Explain the mechanics of drugs.

- Differentiate among drug misuse, abuse, and addiction.

- Compare the biological and psychosocial bases of addiction.

- Describe the effects of nicotine, alcohol, and psychotropic drugs on the body and the brain.

- Relate patterns of substance abuse to gender, age, and ethnicity.

- Discuss substance abuse among nurses.

- Identify the relationship of comorbidity, mental health, physical health, and spirituality to substance abuse and addiction.

- List health promotion and preventive strategies related to tobacco, alcohol, and other drugs.

- Describe the role that nurses have in prevention, abuse, and addiction to drugs.

INTRODUCTION

Human use, abuse, and addiction to drugs in some form or another has always existed. There is reference to alcohol consumption and drunkenness in the Bible. Over 3,000 years ago the Aztec and Toltec Indians used the hallucinogenic flowering head of the peyote cactus during sacred rites and for healing. Perhaps the first drug crisis in America happened in the 16th century when the Spaniards, desiring to keep the Indians subordinate, banned the peyote cactus from the Indians who revered the cactus more than they did the Spaniards (James, 1998). Other drugs, including cocaine and caffeine, have been part of human consumption for centuries.

The use, abuse, and/or addiction to tobacco, alcohol, and other drugs continue to play a major part in the lives of a significant number of individuals in our society, and everyone is susceptible. The short- and long-term effects of tobacco, alcohol, and other drug use and abuse present serious problems for individuals, families, and society. Indeed, two of the 22 priority areas for *Healthy People 2010* target the use of tobacco and alcohol and other drugs as focus areas for improving the health of the nation (U.S. Department of Health and Human Services [USDHHS], 2005).

Many people, including nurses and other health care professionals, have limited knowledge regarding substance use and abuse. In order to promote health, a fundamental understanding of the concepts and issues involved with substance use and abuse is important in nursing practice regardless of the practice area. Promoting healthy behavior is essential whether the nurse is involved in wellness programs aimed at enhancing health, primary prevention services that screen clients for health problems, tertiary care for clients with acute and chronic disease, or programs directly targeted to treat clients with use and abuse problems.

Why do people turn to these substances? Why do people abuse drugs and alcohol to the point of addiction? These are age-old questions and questions whose answers continue to be elusive. Finally, once a person is using, or abusing or is addicted, is there room for health promotion?

This chapter will cover the basic health promotion and prevention strategies related to tobacco, alcohol, and other drugs. A general discussion of drug effects and the bases of addiction will be presented. The effects on the body and the brain of the most commonly used substances will be addressed. Health promotion and prevention strategies are arranged according to the extent of substance use. These strategies are further addressed according to use by gender, age, ethnicity, and presence of **comorbidity** (another disability present in addition to the substance use disability). An additional area of emphasis will be on nurses, their role in prevention, and their use and abuse of and addiction to drugs.

SUBSTANCE USE AND ABUSE

The use and abuse of tobacco, alcohol, and other drugs have been and continue to be devastating to people of all ages in our society. There are over 440,000 smoking-related deaths in the United States each year (Centers for Disease Control and Prevention, 2004). It is estimated that there are an additional 100,000 alcohol-related and 20,000 drug-related deaths each year in the United States as well (Centers for Disease Control and Prevention, 2004).

Death is not the only measure of the devastating effect of drug use and abuse. There are premature infants born with human immunodeficiency virus (HIV) or addiction to cocaine, teenagers with brain cells destroyed by inhalants, adults crippled from drunk drivers, and older adults who suffer liver and kidney problems from unknowingly combining medications. These are just a few examples of the damaging effects of drug use and abuse across the life span. Damages are suffered not only by individuals but also by families, communities, and nations.

WHAT ARE DRUGS?

To understand and discuss substance abuse a certain level of knowledge is necessary. It is important to first have a basic understanding of what drugs are, where they come from, and how they are categorized.

Drugs are any substance that, when taken into a living organism, may modify one or more of its functions (Venes, 2001). More simply, all drugs affect the processes of the mind or the body. They can be taken or administered in many ways as listed in Table 17-1. Drugs are substances that can have either helpful or harmful effects on the body and may be found in ordinary household products as well as medicines and herbal supplements.

SOURCES AND CATEGORIES OF DRUGS

There are four basic sources from which drugs are derived: plants, animals, minerals, and synthetic chemicals. Morphine, which is commonly used to control pain, comes from the opium poppy of the plant kingdom. People with diabetes inject insulin that is manufactured from the pancreas of animals. Aspirin comes from coal

TABLE 17-1 Routes for Drug Administration with Examples

Method	Example
Inhalation	Bronchodilators, tobacco smoke, pollutants
Instillation	Eye drops, ear drops, nose drops
Oral ingestion	Tablets, capsules, teas, alcohol
Mucous membrane absorption	Mouthwashes, dental pastes/gels, rectal suppositories
Intramuscular injection	Antibiotics, illegal drugs
Intravenous injection	Antibiotics, blood transfusions, illegal drugs
Subcutaneous injection	Insulin, immunizations
Transdermal absorption	Hormones, nicotine, deodorants, hair dye

tar, a mineral. Manmade drugs, such as oral contraceptives, are produced in laboratories using various scientific techniques.

There are three major categories of drugs pertinent to discussion of substance use and abuse. These categories are prescription, nonprescription, and psychotropic.

Prescription Drugs

Prescription and nonprescription drugs are taken for health problems that have been diagnosed by a physician or nurse practitioner. Taking these drugs is considered to be within social norms. **Prescription drugs** are prescribed for us by a physician or nurse practitioner and contain substances that aid in the prevention of disease, diagnosis of a condition, or alleviation of symptoms, or help in the recovery from a disease or disorder. The Food and Drug Administration regulates approval for the use of these drugs in the United States. Some examples are antibiotics, narcotics, anticoagulants, diuretics, and cardiovascular drugs.

Nonprescription Drugs

Nonprescription drugs, or **over-the-counter (OTC) drugs,** are those that we can purchase from our pharmacy or supermarket for use when our symptoms are of a minor nature. OTC drugs, like prescription drugs, have gone through testing and approval and are regulated by the U.S. Food and Drug Administration. Examples include analgesics, cold medications, decongestants, vitamins, and sleep aids, to name a few.

Psychotropic Drugs

The third category of drugs relates to those substances that are taken outside the social norm or for the purpose of altering feelings. These drugs are classified as psychotropic drugs and include alcohol. **Psychotropic drugs** affect psychic function, behavior, or experience. Psychotropic drugs modify mental activity and are normally used to treat mental disorders. Many drugs can be classified as intentionally psychotropic, but many other drugs also occasionally may produce undesired psychotropic side effects (Thomas & Taber, 2005). Several classes of psychotropic drugs are used legitimately in treatment, including antidepressants and neuroleptics or tranquilizers. Also in this category are stimulants (caffeine, amphetamines, and cocaine), opiates (morphine, heroin, and methadone), and hallucinogens (marijuana, mescaline, LSD, and PCP), which are not used in the treatment of mental disorders.

DRUG MECHANICS: HOW THEY WORK

Think for a moment about the action of putting a key into a lock, turning the key, and opening the door. Drugs and body cells act much like this. As shown in Figure 17-1, each cell has receptor sites, like keyholes, that are engaged to act when the appropriate key or transmitter fits into it. An example of a naturally occurring transmitter is the hormone epinephrine, that unites with heart muscle cells to stimulate their action, resulting in increased heart rate and blood pressure when more oxygen is needed. Other neurotransmitters, such as serotonin, can slow the body processes, enabling rest and sleep to occur.

Psychotropic drugs act directly on nerve cells and their neurotransmitters to alter brain chemistry and function. Figure 17-3 shows the brain, which is composed of the cerebrum, cerebellum, and brain stem, and the division of the cerebrum into lobes with specialized functions. Inside the brain, and throughout the nervous system, nerve cells transmit information. This involves neurotransmitters (chemicals) that work to facilitate, modify, or cancel normal transmissions between nerve cells at the synapse that exists between the dendrites (Figure 17-2). Psychotropic drugs modify or affect our thoughts and feelings with resulting behaviors by altering the natural physical processes in the body and brain (National Institute on Drug Abuse, 2003).

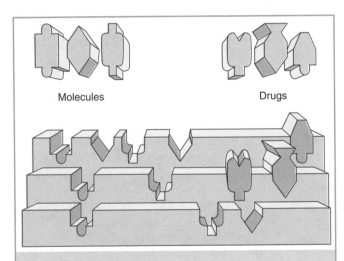

FIGURE 17-1 *Drugs interact with the normal function of the body because they share similar structures with the body's own molecules. As a result, drugs compete for receptor sites on cells.*

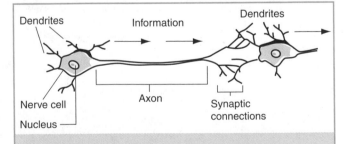

FIGURE 17-2 *The transmission of information among nerve cells along the axon, dendrite, and a synapse.*

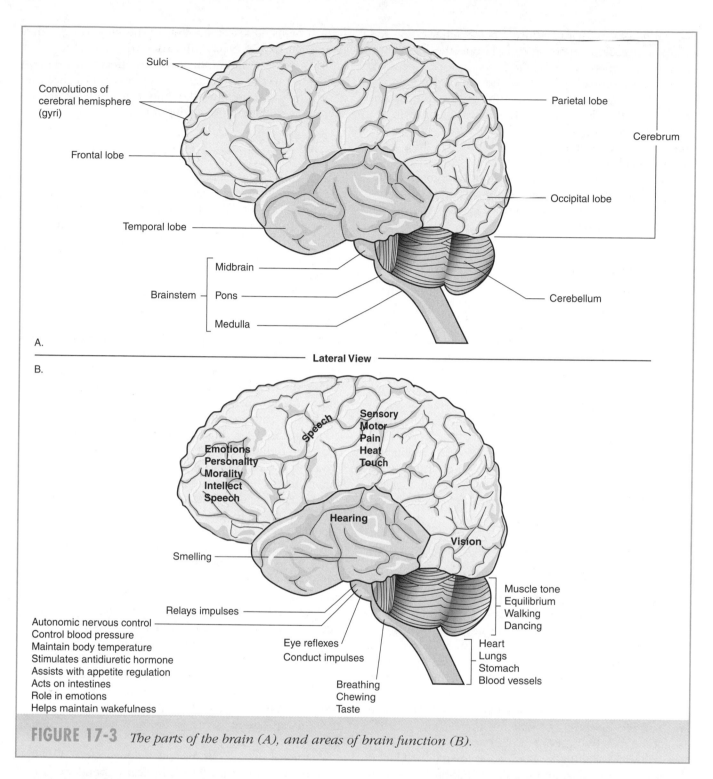

Sulci

Convolutions of
cerebral hemisphere
(gyri)

Frontal lobe

Temporal lobe

Midbrain

Brainstem — Pons

Medulla

Parietal lobe

Cerebrum

Occipital lobe

Cerebellum

A.

Lateral View

B.

Speech

Sensory
Motor
Pain
Heat
Touch

Emotions
Personality
Morality
Intellect
Speech

Hearing

Vision

Smelling

Relays impulses

Autonomic nervous control
Control blood pressure
Maintain body temperature
Stimulates antidiuretic hormone
Assists with appetite regulation
Acts on intestines
Role in emotions
Helps maintain wakefulness

Eye reflexes
Conduct impulses

Breathing
Chewing
Taste

Muscle tone
Equilibrium
Walking
Dancing

Heart
Lungs
Stomach
Blood vessels

FIGURE 17-3 *The parts of the brain (A), and areas of brain function (B).*

DRUG MISUSE, DRUG ABUSE, AND ADDICTION

Prescribed drugs and OTC drugs always have directions for proper use, an explanation or indications for their use, and possible side effects. Drugs are rarely harmful if taken as directed. **Drug misuse**, however, can occur if a drug is used inappropriately. Misuse generally results from a lack of understanding of the directions for use or from polypharmacy. **Polypharmacy** occurs when multiple medications are used without the knowledge of a

supervising physician or nurse practitioner. Seeking health care from more than one care provider, or from self-medication with OTC drugs, or a combination of both of these, can result in polypharmacy.

The result of practicing polypharmacy can be disastrous. For example, decongestants decrease the effectiveness of antihypertensive medications prescribed to prevent strokes in middle-aged and older adult clients.

Drug abuse, or substance abuse, is the use of a drug or drugs inconsistent with social norms, usually to alter feelings or mood, and without relation to medical or health reasons. Drug abuse begins when a person makes a conscious decision to continue the use of the drug or substance for the altered feeling it produces.

Drug abuse leads to deterioration of health in a biological and psychosocial sense. Biologically, the continued use of the drug eventually causes changes in the brain itself creating a need to use the drug, not for the original altered feeling it gives, but for the drug itself. Psychosocially, the drug abuser creates a perpetuation of drug use because of social rejection and guilt. **Addiction** is a gradual process that occurs when a person has developed both a biological and a psychosocial dependence on the substance of use.

Biological Basis of Addiction

The National Institutes of Health (2006) studies have revealed that substances tending to be abused act on brain centers to activate pleasure. The more the pleasure centers are turned on, the more an individual wants to use drugs. This is the reason that individuals use and continue to use drugs.

The more the individual uses a drug the more the brain learns to depend on drugs to bring about the sensation of pleasure. By activating the pleasure circuits, many addictive drugs make the brain act as though the drug itself was as important for survival as food. The continued use of addictive drugs can actually change the way the brain works. They alter the normal process of chemical neurotransmission. This is the biological basis of addiction.

The Effect of Drug Withdrawal

The opposite effects of drugs occur after they are metabolized out of the system. This is known as a withdrawal syndrome (bounce-back effects). Symptoms tend to appear after use is discontinued (e.g., withdrawal symptoms are that depressant drugs result in anxiety; stimulants result in depression). These negative effects perceived by the individual do not seem to be a major deterrent to use, abuse, or addiction. In fact, use, abuse, or addiction often continues in order to avoid the effects of withdrawal.

Drugs have a **half-life,** or what is called a half-time. The half-life of a drug is half the time it takes for the drug to be metabolized out of the system. Different drugs have different half-lives. For example, the half-life of alcohol is 30 minutes, and cocaine's half-life is less than 90 minutes, whereas the half-life of a typical amphetamine is more than four hours, and methadone's half-life is about 15 hours. Basically, during the first part of a drug's half-life, the drug produces its perceived positive effects (altered state of consciousness). In the last half of a drug's half-life, the user perceives the negative (withdrawal) effects.

Detoxification refers to taking an individual who is using drugs off the drug. There are several methods that accomplish detoxification. One method is slow withdrawal by using lesser amounts of the same drug. Other drugs that have a **cross tolerance** (drugs that are similar to each other and produce similar effects on the body and brain) to the drug may be used in a similar fashion. An example is substituting the drug methadone for heroin, thereby eliminating the craving for the narcotic.

Psychosocial Basis of Addiction

Drugs produce emotional states that are initially perceived as pleasurable. Drugs produce these states on demand. It has been well documented that users expect that a drug will produce a perception of well-being (National Institute of Mental Health, 2002). A sense of well-being and the natural highs are more difficult to obtain and happen less frequently without drug inducement. Individuals have difficulty obtaining these states naturally on demand.

Drugs of use, abuse, and addiction produce **tolerance** (Mayo Foundation for Medical Education and Research, 2005). Tolerance to a drug occurs when a progressive increase in the amount of a drug is required to obtain the desired effects. Those individuals who are highly tolerant may be prone to more severe withdrawal symptoms. Thus increased frequency and dose of a drug to obtain the desired results produces physical and psychosocial dependence. For example, cocaine appears to produce psychological dependency because it directly stimulates the pleasure centers of the brain responsible for the reinforcing properties of food, water, and sex (National Institute on Drug Abuse Research Report Series, 2004).

Drugs also can condition and control behaviors by acting as positive and negative reinforcement. Positive reinforcement occurs when an event (a reinforcer) is experienced as positive (e.g., pleasurable effects of drug use) and increases the likelihood that the behavior will occur again. Negative reinforcement occurs when a negative event is taken away when a behavior occurs (e.g., drug use takes away negative feelings), and the removal of the negative event increases the likelihood that the behavior will reoccur. The individual will then seek the drug for reinforcement. Drugs that tend to be abused meet these criteria. This is the psychosocial basis of addiction.

Drugs bring about physical dependence by their very nature. Some produce physical dependence more rapidly than others. For example, heroin produces rapid physical dependence whereas the physical dependence of alcohol is slower.

Physical dependence, however, is not addiction. Although tolerance and physical dependence may be necessary preconditions, addiction must also include psychosocial dependence on the drug. Individuals who are on pain medication, for example, become physically dependent and develop tolerance, but once the need for the drug is past, they are able to give it up.

Individuals who have physical and psychosocial dependence continue to use and abuse because they rely on the drug for their very psychosocial existence. Thus addiction includes physical and psychosocial dependence. Alcohol and heroin are examples of drugs that have both biological and psychosocial addiction processes. Table 17-2 summarizes the biological and psychosocial consequences of drug abuse that result in addiction. It should be noted that all psychotropic drugs do not fit the same pattern for addiction to occur. Controversy exists, for example, regarding a clearly identifiable pattern of tolerance and withdrawal for cocaine and marijuana to be addictive in the biological sense.

COMMONLY ABUSED PSYCHOTROPIC DRUGS

Substances referred to by names such as ecstasy, yellow sunshine, snow, cotton candy, and rainbow sound exciting, comforting, and inviting. This is exactly what some drugs tend to create for their users. For some people, using these substances appears to make life better. The short-term and long-term effects of using these substances, called street-drugs or recreational drugs, pose many dangers.

Opiates

Opiates include opium, morphine, and codeine (naturally occurring opioids) and derivatives such as heroin (synthetic substances). The brain has natural opiate receptors (the endogenous opined system) that operate to regulate mood and the sensation of pain. Opiates bind to these natural receptors and replace the natural opioids. Natural opiate receptors are distributed throughout the brain and body (National Institute on Drug Abuse, 2003). This is why opiates are some of the more powerful chemicals that reduce pain and alter mood.

Opiates act to depress the central nervous system while reducing the ability to experience pain. After-effects (withdrawals) include a heightened sensitivity to pain, chills, and sweating. Perceived positive feelings include a sense of well being, relaxation, and feeling at one with

---

TABLE 17-2 Psychosocial and Biological Progression of Events Leading to Addiction

Psychosocial Progression	Biological Progression
Drug/substance abuse ↓	Drug/substance abuse ↓
Social rejection ↓	Damage to brain cells and neurotransmitters in the central nervous system ↓
Development of guilt and shame ↓	Altered transmission of impulses in brain for normal thought processes ↓
Positive and negative reinforcement leads to increased substance/drug use ↓	Positive and negative reinforcement leads to increased substance/drug use ↓
Reconciliation attempts with family and friends Formation of new peer group associated with drug/substance use ↓	Poor judgment from damaged brain cells and altered neurotransmission ↓
Positive and negative reinforcement leads to increased substance/drug use ↓	Positive and negative reinforcement leads to increased substance/drug use ↓
Social withdrawal from former friends and family Greater acceptance by new peer group of substance users ↓	Physical dependence on drug to avoid effects of withdrawal Development of tolerance leading to increased amount of drug/substance use Development of intensive craving for drug/substance ↓
Psychosocial addiction	Biological addiction

the universe. Many individuals in treatment call heroin the cotton candy drug because it reminds them of when they were children enjoying the sweetness and softness of cotton candy. Several individuals who used or abused heroin have said, "If you ever used heroin or any of the opiates you would not be able to stop because it makes you feel so much in harmony with the world." Signs of opiate use are an appearance of sedation, a decrease in respiratory rate, and a narrowing of the pupils as well as needle marks and nasal discharge. Addiction to heroin is extremely rapid.

In addition to addiction, long-term effects of heroin are very serious and life-threatening. Continued use can cause damage to all major body systems. There can be damage to the skin and veins, bacterial infections, and infections of the lining of the heart and heart valves. Arthritis can develop, as well as kidney and liver disease, and other infectious diseases including acquired immunodeficiency syndrome (AIDS) and hepatitis.

Hallucinogens

Examples of the hallucinogens include lysergic acid diethylamide (LSD), cannabis santiva (marijuana), phencyclidine (PCP), mescaline, peyote, and psilacybe mushrooms. Hallucinogens include a wide variety of responses but the main effect is to produce hallucinations. Some, such as LSD, produce hallucinations in small doses, while others require higher doses of the active ingredient (e.g., marijuana that includes the active ingredient of tetrahydrocannabinol).

These agents, in general, tend to produce visual, auditory, and other sensory hallucinations such as time distortion; short-term memory difficulties, mood changes, and performance problems. In addition to producing hallucinations, PCP is also a stimulant and an anesthetic. PCP is unpredictable in its effects from one batch to the next and can result in long-term cognitive deficits (e.g., schizophrenic symptomology). MDMA (also known as ecstasy) is a hallucinogen with stimulant properties. Tetrahydrocannabinol, the active ingredient in marijuana, in high doses will produce hallucinations. It also has stimulant and depressant effects.

Signs of hallucinogenic use are agitation, increased heart rate, dilated pupils, and altered perceptions of time, sounds, colors, tastes, textures, and patterns. The short-term effects of hallucinogen use can be deadly as users may attempt dangerous feats and can develop severe anxiety leading to panic. Long-term effects include respiratory disease, cancer, altered reproductive abilities, and depressed immune system.

Household Drugs

Household drugs of abuse include agents such as glue, nail polish remover, correction fluid, freon, propellant in spray cans, and some paints and varnishes. Many of these drugs are found in most homes and will produce an altered sense of consciousness when inhaled. Signs of household drug abuse include rash around the mouth or nose, red eyes, and headaches.

Household drugs of abuse enter the blood stream through the lungs and then pass into the brain and nervous system to produce euphoria (Office of National Drug Control Policy, 2003b). The euphoric feeling results because the oxygen in the blood is replaced with the household drug. Parts of the brain then tend to shut down. The resultant physical problems are loss of memory functions and coordination problems.

Stimulants

In addition to nicotine, other drugs that stimulate the nervous system include cocaine, amphetamines, and caffeine. Caffeine, although it is abused and results in addiction, is not discussed here since it does not produce an altered state of consciousness to such a degree that behavior is altered and comes to the attention of health care providers. There may be physical repercussions, but the effects of caffeine on health are inconclusive.

Stimulants increase perceptions of well-being and alertness and decrease perceptions of anxiety and fatigue. They also decrease hunger and are used to reduce weight gain. In contrast to the positive feelings, stimulants also produce negative feelings such as irritability and anxiety. Essentially they act on the body by increasing cardiac output. High doses may cause paranoia and unpredictable violent behavior. Animals will choose stimulants over sex, food, alcohol, sedatives, hallucinogens, and PCP. Human beings appear to respond the same when given free access to all of the above. Stimulants activate the dopaminergic pathways (dopamine is a neurotransmitter) but the neurochemical mechanisms responsible are not clear (Office of National Drug Control Policy, 2003a).

TOBACCO USE AND ADDICTION

Tobacco is an ancient plant that has created many modern problems. Before Columbus set foot on America, only the American Indians knew tobacco and thought it to be a way to connect with the gods. To these ancient Indians, tobacco was the most precious of possessions. The rest of the world was introduced to tobacco only after the Spanish brought it back to Europe in the fifteenth century. And the detriments of tobacco use have been known or suspected for most of the next 400 years.

Tobacco comes in several forms. The two forms most widely used are those that can be inhaled, such as in cigarettes and cigars, and those that may be chewed, as in snuff and chewing tobacco (spit tobacco). The cigarette industry spends billions of dollars on advertising and promotions every year, especially to young people. Children, referred to by cigarette marketing researchers as "consumers in training," are special targets of marketing (Centers for Disease Control and Prevention, 2004).

Addiction to nicotine in tobacco is, by far, the most prevalent, costly, and deadly of all substance abuse addictions. Death from smoking is the most preventable cause of death and disease in our society. It is estimated that each year more than 440,000 deaths in the United States, or one out of every five, are the result of tobacco use. About half of these deaths occur in smokers between the ages of 35 and 69 (American Cancer Society, 2005). In addition to the tragedy of death are the numerous diseases and conditions listed in Box 17-1 that produce untold suffering.

Environmental Tobacco Smoke

Even those who don't use tobacco in any form are at risk for exposure to **environmental tobacco smoke (ETS).**

Also known as involuntary, sidestream, or secondhand smoke, ETS is known to be detrimental to smokers and nonsmokers of all ages. Box 17-2 lists the many health risks for children exposed to secondhand smoke.

Nicotine

The active ingredient in tobacco is nicotine, although the tars, gases, and chemicals that are contained in the cigarette smoke also cause damage to the body (National Institute on Drug Abuse, 2005). Over 5,000 chemicals have been identified in tobacco smoke, 43 of which are known carcinogens (National Institute on Drug Abuse, 2005). Hundreds of the other chemicals are poisonous and cause mutation or cellular changes in body cells. A partial listing of these chemicals and where they are

BOX 17-1	Conditions Linked to Cigarette Smoking

Lung cancer	Atherosclerotic peripheral vascular disease
Laryngeal cancer	
Oral cancer	Gastric ulcers
Esophageal cancer	Fetal growth retardation
Bladder cancer	
Cervical cancer	Low birth weight babies
Stroke	
Coronary heart disease	Sudden infant death syndrome (SIDS) or crib death
Chronic bronchitis	
Chronic obstructive pulmonary disease	Early menopause

Adapted from Cigarette Smoking: Introduction, *American Cancer Society, 2005.*

BOX 17-2	Children and Health Risks from ETS

Conditions that have been linked to exposure of children to ETS include:

Pneumonia	Sinus infections
Bronchitis	Pharyngitis
Asthma	Eye irritation
Influenza	SIDS or crib death
Ear infections	
Upper respiratory infections	

Harmful Effects of Environmental Tobacco Smoke (ETS)

Study Problem/Purpose: To investigate the effect of environmental tobacco smoke (ETS) on lung function and to identify the most sensitive functional parameter for evaluating lung damage. Childhood exposure to ETS adversely affects dynamic spirometric indexes as a result of combined early life (including in utero) and current exposure to parental smoking.

Methods: A cross-sectional health survey was taken of 80 adolescent school-age boys (mean age ± SD, 16 ± 1 years). The participants were classified in three groups: 21 smokers, 30 nonsmokers, and 29 passive smokers. A standardized questionnaire was utilized to document the smoking habits of the subjects and their parents. Lab tests included an assay of urinary cotinine level and measurement of the cotinine/creatine ratio (CCR); lung function tests, including measurements of lung volumes, spirometric dynamic parameters, and the single-breath diffusing capacity of the lung for carbon monoxide (DLCO).

Findings: Passive smokers presented a higher residual volume than nonsmokers, and a lower maximal expiratory flow. Passive smokers whose mothers had smoked during pregnancy had significantly lower maximal expiratory flow rate 25–75 (MEF25) percentage, DLCO, carbon monoxide transfer coefficient, and diffusion capacity of the alveolar-capillary membrane (DM) values than did passive smokers whose mothers had given up smoking during pregnancy. Nevertheless, the MEF25 and DM values of subjects whose mothers had given up smoking during pregnancy were lower than those observed in nonsmokers, suggesting a negative effect of passive smoking independent of the mother's smoking habit during pregnancy. A statistically significant, negative correlation was found between CCR and DLCO in smokers and in passive smokers, but not in nonsmokers, suggesting a dose-effect relationship.

Implications: Current exposure to ETS in healthy male adolescents is associated with lung function impairment independently of the effects of maternal smoking during pregnancy. More information may be obtained from determining static lung volumes and DLCO.

Rizzi, M., et al. (2004). *Environmental tobacco smoke may induce early lung damage in healthy male adolescents.* (Retrieved January 10, 2006, from *http://www.medscape.com*).

commonly found other than in tobacco smoke is in Table 17-3. Although most physical problems attributed to tobacco use (e.g., heart attacks, strokes, and emphysema) are diagnosed many years after exposure, even short-term tobacco use may be harmful.

Nicotine, which is both a stimulant and a sedative, reaches the brain in about eight seconds when inhaled. It activates the area in the brain that initiates a feeling of pleasure. Chewed or inhaled, the nicotine that is in tobacco is an addictive and mood-altering drug. In fact, as Box 17-3 shows, nicotine is as addictive as cocaine and heroin.

Throughout the day, tobacco users maintain a predictable nicotine blood level. They usually have an initial intake of nicotine soon after awakening as the body has depleted its supply of nicotine. Most users of tobacco cannot choose to use one day and not the next.

TABLE 17-3 Harmful Chemicals in Tobacco Smoke and Where They Are Commonly Found

Chemical	Commonly Found In
Acetone	Nail polish
Acetic acid	Vinegar
Ammonia	Floor/toilet cleaner
Arsenic	Rat poison
Butane	Cigarette lighter fluid
Cadmium	Rechargeable batteries
Formaldehyde	Embalming fluid
Methanol	Rocket fuel
Napthalene	Mothballs
Stearic acid	Candle wax

BOX 17-3 Drug Conversion Rates

The percentages of those who convert from using tobacco and illegal drugs to being dependent or addicted to the drug are as follows:

- Cigarettes 23.6%
- Cocaine 24.5%
- Heroin 20.1%

Adapted from Cancer Facts and Figures, *American Cancer Society, 2006, retrieved June 12, 2006, from http://www.cancer.org*

ALCOHOL USE AND ADDICTION

Alcohol (also known as ethanol) is a well-known depressant drug whose effects have been widely studied. Alcohol is considered to be a legal drug and is readily available to adults, illegally obtained by adolescents, and often left unchecked to be misused by children. In small and moderate amounts, alcohol consumption can be associated with benefits. These benefits include protection against heart disease and maintenance of bone density in postmenopausal women. The results of heavy alcohol use, however, can be devastating.

The problems of alcohol abuse and alcoholism affect millions of people world-wide. The social consequences of alcohol abuse are present every day in the form of accidents, violence, crime, and family neglect, just to name a few. Current statistics indicate that almost 14 million Americans, or one in every 13 adults, abuse alcohol or are alcoholic. Sadly, there are several million more adults and adolescents who participate in patterns of drinking alcohol that place them at risk of becoming alcoholics.

The age at onset of drinking appears to correlate with development of alcoholism in later years. The younger the person is when he begins drinking, the more likely it is that he will become alcoholic. A recent survey found that over 40 percent of respondents who started drinking before the age of 15 were later classified as alcoholic later in their lives (National Institutes of Health, 2006).

The harmful effects of alcohol on the body are extensive and often deadly (Box 17-4). When used during pregnancy, alcohol can be detrimental to a developing fetus, causing low birth weight and a syndrome of developmental, cognitive, and behavioral problems. Withdrawal from alcohol, without medical supervision and treatment, may result in severe psychological trauma and potentially fatal seizures.

Why People Drink

There are a number of theories on why people drink. Many people drink during events of happiness and celebration. Although abuse of alcohol may occur, this type

of drinking rarely leads to alcoholism. Those individuals with poor self-esteem who drink out of boredom, when they are stressed, when they are depressed, or just out of habit are most likely to become alcoholic.

An issue of debate is whether psychosocial influences or biological make-up predispose one to becoming an alcoholic. Certainly environment has a great effect on an individual's patterns of behavior. What is learned from one's parents, peer pressure in adolescence, and influences from adult social groups are all influential. There is substantial evidence, however, that alcoholism has a biological basis. This basis for this theory is that some individuals inherit a genetic predisposition for addiction.

There are conflicting views on whether alcoholism is a disease in itself or causes disease. Whatever the case, alcohol addiction can ruin personal and social lives. Alcoholism has been identified as a major factor in dysfunctional families, child abuse, spouse abuse, and impaired job performance. Half of all Americans have someone in their family who abuses alcohol. Multiple drug use often includes alcohol.

BOX 17-4 Physical Effects of Alcohol Abuse

Gastritis	Malnutrition
Gastric ulcer	Nerve damage
Gastric hemorrhage	Hepatitis
Cirrhosis of the liver	Cancer
Liver failure	Stroke
Anemia	Delayed puberty
Osteoporosis	Pancreatitis
Heart disease	

Alcohol and the Central Nervous System

Even with all of the research on alcohol, its action on the central nervous system is still not clearly understood. It probably alters neuron cell membranes to alter neuro-transmission. Certain individuals may be more prone to these neurochemical abnormalities than others. Alcohol tends to stimulate the release of some of the neurotransmitters such as serotonin, dopamine, and noradrenelin in these particular individuals. Minor tranquilizer drugs (e.g., Valium, Librium) and barbiturates (also known as sleeping pills) produce these same kinds of effects. As such, these drugs have a cross tolerance to alcohol.

Depressant drugs, like alcohol, initially produce perceptions of relaxation, well-being, and a decrease in anxiety and insomnia. After effects include nausea, headache, and agitation. Signs of depressant drug use are slurred speech, lack of coordination, difficulty with recent memory, and dilated pupils.

SUBSTANCE ABUSE PATTERNS

Differences in substance use, abuse, and addiction patterns exist or are purported to exist among groups. Some of these groups discussed below are related to gender, age, comorbidity, and ethnicity. Some careers lend themselves to a high level of stress, especially those that require caring for others. Nurses are especially vulnerable to substance use.

Gender

Males and females differ mostly in consumption patterns rather than in an increase in problem behaviors. Females tend to consume drugs in relation to interpersonal dynamics and males tend to consume drugs to maintain their sense of manliness. Females are identified less often than males as having problems because of their protected status in society (i.e., they tend to be shielded from others' gaining knowledge about their use or abuse of substances). Females are also less prone to discuss substance use/abuse/addiction patterns in their lives. Many times it is only at the tertiary prevention stage that a female is identified as having a problem.

Regarding smoking, the group that is reported to have among the lowest smoking rates are white-collar males. Their female counterparts (white-collar female employees), however, have a higher incidence of smoking than do blue-collar female workers. Box 17-5 provides a profile of tobacco users in the United States.

Age

Substance use, abuse, or addiction or all three occur at any age. There are, however, two age groups that are particularly vulnerable: adolescents and the elderly.

Adolescents

Many adolescents do eventually grow out of their use of drugs. The reasons are not totally clear but most tend to move into acceptable roles in society. This acceptance then allows drugs to be replaced by other social and personal reinforcers. Those who continue toward addiction tend to be those who struggle with acceptance by society and with self-value. Peer groups for these individuals tend to be those who continue to use and abuse drugs and engage in antisocial or asocial role modeling. Thus, role identity becomes intricately entwined with drug use and abuse and behaviors that produce conflict.

BOX 17-5 **A Profile of Tobacco Users in the United States**

Current trends of smoking in the United States include the following:

- The prevalence of cigarette smoking among adults age 18 and older declined by nearly half between 1965 and 2002, from 42 percent to 23 percent.
- Although cigarette smoking peaked higher and earlier in men, the gender gap narrowed in the mid-1980s and has since remained constant. As of 2002, the prevalence of smoking in women was 20 percent and in men, 25.2 percent.
- While the percentage of smokers decreased for all levels of educational attainment between 1983 and 2002, college graduates achieved the greatest decline: 41 percent, from 21 percent to 12 percent. Among adults without a high school education, the percentage decreased 24 percent, from 41 percent to 31 percent.
- Per capita consumption of cigarettes continues to decline. After peaking at 4,345 cigarettes per capita in 1963, consumption among Americans 18 and older decreased 56 percent to an estimated 1,903 cigarettes per capita in 2003. Per capita cigarette consumption is currently lower than at any point since the start of World War II.
- Current cigarette smoking among U.S. high school students increased significantly, from 28 percent in 1991 to 36 percent in 1997, then declined to 22 percent in 2003.
- By age 13, 18 percent of students have smoked a whole cigarette, and 58 percent of high school students have tried smoking. This suggests that continued efforts to prevent youth initiation and experimentation are needed.

Adapted from Cancer Facts and Figures, *American Cancer Society, from 2006, retrieved June 12, 2006, from http://www.cancer.org/statistics.*

Tobacco use typically begins prior to the age of 18 primarily in response to peer pressure and to role models, including parents, who use tobacco. There is growing evidence that tobacco use is increasing in the younger age group (Figure 17-4). A recent National Youth Tobacco Survey revealed that among youths 12 to 17 in 2004, an estimated 3.6 million (14.4 percent) used tobacco products in the past month (Substance Abuse and Mental Health Services Administration, 2005).

Elderly

Another age group that is at risk for substance use and addiction are senior citizens. Substances abused in this age group tend to be alcohol and prescription medications.

The senior citizen tends to be in a dependent role with loss of clear role definition, loss of income, and loss of a support system. In addition to misuse as a result of physical problems (such as loss of vision), cognitive problems (misunderstanding of directions), and polypharmacy, drugs may become an avenue to alter perceived negative emotional states resulting from life changes.

Ethnicity

Studies abound that indicate that ethnicity plays an important role in the development and support of substance use, misuse, abuse, and addiction. Perhaps the basis for future problems with substances is more embedded in devaluation and exclusion rather than ethnicity itself.

Drug use, abuse, or addiction or all three appear to be more closely related to the age group than to the ethnic group. Children who have behavioral difficulties are at risk regardless of ethnicity (Substance Abuse and Mental Health Services Administration, 2005). Acceptance by the peer culture is critical to pre-adolescents and adolescents.

The issues of devaluation and exclusion are reflected in the changes in substance use over time. With the exception of tobacco, substance use, misuse, abuse, and/or addiction risk among Whites tends to decrease with age while the risk among African Americans, Hispanics, and Asian Americans tends to increase. In regard to alcohol, however, the Native American tends to have a higher rate of alcohol use and abuse than any other group across age and gender.

Use of tobacco also tends to be higher among Native American adolescents than any other cultural group. African American adolescents have shown lower rates for tobacco use than other ethnic groups except Asian Americans, who have the lowest rates. Smoking rates for White adolescents are usually double the rates found for African American adolescents, yet African American adults have higher prevalence rates than Whites. This suggests that White users as they move into adulthood successfully relinquish tobacco use more often than do African Americans.

Adolescent males have the highest prevalence for smokeless tobacco. The prevalence is greatest for White

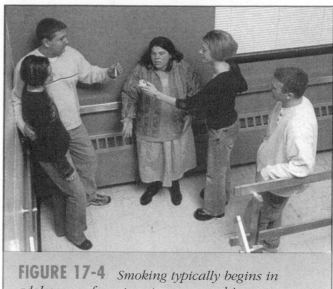

FIGURE 17-4 *Smoking typically begins in adolescence from peer pressure and in response to role models, including parents.*

males at 20 percent, followed by 6 percent among Hispanics, and 4 percent among African Americans (U.S. Department of Health & Human Services, 2003).

Nurses

Beginning in the 1970s and 1980s, much attention was focused on drug abuse among nurses. Because of the stress inherent in their occupation and the availability of drugs, it was believed that nurses were at risk for substance use, misuse, abuse, and addiction to illicit drugs and narcotics. Some nurses were found to have obtained drugs by withholding medications from clients, forging prescriptions, or stealing the drugs from available supplies.

More current research has indicated, however, that abuse of these substances among nurses is no greater than the general population and may, in fact, be even less. Much of the evidence pointing the finger at nurses as addicts was based on individual accounts and not the use of scientific research. Exaggeration of illicit drug use among nurses could have been done to amplify the drug problems of society in order to gain funding for rehabilitation (Taylor, 2003; Dunn, 2005).

This is not to say that there is no problem of drug abuse among nurses. Estimates of drug abuse, or chemical impairment among nurses in the profession, vary from three to five percent. The chemically impaired nurse is at risk of making poor judgments resulting in varying degrees of harm to those in his or her care. In recognition of this, prevention programs have been made available through the State Board of Nursing, the regulating body of the profession, in every state to assist nurses having difficulties with personal drug use. These programs are in place to initiate an intervention, monitor progress, and maintain support for chemically impaired nurses. The National Council of Boards of Nurse Examiners offered the premises listed in Box 17-6 to be considered by each State Board of Nurse Examiners when addressing regulatory issues of peer assistance programs and chemically impaired nurses in their state.

Chemically impaired nurses are less likely to approach and counsel others about drug use, abuse, and/or addiction. Because nurses are in key positions to provide support and counsel to others about drugs it is imperative that their problems are addressed and resolved rather than allowed to progress to the loss or suspension of their licenses because of illegal drug use.

Comorbidity

The effects of drugs on the body will eventually take their toll. An individual in need of treatment for substance abuse problems is many times also in need of treatment for mental, spiritual, and physical health problems. This is called comorbidity, when there is another disability present in addition to the substance use/abuse/addiction. Treating individuals with a **dual diagnosis** (substance abuse along with mental or physical health concerns) or perhaps a **triad diagnosis** (a mental health issue, a physical health issue, and a substance abuse issue) requires a multidisciplinary team approach. Many substance abuse issues come to light only when the individual enters treatment for a mental or spiritual health issue or a physical complaint.

Mental Health Issues

Substance abuse issues and mental health issues are better approached as separate syndromes. Since drugs produce feelings, thoughts, and behaviors that mimic mental health problems, confusion may occur as to which is the primary disability. Also, there may be an underlying mental health issue that preceded and perhaps was exacerbated by substance use.

There are many examples of people with psychological disabilities that may be predisposed to substance use problems. Some of the high-risk groups with mental health problems that are prone to developing substance abuse problems are those with schizophrenia, mood disorders such as depression, anxiety and bipolar disorder, and personality disorders. The three camps of mental health, physical health, and substance abuse issues are divided by philosophy and by physical location. Thus, these individuals are many times bounced from one treatment approach to another without the pooled benefit of the experts most concerned with their well-being.

Physical Health Issues

Physical health issues are related to the detrimental effects of the drugs themselves and injuries from accidents as a result of using the drug. An individual with a physical disability that occurs during drug use or an individual who already has a physical disability is at risk to continue or develop substance abuse problems. An individual's risk for obtaining a physical disability increases with the use of drugs.

Spiritual Health Issues

Drug use, abuse, or addiction or all three create a void in one's spiritual health. It might also be said that poor spiritual health could lead to drug use. It may be debatable to say exactly what is the human spirit; there are a number of various perspectives. It is difficult to define. The human spirit, in essence, may be described as the very depth of the soul. It is the quintessence of the being that we call human. The body, mind, and spirit make up a person, but it is the spirit that seems to maintain the body and the mind. Without the spirit the body and

---

BOX 17-6 Premises of the National Council of State Boards of Nursing for Peer Assistance Programs

Each State Board of Nursing should consider the following premises regarding peer assistance programs.

1. Consumers have the right to receive safe and effective care from nurses licensed in their state.
2. In order to practice, licensed nurses should be physically, mentally, and emotionally capable.
3. Substance abuse or dependency is an illness on the wellness-illness continuum.
4. Because it is an illness, those with substance abuse should be treated rather than punished.
5. It is important that Boards of Nursing be able to reassure the public regarding health, safety, and welfare.
6. State Boards of Nursing have constitutional authority over those they license. In order to obtain or maintain licensure nurses must comply with the requirements of their State Board of Nursing.
7. Privacy and confidentiality of nurses involved in peer assistance programs should be evaluated against the State Board of Nursing's responsibility to protect the health, safety, and welfare of the public and to protect the public from receiving unsafe, incompetent care.

Adapted from Endorsement Issues Related to Peer Assistance/Alternative Programs, 2005, National Council of State Boards of Nursing, Retrieved January, 2006, from http://www.ncsbn.org/files/publications/positions/peerassistance.asp.

Long-Term Effects of Alcohol Abuse

Harry was a 36-year-old male who appeared to be in his 60s. He had abused alcohol since he was 14 years of age. He had never been in treatment. He was independently wealthy and lived alone. His brother, who made weekly visits, found him unconscious one day. When he was admitted to the hospital, his physical health had deteriorated to the point that his system was no longer able to function. He died shortly thereafter. What do you think could have contributed to his alcoholism? What interventions do you think could have changed this scenario?

mind cannot exist. If the spirit is not healthy, the body and the mind may struggle to be.

Drug use, abuse, or addiction or all three appear to rob one of one's spirit. After drugs take their toll, the body and mind may be salvaged to the extent of the damage, but it is the spirit that must heal. The healing of the spirit comes, in part, through the acceptance of oneself and others.

STRATEGIES FOR HEALTH PROMOTION

Promoting health in all individuals involves supporting healthy behaviors which include making healthy choices. Health promotion strategies, therefore, are to prevent individuals from making unhealthy choices including exposure to tobacco, alcohol, and other substances that may lead to use, abuse, and eventually addiction or irresponsible use or both.

Prevention may be arranged according to the degree of substance use and the approaches used to prevent use, continued use, abuse, or addiction. Primary prevention occurs prior to any use. Secondary prevention may be in the form of treatment but most often it targets those who are using and possibly abusing; and tertiary prevention is most often in the form of long-term treatment, the goal of which is to prevent early death and disability.

The evaluation of individuals with substance abuse issues is usually not an easy task, since minimization or secretiveness many times surrounds their relationship with drugs. Few nurses are formally educated or trained to recognize substance use, abuse, and/or addiction, to provide appropriate referrals, and to initiate effective prevention strategies. Yet nurses are in positions that lend the opportunity to provide prevention at all levels. Training nurses to evaluate, refer, and treat substance

use, abuse, and addiction is essential to the overall prevention efforts.

The Agency for Healthcare Research and Quality of the U.S. Department of Health and Human Services has developed guidelines for the health professional to use for smoking cessation (Agency for Healthcare Research and Quality, 2005). Similar guidelines could be helpful for clients with other types of substance abuse as well. The premise behind the development of these guidelines is that health care professionals are in key positions to identify those smokers and plan interventions for smoking cessation. Four basic strategies are identified to guide the health care professional: ask, advise, assist, and arrange. Primarily aimed for use in clinics and medical offices, these strategies involve asking clients about smoking at every office visit, advising the smoker to quit, assisting the smoker in developing a quit plan, and arranging for follow-up contact. Table 17-4 shows how asking, advising, and assisting could be incorporated into substance abuse prevention at the primary and secondary levels in medical offices and hospitals.

Identification of Risk and Protective Factors

Implementation of health promotion strategies for individuals who are at risk for substance use and abuse problems requires that the nurse recognize those factors that place an individual at risk for substance use and those factors that protect an individual from substance abuse. **Risk factors** include situations or conditions or both that increase an individual's vulnerability to substance abuse. **Protective factors** are those factors that build resiliency against substance abuse and increase the likelihood that an individual will resist substance abuse. Research has shown that the more risk factors that are present in an individual, the more likely a substance abuse problem will develop. Scientists have found that both risk and protective factors are critical components in preventing substance abuse. Prevention programs must utilize the body of knowledge related to both risk and protection areas of study. Risk and protective factors extend to all areas of a person's life, and multiple interventions in those areas that increase substance use risk can enhance outcomes (Center for Substance Abuse Prevention, 2001).

There are a number of factors that can protect individuals against substance abuse. Some of these relate to internal factors while some are more externally based. Internal factors that protect individuals from substance abuse include an individual's belief in self and in ability to accomplish meaningful tasks. Other factors include social confidence or the degree to which an individual gets along with others and contributes to a social group. How an individual relates to family and peers, such as in grade school, can assist in protecting against the temptations of substance use. This is especially true during the formative and adolescent years. Research indi-

TABLE 17-4 Substance Abuse Prevention Guidelines for the Health Professional

Strategies	Suggestions for Practice Application
Ask Ask the supervisor in your agency about the existence of a method to identify clients with substance use, misuse, abuse, or addiction problems. Establish a system that assesses for substance use at every office visit or hospital admission.	1. Incorporate asking about use of tobacco, alcohol, or other substance use into the confidential data collection form used at each office visit or admission assessment to the hospital. 2. Denote a special area on the record for documenting these data. 3. Include questions about the use of prescription drugs, nonprescription drugs, herbs, vitamins, tobacco, alcohol, marijuana, cocaine, heroin, and other substances.
Advise Provide professional advice appropriate to the client and in accordance with your agency protocol.	1. If no problem exists, encourage the client to continue healthy behavior. 2. If a problem of use, misuse, abuse, or addiction exists, advise the client of the importance of behavior change.
Assist According to your agency protocol, offer resources available to help with the problem.	1. If change is desired, explain options available for assistance. Options will vary according to resources in the community. 2. If change is not desired, offer motivation and offer continued support for change. 3. Offer educational materials that are culturally sensitive and educationally appropriate.

cates that the risk for substance use during adolescence is strongly related to environmental characteristics in which the adolescent lives. Family supervision, school environment, community opportunities, and the quality of life all influence the development of positive or problem behaviors in youth (Center for Substance Abuse Prevention, 2002). Box 17-7 depicts risk and protective factors associated with substance use. Nurses developing and implementing health promotion strategies for individuals at risk for substance use should familiarize themselves with all of the risk and protective factors associated with substance use and abuse.

Primary Prevention

Primary prevention in regard to substance use is defined as prevention for those who have not used tobacco, alcohol, or other drugs. The goal is to prevent exposure to and experimenting with drugs.

Primary prevention has been touted in the schools, particularly in the early grades, as an effective strategy for prevention of subsequent substance abuse and other high-risk behaviors. Many programs with various approaches have been attempted. There is little scientific evidence that would indicate that school-based preventative pro-

grams are effective in preventing substance abuse problems either in younger children or in adolescents. Studying the effectiveness of these prevention programs is difficult since the individuals in whom primary prevention may be effective would not be identifiable since they would not progress to secondary or tertiary prevention levels.

Tobacco prevention education programs in schools that provide skill-training approaches appear to be effective in reducing the onset of tobacco use (Centers for Disease Control, 2004). To be effective, these programs need to target youth before they initiate tobacco use. Those individuals who develop smoking habits early in life are more likely to become heavy users and to have a greater chance of developing smoking-related diseases due to long-term use.

Are schools expected to replace the family in ethical, moral, and preventive behaviors? Some describe primary prevention as multidimensional with a recommendation that prevention, particularly in the early years, be strategies that promote healthy development (USDHHS, 2005). Schools can be highly influential in building the motivation and social competence children will need as they engage in behaviors that promote health and as they are exposed to risky behaviors such as substance abuse.

- Youth who believe that drugs and cigarettes are harmful are less likely to smoke or use drugs.
- Sensation-seeking personalities are more likely to smoke and do drugs.
- Inappropriate expressions of anger increase the risk of substance use.
- Aggressive and disruptive classroom behavior may predict substance abuse.
- Youths who have conventional values are less likely to abuse substances.
- Poor parenting practices can predict adolescent substance abuse.

- Parental monitoring and supervision protect against substance abuse.
- Outstanding school performance reduces likelihood of drug use.
- Peer substance use is among the strongest predictors of substance use.
- Sustained involvement in structured peer activities is linked to a low level of drug use.
- Ready access to tobacco, alcohol, and other drugs increases use of these substances.
- Stress in the workplace may elevate alcohol consumption.

Adapted from 2001 Annual Report of Science-Based Prevention Programs, *Center for Substance Abuse Prevention, 2001, U.S. Department of Health and Human Services, Substance Abuse and Mental Health Services Administration.*

Primary prevention in adults is aimed primarily at educating them about the unhealthy attributes of drug use and toward responsible use of legal drugs. Prevention programs aimed at increasing self-esteem in adults are probably most effective at the secondary prevention level.

Secondary Prevention

Secondary prevention includes strategies aimed at preventing substance abuse by those considered at risk to develop problems and those who are using substances. Groups of individuals who are considered at risk for substance abuse problems include (but are not limited to) adolescents, elderly, lesbians/gays, minorities, and people with disabilities. The common thread in these groups is exclusion from and devaluation by society. Other high-risk groups are those in vocations that they perceive to be highly stressful. One of these groups is the health care professional.

Those who are users of substances are considered to be at risk for the development of substance abuse and possible subsequent addiction. By experimenting or using, individuals place themselves at risk for abuse and addiction.

Secondary prevention appears to be a tool to identify those individuals prone to develop problems or who have moved into substance use and at times abuse. Many times the potential substance use problems come to light through other avenues during secondary prevention.

Tertiary Prevention

Tertiary prevention in substance use refers to the prevention of death and disability of individuals in long-term treatment. Tertiary prevention is appropriate for two pop-

Spotlight On

Secondary Prevention for Substance Abuse: Troy's Case

Imagine yourself as a school nurse in a local high school. Troy is 18 and a senior in your school. His grades have recently dropped and he is losing weight. His friends are concerned that Troy might be using drugs because he is hanging out with individuals known to use cocaine and speed (amphetamines). The recent death of Troy's older brother has had a devastating effect on his entire family. He no longer feels that his family cares about him, and he is feeling isolated and lonely. Drugs, he feels, make him feel more a part of the human race. What can you do to promote health for Troy?

ulations: those who are considered in need of treatment but still maintain control over their behavior (substance abuse) and those who are considered in need of treatment but who clearly are not in control of their behavior (substance addiction). Many of these individuals tend to use more than one substance. Many use tobacco but do not consider use of this drug as a cause for concern.

The primary treatment goal in tertiary prevention is to learn to live life without drugs. This entails a total change in lifestyle. Education on the effects of drugs may be useful to increase an individual's awareness, but the underlying feelings of self-acceptance and acceptance by others appear to be the more crucial variables in adjustment to a life without drugs. Relapse prevention tends to occur in conjunction with tertiary prevention. Relapse is the return to drug use and **relapse prevention** is the prevention of this behavior. There are several relapse prevention programs that encompass physical and psychosocial addiction processes.

In Control

Individuals who are maintaining control over their behavior but are abusing substances are considered to be in control of their use or, perhaps, abuse of drugs. These individuals have intact families, careers, and physical, mental, and spiritual health, although they may be bordering on the loss of any one or all of these. They are usually identified after the loss of one or more of these areas or they may at times identify themselves prior to any losses. They tend to have a sense of invulnerability to adverse consequences of their substance use or abuse or both. Many use and abuse drugs to provide them with an altered state of consciousness to gain relief from the inner psychological pain.

Out of Control

Individuals who are considered to be out of control of their behavior are considered to have moved into addiction. They have lost their family, friends (other than those who are using or abusing substances), income and career, and their sense of themselves. Their physical, mental, or spiritual health or all three have been compromised. They are usually identified by their family, friends, employers, by law enforcement, and at times by themselves. Drugs have penetrated their every waking moment and have ceased to provide them with a means to seek relief from the internal physical and psycholog-ical turmoil and a sense of well-being. Many have experiences that predispose them to an inability to live life without numbing their memories. Drugs have now become a way of life. The intake of drugs takes on a compulsive nature, and the loss of control is reflected in the frequency, amount, duration, dosage, and behavior of the individual. See the Case Study for an individual with alcohol issues and addiction.

SUMMARY

The overall goals of *Healthy People 2010* are designed to increase quality and years of healthy life and to eliminate health disparities (USDHHS, 2005). As such, strategies aimed at risk-reduction, behavior change, and preventive services are at the core of health promotion of all ages, at varying degrees of health, and in diverse groups.

The prevention of substance use, abuse, and addiction appears complex; but it is no mystery. Whether the underlying reason is psychological, social, or physical, the individual's decision to use substances is based on a desire to alter his perceptions of himself and the world. If an individual feels good and has a sense of belonging to himself and to the world, he will have no need to alter his subjective perceptions and feelings. In an ideal world, a child raised with limits and structure among those who love, respect, and trust that child may have no need to change perceptions of himself and his world. When this occurs, health is promoted and primary prevention is taking place. Secondary prevention relates to preventing a fall into abuse and/or a way to responsible use. Tertiary prevention essentially is to prevent the destruction of the body, mind, and spirit.

CASE STUDY Jane Davey: At Risk for Alcohol Abuse and Addiction

Objectives/Goals: Through participation in discussion of this case study, participants will have the opportunity to:
1. Identify factors that can lead to alcohol abuse and addiction.
2. Describe physical effects of alcohol abuse and addiction.
3. Describe psychosocial effects of alcohol abuse and addiction.

Health Promotion Concern, History and Physical, Present Health Status, Past Health Status, Family History, and Social History

Jane Davey is a 29-year-old Caucasian female who is currently a stay-at-home mom. Her day includes homeschooling her three young boys, maintaining the family home, and shopping and cooking for the family. She has a college degree in business and always thought she would someday develop her own company. Jane's husband of six years is a successful lawyer who works 14+ hours a day with hopes of making partner within the next five years. He is home less and less due to his demanding career. Jane starts drinking alcohol early in the day to "relax and get through her very long days." Jane thinks she has been able to hide her drinking for several months now.

Review of Pertinent Domains

Biological Domain

Physical exam reveals an overweight individual who is 66 inches tall and weighs 205 pounds with a previous weight of 230 pounds.

Gastrointestinal: Ms. Davey has a history of unexplained weight loss. Her dietary patterns have not changed. She usually tries to eat three well-balanced meals a day but admits to drinking at least one soft drink with her meals and snacking and drinking in the evening. She has been feeling very tired lately.

Diagnostic testing: Glucose and cholesterol readings are significantly above normal.

Psychological Domain

Ms. Davey was diagnosed with postpartum depression shortly after her third birth. She discontinued the prescription treatment against medical advice. Jane feels she has become more isolated since the birth of the children.

Social Domain

Ms. Davey dedicates her entire day to homeschooling the children as well as taking care of the home environment. She no longer has social contact with family and friends; however, she does attend her husband's occasional social events with the law firm. She is isolated and has feelings of decreased self-esteem.

Environmental Domain

Ms. Davey finds her environment stressful and non-stimulating intellectually. Although she homeschools the children, she is also responsible for taking care of all the household chores and making dinner daily.

Questions for Discussion

1. What are the signs of depressant drug use such as alcohol?
2. What are the social consequences of alcohol abuse?
3. Develop a plan to help Ms. Davey with her social isolation and reliance on alcohol.

Key Concepts

1. The misuse, abuse, and addiction to substances such as tobacco, alcohol, and psychotropic drugs affect the well-being of individuals, families, communities, and nations. The effects range from destruction of personal lives and relationships, to millions of dollars spent in health care and treatment, and to hundreds of thousands of lives lost nationwide.

2. Use of prescription, nonprescription, and psychotropic drugs each can lead to misuse, abuse, and addiction.

3. All drugs are designed for specific actions and interactions with our body cells. Drugs that tend to be abused alter the normal body processes specific to the brain at the level of the neurotransmitters.

4. It is possible for individuals to become addicted biologically, psychosocially, or a combination of both.

5. Nicotine, alcohol, and psychotropic drugs act on the pleasure centers of the brain, altering mood and, in some instances, perceptions.

6. Diversity exists in patterns of substance use according to gender, age groups, and ethnicity, and according to the particular substance.

7. Comorbidity, mental health, physical health, and spirituality are issues influencing drug use among individuals.

8. Knowledge about drugs and substance abuse is powerful for promoting health and in prevention of use and abuse among those at risk.

9. Nurses are in key positions to ask about substance use, to advise individuals of the health risks of using, and to assist those who are using and desire to quit.

Learning Activities

1. Describe the difference between drug misuse and drug abuse.

2. List at least five ways that drugs may enter the body.

3. How is physical dependence different from psychosocial dependence?

4. Describe the effects of environmental tobacco smoke (ETS).

5. How can nurses be effective in primary and secondary drug abuse prevention efforts?

6. How can nurses get help if they have a problem with substance abuse?

True/False Questions

1. T or F   Nonprescription drugs are those that can be taken outside of the social norm or for the purpose of altering feelings.

2. T or F The biological basis for addiction is in the alteration of the normal process of chemical neurotransmission.

3. T or F Daily deaths related to alcohol use are more than those for tobacco and illegal drug use combined.

4. T or F Alcohol is a legal drug.

5. T or F Drug use, abuse, or addiction or all three appear to be more closely related to age group than to ethnic group.

Multiple Choice Questions

1. Which of the following may be an effect of drug use and abuse?
   a. Cerebral palsy
   b. Early puberty onset
   c. Eczema
   d. Prematurity

2. All of the following are basic sources from which drugs are derived except:
   a. Animals
   b. Minerals
   c. Plants
   d. Soil

3. Psychotropic drugs do which of the following?
   a. Act by affecting the stomach lining, increasing absorption.
   b. Affect respiratory function.
   c. Alter mental activity and are used to treat mental disorders.
   d. Do not affect thoughts and feelings.

4. Bladder cancer is a condition linked to which of the following?
   a. Cigarette smoking
   b. Drug inhalants
   c. Opiate drug use
   d. Psychotropic drug use

5. Which of the following statements is true?
   a. Ethnicity does not play a role in development of substance abuse.
   b. Drug use and drug abuse in nurses are no greater than in the general population.
   c. Men and women do not differ in drug consumption patterns.
   d. There are no age groups that are particularly vulnerable to drug abuse.

Websites

http://www.ash.org Provides information for people concerned about smoking and nonsmokers' rights, smoking statistics, quitting smoking, smoking risks, and other smoking information.

http://www.cdc.gov/tobacco Tobacco Information and Prevention Source, Centers for Disease Control and Prevention. Information on smoking statistics, smoking cessation, and other tobacco-related health problems.

http://www.drugfree.org Provides information on child drug use and keeping children off drugs. Includes intervention and treatment information.

Organizations

Centers for Disease Control and Prevention (CDC)

1600 Clifton Road
Atlanta, GA 30333
Tel: (404) 639-3311; (404) 639-3534; (800) 311-3435

The CDC is one of the 13 major operating components of the U.S. Department of Health and Human Services, which is the principal agency in the U.S. government for protecting the health and safety of all Americans and for providing essential human services, especially for those people who are least able to help themselves. The CDC is committed to achieving true improvements in people's health.

The United States Food and Drug Administration (FDA)

1500 Fishers Lane
Rockville, MD 20857-0001
Tel: (888) INFO-FDA; (888) 463-6332

The FDA is responsible for protecting the public health by assuring the safety, efficacy, and security of human and veterinary drugs, biological products, medical devices, our nation's food supply, cosmetics, and products that emit radiation. The FDA is also responsible for advancing the public health by helping to speed innovations that make medicines and foods more effective, safer, and more affordable, and for helping the public get accurate, science-based information about medicines and foods to improve their health.

The National Institutes of Health (NIH)

9000 Rockville Pike
Rockville, MD 20892
Tel: (301) 496-4000

The NIH is a part of the U.S. Department of Health and Human Services and is the primary federal agency for conducting and supporting medical research. NIH scientists investigate ways to prevent disease as well as the causes, treatments, and even cures for common and rare diseases.

National Institute on Drug Abuse (NIDA)

6001 Executive Boulevard, Room 5213
Bethesda, MD 20892-9561
Tel: (301) 443-1124

NIDA leads the nation in bringing the power of science to bear on drug abuse and addiction. NIDA-supported research addresses the most fundamental and essential questions about drug abuse, ranging from the molecule to managed care and from DNA to community outreach.

References

Agency for Healthcare Research and Quality (2005). *Treating tobacco use and dependence.* Retrieved January 1, 2006, from http://www.ahrq.gov

American Cancer Society. (2006). *Cancer facts and figures.* Retrieved June 12, 2006, from http://www.cancer.org

American Cancer Society (2005). *Cigarette smoking: Introduction.* Retrieved December 30, 2005, from http://www.cancer.org

Center for Substance Abuse Prevention (2001). *2001 annual report of science-based prevention programs.* U.S. Department of Health and Human Services, Substance Abuse and Mental Health Services Administration.

Center for Substance Abuse Prevention. (2002). *The national cross-site evaluation of high-risk youth programs: Understanding risk, protection, and substance use among high-risk youth.* Monograph Series No. 2. U.S Department of Health and Human Services, Substance Abuse and Mental Health Services Administration. Retrieved June 12, 2006, from http://www.samhsa.gov

Centers for Disease Control and Prevention. (2004). *Health effects of cigarette smoking fact sheet.* February 2004. Retrieved January 1, 2006, from http://www.medofficeinc.com

Dunn, D. (2005). Substance abuse among nurses—Intercession and intervention. *AORN Journal* (November 2005).

James, J. (1998). *Peyote & mescaline: History & uses of the 'divine cactus.'* Tempe, Arizona: Do It Now Foundation.

Mayo Foundation for Medical Education and Research. (2005). *Pain pill-addiction: What's the risk?* Retrieved June, 12, 2006, from http://mayoclinic.com/

National Council of State Boards of Nursing. (2005). Retrieved January 1, 2006, from http://www.ncsbn.org

National Institute on Drug Abuse Research Report Series. (2004). *Cocaine abuse and addiction.* Retrieved June 12, 2006, from http://www.drugabuse.gov/

National Institute on Drug Abuse. (2003). *Stress and the brain: Developmental, neurobiological, and clinical implications.* Retrieved June 12, 2006, from http://www.drugabuse.gov/

National Institute on Drug Abuse. (2005). *Smoking/nicotine.* Retrieved June 12, 2006, from http://www.drugabuse.gov

National Institute of Mental Health. (2002). *Medications publication 2002.* Retrieved December 25, 2005, from http://nimh.nih.gov

National Institutes of Health. (2006). *The brain—Lesson 4—Longterm effects of drugs on the brain.* Retrieved on January 4, 2007, from http://science.education.nih/

Office of National Drug Control Policy. (2003a). *Drug czar unveils new resource for youth drug prevention.* Retrieved June 12, 2006, from http://www.whitehousedrugpolicy.gov

Office of National Drug Control Policy. (2003b). *Inhalants.* Retrieved June 12, 2006, from http://www.whitehousedrugpolicy.gov

Rizzi, M., Sergi, M., Andreoli, A., Pecis, M., Bruschi, C., & Fanfulia, F. (2004). Environmental tobacco smoke may induce early lung damage in healthy male adolescents. Retrieved January 10, 2006, from http://www.medscape.com

Substance Abuse and Mental Health Services Administration. (2005). *The 2004 National Survey on Drug Use and Health.* Office of Applied Studies, NSDUH Series H-27, DHHS Publication No. SMA 05-4061. Rockville, MD. Retrieved June 12, 2006, from http://oas.samhsa.gov/

Taylor, A. (2003). Support for nurses with addictions often lacking among colleagues. *American Nurse, 35* (September/October 2003): 10–11.

Thomas, C. L., & Taber, C. W. (Eds.). (2005). *Taber's cyclopedic medical dictionary.* Philadelphia: F. A. Davis.

U.S. Department of Health and Human Services (USDHHS). (2005). Health promotion and disease prevention objectives for 2010. Retrieved January 1, 2006, from http://www.os.dhhs.gov

U.S. Department of Health and Human Services, National Institutes of Health, National Institute on Drug Abuse. *Preventing drug abuse among children and adolescents.* (2003). Retrieved January 1, 2006, from http://www.drugabuse.gov/prevention/

Venes, D. (Ed.). (2001). Taber's cyclopedic medical dictionary, thumb-indexed version. Philadelphia: F. A. Davis.

Bibliography

Boles, S. M., Joshi, V., Grella, C., & Wellisch, J. (2005). Childhood sexual abuse patterns, psychosocial correlates, and treatment outcomes among adults in drug abuse treatment. *Journal of Child Sexual Abuse, 14*(1), 39–55.

Krowchuk, H. V. (2005). Effectiveness of adolescent smoking prevention strategies. *American Journal of Maternal-Child Nursing, 30*(6), 366–372.

Kuper, H. (2002). Tobacco use and cancer causation: Association by tumour type. *Journal of Internal Medicine, 252,* 206–224.

Rea, T. D. (2002). Smoking status and risk for recurrent coronary events after myocardial infarction. *Annals of Internal Medicine, 137,* 494–500.

Usher, K., Jackson, D., & O'Brien, L. (2005). Adolescent drug abuse: Helping families survive. *International Journal of Mental Health Nursing, 14*(3), 209–214.

Williams, C. M. (2002). Using medications appropriately in older adults. *American Family Physician, 66*(10), 1917–1924.

Chapter 18

ENHANCING HOLISTIC CARE

Marsha Walker, MSN, RMT, HNC, RN
Janice A. Maville, EdD, MSN, RN

KEY TERMS

ayurveda
CAM
capacity building
chakras
energy
energy field

grounding
heliotherapy
holistic care
holistic healing
holistic nursing
imagery

learned helplessness
meditation
modeling and role
  modeling
nurse healer
phytochemicals

presence
reflexology
relaxation response
therapeutic touch

OBJECTIVES

Upon completion of this chapter, the reader should be able to:

- Create a personal definition of a healing nurse.
- Discuss how the nurse can help the client discover and meet health needs.
- Explore the concept of the human energy field and its relevance to nursing.
- List two ways to become conscious of and change unwanted thoughts.
- Discuss how imagery can be used to promote health.
- Practice and teach the Relaxation Response technique.
- List two ways the nurse can use light and sound for health promotion.
- Demonstrate the use of Centering and Grounding as used in Therapeutic Touch and Healing Touch.
- Demonstrate the use of touch therapy by using reflexology or massage to help balance the body for relaxation and healing.
- Choose among methods of nurturing the self and managing stress and describe how they can be used for health promotion.
- Describe how healing and health can be promoted through human caring and love.

INTRODUCTION

Today, there are a wide variety of methods that people use to help heal themselves, and these and other methods are finding their way into professional health care practice. With the growing concern in the health professions and health care delivery systems about the cost of health care, greater emphasis must be placed on promoting health and finding alternatives to traditional health care.

This chapter will discuss what is meant by holistic healing, what a nurse healer is, and how incorporating holistic care can enhance health promotion. The importance of the relationship of a nurse with her own inner being as well as with the client will be explored. Ways will be suggested to help the client and nurse discover what each needs to allow healing to occur, and how to meet those needs. Many holistic healing modalities will be introduced, and ways the nurse can incorporate them into nursing practice will be discussed. The goal of this chapter is to offer new tools and new points of view that you as a nurse can use in the ongoing quest to help your clients and yourself to be healthy.

WHAT IS HOLISTIC CARE?

Providing nursing care is more than giving medicines, changing dressings, and charting. It is eye contact, smiles, touch, time, and caring. It is considering clients as individuals with unique needs and fears. It is helping them to feel in control by meeting those needs and comforting those fears. In vulnerable moments it is helping others with private activities of daily living when they cannot help themselves. It is looking at, and interacting with, clients holistically.

Nursing has always been holistic. **Holistic healing** means considering all aspects of a person's internal and external environment that may contribute to her health and well-being, and being willing to entertain a wide variety of options to help that person heal. Nurses view this total picture when suggesting which modalities clients might use to help correct imbalances in their state of health. **Holistic nursing** is looking at a person as a whole greater than the sum of the parts. Another view of holism is that human beings are holograms, which means that each part reflects the whole (Eliopoulos, 2004).

What are these aspects of the human being? They are both the physical and energetic aspects of the body, the mind or thoughts, the emotions and feelings, and the spirit. Central to the holistic health philosophy are the following:

- Holism of the person (body, mind, and spirit) is in interaction with the environment.

- Health promotion and disease prevention are the focus rather than treatment of symptoms.

- Disease, illness, or imbalance are opportunities for positive growth.

- Clients are responsible and active participants in their own health.

- Collaborative relationships among clients and practitioners are emphasized.

- Cultural diversity is a highly valued component.

- Complementary and alternative modalities are part of a worldview perspective. (Bright, Andrus, & Lunt, 2004)

Holistic nursing considers a person's total environment whether at work, home, school, or in the community. A person's environment includes everything. It includes feelings of social support, stressors and how they are handled, the quality of air and water, the food ingested, type and location of home, presence of animals or pets, and habits of daily living such as sleep, exercise, and play. Holistic nursing care means considering the whole person. It looks at all that contributes, or has contributed in the past, to make clients who they are, and it discovers how all those factors affect health and the disease process. Nurses consider these factors when assessing, planning interventions, and evaluating progress. Nursing is inherently holistic. Very few nurses consider the state of a person merely by her physical body. Because nurses are intuitive and caring, they consider a person's thoughts, feelings, and family life to one degree or another.

People are multifaceted beings with all aspects of their selves and their lives constantly interacting to produce all degrees of health and illness. To help clients discover and achieve their unique desired level of wellness, all of these facets must be considered.

What Is Healing?

A core component to nursing is helping people to heal. What it means to heal is unique to each individual.

The words *healing* and *holy* both come from the root word *hal* (hale), which means to make whole. As people begin to feel the connection between spirit, thoughts, feelings, and bodies, healing happens. Those who are conscious of their total being make changes that create lives that are fun and fulfilling. This is healing.

In the heart of each person, people are, and always have been, whole and complete. Events in life such as childhoods that were less than supportive, disappointing relationships, anger, and even lack of sleep can cause individuals to forget their inherent state of wholeness. Healing is remembering one's true nature. Nurses use many tools to help people remember, such as prescription drugs, surgery, prayer, massage, exercise, play, and many, many others.

It is the natural state of the body to heal itself, to have abundant energy, and to have no pain. Disease or imbalance occurs when people deprive themselves of physical, mental, emotional, or spiritual needs. Symptoms such as constipation, headaches, pain, depression, and low energy are wake-up calls. If an individual makes the necessary changes, she may prevent both acute and chronic illness. By removing the resistances that are self-inflicted and by providing needed nourishment instead, the mind and immune system can become powerful allies for health maintenance and restoration.

What Is a Nurse Healer?

Nurses are health professionals who provide services for health promotion, restoration, maintenance, and general well-being. Nurses support, nurture, cherish, and care to enable healthy growth and development throughout the lifespan. Involving clients and their families in decision-making for health and well-being is an important part of nursing. Two terms associated with facilitative decision making are *empowerment* and *capacity building*. Empowered clients have control over and confidence in their decision making, which is central to health promotion and healing. It is important to note that nurses do not empower clients. Clients become empowered through mobilization of their own strengths, abilities, and resources. This is called capacity building. **Capacity building** is a developmental process that results in independence and self-confidence. Nurses facilitate the capacity of clients to empower themselves through trust, support, guidance, and education.

Nurse healers help clients discover what they need to heal and meet those needs. Nurses help clients find their own definition of health and set their own goals for healing. They are empowered to help themselves by helping themselves feel worthwhile and capable, in control of their lives. Furthermore, by learning how to care for themselves they make positive change in their lives.

Being a nurse healer means many things. It is about **presence,** or being with another in a meaningful way, giving of one's self in the current moment; listening, and providing unconditional acceptance (McKivergin, 2004). These are the most important qualities. The nurse who puts presence into her practice helps her clients feel cared for and safe and may assist them in listening to their own inner voice to discover what they need to heal.

The nurse healer speaks with the client and/or family about their health goals, needs, and strategies for meeting needs. She may choose to practice and teach holistic healing techniques she finds effective. Some of these may include Therapeutic Touch, massage, Healing Touch, or reflexology. The nurse teaches the client and/or the client's family about self-care, and may give them information about nutrition, herbs, communication, exercise, meditation, visualization, and prayer.

Finally, the nurse healer begins to apply holistic principles in her own life. These holistic principles include:

- examining thoughts and feelings about healing and nursing;

- being aware of thoughts, tones of voice, and words used when with the client; and

- incorporating the use of holistic healing techniques into the nurse's own life.

Nurses are much more effective in teaching clients about the benefits of holistic health care when they speak from personal experience. They can choose how and where they want to begin to try some holistic ideas. It is not necessary to wait until all of these ideas have been fully incorporated into life to begin sharing them with clients. Nurses can teach as they learn.

HOLISTIC NURSING: PAST, PRESENT, AND FUTURE

Where did this "new" form of healing begin? It may be helpful to look at the history of holistic healing and its place in nursing to answer this question.

The Past

Holistic healing is as old as humankind. Early tribes all over the world believed that all things in the universe were connected. Humankind, the animals, sky, rocks, sun, rain, plants—all had spirits that affected and were intimately related to each other. These cultures had shamans or medicine men and women to help them in the healing process. As described in Chapter 1, the healing practices of the Greeks of 700 BC–AD 300 centered on the ideals of holism. They believed that the ideal was to have balance in all areas of life with a strong mind, body, and spirit. There were many healing temples which existed for hundreds of years that incorporated many healing techniques including looking at dreams, music, art, massage, rest, laughter, hot baths, herbs, diet, and feelings of love and kindness. The primary belief of Hippocrates, the father of modern medicine, was that the purpose of the healer was to help the body heal itself.

Beginning as early as 2000 BC, and continuing to the present, a very holistic form of medicine has been practiced in India called **Ayurveda.** Ayurveda as a healing modality recognizes the holistic concept of body, mind, and soul connectedness and covers all aspects of health and wellness in life from birth to death (Qutab, 2005). This form of healing focuses on physical health and spiritual growth, using meditation, sound, massage, herbs, the breath, and types of food specific to the individual to help balance the body and its energy field.

Fabiola, considered a patron saint of nursing, established the first free Christian hospital in Rome in AD 390. In approximately AD 800, nursing came to be regarded as the work of God, as it was caring for the sick with no expectation of earthly reward. By the 1300s there were orders of nursing nuns who had begun using caring, nurturing, prayers, songs, and herbs for healing. In the 1700s the religious hospitals began to close, leaving only city hospitals. The religious hospitals had gardens, clean water, and lots of room, with nurses who ministered to the spirit of the clients.

At the time when hospitals were places to go to die instead of to get better, Florence Nightingale entered the world of health care. In 1854, at the age of 38, she became the head of the nurses in a hospital during the Crimean War. She and her 39 nurses cleaned the filthy sickrooms, fixed nutritious meals, opened windows, and cared for wounds. Nightingale believed that if the nurse could provide the basics for the mind, body, and spirit, nature could do the healing. When she arrived at the hospital, the mortality rate was 60 percent. When she left it was 1 percent. She was the first nurse to prove that quality nursing care could affect healing (Joel, 2006).

Until the discovery of sulfa in the 1930s, America was on its way to creating a very holistic health care system. There were homeopathic medical schools in America, physicians in their practices were using reflexology, and light and color were being used in hospitals. With the advent of drugs, these modalities were considered nonscientific.

In the 1940s Scherrer discovered that experiencing stress affected the endocrine system. In 1956 Hans Selye proposed his General Adaptation Theory. Many nursing theories are built upon this theory that states that if organisms do not cope well with the stressors of life, physical and mental imbalance and disease will result (Selye, 1956). This was the beginning of research into the connections between the thoughts of the mind, the feelings, and the health of the body.

The Present

Two important nurse theorists made great contributions to holistic healing. In the 1970s, Dr. Martha Rogers, R.N., introduced the idea that the nurse, the client, and everything in their environments are interconnected and constantly interacting. In the mid-1970s, Dr. Dolores Krieger, R.N., began doing research on her technique Therapeutic Touch, which uses the hands to help balance the energy field to aid healing.

It was during the 1970s that holistic healing centers sprang up in many cities in America. The majority of the health care community, including physicians and nurses, did not yet believe that the philosophies and techniques of holistic healing were sound or had much to do with health. At that time little research had been done in America on the mind-body-spirit health connection, or on holistic techniques. Much of the rest of the world was using both traditional holistic techniques and "modern" medicine.

There were pioneers, however, among physicians, nurses, psychologists, and other health care providers who supported the benefits and practices of holistic healing. They began giving seminars and writing books for the public, providing testimony in favor of holistic techniques. By 1975, reflexology, massage, Therapeutic Touch, polarity, color, sound, music, fasting, herbs, diet, yoga, and meditation were all becoming more popular.

From all walks of life people were beginning to search for and find answers to how they could understand the body-mind-spirit connection and heal themselves. This popularity was evidenced in 1998, when the National Center for Complementary and Alternative Medicine (NCCAM) became one of the 27 institutes and centers that make up the National Institutes of Health (NIH). NCCAM recently reported on a nationwide government survey conducted in 2002, revealing that 36 percent of U.S. adults age 18 years and over use some form of complementary and alternative medicine, **CAM** (see Figure 18-1; Barnes, Powell-Griner, McFann, & Nahin, 2004).

Interestingly, the survey results indicated that when prayer, specifically for health reasons, was included in the definition of CAM, the number of U.S. adults using some form of CAM in the past year rose to 62 percent (see Figure 18-1). NCCAM defines CAM as a group of diverse medical and health care systems, practices, and products that are not currently considered to be conventional medicine or that which is practiced by medical doctors or other health professionals, such as physical therapists, psychologists, and registered nurses (NCCAM, 2004). More specifically, complementary modalities are used as an adjunct to conventional medicine, while alternative modalities are used instead of conventional medicine.

Reflective of the growing interest in holistic healing, the American Holistic Nurses Association (AHNA) and the American Holistic Medical Association were established in the early 1980s by Charlotte McGuire, R.N. and Norm Shealy, M.D. (cofounder), respectively. By the late 1980s, membership in AHNA was growing and the organization was defining itself. Nurse researchers such as Erickson, Parse, Newman, and others were proposing nursing theories that addressed body-mind-spirit environment. Nurses all over the world are now researching, practicing and teaching Therapeutic Touch, Healing Touch, and Holistic Nursing in hospitals, universities, clinics, private practices, and with families and friends. It is now possible to

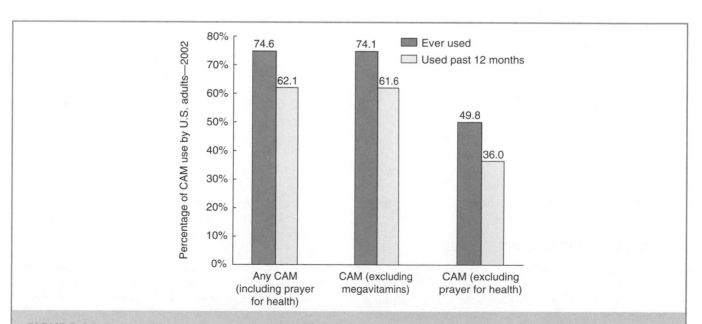

FIGURE 18-1 *CAM Use by U.S. Adults, 2002. From* Complementary and Alternative Medicine Use Among Adults: United States, 2002 *(CDC Advance Data Report #343), by P. Barnes, E. Powell-Griner, K. McFann, & R. Nahin, 2004, National Center for Complementary and Alternative Medicine, National Institutes of Health, Bethesda, MD: National Institutes of Health, Department of Health and Human Services.*

become a Certified Holistic Nurse. The AHNA endorses certificate programs in aromatherapy, guided imagery and visualization, and holistic nursing.

The Future

Nurses have always been holistic healers in theory and practice. What makes nurses unique, with regard to other health care professionals, is that they have always looked at the client's total inner and outer environment, and its relationship to body, mind, and spirit. Martha Rogers brought the study of energy fields to nursing before they were part of popular conversation.

Now many health professionals are realizing that people are not happy and healthy if only the body or only the mind or only the environments are taken into consideration. Nurses have been doing this all along. Holistic care fits well within the nursing model of practice that emphasizes disease prevention and health promotion, health restoration, and health maintenance.

In the future, nurses will be primary consultants, teachers, and practitioners of holistic healing in the hospital, home health, private practice, and educational settings. Nurses are already leading practitioners of holistic modalities. The potential exists for holistic healing clinics in every state with nurses as directors and practitioners. It is time for nurses to take leadership roles in the research, teaching, and practice of holistic healing as a unique role in the emerging new paradigm of health care.

THE NURSE-CLIENT RELATIONSHIP

Attitudes about healing that allow the individual her own unique view of health and to explore all avenues toward that health create an open mind and heart where many possibilities can emerge. The nurse's attitude about healing, and about herself, influences the type and quality of the nurse-client relationship. Since holistic nursing involves the entire world of the client, the nurse becomes a part of that world. The way the nurse views herself, the thoughts and feelings she has, and how she thinks and feels about clients when she is with them all play a part in the quality of the healing relationship.

The Nurse's Attitude About Healing

Healing does not always mean a perfectly functioning body, a totally clear mind, or being completely happy. As nurses begin working with clients, it is helpful to examine their personal definitions of healing. This definition will greatly affect how one interacts with clients. Since the word heal comes from the word hal which means whole, what does wholeness mean? Nurses can ask what is needed to feel whole, or to heal. Wholeness or health is a balance of body, mind, emotions, and

spirit that is unique to each individual. Often healing requires making change of some kind. The nurse's attitude about what healing is will color all interactions with clients and can enhance or hinder their healing.

The Nurse's Attitude About Self

A characteristic of a great nurse is the presence with which the nurse moves through all aspects of life, especially when with clients. To contemplate presence, or being, the nurse can look within and explore the inner self.

For nurses to fully practice holistic healing they must be willing to look at themselves—their comfort in body, feelings, thoughts, and world; discovering where they are happy and where they are not. In the areas where they are not happy, they must begin to choose changes in thoughts, feelings, and actions. To be the most effective healer possible, nurses must be able to choose their responses to the unpleasant as well as the pleasant circumstances in life.

Everyone is in a constant state of Becoming. The healing work is creating the balance between Being and Becoming. As people are more conscious or awake in each moment, they realize that healing is the balance between Being present in the moment, just observing; and Becoming, which is learning, changing, and growing. When people are still, they feel their feelings, discover their needs, listen to others, and create an open space for intuition to arise. When people are Becoming, they are open to pursuing opportunities that come their way for growth, learning, and service. These opportunities are constantly leading all people along their own unique healing journey. Whichever area is focused on most will eventually lead to the balance of both. The path is different for each one. Some begin with great personal awareness and few techniques to share with clients. Others know many techniques but have not yet become comfortable with themselves.

Nurses who desire to enhance their healing abilities must become conscious in the moment. All people are responsible for the thoughts and tones of voice they choose to have and the words they choose to speak. Positive thoughts or affirmations increase confidence, energy, and hope while those that are negative result in tightening of the body as well as increases in blood pressure, breathing, and heart rate (Dossey & Keegan, 2005). Assessing and analyzing our thoughts enhances our ability to clarify our goals, examine our options, and gain control of situations we encounter.

Negative emotions experienced by the nurse, including such feelings as inferiority, frustration, sadness, or anger, should be recognized as a red flag to stop and reflect. The nurse's environment away from work affects the type of person the nurse is with clients. If events of life are stressful, there are many techniques the nurse may use to create an outer world that is healing.

Interaction Between Nurse and Client

There are three parts to the nurse-client relationship as depicted in Figure 18-2. The role of the nurse has been explored. It is impossible to directly change the client. Only the client can do that. What the nurse may do is look at the interaction between the nurse and client. As a health care professional the nurse should be able to be more conscious in the interactions between the self and the world, and discover that transforming relationships can occur—helping to get both the nurse's and the client's needs met, so all parties benefit.

Being conscious in the moment, or choosing responses to others, may be more difficult than it sounds. As a nurse enters a client's room with every intention of being kind and caring, the client may react negatively because the call light was not answered fast enough, or the pillow is not in the right place. This may create a negative feeling in the nurse, but if the nurse is conscious in the moment, there will be realization of the emotion that is felt, analysis as to why it is being felt, and choice of a caring response.

Questions that often cut through the exterior gruffness and get to the heart connection are: "What can I do for you?" "What do you need?" If a nurse views all people and clients as precious beings, then the actions selected will help everyone heal.

Words, tone of voice, and body language help to create a feeling of trust and caring. Eye contact, soft, low tones of voice, sitting close to a person, touching or holding their hand, really listening to what is being said and not being said, and smiling are all behaviors that help people feel safe. The nurse must use judgment to decide which of these would be most effective with different clients.

When a person feels safe, it is easier to open up and explore what is needed to heal. This varies with each individual. The nurse must ask each client what he thinks he needs to heal. One client who is an athlete with a broken leg may want to be able to run again, a

client with emphysema may want to breath without having to think about it, and another may want to make it through a day without grieving for a deceased child. Dr. Helen Erickson, R.N. developed the Theory of Modeling and Role Modeling, which says that for people to heal their needs must be met. Sometimes nurses or family members can meet those needs for the client. Sometimes the nurse helps clients discover their needs and how to meet them. To meet those needs, clients must look at the stressors in their lives and resources for coping with those stressors. Nurses can be most facilitative when they have made the effort to acknowledge and understand clients as individuals and to see situations through the world of the client (**modeling**)—a world reflective of life's experiences, values, culture, knowledge, and so forth. In **role modeling,** the nurse plans interventions that facilitate growth, development, and healing at the client's own pace based on the unique model of the client's world (Erickson, 2002; Frisch & Bowman, 2002). When needs are met, healing is facilitated. Table 18-1 provides a framework to help clients discover and meet their needs. This framework is applicable to clients as individuals, families, groups, or communities. Inherent is the interaction between the nurse and client whereby

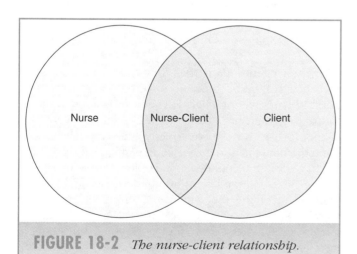

FIGURE 18-2 *The nurse-client relationship.*

TABLE 18-1 Helping Clients Discover Their Needs: A Framework

Questions and statements that follow are related to five major areas that could help the nurse and client identify needs and plan for meeting them.

1. Description	How do you describe what is happening?
	What do you think it is related to, or what caused it?
2. Needs	What has helped you feel better in the past?
	What will help you feel better now?
	You know best what you need to heal.
3. Expectations	What do you think is going to happen?
4. Resources	How can I help you to help yourself?
	Who else can help you?
5. Goal	When do you think you will feel better?
	What would you like to have happen?
	What would it take to have that happen?

Adapted from Interactive Communication Strategies: Tools That Transform and Heal, *by H. Erickson, 1998, workshop presented at the University of Texas at Austin, April 15–17, 1998.*

the nurse creates a safe, comfortable, and caring space allowing the discovery of the client's needs, strengths, and resources needed to create goals and plan interventions that promote health and well-being.

HOLISTIC TECHNIQUES FOR HEALTH PROMOTION

Having explored the importance of the nurse's relationship with healing, and the client, it is important to briefly discuss several holistic healing modalities or tools that may be incorporated into nursing practice. The focus of these tools is to establish and maintain health and well-being rather than to treat a specific illness. These tools may be used by a nurse for personal growth and healing, and can be shared with family and friends. The nurse can choose those that are appropriate in the practice setting or taught to clients and their families for self-

care and health promotion at home. Nurses may teach these techniques to students, other nurses, and health care providers to use in their practices. This chapter is intended to provide an introduction to these tools and some simple ways to use them in nursing practice.

Very often it is an imbalance or illness that inspires a person to seek any kind of health care, including holistic care. Holistic modalities may be used when there is illness to help restore balance and health to the system. Just as importantly, however, they may maintain health so that disease or illness occurs much less frequently. That is the goal.

As discussed earlier in this chapter, many people incorporate complementary and alternative medicine (CAM) into their lives for health and healing. NCCAM (2004) has noted that the list of what is considered CAM is in constant change as evidence grows regarding the safety and effectiveness of tested therapies and as new approaches to health care are adopted. Table 18-2 identifies five major categories of CAM recognized by NCCAM and examples of modalities associated with each.

The Teaching and Learning of Healing Techniques

Since many of these techniques or modalities involve teaching in one way or another, it is necessary to examine teaching for a moment. First there has to be a learner. This means that clients must want the information, connect with how it will meet their needs, and fit with their view of health. Nurses often project onto people their own definition of health and their own health goals. If they are not the same as the learner's, even the best teaching is ineffective.

By listening carefully, the nurse will hear exactly what is needed by clients, and how best to proceed with teaching.

People are ready for different levels of learning at different times. If many new things are going on in life at the same time, positive or negative, only a small amount of information may be absorbed. Sometimes the nurse must teach in short increments for the client to learn effectively. Sometimes only one thing can be changed at a time.

When clients learn that they can have control in their health they become empowered. How can nurses assist in empowering clients? They can teach them tools to use for health promotion. How can nurses encourage clients to use those tools? Briefly, they can share with them the benefits of the tools, and results that other people have gotten using these modalities. Nurses must help them realize that the body and mind are designed to feel good most of the time. Pain and emotional upset are warning signals to change something. Nurses can remind clients that they deserve to feel good. Sometimes people have learned from childhood not to expect good health,

CAM Category and Descriptor	Associated Modalities Examples	
Biologically based practices use natural substances, special diets, or vitamins (in doses outside those used in conventional medicine).	Herbal medicine (unrefined plant-based products) Phytotherapy (plant derivatives) Botanical medicine (herbs and plants) Orthomolecular medicine (other nutritional supplements)	
Energy medicine based on energy fields (magnetic or biofields) subcategorized as veritable, which can be measured and putative, which have yet to be measured.	Reiki and Johrei (Japanese) Qi Gong (Chinese) Healing Touch Therapeutic Touch	Huna (Hawaiian) Bioelectromagnetics Intercessory prayer (prayer on behalf of another)
Manipulative and body-based practices based on manipulation or movement of one or more body parts.	Chiropractic manipulation Craniosacral therapy (skull massage) Feldenkrais method (movement) Massage therapy (pressure and movement) Reflexology (foot and hand massage)	Rolfing (deep tissue massage) Trager bodywork (slight rhythmic rocking and shaking of the body) Tui Na (pressure on acupoints) Pilates exercise
Mind-body medicine uses techniques for enhancing the mind's ability to affect bodily functions and symptoms.	Relaxation hypnosis Visual imagery Meditation Yoga Biofeedback Tai Chi	Qi Gong Cognitive-behavioral therapies Group support Autogenic training Spirituality
Whole medical systems based on complete theory and practice developed apart from conventional Western medical practice.	Traditional Chinese medicine (TCM) Ayurvedic medicine (India) Homeopathy Naturopathy	Other systems from various cultures (Native American, African, Middle Eastern, Tibetan, and Central and South American)

From The Use of Complementary and Alternative Medicine in the United States, *by National Center for Complementary and Alternative Medicine (NCCAM), 2004, retrieved June 17, 2006, from nccam.nih.gov; and* Nursing Now! Today's Issues, Tomorrow's Trends, *by J. T. Catalano, 2006, Philadelphia: F. A. Davis.*

or that individuals have no control over their health. Sometimes people have learned that they are not capable and cannot learn new things, or that they do not deserve to be happy and healthy. These are issues of self-esteem. Cognitive learning theories from educational psychology present effective methods for teaching people new information.

To learn and to change, people must feel they are in control of their environment, or have the ability to choose and affect their environment. If individuals feel safe and are asked, they know best what they need to create health and happiness in their lives, or at least to take a first step. The nurse can ask these questions, help the client explore choices, and become a key figure in the empowerment of clients.

Using Energy as a Healing Tool

What is energy? **Energy** is a dynamic quality or power that has the capacity for doing work. The concept of the energy field in nursing is not a new one. Martha Rogers, considered to be one of the first nurse theorists, proposed her theory, the Science of Unitary Human Beings, in 1970. This theory suggests that all living things are continually interacting energy fields, and that these fields are infinite in space and time connecting all things, even at great distances. Some say the **energy field** is a field of energy composed of constantly changing vibrational frequencies that surrounds and connects all matter. According to Dr. Rogers, people and all living things are energy fields that affect and are affected by all other

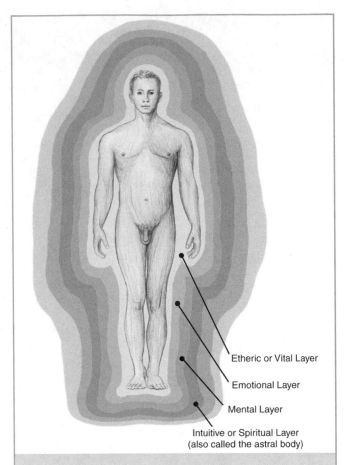

FIGURE 18-3 *Layers of the human energy field extending beyond the physical boundaries.*

forms of energy, creating health and disease. Rogers based much of her theory on Albert Einstein's work in physics. He found that all matter is energy in motion. Therefore, the nurse, client, family, and the total environment of all of them are continually affecting each other.

Dr. Dolores Krieger, RN, used Martha Rogers's theory as the foundation of her work on therapeutic touch (TT) (Krieger, 2002). **Therapeutic touch** uses the hands to facilitate balance of the energy field to enhance relaxation and healing. TT is used by thousands of nurses worldwide in all types of nursing scenarios.

Dora Kunz, the co-originator of TT, was born with the ability to see energy fields of living objects and used her perceptions as a guide for the hands-on healing of TT (Eliopoulos, 2004). The energy field contains several layers of varying frequencies of vibration, one corresponding to the body, one to thoughts, one to feelings, and one to spirit, with the physical body being the most dense area of the field. She reports that the human field extends from two inches to three feet around the body. It is composed of layers of different vibrational frequencies, colors, and patterns that respond very quickly to thoughts and feelings, especially those held over long periods of time. Figure 18-3 depicts the four major layers of the human energy field, and Figure 18-4 shows how human energy fields can interact.

Human energy fields are not separate, but are part of, or connected with, the universal field, or Higher Power, as understood by the individual. Within the energy field layers are **chakras,** which are spinning wheels of energy that help move healing energy from the universal field through the layers of the individual field (spiritual, mental, emotional, etheric) to the human body. This can be visualized in Figure 18-5. The body uses this energy for the maintenance of health.

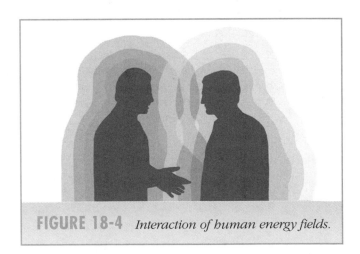

FIGURE 18-4 *Interaction of human energy fields.*

Many researchers have studied, and continue to study, the characteristics of the energy field around living things, how it changes in health and disease, and what can be done to promote health (Jobst, Niemtzow, Curtis, & Curtis, 2004; Hover-Kramer, 2002; Krieger, 2002; Kreitzer & Snyder, 2002; Leigh, 2004; Nelson & Schwartz, 2005).

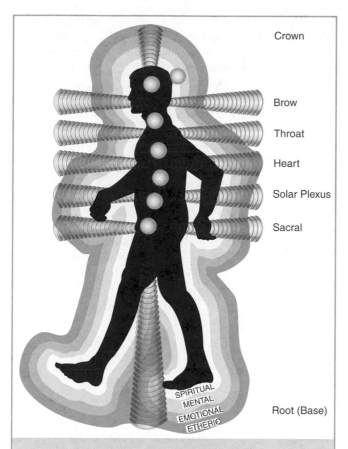

FIGURE 18-5 *The Chakras in relation to the human energy fields.*

Crown

Brow

Throat

Heart

Solar Plexus

Sacral

SPIRITUAL
MENTAL
EMOTIONAL
ETHERIC

Root (Base)

Research Note

Therapeutic Touch and Quality of Life in Women Receiving Cancer Radiation Treatment

Study Problem/Purpose: To investigate the effect of Healing Touch therapy on the quality of life of women receiving radiation treatment for gynecologic or breast cancer.

Methods: A clinical trial using a two-arm single-blind study design was conducted with 62 female participants newly diagnosed with cervical, endometrial, or breast cancer and receiving radiation treatment. The setting was a large midwestern university–affiliated hospital. Women who had experienced Healing Touch in the past were excluded. All participants completed the Mini-Mental Status Exam to assure mental stability and confirm the ability to read and understand English in order to complete questionnaires. The participants were randomly assigned to either a Healing Touch (HT) or Mock Treatment (MT) group. The

majority were Caucasian, with median age of 50 and education level of 12.3 years. There were 61.3 percent with either cervical or endometrial cancer and 38.7 percent with breast cancer.

Trained providers administered Healing Touch and laypersons with no experience or training with Healing Touch conducted the mock treatment sessions. An opaque screen was placed between the head and body of each participant to obscure vision. The mock providers walked about, without passing hands on or near the participant, and were directed to divert thoughts from healing by doing simple math mentally.

The HT providers used techniques on or near the body and focused on healing intentions. Six treatments were provided to each group over a period of four to six weeks. Measurements were taken to determine socioeconomic and medical status; attitude about Healing Touch and beliefs about group assignment; and subjective evaluation of Healing Touch and Quality of Life. Quality of Life was evaluated using the SF-36 Quality of Life instrument from the Medical Outcomes Study at Rand Corporation that addresses nine domains via 36 questions. The domains include: physical functioning, physical role functioning, pain, general health, vitality, social function, emotional role function, mental health, and health transition. The SF-36 has a reliability coefficient of .80 and test-retest reliability between .73 and .90.

Findings: There was no difference in attitude toward Healing Touch between groups. The majority of participants felt they were in the HT group. The HT group had better outcomes in all nine domains with statistically significant results obtained for physical functioning, pain, and vitality. A within-groups-over-time measure found that the HT group had the most pronounced change in emotional role function, mental health, and health transition.

Implications: This study found that there was value in the use of Healing Touch on women with gynecologic or breast cancer receiving radiation treatment. Generalization to other populations is limited due to the small sample size of 62 and the fact that the study was conducted in one hospital in the Midwest.

Cook, C. A. L., Guerrerio, J. R., and Slater, V. E. (2004). Healing touch and quality of life on women during radiation treatment. *Alternative Therapies in Health and Medicine, 10*(3), 34-41.

The energy field, including the functions of the chakras, have been part of Ayurvedic medicine for hundreds of years. The fields and chakras have specific connections to feelings, thoughts, endocrine glands, and nerve plexus. Balancing the chakras and energy field can aid the healing and maintain balance in areas of the body that correspond to the chakra areas (Hover-Kramer, 2002; Krieger, 2002; Wauters, 2002). For example, the second chakra, sacral, is below the navel, and balancing it aids in the function of the intestines.

The energy field is constantly vibrating because it is constantly moving when the person is healthy and in balance. When there is imbalance in the mind, body, or spirit, it is reflected in the energy field and can be perceived by the hands as an area in the field that is not moving, as it should. The Law of Resonance in physics says anything that vibrates is affected by all other vibrations. When nurses look at what may help to balance the energy field, they consider light, color, sound, music, and thought because all of these are forms of energy waves or vibrations. The energy coming from the hands is also a form of vibration affecting the field.

Considered controversial by some, the North American Nursing Diagnosis Association (NANDA, 2007) has included "Disturbed Energy Field" as a diagnostic domain in Taxonomy II: Activity/Rest—Class 3 Energy Balance. NANDA addresses the definition of this diagnostic domain as well as the following areas: related factors, defining characteristics, desired outcomes/evaluation criteria, actions/interventions, and documentation focus. Nursing interventions such as Therapeutic Touch and Healing Touch address this diagnosis.

The Power of Thoughts and Feelings

Thoughts and feelings are forms of energy with vibrations that affect personal energy fields and those of others near and far. It has only been within the last 25 years that people have begun to realize that what is thought and felt is a strong determinant of health or illness. Prior to this time thoughts and feelings were considered unimportant to health, perhaps because they seem to have no material substance, are fleeting, and are "only in the mind."

Almost 20 years ago, the formalized study of the body-mind connection called psychoneuroimmunology (PNI) was born. PNI, discussed in detail in Chapter 8, is the study of how thoughts and feelings affect the body. Much research has been done to discover the effects of different thoughts and feelings on the health of the body. Emotional states such as anger, fear, depression, learned helplessness, joy, and perceived control have been examined to determine their effects on different aspects of physiology, such as the immune, cardiovascular, digestive, and endocrine systems.

One very important example of PNI is **learned helplessness** (Abramson, Seligman, & Teasdale, 1978). This phenomenon is basically, if one believes one has no control over one's experience (whether positive or negative), or that what one does cannot get a positive outcome, one learns to become helpless. Some characteristics of learned helplessness are decreased immune function, lack of motivation and creativity, and depression. It affects health, and success in school, job, and relationships. Learned helplessness may be reversed when persons learn that they can affect their world.

Thoughts and feelings cause chemicals to be released from the brain and the organs of the immune and endocrine systems. These chemicals travel through the bloodstream and enhance or depress the functions of all the others. What people habitually think and feel, or worry about, does cause physiologic change in the body.

Knowing about PNI is important for nurses who may feel out of control, angry, frustrated, or depressed in the work setting. These feelings can lead to stress and the burnout syndrome. If the nurse feels out of control at work, this may often be balanced by incorporating even one regularly practiced stress management technique into work or home life.

Clients often feel helpless when they are in a health care setting. Realizing the deleterious effects on health that these feelings can create, the nurse can find ways to help clients feel more in control of their experiences. Some of these ways might include choosing what they want to eat and when, what they wear, when visitors come, when activities are scheduled, and any other choices they can possibly make. The nurse may also encourage clients to focus on being hopeful and appreciative because both of these have positive effects on the body.

Thoughts are also very powerful in the area of stress. It is not what happens, but how events are perceived, that creates a physiological stress response. A situation occurs and a reaction results before the situation is fully assessed. This reaction is often anger, fear, resentment, guilt, or another emotion. Those feelings and words set the stress response in motion with all of its physiologic, mental, and emotional outcomes. In communication with others, words often happen so fast that they may go from being kind and friendly one moment to being curt and angry the next.

How can one learn to be aware of thoughts and therefore be selective over responses? Box 18-1 describes techniques for recognizing and changing thoughts. Nurses may use these suggestions for themselves and teach their clients self-care.

One approach to changing responses to stressful situations involves a method called Freeze Frame (Childre, 1998). In this model, when a stressful feeling is noticed, a person should freeze the moment. The individual should take a mental time-out for 30 seconds, focusing on a positive person or feeling, finally returning to the present situation. Most often one will have a changed perspective and be able to choose different, more constructive thoughts and responses.

People's perceptions of and responses to stress are considered to contribute to the majority of all disease. Nurses can therefore no longer dismiss symptoms as, "Oh, it's just stress." They must address the causes of stress.

The problem is never only one event for a short time. When many stressful events continue for prolonged periods, health problems result. Nurses can help clients look at all of the factors in their lives that are

BOX 18-1 Techniques for Recognizing and Changing Thoughts

- **Thought check**—Once each hour, check your thoughts. If there are thoughts that are not serving life, substitute the thoughts that will focus on what you want to happen in your life. Energy follows thought. What we think about over and over again emerges in our lives.
- **Red flag your feelings**—Feelings are wake-up calls. When you feel a feeling, use it as a red flag. Thoughts precede feelings. Stop and look at the thoughts you are having—what is your self telling you? Decide if those thoughts are really serving you well.
- **Notice the breath**—Taking a few deep breaths stops the clock and helps us become aware of what we are thinking at that moment.
- **Notice physical cues**—"Knots in the stomach," "lumps in the throat," headache, or neck ache. Take a moment and breathe into that spot, let your exhale go there. What thoughts come to you?
- **Listen to yourself**—Notice what your self is telling you, how you explain the times when you fail or have misfortune. If you think it is always your fault, or the problem will probably last a long time, and all areas of your life look pretty bad, these are characteristics of learned helplessness, as mentioned earlier.
- **Use humor**—Humor or laughing can create new perspective on a situation. When you feel depressed or angry, look at yourself in the mirror and smile. You can't help but laugh. Sound ridiculous? Smiling causes the release of endorphins from the brain that help to create a sense of pleasure.

Adapted from Using Energy to Enhance Nursing Practice Through the Use of Color, Music, Touch, and Movement, *M. Walker, 1996, Holistic Nursing Series workshop presented at the University of Texas School of Nursing, Austin, TX.*

stressful over a long period, and help them see how and where they can make changes.

The Breath

The breath is a powerful tool for balancing the body for healing and promoting health. It is the one part of the autonomic nervous system that may easily be controlled. The autonomic nervous system affects all automatic functions such as the immune system for healing, digestion and assimilation, heart rate, etc. The breath usually occurs automatically, but it may be consciously changed, either the rate or the depth. The rate of breath affects heart rate and brainwaves. Slowing the breath creates relaxation and speeding it up is stimulating.

There are physical, mental, and emotional benefits of slow, deep, continual breathing. In the stress response the body shifts to chest breathing. Chest breathing is shallow and quick. Chronic chest breathing can re-create feelings of stress in the body. Slow breaths can create feelings of relaxation and clarity. The lungs can hold two pints of air, but the average breath is less than one pint. Adequate oxygen is crucial for combining with food to produce heat and energy for the body. Deep breathing can enhance the oxidation of lactic acid in sore muscles, increase physical energy levels, and lead to more efficient metabolism. Slow, diaphragmatic breathing allows the abdomen to expand with the inhale and contract with the exhale. This allows the greatest filling of the lungs and is the most relaxing breath. It is generally accepted that slow, diaphragmatic breathing can help to decrease anxiety, release negative emotions, and diminish the

stress response. There are many variations of diaphragmatic breathing exercise. Try the breathing exercise suggested in Box 18-2.

Changes in feelings are reflected by changes in breathing. Anger, fear, and sorrow have specific patterns

BOX 18-2 Breathing Exercise for Well-being

1. Find a quiet place.
2. Sit comfortably, extremities uncrossed, and rest your arms in your lap.
3. Focus on how you feel in the moment (mentally, physically, emotionally).
4. Exhale deeply and contract your stomach muscles at the same time.
5. Inhale slowly and think about your abdomen expanding.
6. Inhale further, more deeply, expanding your chest and raising your shoulders up toward your ears.
7. Hold the inhaled breath for a few seconds.
8. Slowly exhale, reversing the process: relaxing the shoulders, relaxing the chest, and contracting the stomach muscles until all air is exhaled and your body feels limp.
9. Repeat the process two or three times with increasing ease.
10. Reexamine how you feel in the moment.

of breathing. Often unpleasant emotions create a constriction of energy and a holding of the breath. Unconscious reactive decisions and actions often follow. Consciously changing breathing patterns changes the emotion being felt. Full breaths relax the mind and allow a flow of energy to occur that fosters greater choice of word and deed. Deep, slow continual breaths can bring conscious awareness to the present moment, and they offer an opportunity to examine and choose thoughts and feelings.

The spirit and breath have much in common. In fact, the word breath is a derivative of the Latin word *spiritus,* which comes from the verb *spirare,* which means to breathe. The breath is our vehicle to consciously still the thoughts of the mind, allowing an experience of our spirit and a connection with a Higher Power.

When nurses have been very busy for the entire shift, "out of breath" and stressed, then can immediately become more still and calm, and reduce stress levels, by taking a few deep breaths. Before entering a client's room, taking a few deep breaths allows the nurse to bring about an awareness to the present and be better able to choose the feelings and words with which to interact with the client. Taking five minutes at lunch to sit and breathe lets confusion and mental tension drift away and invites a sense of calm and peacefulness.

Learning about the power of the breath for relaxation and the ease with which breathing patterns may be changed is a valuable tool for clients. They may use this tool at any moment to help reduce muscle tension, pain, the anxiety, fear, and depression that often accompany illness.

For health promotion, in the absence of illness, continued deep breathing is energizing, stress reducing, and calming for the ever restless mind and emotions. Focusing on the breath is a beginning step to practicing meditation and imagery because it quiets the mind and brings the person's awareness to the present moment.

Imagery

Imagery is another method by which a person may consciously use thoughts and feelings to create a variety of desired physiologic conditions such as relaxation, increased sports performance, or decreased blood pressure. One can focus on the desired outcome and/or the steps that need to be taken to achieve that outcome. **Imagery** focuses on thoughts and feelings and then uses them to create images that are desired to make changes in life. When an image is held in the mind the body begins responding to it to try to make it happen. Imagery is a communication mechanism between perception, emotion, and bodily change.

The most effective images for creating physical change are those that use all five senses plus movement and emotion. Imagery gives the subconscious mind a plan for constructing reality.

Nursing Alert

Breathe for Relaxation

- At least once every hour remember to take five or six deep, slow, continuous breaths, like long sighs.
- In times of emotional or mental stress, noticing and changing the breathing pattern to a slower, deeper pattern will change the emotional or mental outlook.

Research Note

Guided Imagery

Study Problem/Purpose: To investigate the effectiveness of guided imagery for immediate smoking cessation and long-term abstinence in adult smokers. The national objective of *Healthy People 2010* is to decrease the percentage of adult cigarette smokers to no more than 12 percent. Currently, however, 22 percent of adults continue to smoke.

Methods: Study participants included 71 smokers from an outpatient hospital clinic who smoked five or more cigarettes a day for at least a year. Participants were randomly assigned to a control or an intervention group. Over a 24-week period both groups received counseling and educational sessions. The intervention group was taught guided health imagery and provided with a relaxation audiotape. Smoking rates were monitored via self-reports of participants and validated by corroborating family members. The intervention group was taught a guided imagery technique and a diaphragmatic breathing exercise. The Creative Imagination Scale was used to evaluate use of guided imagery. Data on smoking rates were collected at 3, 6, 12, and 24 months.

Findings: Abstinence was greater among the guided imagery intervention group. There was a 26 percent abstinence rate for this group compared to a 12 percent abstinence rate for those who did not receive the guided imagery intervention.

Implications: It is possible that nurses prepared in the use of guided imagery can assist clients with smoking cessation. Other factors that might have influenced the participants' rates of smoking abstinence, such as intention and social support, were not evaluated and could have had an effect. Nonetheless, guided imagery can be a useful tool.

Wynd, C. A. (2005). Guided health imagery for smoking cessation and long-term abstinence. *Journal of Nursing Scholarship, 37*(3), 245-250.

A Case Study for Imagery

A nurse named Lou was preparing her client, Mr. B, for surgery. Mr. B was very afraid and did not want to go. Lou asked him to think about his favorite place, a place where he felt safe and comfortable. He told Lou about the flowers, the trees, the weather, the road, the location, and the breeze near the lake he was imaging. Lou handed him a pencil and said, "Take this to surgery and when you feel afraid, hold it, and think of this moment." Mr. B came through surgery just fine. Later he found Lou and told her that the pencil helped him remember his safe place and he wasn't afraid. He still comes to see her, a year later.

Using Meditation

Meditation is taking a moment to become conscious of who one is. One simple way for anyone to do this is to set a timer for five minutes and sit down, be still, and focus on happy times or thoughts.

It is also possible to use thoughts to scan the body from head to toe. By focusing in an area, it is possible to note if the area is holding tension. By directing a breath or two to each area, the tension can melt away with each exhale. Nurses can teach clients and families to use imagery for specific health improvements and for relaxation.

To enhance the effects of imagery, it is helpful to relax first. Progressive relaxation is a very effective technique for becoming aware of, and releasing, tension. Tighten and relax each muscle group from feet to head, one at a time. This can be practiced before imagery or by itself to relax tight areas.

Meditation

There are many forms of meditation such as Transcendental Meditation, Siddha Yoga, Mindfulness Meditation, and many others. What most have in common is bringing awareness of the everyday, rampant thoughts of the mind. When not focused on hectic or troubling thoughts, the body relaxes, and the stress response ceases. People have the opportunity to experience greater peace and creativity and they may get in touch with a Higher Power.

Meditation may be done with the body in a stationary position or with movement. Examples of both types will be discussed here.

Herbert Benson, M.D. (1975, 1996), studied many forms of meditation and noticed two steps that most of them have in common. When people practice these steps, which he calls the **Relaxation Response,** they notice a sense of relaxation that interrupts the stress response. Benson has been researching The Relaxation Response since 1975. Box 18-3 describes the two steps involved in practicing this technique. The benefits of using the Relaxation Response technique include decreased blood pressure, heart rate, muscle tension, and cardiac dysrhythmias, and increased alpha brain

waves (produced during relaxation and creativity), concentration, ability to cope with stressors, and stimulation of the immune system. It is recommended to practice this 10 minutes, twice a day. If that is impractical, it is suggested to try five minutes once a day. It is an easy technique that may be taught to clients, practiced anywhere, and can have many physiologic benefits.

T'ai Chi, Qi Gong, and Yoga are three forms of moving meditations. They have been practiced for hundreds of years in China and India for relaxation, balance, and healing of the body, mind, emotions, and spirit. They focus on the breath and slow precise movements designed to connect and balance all areas of the physical body, energy field, and the life force or chi (chee) or prana.

As the life force begins to flow freely through the body, benefits include:

- stress reduction

- deeper respirations

- relaxation of spine and muscles

- increased energy to the nervous system

- stimulation of internal organs

These techniques may be learned by watching videotapes, but it is recommended to take classes from teachers who have practiced and taught these techniques for some time. There are classes for all levels of expertise, physical condition, and age.

BOX 18-3 Relaxation Response Technique

Step 1 Focus on repetition. Choose a word, phrase, prayer, or movement (breathing, walking, knitting) that is repetitive.

Step 2 If you notice you are having thoughts about your life, return your focus to your repetition.

Adapted from The Relaxation Response, *by H. Benson, 1975, New York: Avon.*

The Power of Prayer

Religions the world over believe in the power of prayer. Since humankind began, prayer has been viewed as a way to communicate with a Higher Power and to aid one's self and others. The reports of healing with prayer became so numerous that scientists finally became interested. Spiritual practices such as prayer have been found to positively affect many kinds of living entities such as enzymes, red blood cells, plants, cancer cells, and bacteria ("The Proof That Prayer Works," n.d.). Epidemiological and medical literature documents hundreds of studies in which spiritual and religious practices have been statistically associated with positive health outcomes. Opposing views also exist on the merits of prayer on effecting positive health outcomes. Nonetheless, the role of religious involvement in the promotion of health and well-being is receiving increasing attention from researchers and is integral to providing holistic nursing care.

Prayer has been found to have an effect on one's self as well as on others who are nearby or at great distances. Studies indicate that it does not seem to matter what religion or type of prayer is used. Each person may be inspired to pray in different ways at different times for different reasons: by speaking, singing, chanting, or in silence; individually or in groups; in public or in private; for forgiveness, direction, thanks, concern for others. In fact, prayer has been categorized into four distinct types: (1) adoration (worship and praise for God), (2) confession (faults, misdeeds, sins acknowledged), (3) supplication (requests for divine intervention in a life event), and (4) reception (awaiting divine wisdom, understanding, or guidance) (Laird, Snyder, Rapoff, & Green, 2004). Some people include techniques such as visualization, guided imagery, or relaxation, and movement such as walking, dancing, or drumming (Burkhardt & Nagai-Jacobson, 2005).

Dr. Larry Dossey (1994), physician and co-chair of the Panel on Mind-Body Interventions of the Office of Alternative Medicine at the National Institutes of Health in Washington, D.C., reported on over 100 studies on the effects of prayer/visualization in his 1994 book, *Healing Words*. More than half showed an effect on everything from seed germination to wound healing and positive effects on hypertension, heart attacks, headaches, and anxiety. Dr. Dossey summarized that the results occurred not only when people prayed for explicit outcomes but also when they prayed for nothing specific.

How does prayer work? No one really knows. Although studies show that people receive images or physical sensations at great distances that others are imaging, there is no energy in the classical physical sense recorded as being sent or received. Physics has discovered through research that a field of energy connects all things in the universe. In this field, nonlocal connections are events that happen between subatomic particles. Nonlocal connections happen instantaneously, where the activity of one particle affects the activity of another even at great distances.

A Higher Power and all things in the universe may be connected by this pervasive field with prayer as a vibrational frequency that helps to amplify the vibrations of health and balance in self and others. Prayer may be letting the mind or daily thoughts go while connecting with, and lending support to, the Universal Whole that connects all things.

The nurse, if she is so inclined, may pray for and with clients, holding the clients in her thoughts and wishing them the best possible outcome. The nurse may educate the clients on the power of prayer as a tool for self-healing.

Spotlight On

Using Prayer for Client Health

Choose a specific client in your practice to pray for. In three or four 30-second intervals over two to three days, offer prayers for that person or send positive thoughts and feelings, wishing the best possible outcome. Assess changes in body, mind, and/or spirit that occur.

Light and Color

Light and color have been used for promoting health since ancient times. Around 500 BC the Greeks used **heliotherapy,** the use of sunlight for healing. In the early 1900s, hospitals used ultraviolet (UV) light with clients to kill bacteria up to eight feet away at a strength that would not create redness even on fair skin. UV light has been used as a treatment for tuberculosis, streptococcal infections, viral pneumonia, mumps, the flu virus, and fungal infection of the skin.

Light is energy that is constantly moving in vibrating waves. Colors are the different frequencies (some fast, some slow) of light. Sunlight contains the full visible spectrum of the rainbow plus UV light and many other frequencies.

Sunlight, or full-spectrum light, is nourishing to the human body. Until recent times, humankind lived outside bathed by sunlight. Everyone needs exposure to full-spectrum light every day. The healing effects of sunlight in Box 18-4 can be obtained with as little as five minutes a day without UV protection on the eyes or skin. More is not, however, better. In homes or hospitals clients may greatly benefit by sitting by windows or in sun rooms, by going out on porches to look at sunlight, or having sun shine on them for short periods of time.

Dr. John Ott, a pioneer in light research, studied the health effects of full-spectrum light and suggested that

BOX 18-4 Healing Effects of Consistent Normal Exposure to Sunlight

Enhances:	Decreases:
Tolerance to stress	Lactic acid in the blood
Energy, strength, and	following exercise
endurance	Blood pressure
Ability of the blood	Respiratory rate
to carry oxygen	Blood sugar
Ability of the blood	Resting heart rate
to absorb oxygen	
Mood	

Spotlight On

Sunlight

In our daily lives, in all seasons, most of us are outside very little. We wear sunglasses and sunscreen when we do go outside. We spend much of our time inside, often in rooms that have limited or no outside light. Many of our inside environments have fluorescent lights or incandescent lightbulbs. Could we be creating our own seasonal affective disorder (SAD)?

malillumination, or lack of adequate full-spectrum light, may be the cause of many physical health problems (Ott, 1973). Today, we know that seasonal affective disorder (SAD) is a type of depression that occurs more commonly in winter when exposure to full-spectrum light is decreased.

Researchers have connected the development of SAD to the regulation of serotonin (wakefulness) and melatonin (sleep-inducing), two hormones regulated by the pineal gland in the brain (Miller, 2005). It is suggested that melatonin contributes to the development of SAD in individuals deprived of sunlight. Sunlight, as

shown in Figure 18-6, has a direct neurological pathway via the retina (optic nerve) to the pineal gland. Stimulation by sunlight prevents the pineal gland from converting serotonin to melatonin. When possible, using full-spectrum fluorescent bulbs can create a healthier environment especially for people who cannot go outside and for nurses working inside. Box 18-5 provides further suggestions for enhancing the healthful benefits from natural light.

Just as people need a wide variety of foods, they also need a wide variety of colors. The ancient Egyptians were the first to have temples of light in which color was used for healing. Physicians, nurses, optometrists, and chemists have researched the specific effects of the individual

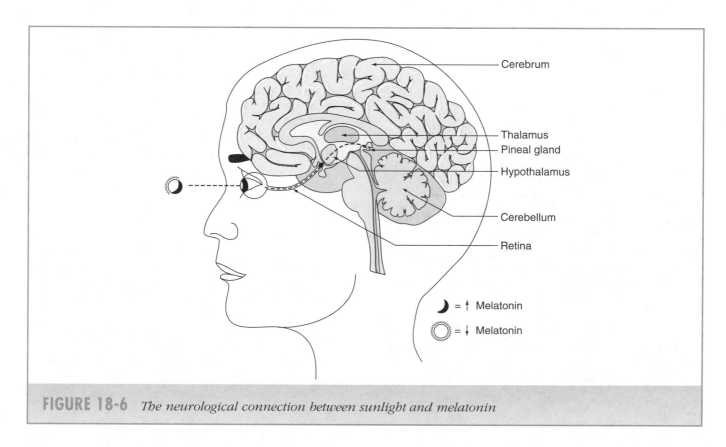

FIGURE 18-6 *The neurological connection between sunlight and melatonin*

Spotlight On

Using Color in Practice

- Incorporate all colors into your life for balance.
- Use blue for relaxation and for aiding pain relief.
- Imagine yourself or your client surrounded by a wash of color that corresponds to the need.

Nursing Alert

Using Care with the Color Red

The color red is stimulating in small amounts but can be energetically overwhelming in large amounts. Red is known to stimulate heart rate, blood pressure, and appetite. Many restaurants use red tablecloths for appetite stimulation. If you are trying to limit food intake, a dark blue or black tablecloth or placemat would be a better color choice.

colors on the body and mind (Demarco, 1998; Lieberman, 1990; McDonald, 1982). Many health practitioners throughout the 20th century have used color as therapy, alone and in combination with other therapies.

It has been observed that different colors may also aid the healing of different parts of the body and the mind. Nurses can use the principles of light and color to help themselves, their clients, and clients' families. Table 18-3 lists general effects of the color spectrum for promoting health. The warm colors are used to stimulate the body, including the function of the liver, pancreas, sinuses, and intestines for digestion, assimilation, and elimination. They can help to loosen chronic congestion. Green can aid the healing of muscles and tissue and balance physical conditions. Magenta (a combination of red and violet) is effective in balancing emotions and physical and emotional heartache. The cool colors are relax-

ing and used to calm acute conditions. They are effective for anxiety, pain relief, insomnia, boosting immune function, fevers, and skin conditions, and to enhance meditation.

Color can be added to the nursing environment in many creative ways. Pieces of cloth can be put in the client's field of vision, or she can wear colored clothing. Nurses can wear colored uniforms or jackets or pins. Flowers, curtains, and pictures can add color. Visualizing a particular area of the body filled with a color or seeing one's entire person surrounded by a color is also an effective way to use color to promote health. Color may be projected onto the body using colored light bulbs, and plastic or cloth can be put on a window or lamp.

Sound

Many cultures and religions believe that the world was created by sound. Some American Indian tribes believe that the spoken word "Inyan" was the creative word. In the Ayurvedic tradition of India "om" is a primordial sound believed to be the first breath of creation. The Christian tradition says that in the beginning was the Word. Hans Jenny, M.D., and Peter Manners, M.D., performed experiments showing that sound creates three-dimensional form. Using sounds from the voice, musical instruments, and other tones, particles of various types of inert matter (such as iron filings suspended in water and oil) formed different three-dimensional shapes and patterns in response to the different sounds. These

TABLE 18-3 Colors and Associated Energies and Emotions

Red	Survival, security
Orange	Nurturance, creativity, passion
Yellow	Personal power, goals, intellect
Green	Healing, emotions, confidence, compassion
Blue	Calming, communication, mental creativity
Indigo	Intuition, insight
Violet	Spiritual energy, connection to a higher power, healing

From Invitation to Holistic Health: A Guide to Living a Balanced Life, by C. Eliopoulos, 2004, Sudbury, MA: Jones and Bartlett.

shapes and patterns were very similar to many patterns found in nature. Mandala patterns formed by the sound "om" resemble patterns in snowflakes. Certain sounds produce shapes that resemble the spinal column. Spiral patterns like those seen in sea shells, human finger prints, the human red blood cell, and many other places are created by certain sounds. Cymatics, the study of patterns of shapes evoked by sound, has shown how sound affects shapes and influences change in shapes (Volk, 2002).

Using one's voice is the most effective way to use sound to balance one's own energy field. The voice may also be used to help balance the energy field of others. Toning is one way to use the voice for healing. When toning, people get comfortable, take a breath, and let sounds come spontaneously. The body knows what sound vibrations it needs to balance or heal itself. Sounds can be made quietly if in a public place. At home, let the sound come out in whatever tone or volume it emerges. Spending 1 to 60 minutes per day toning can be relaxing, rejuvenating, healing, and can aid in pain relief.

The vagus nerve is one way that the effects of sound are carried throughout the body. The vibrations of sound are also transmitted through the bones of the skeleton.

The tones of words can greatly affect the listener and the tension level of muscles. Sound activates memory and feeling. Primordial sounds that are used in Ayurvedic medicine are thought to vibrate certain areas of the body, bringing them into balance. Table 18-4 offers some healing sounds for specific body areas used in Qi Gong (pronounced "chee-GUNG"), which is a component of traditional Chinese medicine that combines movement, meditation, breathing, and sound to enhance the flow of qi, or vital energy, in the body to improve blood circulation and enhance immune function.

Environmental sounds, those within and those beyond people's control, can create states of relaxation or tension. Sounds of nature such as running water, rain, the ocean, birds, and frogs can create relaxation. Sounds like motorcycles, lawn mowers, airplanes, traffic, and machines can cause the body and mind to feel tense.

Music

Sound in the form of music has been a part of healing rituals as revealed in some of the oldest accounts of medical practices. Its effect on health can be explained by modern physics.

According to physics, all vibrations are rhythm, or repeated patterns. Vibrations are waveforms. In passive resonance a waveform triggers a vibration in a resting source. Active resonance or entrainment happens when one vibrating source changes the vibration of another vibrating object. Music is vibrations with rhythm or repeated patterns. Music with 60 beats per minute, such as some Mozart largos, have been found to entrain the heartbeat, lowering it from 72 to 68, and to entrain brain waves, lowering them to alpha frequencies of three to seven cycles per second. Alpha frequencies are those of

Spotlight On

Using Sound and Music in Nursing Practice

Here are some suggestions for using music for yourself and for your clients.

1. For stress relief, start with music that matches your current feelings. If you are stressed, pick something with a fast rhythm. After five minutes switch to something slower and more relaxing.
2. Be mindful of your tone of voice when speaking to clients. A lower-pitched voice at a slower pace can be very calming.
3. Teach clients and families about toning techniques for release and balancing of feelings and tension in the body.
4. Encourage the family to bring a recording of the client's favorite music. If they do not know what the client likes, you can suggest some of the following for balancing the entire body:
   a. Nature sounds—frogs, waves
   b. Indian Ragas—Tabla and sitar, Ravi Shankar, for example
   c. Gregorian chants—church music of medieval origin
   d. Largos—a type of classical music such as in Mozart largos
5. Take five minutes of silence and stillness each day, even if you must use earplugs.

TABLE 18-4 Qi Gong Healing Sounds for the Body

Practiced daily, the following sounds benefit certain parts of the body by enhancing the flow of chi, or energy.

1. ah	lungs
2. n	ears
3. hum	sinuses and head
4. ha	heart
5. ma	nasal passages and sinuses
6. heng	kidneys
7. ya	jaw (migraine and tension headaches)
8. shhhh	liver
9. huh	stomach (indigestion, heartburn)
10. merrr	spleen

Adapted from Healing Sounds, *retrieved January 22, 2006, from www.geocities.com.*

meditation, relaxation, and creativity. Lullabies played in neonatal intensive care nurseries have been found to entrain the breathing rhythms of babies to the rhythm of the music, resulting in a decrease in the amount of time needed for discharge of premature babies.

Many studies have been done on the beneficial effects of music to promote the health of the body. Some of the effects range from decreasing blood pressure, respirations, blood levels of ACTH, pulse, and heart rate, to increasing beta endorphins that promote feelings of well-being. These beneficial results are most often found when the music is of the client's choosing (Dunn, 2004).

Energy-Based Therapies: Therapeutic Touch and Healing Touch

Energy as a healing tool was discussed earlier in this chapter. Two specific modalities originated by nurses that use energy as a healing tool are Therapeutic Touch (TT) and Healing Touch (HT). With these modalities the hands are used to perceive and help to balance the energy field that exists around all living things. TT focuses on balancing the entire field with attention to areas in the field where the energy is not moving. HT addresses the entire field with attention to these areas and the chakras also. Nurses may use both techniques on themselves as well as on clients.

Kunz and Krieger began teaching TT to nurses in the early 1970s. Dr. Krieger's early study of TT indicated that it could raise hemoglobin levels. This became the foundation for the research that has followed. Nurses have studied the effects of TT and found it to be beneficial with premature and full-term infants in the neonatal nursery who had respiratory distress, and it helped them gain weight. Studies have been done indicating that TT aids in pain relief after surgery, is helpful for headaches, and for wound healing. TT has also been shown to decrease respiratory and heart rates, pain, anxiety, nausea, and shortness of breath. It has been shown to increase warmth in extremities and to enhance immune function in both the practitioner and the recipient. TT may be done in 3 to 20 minutes, is very effective, and is easy to learn and teach to clients and their families.

Healing Touch was founded in 1989 by Janet Mentgen, R.N. HT incorporates several energy-based healing techniques including TT, and many of Janet Mentgen's original techniques. HT techniques include balancing the entire field, working with specific techniques for chakra balancing, and working with specific pain problems such as in the spine and migraines.

Energy-based therapies do not require many classes. Legitimacy of the practitioner, however, is provided through certification for some therapies. For example, Healing Touch certification is achieved through completion of a sequence of five courses in addition to documented evidence of practice and mentorship. Almost anyone can learn to feel the energy field and its distur-

Ask Yourself

The Energy Field and Nursing

Have you ever walked into a room with people and noticed a particular feeling to the room? If we are connected to others through the interconnections of energy fields, how might our thoughts affect our own and another's field?

bance with the hands with practice. Practicing the techniques sensitizes the hands and allows the brain to better interpret the signals the hands receive. The brain is not familiar with interpreting non-three–dimensional stimuli. Also in a short time one can learn to help balance the field using TT and HT. For these reasons, both techniques are ideal for teaching to clients and their families for relaxation, pain relief, and wound healing. The Krieger-Kunz method of TT includes four basic phases: (1) centering and grounding; (2) assessment; (3) unruffling; and (4) directing and modulating energy (Bright, 2004).

Touch Therapies—Reflexology, Massage, and Acupressure

One of the most healing things a nurse can ever do for a client is to touch her. Touch conveys more than words ever may. A touch on the arm can say, "I understand, I'm here, I care." Of course, the nurse must use her professional judgment to determine whether a client is receptive to being touched.

Some nurses may be uncomfortable with simply sitting and holding a client's hand. Many types of touch can be therapeutic. All nurses should be aware of the importance and use of touch as a therapy. Some techniques, however, require special training, licensure, or certification. With any touch therapy, it is important for nurses to observe the following general guidelines:

1. Examine personal feelings about touch.

2. Understand the client's culture in relation to touch.

3. Obtain the client's permission to use touch therapy.

4. Respect the client's privacy.

5. Offer explanations before and during the session.

6. Move slowly.

7. Exercise extra care and gentleness with the frail, elderly, and critically ill, and with infants.

8. Inform the client when the session is over, allowing time for reorientation.

9. Obtain feedback from the client.

Ask Yourself

Touching a Client

Have you experienced touch as being especially comforting? How do you feel about touching a client in a caring way? What does it mean to you to touch a client in a caring way? How would you feel about sitting down on the bed and holding a client's hand?

Spotlight On

Reflexology in Nursing Practice

To help someone sleep, work on all points of both feet, very slowly. If someone has back pain, find the bone that goes from the heel along the arch on the inside of the foot to the bunion joint. Rub along the entire bone on both feet.

Reflexology

Reflexology is an ancient healing technique based on the belief that the entire body is reflected in the ears, eyes, palms of the hands, and soles of the feet. When the pad of the thumb is used to apply pressure to specific points in these areas, it increases circulation and relaxation of the corresponding areas of the body. The right hand and foot correspond to the right side of the body. Applying the reflexology technique to the entire foot, even if the exact points are missed, can provide a feeling of relaxation and well-being for clients. At this time, there is no certification required, so reflexology may be practiced by anyone who feels she is competent.

There are many anecdotal accounts of the benefits of reflexology. Although there are few scientific studies on this practice in the United States, extensive research has been done in China and Denmark. Pressing a reflexology point is thought to increase circulation to the corresponding areas, bringing nutrients and oxygen and carrying off waste, increasing nerve flow, and removing blockages in the energy field, helping to restore balance to the body. This balance enhances the healing process.

There are hieroglyphs in the Physician's Tomb in Egypt from 4000 years ago of physicians pressing on the feet of clients. Around 1900 William Fitzgerald, M.D., used pressure point therapy for anesthesia in his medical practice. In 1925 Joe Riley, M.D., wrote a reflexology book for physicians based on Fitzgerald's findings. Eunice Ingham worked in Riley's office and began using these points on the feet and hands of all Dr. Riley's clients. She coined the term *reflexology* and is considered the originator of modern-day practice. After 17 years of mapping the feet and hands and coordinating points with clients' experiences, she wrote *Stories the Feet Can Tell* (Ingham, 1959) and *Stories the Feet Have Told* (Ingham, 1963). Reflexology is practiced and taught globally, with other people adding their own flavor and changing the name somewhat. It should be noted that reflexology is not for diagnosing, but only for helping the body rebalance itself for healing.

Reflexology is an excellent tool for nurses because usually no matter how restricted a person is the nurse can always get to the feet or hands. Having the feet touched feels wonderful and relaxes the whole body. Much benefit can be gained with just one to two minutes of work, making it perfect for nurses. The basic technique is described in Box 18-6.

Reflexology can be used for overall relaxation by working on the entire foot. If someone has pain or has a particular health problem, focus on the part of the foot or hand corresponding to that part of the body in addition to the entire foot.

Some advantages of knowing reflexology are that it may be used to help people with conditions that cannot be touched, like burns, broken bones, internal organs, the immune system, skin rashes, and the eyes and ears.

Reflexology may be used on most people with most conditions. It can be done with socks or on bare feet. If someone is ticklish, just hold the foot for a moment before beginning. This can be taught to clients to do on themselves or to families to do for the client and each other.

Massage

Massage is another ancient healing art. As early as 1800 BC, mention of rubbing is found in the healing practices of China and in Ayurvedic medicine in India. Hippocrates, the father of modern medicine, said that massage and exercise were crucial parts of medicine. In the 1800s the word *massage* was first used by the French for rubbing the body. In the early 1800s Ling and Mesger of Sweden

BOX 18-6 Reflexology Technique

The technique for reflexology involves three basic actions. With the pad of the thumb, press on the area of the foot desired and perform one or more of the following:

1. Hold steady firm pressure.
2. Make small clockwise circles.
3. Inch the tip of the thumb along the foot by bending and straightening the first thumb joint.

Can I Do Massage?

Deep tissue massage may activate the lymphatic system, which may be undesirable for some clients with conditions such as cancer. If clients have varicose veins or a history of blood clots, those areas should not be massaged. If you want to use massage but question whether it is appropriate or contraindicated, just do a one- to two-minute massage on the feet or hands to promote relaxation and a sense of well-being.

Simple Massage for Relaxation

1. Massage for the back with lotion:
   a. Apply *warmed* lotion to the back, slowly, from the base of the neck to the tailbone using long smooth strokes with your palm.
   b. Press with the heel of your palm starting in the sacrum area (below the waist by the tailbone) along the side of the spine (*not on it*) from the sacrum to the top of the shoulder.
   c. Repeat slowly several times to both sides of the spine.
2. Massage without lotion for headaches and neckaches:
   a. Make slow circular movements with your fingers and thumb.
   b. Press up under the occipital ridge (where the neck connects to the skull) starting behind the ears and rub with the fingers and thumb, simultaneously, in toward the spine.
   c. If the person is sitting, hold the forehead in the palm of one of your hands for support.
   d. Rub the entire scalp with the pads of the fingers using fast or slow motions according to the client's preference.

created Swedish massage and named the specific strokes of that form of massage. They founded the first massage schools. In 1871, George Taylor, M.D., wrote a book on massage and its effects on the physiology of the body.

Currently, every state in the United States has its own massage laws. In some states, to be called a Massage Therapist, one must graduate from a massage school licensed by the Department of Health. Nurses can do massage within the scope of their practice, whether in the hospital or in private practice under their nursing license, but cannot use the term Massage Therapist. It is essential for a nurse to find out what the regulations are in her or his state.

Massage has been part of nursing care since the beginning of nursing. It was taught in nursing schools and was a standard part of evening care until the late 1960s. Nurses who do massage for clients find the client needs less medication for sleep and for pain. Clients report feeling happier and cared for after receiving a massage.

Massage can enhance circulation, lymph flow, digestion, and elimination. It can help reduce swelling of joints, speed healing of fractures, and improve the quality of the skin. Massage is not just for relaxation, although in today's world, the reduction of the stress response may be its most useful characteristic. There is nothing better at relieving muscular tension and pain than a massage. Often tight muscles press on the nerves, creating pain and numbness. Tight muscles can cause headache and neck pain. When the back muscles are tight, they interfere with nerve and blood flow from the spine to the rest of the body. Dr. Tiffany Field, of the Touch Research Institutes, is currently one of the leading researchers of the physical and emotional benefits of massage. She has found that massage greatly benefits preterm and full-term infants, reduces pain of arthritis, headaches, and lower back, and enhances immune function. It also alleviates depression and anxiety (Aukett, 2004).

Massage interrupts the stress response. The stress response is covered in detail in the chapters on stress

and psychoneuroimmunology. In brief, it is understood that when people perceive something as a stressor over a long period of time the immune system and endocrine system are compromised. By affecting the stress response, massage aids healing on the physical as well as mental and emotional levels.

The healing effects of massage benefit all areas of nursing including maternity, pediatrics, gerontology, cardiovascular, rehabilitation, orthopedic, and home health. Nurses can teach these techniques to families to use on each other. Nurses can also treat each other to a shoulder rub to promote health in the workplace.

Massage may be done in a chair, on a bed, or on a massage table. Massage may be with or without lotion, and it may cover just the back, feet, head, or the entire body. It can last for one hour or be very beneficial in just three to four minutes. It is easily adapted to a nurse's schedule. Figure 18-7 shows a therapeutic back massage.

Acupressure

Acupressure is a touch therapy that may be very useful to nurses and easy to teach clients. The technique of acupressure involves firm pressure that is applied with the pad of the thumb, in most cases, to specific points to help balance the body and stimulate healing.

In the ancient Chinese healing system of acupuncture, needles are put into the points that are located

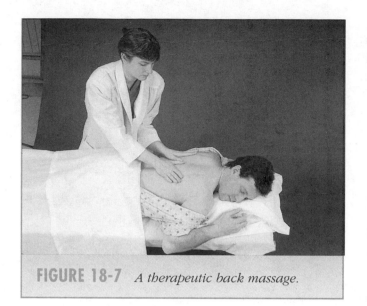

FIGURE 18-7 *A therapeutic back massage.*

Nursing Alert

Using Acupressure in Nursing Practice

The following method of acupressure has been used to enhance immune function and to help relieve headaches, constipation, vertigo, allergies, sinus problems, toothache, and menstrual cramps.
1. Using the pad of the thumb and first finger, apply pressure to both sides of the web between the thumb and forefinger of one hand of your client.
2. Hold the pressure steady or rub gently in a circle.
3. Continue for one to five minutes or until the pain subsides.

along meridians, or lines of energy, that flow from the head to toe. Each meridian corresponds to a different organ of the body. In acupressure, pressing on these points also helps the energy to flow through these meridians, energizing and balancing the corresponding organ. When the energy is properly flowing through all meridians, the body is in balance and able to maintain health.

Much detail may be learned and practiced for working with complex situations. However, there are points that the nurse can begin to use. The complete system of acupressure is best learned from an experienced practitioner and teacher.

The nurse must also recognize that with any therapy there are liabilities. Box 18-7 identifies areas of legal risks to consider for integrative therapies.

Nurturing the Self

This section will briefly mention areas that are covered in greater depth elsewhere in this book. These areas are mentioned here because no discussion of holistic healing and promotion of health would be complete without mentioning the importance of caring for the self.

Environment

The environment is often taken for granted. Noise levels, the cleanliness of the air, water, chemicals emitted from central air ducts, carpets, paint, perfumes—all affect the health of the body. When only one exists, and only occasionally, the immune system can cope. When the immune system has to handle an environment with multiple toxins, plus stress, plus viruses and bacteria, it

---

BOX 18-7 Integrative Therapy and Legal Risks

Therapeutic touch, massage, and acupressure are among many modalities in integrative health care. Nurses who choose to practice any of these need to know about the following.

1. **Standards and scope of practice:** Do the standards and scope of nursing practice in your state allow for the inclusion of the integrative therapy on and off duty?
2. **State laws regulating integrative therapy:** Is a license required?
3. **Employer policies and job description:** Does the scope of employment include the use of the integrative therapy?
4. **Financial risk:** Are your actions covered by your employer's insurance? Does your own liability insurance cover the integrative therapy you choose to practice?
5. **Consent:** Did you obtain verbal permission from the client for the integrative therapy to be used such as therapeutic touch, massage, or acupressure?
6. **Documentation:** If you practice an integrative therapy, have you properly documented the date, permission granted from the client, any teaching provided, the nature of the treatment, and the client's response?

Adapted from "Legal Risks of Alternative Therapies," by P. S. Brooke, 1998, RN, 61(5), pp. 53–58.

often becomes overloaded and cannot perform its function of keeping the body healthy. Allergies, asthma, fatigue, rheumatoid arthritis, infections, colds, skin eruptions, and other diseases may occur or become exacerbated by the environment.

What can nurses do themselves and suggest to clients? Box 18-8 lists suggestions for coping with environmental stressors.

Sleep

Sleep is often the first thing to go when persons' lives become hectic. When feeling confused, irritable, depressed, sleep is often a good first step. All of these are symptoms of sleep deprivation. While we sleep the body repairs itself. The immune system is repaired at night, memories are processed and preserved, and internal pacemakers are set that regulate the circadian rhythms of the body—like the release of hormones, and the sleep-wake cycle. The room should be as dark as possible for proper secretion of the hormone melatonin, which aids sleep. Often eight hours of sleep for three days in a row will improve one's outlook.

Exercise

Exercise is often a dreaded word. For some clients exercise may be holding a can of peas in each hand and raising and lowering their arms. Walking is considered to be a form of exercise that is the most beneficial with few side effects. Whatever the exercise, doing 20 minutes of it two to three times a week is recommended. The body was made to move. When we do not move it, or do repetitive tasks, the muscles, nerves, circulation, and lymph system do not function in the most healthy way.

Communication

Just a word or two must be said about communicating. Communicating in relationships is one of the most challenging and potentially stressful and difficult things we humans do. If you watch other animals like dogs, cats, horses, insects, and fish, they all have very clear signals and methods of conveying their needs, wants, and ideas. In childhood people learn the meaning of tone of voice and facial expressions. Because all childhoods were different, people attach different meanings to these cues.

Most people were never taught to communicate their needs, wants, and ideas clearly, especially in situations with high levels of emotion. Assuming that another person knows how one feels often causes big trouble. To help clients heal, nurses must ask, "What do you need right now?" For more detailed information on communication refer to Chapter 5.

Nutrition

Nutrition is vital to enhancing holistic care. There are more opinions on how people should eat, and books written on it, than can even begin to be cited. Opinions vary from pure vegetarianism, to vegetarian with dairy and eggs, to high protein including meat.

BOX 18-8 Coping with Environmental Stressors

1. Wear earplugs if noise is inevitable.
2. Create a few minutes, or a day, of silence.
3. Use a good water filter on the tap for all water you drink, and use a good air filter in a central system.
4. Get away from town frequently into a place with lots of trees to breathe fresh air.
5. Minimize exposure to perfumes and chemicals. They are often where you least expect them (even in commercial bedding).
6. Minimize exposure to electromagnetic fields such as microwaves, electric blankets, and alarm clocks.
7. Have your sleeping space free of electric devices.

Adapted from Using Energy to Enhance Nursing Practice Through the Use of Color, Music, Touch, and Movement, *by M. Walker, 1996, Holistic Nursing Series workshop presented at the University of Texas School of Nursing, Austin, TX.*

Different diets are needed because people are unique. Humans require nutrients from the six food groupings, but how these nutrients are consumed is open to debate. Two things that can benefit all people are to drink at least one quart of water a day, and to enjoy the food eaten. The main thing is to choose foods that help one feel healthy, relaxed, have plenty of energy and maintain a comfortable weight. See Chapter 14 for more information on nutrition.

Herbs

The use of **phytochemicals** from herbs or plants to promote and maintain health and cure disease is an ancient art. Every traditional culture has had a medicine man or woman who knew which plants to pick, when to pick them, what part of the plant had which effects, and how to prepare the herbs. For some situations the entire plant is used, and in others, just the flower, leaf, root, or berry. Herbs may be grown at home, bought in health food stores, and even ordered by mail. They can be ingested as a tea, capsule, or liquid tincture (herb extracted in alcohol). Salves and creams containing herbs can be rubbed on the body. Many of our drugs today are made from plants. A growing concern over the loss of the rainforests is that plants that could be cures for disease and enhancers of health may be lost.

The study and practice of herbology is enjoying renewed popularity. A few simple herbs can be part of any medicine cabinet, or the study can become complex with combinations of herbs to address all health situations. These situations include enhancing the immune system, helping women cope with menopause, aiding in prevention of colds and flu, aiding sinus and allergy conditions, decreasing blood pressure, and enhancing the digestive and eliminative functions. There are stimulating, calming, nutritive, and cleansing herbs. In fact, the number and combinations of herbs are so extensive that almost all health situations can be addressed through the proper use of herbology. For example, aloe vera is extremely effective for healing minor burns. Peppermint in any form is excellent to promote calmness and digestion and ease an upset stomach. Arnica oil is beneficial when rubbed into muscles and tissues affected by sprains, strains, and tension. Black cohosh is used for menstrual cramps and menopausal symptoms.

The most popular legal herbal products purchased and used are ginkgo biloba, St. John's wort, ginseng, garlic, echinacea, saw palmetto, and kava (Bayer, 2002; Sand-Jecklin & Badzek, 2004). Benefits and risks of these are described in Table 18-5. It should be noted that herbal supplements are not regulated by the U.S. Food and Drug Administration and the strengths and dosages are not standardized. Studies on the benefits, risks, and dosages of herbal therapies are inconclusive, and, therefore, they must be used with knowledge by the consumer. Although millions of people use herbal therapies

for health-related reasons, many of these individuals, along with physicians and nurses, lack knowledge about their benefits and risks (Sand-Jecklin & Badzek, 2003, 2004; Sohn & Loveland-Cook, 2002). It is important that health care professionals become educated on herbal therapies in order to promote, protect, and preserve the health of their clientele. Workshops are available for both the beginner and the advanced practitioner.

★ **Nursing Alert**

Use Caution with Herbal Supplements

Just because a product is labeled "natural" does not mean it cannot be harmful. Interaction with other medications must be considered. Dosages for children should be reduced. Pregnant women and infants should not take or be given herbal supplements. Consultation with a health care practitioner knowledgeable in the use of herbs is important.

TABLE 18-5 Benefits, Risks, and Cautions for Seven Commonly Used Herbs

Herb	Major Benefits	Identified Risks
1. Echinacea	Enhances immune system, anti-inflammatory, antibacterial, prevents/reduces colds, flu	Rare. Can cause flare-ups in some autoimmune diseases such as lupus, some forms of arthritis, and AIDS
2. Garlic	Improves circulation, enhances cholesterol levels and blood pressure, thins blood	Odor, indigestion; interacts with vitamin E and other medications used for blood thinning
3. Ginkgo Biloba	Improves memory in dementia, reduces ringing in the ears, reduces blood clots	Inhibits clotting (like aspirin), interacts with other medications used for blood thinning
4. Ginseng	Sold as energy booster or aphrodisiac (studies inconclusive)	Interacts with other medications used for blood thinning, may cause breast tenderness in women, increases blood pressure
5. Kava	Reduces anxiety	Toxic to liver, interacts with alcohol, damage to central nervous system
6. Saw Palmetto	Reduces enlarged prostate, also used in the treatment of upper respiratory infections, ovarian pain and cysts, and infertility	None known
7. St. John's Wort	Reduces anxiety and depression, menopausal symptoms, gastrointestinal inflammation, and peptic ulcers	Sensitivity to light, interacts with other drugs such as blood thinners and oral contraceptives

From Bayer, R. (2002, June). "Risk-Benefit Profile of Commonly Used Herbs—Legal and Otherwise," by R. Bayer, June 2002, Alternatives Magazine, 22, retrieved January 24, 2006, from http://alternativesmagazine.com; Invitation to Holistic Health: A Guide to Living a Balanced Life, by C. Eliopoulos, 2004, Sudbury, MA: Jones & Bartlett.

Aromatherapy

Aromatherapy is the use of the essential oils from plants for beneficial effects on body, mind, emotions, and spirit. The essential oils are steam distilled from plants and flowers. Oils are 75 to 100 percent more potent than the plants from which they are distilled. The term *aromatherapy* implies that a scent is inhaled; however, it also includes the application of essential oils in massage and in bathing (Buckle, 2003).

Whether used in a bath, massage, or inhaled as a scent, aromatic oils have long been known for their therapeutic effects. Babylonian clay tablets and Egyptian tombs indicate that as long as 7,000 years ago oils and scents were used for healing. The term *aromatherapy* was coined in 1928 by a French chemist named Gatefossse. He badly burned his arm and plunged it into a vat of lavender. The pain was immediately reduced, and there was minimal scarring (Buckle, 2003). Jane Buckle, R.N., is currently a leader in the teaching of aromatherapy for nurses and other health care professionals.

Our brain recognizes approximately 10,000 scents. When one inhales a scent, tiny molecules of the substance travel from the nose to the olfactory part of the brain, which is directly connected with the limbic area of the brain. The limbic area affects memory, emotions, and learning and is connected to the hypothalamus, which controls the autonomic nervous system. People react immediately and involuntarily to scent.

These oils have healing properties such as being calming, analgesic, stimulating, antibacterial, deodorizing, and antiviral (Buckle, 2003; Thomas, 2002). Combinations of oils may increase the circulation of endorphins, which aid in pain reduction; enkephalins, which can cause us to feel happy; serotonin, which helps to reduce insomnia; and noradrenalin, which can be stimulating.

Because essential oils can be very effective and some are not advised with certain conditions, the advice of an experienced practitioner is recommended. There are some, however, that the beginner can use. For example, French lavender is very safe, calming, sleep inducing, healing, and antibacterial, and peppermint aids in digestion.

Since essential oils can be so powerful, they should not be applied directly to the skin. One to two drops on a pillow (not pillowcase), cottonball, or handkerchief can be inhaled. The essential oil can be poured into a porous clay pot and it will diffuse into the room. There are diffusers that use a heat source. Essential oils can also be absorbed through the skin and travel via the blood to the organ on which they have an effect. There are about 150 essential oils (Thomas, 2002). Table 18-6 provides a sample of some of these and their reported effects.

Love and Healing

This world is much more than meets the eye. People are not just three-dimensional conglomerates of matter that operate *only* according to all the physical laws we have

TABLE 18-6	Some Essential Oils and Their Effects
Essential Oil	**Effects**
Basil	refreshing, clarifying, concentration enhancing
Chamomile	refreshing, relaxing, calming
Frankincense	relaxing, rejuvenating, rids fears
Jasmine	relaxing, confidence-building
Lavender	refreshing, relaxing, calming
Lemon	stimulating, motivating
Lemongrass	toning, fortifying
Marjoram	warming, sedating
Myrrh	toning, strengthening, rejuvenating
Orange	refreshing, relaxing
Peppermint	cooling, refreshing, head clearing
Thyme	antiseptic, immune strengthening

up to this moment accepted in science. Humans are on the brink of new discoveries of how the universe works and what it is to be human.

There is evidence suggesting that humans and all animals, plants, and all matter in the universe are beings of energy, vibrating at different frequencies. All other forms of vibrating energy, such as sound, light, thoughts, and feelings, affect these bodies of energy. A field of energy connects us all. There is no separation.

Many researchers in the arts and sciences are now studying exactly how all of this is connected. Human beings, animals, and plants heal and thrive in the presence of caring and loving. Many healers say that love is the power that allows healing to happen at a distance. For so long in nursing it was recommended not to touch clients except to do necessary procedures, and not to get "emotionally involved" with clients. Hundreds of studies on social support and touch are now telling us what common sense has always known. Humans need to be touched, physically and emotionally. They need each other to be healthy and happy. Social support can be a friend who listens, a pet, a church group, family, a feeling of connection to a Higher Power, plants people care for, a social group, or wherever one feels loved and accepted.

The literature abounds with studies on social support and the positive effects it can have. These effects include increasing feelings of self-esteem, self-identity, and control over one's environment (which tends to result in enhanced immune function), higher life expectancy, low incidence of heart disease, faster recovery from surgery, decreased blood pressure, and decreased anxiety levels (Buckle, 2003).

Spotlight On

Love and Caring in Nursing Practice

Take a moment with a client who perhaps seems difficult for you to work with. Take a breath. Feel love, appreciation, or caring for the client or for someone or something in your life. Imagine the two of you being surrounded by a warm light. Come back to your client. Notice if you feel differently about her. View her as a precious thing, someone that may feel very vulnerable and afraid. How would you feel in her shoes?

A lack of social support has been linked to general mortality rate, the onset and progression of disease, decreased ability to learn and remember information, increased asthma, pregnancy complications, arthritis, hypertension, depression, coronary disease, cancer, autoimmune disease, and infectious disease.

Love is a very powerful force. Research studies and anecdotal accounts indicate that love and caring create connection over time and great distances, affecting physical change (Watson, 2002a, 2002b, 2005). If one doesn't have love, one continually seeks it. Yet no one can say exactly what love is or how to get it or how it is lost. Love is an energy that promotes health and facilitates healing.

What does this imply for nurses? Love, caring, and empathy are energies that create healing in ways not fully understood at this time. Nurses need to create ways to support each other. Clients need their loved ones around them to facilitate healing. When a loved one cannot be present, a picture or object can help the client feel loved and supported. Sometimes the nurse is the only person in a client's experience to help her feel loved and cared for. No words are needed. Sitting down for a moment or holding a hand can create a heart connection that opens a space for the mystery of healing.

SUMMARY

Each nurse has a personal definition of what healing is, and what it means to be a nurse. For most nurses some part of the decision to be a nurse had to do with wanting to help people feel better. The days are gone when people believed that the health of the body is separate from the health of the mind and the fullness of the spirit. For human beings to realize their full potential, it is necessary to consider their whole nature as body, mind, feelings, spirit, and energy field, and how all of these aspects interact with each other and with all other living things in this universe.

Enhancing health promotion by incorporating holistic principles and modalities into nursing practice gives nurses new tools for embracing the entire human nature and helping clients do the same to achieve maximum desired individual health goals. Holding clients and ourselves as nurses as the most precious of beings helps the heart to open, promotes health, and allows for healing to happen.

CASE STUDY Charles Fowler: Living with Painful Arthritis

Objectives/Goals: Through participation in discussion of this case study, participants will have the opportunity to:

1. Discuss the effect of the nurse's attitude toward healing on client outcomes.
2. Describe a holistic approach to healing.

Health Promotion Concern, History and Physical, Present Health Status, Past Health Status, Family History, and Social History

Charles (Charlie) Fowler is a 75-year-old white non-Hispanic male with painful arthritis in both knees. He is a retired farmer, has been married 48 years to his wife, Helen, and has four adult sons. Two years ago he sold his farm when the pain in his knees was so great that he could no longer physically perform the work required. He and Helen recently moved into a small home in a nearby town. He is 5 feet 9 inches tall and weighs 164 pounds. As prescribed, he is currently taking acetaminophen 650 mg q four hrs and capsaicin cream 0.025 percent applied twice daily to both knees. He is emphatic about avoiding knee replacement surgery. He would like to know what nonmedical methods or treatments are available for help in easing his knee pain. He has also asked about using saw palmetto, which he read was good for prostate problems.

Review of Pertinent Domains

Biological Domain

Physical exam reveals an elderly male of appropriate weight for body stature who is experiencing moderate pain to both knees. There is varus (turned inward) deformity of both knees as well as moderate inflammation. His vital signs were: B/P 132/62, pulse 78 and regular, respirations 12, and temperature 98.2 degrees.

Gastrointestinal: Reports no problems in this area. He has regular bowel movements. His diet is well balanced with fruits and vegetables and he rarely eats at fast-food restaurants.

Genitourinary: He reports having "spells" within the past year of frequent urge to urinate with sometimes only a small stream of urine produced. There is no history of urinary tract or reproductive problems, but he thinks it is his prostate that is "getting old, like me."

Musculoskeletal: Complains of pain in the joints of both knees and knee joint stiffness when sitting too long and upon rising in the morning.

Psychological Domain

Charlie graduated from high school and says he enjoys reading science and agriculture magazines. He also reports reading more and taking a greater interest in personal wellness to "keep away" from taking medication. Charlie states he has lived a fulfilled life and feels blessed with the love of his wife and children. He says he has tried to be a "good" person and feels rewarded that his farming has made a difference in the lives of many. He has a great sense of humor and enjoys telling jokes and stories to make his wife laugh.

Social Domain

Charlie plays shuffleboard at the local senior citizen center when his knees aren't "acting up." He also enjoys sitting with his retiree friends, just "gabbing" about life. He and Helen have taken many trips to visit their four children, who live 50 to 750 miles away, but driving has become a painful experience because of his knees.

Environmental Domain

Charlie lives in a one-story home with five steps leading up to the front door. He says that using steps is painful at times. He loves to attend to the small garden in the back yard.

Spiritual Domain

Charlie is a member of the local Presbyterian church and attends services weekly. He believes in a "higher power" and says he prays for good health for his family first and then himself. He says his great-great grandfather was a Cherokee Indian and feels that his "Indian blood" is why he feels a connection with nature.

Technological Domain

Charlie's younger son purchased a computer and software for Charlie and Helen and gave them basic instructions on how to access the Internet and use email. Charlie says he gets a "kick" out of "surfing the Web without ever getting wet."

Questions for Discussion

1. How can the nurse's attitude toward healing affect Charlie's desire for alternative or complementary health care or both?
2. How can the nurse help Charlie discover what his needs are and develop a plan to meet them?
3. Identify two areas of caution for Charlie and how the nurse should address them.

Key Concepts

1. What it means to be a healing nurse is unique to each individual. To help the nurse discover a personal definition, she can consider what healing means to her, what her goals for self-healing are, and what her role is in helping clients heal.

2. When people's needs are met, the body, mind, and spirit can heal. Nurses can help clients discover needs and create strategies to meet them by asking them to: describe their health now; what they think they need to heal; what they expect to happen; how they or others can help them; and what their goals are and what has to happen to reach those goals.

3. Energy fields are part of and surround all living things. Balance in the field affects the health of the body. The nurse can use energy-based therapies such as TT, HT, light, color, sound and music, and thought to help create balance in the field.

4. The thoughts people think affect their physiology and their energy fields. By consciously choosing their thoughts, people can affect health and relationships. They can become conscious of thoughts by using feelings to wake them up to their thoughts. Individuals begin to change thoughts by substituting a thought about what they want in life for a thought that is not about what they want.

5. Imaging is creating a picture in the mind that incorporates the five senses. The picture is what a person wants to occur in the body or events in life. Imagery is used for relaxation, stress reduction, and enhancing healing of the body.

6. The Relaxation Response relaxes the autonomic nervous system, counterbalancing the stress response. It is a technique utilizing principles from various types of meditation.

7. The nurse can teach clients to visualize a blue color to enhance relaxation and pain relief. Other colors have different effects on humans. Music of the client's choosing has been shown to increase immune function and decrease the stress response.

8. Centering and grounding are techniques to use before working with clients in any way, especially energy-based therapies like HT and TT. Centering encourages the nurse to clear the mind, bringing her attention to the present. Grounding connects the nurse to the Earth as a steady source of energy and to the universal source of healing energy.

9. Reflexology points on the feet can be pressed to help relieve pain and encourage relaxation in corresponding parts of the body. Simple massage to the head, neck, and shoulders can relieve pain and promote sleep and a feeling of being cared for.

10. Techniques for nurturing the self can be used by nurses and taught to clients. There are many to choose from, and they are effective primarily because they reduce stress and increase feelings of health and happiness. Among them are communication, sleep, nutrition, and love.

11. Because of people's energy nature, all are connected in very real ways. The unique role of the nurse is to help to promote health and to heal by appreciating each client, providing direction and support, and by helping when clients cannot help themselves in the most vulnerable of times.

Learning Activities

1. What are the qualities that you have, or that you want to learn, that would make you feel that you are a nurse healer?

2. A client tells you he is having headaches and pain in his neck, shoulders, and back, is unusually irritated, is having diarrhea, and is not sleeping well. Using your knowledge of holistic principles, you believe he is experiencing more stress than he can handle. Discuss how you would help him discover the causes of his stress and what he might do about it using the Modeling and Role Modeling techniques presented in this chapter.

3. A client has had a mild heart attack and wants to create a health promotion plan to prevent future health problems. She has heard of holistic healing and wants you to help her incorporate it into her plan. Use the holistic modalities presented in this chapter and create a plan for this client.

True/False Questions

1. **T or F** Holistic healing modalities and Western medicine should both be considered when helping a client create a health promotion plan.

2. **T or F** It is safe to administer massage strokes deeply and slowly all over the body.

3. **T or F** Massage is always contraindicated for clients who have had cardiac surgery.

4. **T or F** The nurse's judgment about what is best for a client is more important than what the client thinks is needed to heal.

5. **T or F** It is possible for the nurse to use prayer to affect the health of a client from a distance.

6. **T or F** With Therapeutic Touch, the nurse can aid the healing process of the client without ever touching the client's body.

Multiple Choice Questions

1. Which of the following is central to the holistic philosophy?
   a. Cultural diversity is more important than any other component.
   b. Disease, illness, or imbalance are opportunities for positive growth.
   c. Environment is separate and distinct from the person.
   d. Treatment of symptoms is the focus for health promotion and disease prevention.

2. A recent survey of adults in the United States found the use of complementary and alternative medicine, excluding prayer, to be prevalent in:
   a. 1 of 6 adults
   b. 1 of 3 adults
   c. 2 of 3 adults
   d. 2 of 10 adults

3. Reiki, Healing Touch, and Therapeutic Touch are examples of which one of the following categories of complementary and alternative medicine identified by the National Center for Complementary and Alternative Medicine?
   a. Biologically based practices
   b. Energy medicine
   c. Manipulative and body-based practices
   d. Mind-body medicine

4. Which one of the following colors can be overwhelming in large amounts and is known to stimulate heart rate, blood pressure, and appetite?
   a. Blue
   b. Green
   c. Red
   d. Yellow

5. Which of the following sounds can benefit the sinuses?
   a. ah
   b. hum
   c. shhhh
   d. ya

6. Which of the following terms is a developmental process that results in independence and self-confidence of the client for health promotion?
   a. Capacity building
   b. Empowerment
   c. Grounding
   d. Heliotherapy

Websites

http://www.healthy.net Offers a general overview of mind/body medicine, including articles on Introduction to Mind/Body Medicine, Mind/Body Therapies, and Mind/Body Approaches to Health Disorders. Includes links to interviews with Larry Dossey, M.D., Deepak Chopra, M.D., and James Gordon, M.D.

http://www.nicabm.com National Institute for Clinical Applications of Behavioral Medicine. Site offers continuing education on mind-body topics for health care practitioners.

http://www.rosenthal.hs.columbia.edu Excellent source for a listing of reliable links for therapies, health issues, information and research, professional associations, education, training and certifications, and legal issues related to complementary and alternative medicine.

http://www.herbs.org Herb Research Foundation. The Foundation is considered a reliable source of accurate, science-based information on the health benefits and safety of herbs, and expertise in sustainable botanical resource development.

http://www.reiki.org Offers a wealth of information about Reiki practice and teaching. There is a free download for articles, including free Reiki practice and teaching materials. Streaming audio files, a slide show, and a free online newsletter are also available as well as the opportunity to purchase materials.

http://www.amfoundation.org Alternative Medicine Foundation. This nonprofit organization provides consumers and professionals with responsible, evidence-based information on the integration of alternative and conventional medicine. Resource guides on a variety of alternative treatment modalities and health issues and a primer on medical research studies are provided.

Organizations

Healing Touch International Inc.
445 Union Blvd., Suite 105
Lakewood, CO 80228
Tel: (303) 989-7982
This is a nonprofit membership and educational corporation established in 1996 to administer the certification process and facilitate healing through the practice, teaching, and research of Healing Touch.

NCCAM Clearinghouse
P.O. Box 7923
Gaithersburg, MD 20898-7923
Toll-free in the U.S.: (888) 644-6226
International: (301) 519-3153
TTY (for deaf or hard-of-hearing callers):
  (866) 464-3615
http://www.nccam.nih.gov
Email: info@nccam.nih.gov
National Center for Complementary and Alternative Medicine (NCCAM) is one of the 27 institutes and centers that make up the National Institutes of Health (NIH). The NIH is one of eight agencies under the Public Health Service (PHS) in the Department of Health and Human Services (DHHS). NCCAM exists to explore complementary and alternative healing practices in the context of rigorous science, train complementary and alternative medicine (CAM) researchers, and disseminate authoritative information to the public and professionals.

National Institute for Clinical Applications of Behavioral Medicine
P.O. Box 523
6D Ledgebrook Drive
Mansfield Center, CT 06250
Tel: (203) 456-1153
http://www.nicabm.com/
This organization offers training for mind-body practices and techniques for health practitioners.

Center for the Study of Complementary and Alternative Therapies (CSCAT)
P.O. Box 800905
Charlottesville, VA 22908-0905
Tel: (434) 924-0113
http://www.Healthsystem.virginia.edu
CSCAT is located at the University of Virginia and was established in 1995 as one of the original NIH-funded centers for research, collaboration, and information about complementary and alternative medicine (CAM).

Ayurvedic Institute
P.O. Box 23445
Albuquerque, NM 87192-1445
Tel: (505) 291-9698

The Institute is a recognized school and Ayurveda health spa established in 1984 to teach and provide the traditional Ayurvedic medicine of India, including herbs, nutrition, panchakarma, cleansing, acupressure massage, yoga, Sanskrit, and Jyotish (Vedic astrology).

The Nurse Healers-Professional Associates International (NH-PAI, Inc.)
P.O. Box 158
Warnerville, NY 12187-0158
Tel: (518) 325-1185; (877) 32N-HPAI
Fax: (509) 693-3537
NH-PAI is the official organization of Therapeutic Touch whose mission is to inspire and advance

excellence in Krieger and Kunz Therapeutic Touch as a healing practice.

Therapeutic Touch: A Video Course for Health Care Professionals by Janet Quinn is a three-part series addressing theory, research, and application of Therapeutic Touch. Offered through the Nurse Healers-Professional Associates International. More information is available at http//:www.therapeutic-touch.org, or email nhpai@therapeutic-touching.org

References

Abramson, L. Y., Seligman, M. E. P., & Teasdale, J. D. (1978). Learned helplessness in humans: Critique and reformulation. *Journal of Abnormal Psychology, 87*, 49–74.

Auckett, A. (2004). *Baby massage: Parent-child bonding through touch.* New York: Newmarket Press.

Barnes, P., Powell-Griner, E., McFann, K., & Nahin, R. (2004, May 27). *Complementary and alternative medicine use among adults: United States, 2002.* (CDC Advance Data Report #343). National Center for Complementary and Alternative Medicine, National Institutes of Health, Bethesda, MD: National Institutes of Health, Department of Health and Human Services.

Bayer, R. (2002, June). Risk-benefit profile of commonly used herbs—legal and otherwise. *Alternatives Magazine, 22.* Retrieved January 24, 2006, from http://alternativesmagazine.com

Benson, H. (1975). *The relaxation response.* New York: Avon.

Benson, H. (1996). *Timeless healing.* New York: Simon and Schuster.

Bright, M. A., Andrus, V., & Lunt, Y. (2004). Health, healing, and holistic nursing. In M. A. Bright (Ed.), *Holistic health and healing* (pp. 31–46). Philadelphia: F. A. Davis.

Bright, M. A. (2004). Therapeutic touch. In M. A. Bright (Ed.), *Holistic health and healing* (pp. 171–179). Philadelphia: F. A. Davis.

Buckle, J. (2003). *Clinical aromatherapy: Essential oils in practice.* New York: Churchill-Livingstone.

Burkhardt, M. A., & Nagai-Jacobson, M. G. (2005). Spirituality and health. In B. M. Dossey, L. Keegan, & C. E. Guzzetta (Eds.), *Holistic nursing: A handbook for practice* (4th ed.), pp. 137–172. Sudbury, MA: Jones & Bartlett.

Catalano, J. T. (2006). *Nursing now! Today's issues, tomorrow's trends.* Philadelphia: F. A. Davis.

Childre, D. (1998). *Freeze frame: One minute stress management.* Boulder Creek, CA: Planetary Publications.

Cook, C. A. L., Guerrerio, J. R., & Slater, V. E. (2004). Healing touch and quality of life on women during radiation treatment. *Alternative Therapies in Health and Medicine, 10*(3), 34–41.

Dossey, B. M., & Keegan, L. (2005). Self-assessments: Facilitating healing in self and others. In B. M. Dossey, L. Keegan, & C. E. Guzzetta (Eds.), *Holistic nursing: A handbook for practice* (4th ed.), pp. 379–393. Sudbury, MA: Jones & Bartlett.

Dossey, L. (1994). *Healing words.* San Francisco: HarperCollins.

Dunn, K. (2004). Music and the reduction of post-operative pain. *Nursing Standard, 18*(36), 33–39.

Eliopoulos, C. (2004). *Invitation to holistic health: A guide to living a balanced life.* Sudbury, MA: Jones & Bartlett.

Erickson, M. E. (2002). Modeling and role-modeling. In A. M. Tomey & M. R. Alligood, *Nursing theorists and their work* (5th ed.), pp. 443–464. St. Louis: Mosby.

Frisch, N. C., & Bowman, S. S. (2002). The modeling and role-modeling theory. In J. B. George, *Nursing theories: The base for professional nursing practice* (5th ed.), pp. 463–487. Upper Saddle River, NJ: Prentice Hall.

Hover-Kramer, D. (2002). *Healing touch: A guide book for practitioners* (2nd ed.). Albany, NY: Delmar.

Ingham, E. (1959). *Stories the feet can tell.* Rochester, NY: Ingham Publishing.

Ingham, E. (1963). *Stories the feet have told.* St. Petersburg, FL: Ingham Publishing.

Jobst, K. A., Niemtzow, R. C., Curtis, B. D., & Curtis, M. L. (2004). Special issue on science and healing: From bioelectromagnetics to the medicine of light. *Journal of Alternative and Complementary Medicine, 10*, 1–222.

Joel, L. A. (2006). *The nursing experience: Trends, challenges, and transitions* (5th ed.). New York: McGraw-Hill.

Kreitzer, M. J., & Snyder, M. (2002). Healing the heart: Integrating complementary therapies and healing practices into the care of cardiovascular patients. *Progress in Cardiovascular Nursing, 17*(2), 73–80.

Krieger, D. (2002). *Therapeutic touch as transpersonal healing.* New York: Lantern Books.

Laird, S. P., Snyder, C. R., Rapoff, M. A., & Green, S. (2004). Measuring private prayer: Development, validation, and clinical application of the multidimensional prayer inventory. *International Journal for the Psychology of Religion, 14*(4), 251–272.

Leigh, B. K. (2004). Incorporating human energy fields into studies of family communication. *Journal of Family Communication, 4*(3/4), 319–335.

McKivergin, M. (2005). The nurse as an instrument of healing. In B. M. Dossey, L. Keegan, & C. E. Guzzetta (Eds.), *Holistic nursing: A handbook for practice* (4th ed.), pp. 233–254. Sudbury, MA: Jones & Bartlett.

Miller, A. L. (2005). Epidemiology, etiology, and natural treatment of seasonal affective disorder. *Alternative Medicine Review, 10*(1), 5–13.

National Center for Complementary and Alternative Medicine (NCCAM). (2004, September). *The use of complementary and alternative medicine in the United States.* Retrieved June 17, 2006, from http://www.nccam.nih.gov

NANDA (2007). *Nursing diagnoses: Definitions and classification 2007–2008*. Philadelphia: NANDA International.

Ott, J. N. (1973). *Health and light: The effects of natural and artificial light on man and other living things*. Old Greenwich, CT: Devin-Adair.

The Proof That Prayer Works. (n.d.). Retrieved January 21, 2006, from http://www.1stholistic.com/Prayer/hol_prayer_proof.htm

Qutab, A. (2005). Ayurveda. In B. M. Dossey, L. Keegan, & C. E. Guzzetta (Eds.), *Holistic nursing: A handbook for practice* (4th ed.), pp. 273–283. Sudbury, MA: Jones & Bartlett.

Sand-Jecklin, K., & Badzek, L. (2004). Know the benefits and risks of using common herbal therapies. *Holistic Nursing Practice, 18*(4), 192–198.

Sand-Jecklin, K., & Badzek, L. (2003). Nurses and nutraceuticals: Knowledge and use. *Holistic Nursing Practice, 21*(4), 384–397.

Selye, H. (1956). *The stress of life*. New York: McGraw-Hill.

Sohn, P. M., & Loveland-Cook, C. A. (2002). Nurse practitioner knowledge of complementary health care: Foundation for practice. *Journal of Advanced Nursing, 39*(1), 9–16.

Thomas, D. V. (2002). Aromatherapy: Mythical, magical or medicinal? *Holistic Nursing Practice, 17*(1), 8–16.

Volk, J. (2002). Sound insights. *Kindred Spirit, 60*, 14–17.

Watson, J. (2005). *Caring science as sacred science*. Philadelphia: F. A. Davis.

Watson, J. (2002a). *Instruments for assessing and measuring caring in nursing and health sciences*. New York: Springer.

Watson, J. (2002b). Intentionality and caring-healing consciousness: A theory of transpersonal nursing. *Holistic Nursing Practice, 16*(4), 12–19.

Bibliography

Dossey, B. M., Keegan, L., & Guzzetta, C. E. (Eds.). (2005). *Holistic nursing: A handbook for practice*. Sudbury, MA: Jones & Bartlett.

Faass, N. (2001). *Integrating complementary medicine into health systems*. Gaithersburg, MD: Aspen Publishers.

Fontaine, K. L. (2000). *Healing practices: Alternative therapies for nursing*. Upper Saddle River, NJ: Prentice Hall.

Jonas, W., & Crawford, C. (2003). *Healing, intention, and energy medicine*. London: Churchill-Livingstone.

Keegan, L. (2001). *Healing with complementary and alternative therapies*. Albany, NY: Thomson Delmar Learning.

Peters, D., Chaitow, L., Harris, G., & Morrison, S. (2002). *Integrating complementary therapies in primary care: A practical guide for healthcare professionals*. Edinburgh, UK: Harcourt Publishers.

SECTION V

HEALTH PROMOTION CONCERNS

CHAPTER 19
Concerns of the Health Professional

CHAPTER 20
Economic and Quality Concerns

CHAPTER 21
Ethical, Legal, and Political Concerns

Chapter 19

CONCERNS OF THE HEALTH PROFESSIONAL

Carolina G. Huerta, EdD, MSN, RN
Kathie Rickman, LCDC, CARN, DRPH, RN
Susan Uecker, CS, MSN, RN

KEY TERMS

burnout	**genogram**	**health behavior patterns**	**spirituality**
ergonomics	**hardiness**	**occupational stress**	**stressors**

OBJECTIVES

Upon completion of this chapter, the reader should be able to:

- Identify current issues that have an impact on the health care professional.
- Recognize specific factors that affect the nursing profession.
- Discuss health behavior patterns and their implications for the health professional.
- Describe how a health care professional's health promotion practices influence the biological, psychological, spiritual, sociocultural, environmental, and technological domains.
- Identify strategies for positive health promotion for health professionals.
- Utilize the steps of the nursing process to develop a health promotion plan for the health care professional.

INTRODUCTION

Health professionals most often overlook their most important clients—themselves. That is, busy health professionals concentrate all of their energies on their responsibilities to help the sick, and they ignore basic health promotion principles essential for achieving their own maximum wellness. Although researchers from a variety of professions study health care professionals, primarily in relation to issues affecting job performance, the outcomes of such studies have had little impact in alleviating these problems. Master's theses and doctoral dissertations have produced a number of scholarly papers on this topic; however, there is no evidence that the issues affecting the health of health care professionals have been adequately resolved (Gillespie & Melby, 2003; Reineck & Furino, 2005). At a time when radical changes in health care services are taking place, it is important to focus on those **stressors,** or stress-provoking factors, that can impact the health of those who provide health care to others.

Nursing, for example, has become increasingly concerned about the health-related stressors affecting the profession. The *American Journal of Nursing*, the official journal of the American Nurses Association, dedicates a section in each issue of the monthly journal to Health and Safety. This section responds to issues raised by practicing nurses on the impact of nursing work on personal health. Nursing students and professionals read this section in the journal with concern about the reality of the profession. To some, it appears that at times the health care professions seem obsessed with the negative consequences of the work and seem to blame the individual professions. These findings need to be looked at with objectivity and cool detachment. How different is nursing or occupational therapy, for example, from other helping professions such as social work or teaching? Although health care professionals are well paid and usually have job flexibility and career opportunities, they are exposed to a great amount of stress dealing with human frailty and life and death situations.

Classroom teachers and social workers, however, may argue that they too are exposed to major stressors in their workplace environment. In all instances, factors in the ever-changing workplace environment, no doubt, do contribute to professionals' neglect of their own health promotion needs. Previous chapters have focused on the concept of health promotion from the point of view of the professional health care giver providing care for the client. This chapter will focus on the health promotion needs of health professionals, specifically nurses, who often ignore these needs and consequently suffer deleterious effects. Issues impacting the health care professional as well as strategies that enhance health will also be discussed.

CHANGE AND ITS IMPACT ON THE HEALTH PROFESSIONAL

Change sometimes seems to be the one constant in this high-tech information age. In the frenzy to "fit" into the current and future forms of health care, health care professionals find themselves returning to academic settings for additional education or moving from acute care settings to community or home-health environments. If a health care professional chooses to exit the workforce to spend time raising a family or caring for an elderly relative, he or she may find numerous technological and pharmacological advances upon reentering the profession (see Figure 19-1). A refresher course may be required in order to become current. For example, data collection and recording options change almost daily with bedside or handheld computers for inputting information. In this day of specialty focused care, time is spent learning new things, adapting to changes, hurrying to meet deadlines, and fulfilling responsibilities to others who depend on nurses. No wonder today's caregivers perceive that they have little time to relax, exercise, or play. When inexperienced workers enter the profession, they do so with enthusiasm and gusto. As core workers, they are expected to work hard for a period of time, experience **burnout,** and be replaced by other more energetic core workers. Burnout is the state of physical and emotional exhaustion that occurs when health care givers deplete their adaptive energy sources (Ekstedt & Fagerbert, 2005). Unfortunately, burnout occurs frequently among health care professionals who are trying desperately to adapt to the technological and social changes that are occurring in a fast-paced world. Burnout in nursing depletes the professional workforce and its resources. (See Technological Domain at the end of the chapter).

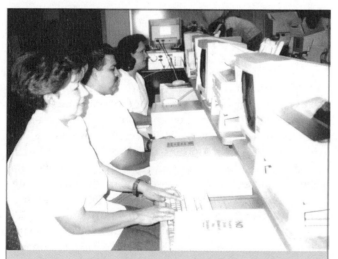

FIGURE 19-1 *Becoming technologically competent can also be stressful.*

ISSUES IMPACTING THE HEALTH CARE PROFESSIONAL

Health care professionals do differ from other types of workers. They are faced with illness and death on a daily basis and are prone to experience **occupational stress,** or stress that is job related, which leads to extreme tension, anxiety, and possibly even physical symptoms (Layne, Hohenshil, & Singh, 2004). They are expected to find out what the clients' needs are as well as provide comfort and support for all who are in their care. They come face-to-face with human suffering and emotional turmoil. They are expected to respond to stress and suffering with compassion and control (Stacciarini & Tróccoli, 2004). Health care professionals are given an enormous amount of responsibility and, with the exception of physicians, very little autonomy. Additionally, the population that they serve is ever changing. A mobile society with an increasing aging clientele presents new challenges to primary, secondary, and tertiary health care providers. These challenges are tremendous and impact the professional caregiver's ability to experience job satisfaction and provide optimum care (Cohen-Katz, et al., 2004).

Several research studies have been done on the stressful issues experienced by physicians, nurses, and other health care workers (McVicar, 2003; Rosenstein, 2005). As a result of the exhausting stresses encountered in the health care environment, nurses, physicians, and other health care workers are at high risk for chronic stress and burnout. The consequences of stress and burnout are numerous and devastating. These may include physical as well as psychological problems that can lead to inappropriate coping behaviors such as excessive drinking of alcohol (Cohen-Katz et al., 2004). (Chapter 17 provides an in-depth overview of the health risks associated with alcohol.) Study results indicate that professionals experience increasing levels of stress and burnout. They experience stress in relation to lines of authority, restructuring initiatives, staffing levels, and managed care (Friese, 2005).

Nursing literature has also identified issues affecting nurses in their work. This literature reports that nurses are leaving the nursing profession because of workplace issues such as the hospital environment, increased client acuity, excessive workloads, and the lack of support for maintaining the quality and safety of client care (Milstein, Gerstenberger, & Barton, 2002). Tinsley and France (2004), for example, in their study on why experienced nurses leave nursing, found that nurses described nurse abuse, burnout, and lack of their original feelings of love for nursing as the three prevalent themes for exiting the nursing profession. Although Buerhaus, Donelan, Ulrich, Kirby, Norman, and Dittus (2005) found that nurses' satisfaction with their jobs increased from 21 percent in 2002 to 34 percent in 2004, they also note that over 50 percent of nurses agreed that nursing was not a good career for individuals seeking respect in their career. In addition, overwhelming paperwork, staffing shortages, and hassles at the workplace have been cited by nurses unhappy with their jobs and thinking of leaving the profession (Egglefield-Beaudoin & Edgar, 2003).

New nursing graduates also face stresses associated with their new position. The first few months have the potential to be the most stressful and challenging for the newly graduated nurse. Role stress in new nursing graduates has been found to be relevant to nursing education and practice. The first six months, in particular, have been shown to be the most stressful period of adjustment for the registered nurse (Greenwood, 2000). Role ambiguity, lack of clarity in terms of the behavior expected, unrealistic expectations, and anxiety have been found to produce stress in the new graduate. Chang and Hancock (2003) studied new nursing graduates employed for one year or less and found that role stress was affected by role ambiguity and role overload. As nurses gained experience, role overload was a greater contributor to stress than role ambiguity.

It is interesting to note that nursing students are not immune to some of the same stressors experienced by the professional health care employee. Findings from research studies suggest that students experience stress in their clinical practice and in their nursing education

Spotlight On

Issues Impacting a Nursing Student

Elizabeth, a 32-year-old mother of a 6-year-old and a 4-year-old, has decided to return to college after being out of school for six years. She has already completed all her prerequisite courses and is now ready to enter the registered nurse program. Her mother and mother-in-law both believe in the traditional role of the mother staying home to care for her young children. They have both been very verbal about that. Although this is stressful to Elizabeth, she is intent on being the first in her family to complete college. She does find herself in conflict sometimes with her parents and her in-laws over her lifestyle choices. Elizabeth finds herself preoccupied with her current situation and worries that her husband will resent her for returning to school. She is aware that she will have little time for fun due to the demands of school and her mothering responsibilities.

program (Nicholls & Timmings, 2005). These stresses, of course, can also have deleterious effects on students' health and can impact academic outcomes. In addition to the stresses experienced by students in general, nursing students are faced with the demands of clinical contact with clients and the urgency to master clinical competencies (Baldwin, 1999). See Box 19-1 for a summary of the issues impacting the health care professional that might also impact the student nurse.

FACTORS AFFECTING THE NURSING PROFESSION

The face of nursing is changing rapidly, both for students and for practitioners. The myriad responsibilities that professional nurses assume in the workplace has the potential for affecting their personal and professional functioning. These responsibilities may cause individuals to seek other career options or drop out of the health care arena totally. In fact, recent surveys indicate that health care institutions are experiencing difficulty recruiting registered nurses. In May 2005, the National Commission on Nursing Workforce for Long-Term Care released its report, which found that there are nearly 100,000 vacant nursing positions in health care facilities on any given day. The report also found that the current nurse turnover rate exceeds 50 percent. This shortage is costing health care facilities an estimated $4 billion a year in recruitment and training expenses (American Association

---

BOX 19-1   Issues Affecting the Health Care Professional

- Aging clientele
- Aging workforce
- Heavy workload
- Human suffering
- Managed care
- Outcomes measurement
- Role conflict
- Role ambiguity
- Technological change
- Stress

Research Note

Nursing Students' Perceived Stressors

Study Problem/Purpose: To examine the perceived stressors in a group of nursing students undertaking a part-time bachelor of nursing science program. Stress among the nurses is evident within the nursing literature, but little information is available on the specific stressors that affect nursing students.

Methods: The sample consisted of 70 students present in the final week of the program. A specific tool was developed for the study in order to identify the program areas that the students perceived affected their experience. The students filled out the 45-item questionnaire which was analyzed using a Spearman's rank order correlation coefficient.

Findings: The major stressors identified by the students included writing assignments at degree level and fulfilling personal and academic needs. Trying to balance work commitments and study requirements and the prospect of a final examination were also high stress-inducing factors.

Implications: This study has implications for those involved in nursing education programs. Consideration should be given to the impact of workload on student welfare, and curriculum approaches that reduce stress should be adopted. The incorporation of stress management programs in nursing schools should also be considered.

Nicholls, H., and Timmins, F. (2005). Programme-related stressors among part-time undergraduate nursing students. *Journal of Advanced Nursing*, 50(1), 93-100.

of Colleges of Nursing [AACN], 2005). This shortage is predicted to become even more severe by the year 2010 (Buerhaus, 2005). Registered nurses identify understaffing, nursing staff turnover, client acuity, few new graduates, and client volume increases as the most likely reasons for the current and anticipated shortage. Several factors such as those described impact professional nursing today. These factors are primarily related to the nursing supply and demand. Unless they are adequately examined by the profession itself, nurses will continue to experience stress, poor health, and, eventually, job burnout. Until the nursing shortage is resolved through strategies that encourage chief nurse officers to work with nurses to alleviate some of the issues affecting nursing, strategies for improving the quality of client care will not be accomplished (Buerhaus, 2005). Factors include current nursing student characteristics, the supply of professional nurses, and the impact of managed care.

Nursing Student Characteristics

Nursing students are a large group, primarily enrolled in technical-level nursing programs, and comprise more than half of all health professions students AACN, 2004a. These students bring a variety of assets and experiences with them as they prepare for their nursing career. Statistics published by the national Sample Survey of Registered Nurses (U.S. Department of Health and Human Services [USDHHS], 2000) indicate that the average age for the associate degree nursing program graduate is 33.2 years and the average age for the baccalaureate degree nursing program graduate is 27.5 years. A large percentage of all nursing students have worked in other areas of health care before entering nursing school. Many of these students also have other academic degrees prior to enrolling in nursing courses. The majority of nursing students enroll in programs that do not lead to an academic degree. It has been reported that 34.4 percent of all registered nurses have an associate degree as their highest level of education and 32.7 percent have a baccalaureate degree as the highest degree (Health Resources and Services Administration, 2001).

The preceding statistics are significant in that the wider age ranges as well as previous careers indicate that today's nursing student may be involved in more diverse life tasks such as caring for aging parents and raising children while juggling other multiple roles. Students may also be spouses, parents, single or married, and employed part-time or full-time while in school. Juggling multiple roles presents life challenges that are overwhelming at times and may lead to neglecting personal health practices and needs. In addition, the age at which a student graduates from nursing school is of concern since older graduates become older nurses in the workforce. Older nurses usually have a shorter career life expectancy. The fact that the majority of nursing students are enrolled in technical programs impacts the health care delivery system and the nursing profession as well. An inadequate health care system and fewer years of academic preparation may provoke stress and burnout in those delivering care.

Nursing Student Stress

Many students in nursing are described as overachievers who have difficulty setting priorities that include play and having fun. These students are faced with a demanding scientific curriculum that dictates the establishment of new priorities and alterations in lifestyle. Nursing students are faced with many of the same problems encountered by nurses in the profession. They must adjust to shift changes, heavy workloads, and death and dying situations. For these students, anything less than the highest grade signifies failure and may lead to demoralization and stress. Stress can have a major impact on academic outcomes since it has been found to lower academic achievement and increase attrition rates (Huerta, 1990).

It is important for students to recognize that good grades are important, but not at the cost they often demand. Perfectionism is an unrealistic goal with a big price tag attached. No goal justifies the loss of physical or emotional health. Being the class hero may be a reenactment of being the family hero attempting to meet all the needs of the family growing up, or to gain personal recognition in order to feel significant. The above is also true of other health care students who have begun in a highly competitive field. Sadly, many of the health care professions including nursing reinforce these behaviors. These professionals are taught to nurture, comfort, and "fix" those who come to them for help. Unfortunately, students are not taught how to "fix" themselves as well.

Professional Nursing Supply

The demand for professional nurses is very market driven and shortages have occurred periodically over the years. Nursing shortages were evident in the late 1980s and early 1990s. Most recently, the nursing shortage in the United States has become quite severe and is predicted to become even more so. It is estimated that if current trends continue, the gap between supply and demand for professional nurses will expand to between 400,000 and 800,000 by 2020 (Buerhaus, 2005). The current shortage is much more acute than in years past.

This current and anticipated lack of an adequate nursing supply is predicted to be more resistant to short-term economic strategies that have previously worked (Heller, Oros, & Durney-Crowley, 2000). Nursing shortages have a negative impact on nursing professionals who are attempting to provide quality client care.

Lack of the necessary manpower to provide this care will result in workload-related stress; poor health practices such as skipping meals, overeating, or excessive drinking of alcohol; working long hours; and possibly job burnout or profession dropout. To adequately understand the demands placed on nurses and the impact these demands have on nurses' own health care needs, it is important to look at the make-up of professional nurses today in terms of gender, age, ethnicity, and educational diversity.

Gender

Gender inequities certainly exist in the nursing profession. Between 85 and 95 percent of all nursing students are female (USDHHS, 2000). This lack of diversity is, of course, then reflected in the general nursing population. Trends, however, are showing that more males (see Figure 19-2) are entering the nursing profession than previously. Men enter nursing for a variety of reasons but it seems that, according to the literature, their primary motivations are job security and career opportunities. The majority of the men in nursing are concentrated in certain types of jobs such as hospital administration and areas of specialty such as emergency room, psychiatric, and intensive care nursing.

Although current trends may indicate that the male registered nurse population is increasing, these statistics are still of concern since the majority of registered nurses are married females with children who still live at home. Traditionally, women have been charged with the additional responsibilities of child rearing and making

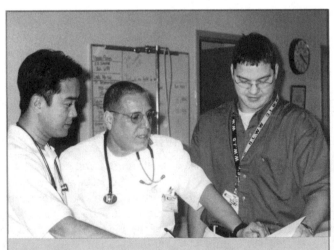

FIGURE 19-2 *Men are a growing presence in nursing.*

sure that the family life runs smoothly. Fortunately, nursing is a profession that can be exited and reentered based on personal and family needs. This too may sometimes be viewed as a limit in career development. But because nursing is primarily a female workforce, the inherent strengths of women predominate. Women nurture relationships and are able to multitask. The skills are vital for shaping the health care environment of the future. It is important to note, though, that a gender-diverse profession has all the benefits of balance within the profession (Christman, 1998)

Age

Registered nurses in the United States number 2.5 million, with approximately 60 percent of these nurses employed in direct client care. Nurses comprise the largest single component of hospital staff employees. The majority of health care services today involves caring for the growing population of elderly clients and usually includes some form of care by nurses (AACN, 2004b). These statistics are frightening in view of the fact that nurses are growing older along with the general population. An aging workforce can result in negative health outcomes both for the client and for the nurse providing the care.

The average age of the registered nurse in this country is 43.2 years, up from 42.3 years in 1996. It is estimated that 40 percent of all registered nurses will be older than 50 in 2010 and will leave the workforce within the next 10 years. In 1980, 25 percent of all nurses were under the age of 30. Current statistics reveal that only 9 percent of all nurses are under the age of 30 (AACN, 2005).

It is obvious that an aging registered nurse workforce will be less mobile and more resistant to change, and may be unable to adequately care for the acutely ill clients receiving nursing services today. This is especially true if the nurse caregiver is dealing with personal

health problems that occur as a result of aging. Issues such as health care insurance, retirement prospects, workloads, and career benefits will surely impact the nursing supply, especially when considering the aging of the nursing population. Excessive workloads, increasing stress in providing client care, and the demands of ever-changing technology can all have a deleterious effect on the health-promoting behaviors and health status of the professional caregiver.

Ethnicity

In assessing the professional nursing supply, it is important to note that there is a definite lack of ethnic diversity. In fact, the Sullivan Commission on Diversity in the Healthcare Workforce (2004) reports that there is an imbalance in the makeup of the nation's health care workforce in general. Many barriers have been identified as deterrents to enrolling and succeeding in the nursing and health care professions. This lack of ethnic diversity among nurses contributes to the gap in health status and lack of access to health care for many in our population (Sullivan Commission, 2004, p. iv). Although enrollment of minorities in nursing has shown a slight increase, the number of nurses from minorities has failed to keep up with the growth of the minority population. According to data collected by the National Sample Survey of Registered Nurses, only a small percentage of all registered nurses come from a racial or ethnic minority background (USDHHS, 2000). The data indicate that the number of minority nurses is substantially less than the number of minorities in the United States.

The numbers of minority populations are increasing rapidly in the United States. Many of these minority populations are first-generation Americans who may be living in poverty, lack access to health care, and be undereducated. Nurses are called upon daily to deliver nursing care to these minority populations with their complex health care needs. Nurses who are predominantly White and not from an ethnic minority may not understand a client's culture, values, and beliefs but are still expected to provide culturally sensitive care. There is the expectation that professional nurses must provide cultural congruent care. This added responsibility may provoke stress in the nurse and may eventually lead to job burnout or dropping out of the nursing profession.

Education

Registered nurses are educated either at the technical level, such as the associate degree and nursing diploma, or at the baccalaureate (BSN) level. Associate, diploma, and baccalaureate prepared nurses all take the same licensing exam but are prepared to function at different levels. Baccalaureate graduates are prepared to practice in all health care settings since their education includes a broad spectrum of courses in the sciences and humanities, as well as courses in critical thinking, community health, and leadership (AACN, 2000). Unfortunately, only 31 percent of all nurses hold a baccalaureate degree in nursing as their highest degree, while close to 60 percent of all nurses are prepared at the associate or diploma level. It is also important to note that fewer than 10 percent have graduate nursing degrees (Peterson, 1999).

While the preceding statistics may not be alarming to many, this lack of educational preparation may be reflected in the quality of care received by clients. It is also reflected in the amount of responsibility placed on the nurse, especially one who possesses a baccalaureate degree and is responsible for supervising client care. Technical nurses provide the majority of the client care with the vast majority of nurses with a university degree working in management settings. Managing a poorly prepared workforce, assuming excessive responsibility when inadequately educated, and dealing with the multitude of issues associated with today's nursing environment may lead to unhealthy behavior patterns in the nursing workforce.

Impact of Managed Care on Nursing

Traditionally, health care was delivered by the health care provider only when people sought care for an illness. This lack of emphasis on prevention has been replaced by current health models that focus mainly on levels of prevention. Managed care, however, is a different approach to the use of health services. This model of health care delivery looks at providing services from a cost-containment perspective (Black & Hawks, 2005).

Although there are acknowledged benefits to managed care, primarily in terms of access to health care, cost containment, and the emphasis on disease prevention, managed care has also become a source of stress and discontent for the professional workforce. Criticism of managed care revolves around the issue of short-term cost containment with little emphasis on quality client care. The discipline of nursing is centered around core values such as caring, empathy, and preservation of integrity. Taking the time to treat clients holistically is also central to the profession.

Unfortunately, managed care promotes cost containment at the physical expense of the client. These clients are admitted to health care institutions in a sicker state and dismissed earlier than ever before. In the effort to reduce expenses, institutions that function under managed care have had to cut back on professional nursing personnel and increase the number of unlicensed health care personnel. These actions only add to the workload stress experienced by nurses working for these institutions. Nurses working under these adverse conditions may also develop unhealthy ways to cope with the stressful environment and suffer dire health-related consequences.

HEALTH BEHAVIOR PATTERNS

People face important decisions about healthy eating, alcohol abuse, sexual practices, and exercise patterns. Eating disorders run rampant in our society, which appears fixated on a perfect, thin body. As students enrolled in health care courses learn about disease and health in others, opportunities will arise to evaluate and perhaps change their own health patterns. One way for students to learn about their propensity for future health concerns is to draw their family health **genogram** and observe their family health patterns. A genogram is a useful tool that diagrams and depicts family relationships over a period of several generations, usually at least three (Allender & Spradley, 2001). See Figure 19-3 for an example of how to construct a genogram.

Most health care professionals have established **health behavior patterns** by the time they become college students. These are health habits that may relate to physical functioning, such as exercise, food, and routine maintenance, or to the person's psychological, spiritual, and/or professional life. The choices made in the early adult years about diet and exercise have a lasting effect. If a person continues to eat junk food and plans to start exercising "tomorrow," that person may wake up 30 years later still planning to do something about his or her own health. Health care professionals who ignore their psychological well-being, physical and spiritual needs, and professional health needs lose both individually and collectively.

Health care professionals are very aware of the fact that people's needs change with each life stage and that they, as health care providers, are not immune to these changes. Many times, however, they are more in tune with their clients' changing needs than their own and forget to apply special health care knowledge and prin-

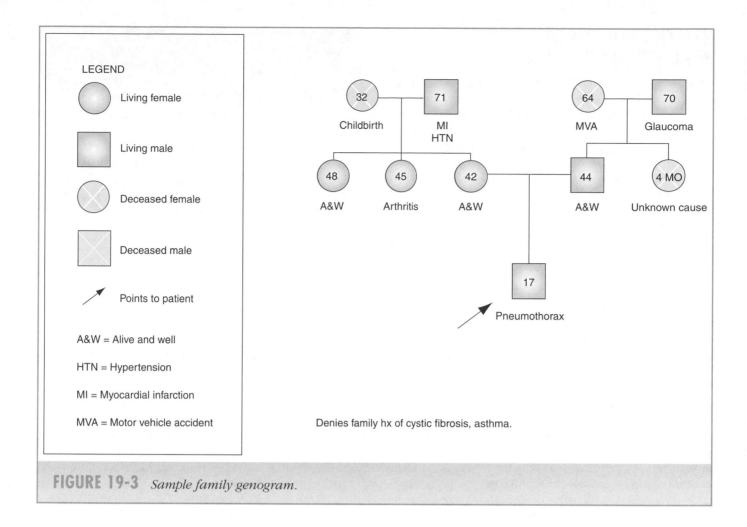

LEGEND

⬤ Living female

⬛ Living male

⊗ Deceased female

⊠ Deceased male

↗ Points to patient

A&W = Alive and well

HTN = Hypertension

MI = Myocardial infarction

MVA = Motor vehicle accident

Denies family hx of cystic fibrosis, asthma.

FIGURE 19-3 *Sample family genogram.*

ciples to themselves. These professionals have a rich source of information about health and health behavior patterns that can improve general health. This information is gleaned from years of study, professional journals, and personal experiences. For example, nursing and medical professionals know that mortality increases with increased body weight and that being substantially over the recommended body weight increases the chance of death from cardiovascular disease and even from cancer. Yet many of these individuals choose to overlook these facts rather than make the necessary health promotion changes.

Nurses, of course, are no exception. They have a rich source of information about nurses' health in the Nurses' Health Study, a major research study conducted by the Harvard School of Public Health. There are 120,000 nurses in this study, which is close to 30 years old. This research study has found an increased risk of coronary disease with six or more years of rotating shift work. There are also complex findings in the study regarding alcohol, indicating that light-to-moderate alcohol intake is associated with a lower rate of coronary heart disease, but that these same levels are associated with increased risk for breast cancer. The findings also indicate that light-to-moderate alcohol intake is associ-

Spotlight On

Personal Decision Making

Although nurses know the benefits and risks of hormone replacement therapy, female nurses must still weigh the pros and cons of estrogen replacement therapy or postmenopausal hormone replacement for themselves in the same way as any female client.

ated with an overall reduction in mortality, but only in the subpopulation of women 50 or older who have additional risk factors for coronary disease. These findings and many others related to general health, diet, exercise, family planning, and various risk factors are readily available to nurses, yet many choose to continue with their unhealthy behaviors. Unless nurses and other members of the health care professional workforce adopt behaviors that are health promoting, they will continue to experience the physical, psychological, and spiritual stress that ultimately leads to burnout or dropout from the profession.

HEALTH PROMOTION PRACTICES BY DOMAIN

Of all occupations, health care ranks as the second highest for occupational injury and illness in the United States. Many major concerns must be addressed in order to ensure a healthy and productive nursing population. These concerns include needlestick and back injuries, workplace violence, and exposure to respiratory agents, among others (Hess, 2005). It is vital for health care professionals to be in control of their physical, emotional, spiritual, and professional health to be effective as well as healthier individuals. The first step is assessing overall health and then determining future goals. The domains provide a framework for assessing overall health in the health professional and for planning strategies that will improve health status. Not only do these domains highlight areas that need addressing, they also provide a system for performing a personal evaluation in a holistic manner. It is important to note that when any domain is neglected, ill or unwanted effects may result.

The domains that are of concern are the same as those previously discussed and include the biological, psychological, spiritual, sociocultural, environmental, and technological domains. It is important to note that change in one domain causes change in other domains. This idea is similar to that of different ingredients being mixed in a punch bowl, in which a variety of flavors intermingle and saturate each other to produce a single taste. One-sided growth or deterioration in part of the system is dangerous at any period of life. The demands of working in a high-pressure profession can cause imbalance that may result in serious health concerns.

Biological Domain

In thinking about ways to prevent illnesses that affect the physical or biological domain, it is obvious that there are many simple things that nurses and other health care professionals can do for themselves to promote their own physical health. For example, it is useful to follow established guidelines on routine immunizations such as tetanus and hepatitis B, which may be overlooked after school days are over. Regular dental care impacts future health of teeth and gums. All health care professionals can recall clients with poor dental hygiene, a problem that develops over time.

There are also other work-related factors that can seriously affect the biological domain and that can have lifelong health-related consequences. All health care providers, for instance, who are actually providing bedside care are prone to injuries involved with lifting and moving clients. Major injuries are well documented in health care workers. Nurses may be on their feet all day, moving their hands, keeping their arms busy doing procedures. These activities may result in many musculoskeletal aches and pains that could eventually force

them to drop out of the nursing profession. Close to 70 percent of all disabling injuries suffered by nurses are caused by overexertion to the back or trunk. It is estimated that back injuries affect up to 38 percent of all nurses and that nurses have 30 percent more absenteeism due to back injuries than the rest of the population (Nawar, 2000). Although client handling and manual lifting of objects are factors that place nurses and other health care professionals at risk, the majority of these injuries are attributed to the act of lifting clients. The American Nurses Association is so concerned about the musculoskeletal injuries that occur in the workplace that it has published a position statement on elimination of manual client handling and advocacy of assistive devices for nurses (ANA, 2003). Effective and safe client handling programs using assistive devices greatly reduce back injury risks. Use of safe equipment also offers a more secure, comfortable, and dignified way to handle clients (Hess, 2005).

Health care disciplines have shown a lot of interest in the field of ergonomics and its application to the workforce. **Ergonomics** involves the study and analysis of human work particularly as it relates to an individual's anatomy and other human characteristics (Nawar, 2000). Following appropriate ergonomic principles and pushing for ergonomic standards are strategies that can decrease the risk of injury. Discovering what lifting devices are commercially available and working only in institutions that use these are also strategies that might be helpful in decreasing this type of work-related injury.

Another area of concern affecting the biological domain is risk for chemical hazards. Serious chemical exposures can result from use of sterilizing agents and chemotherapeutic agents. Reactive airway symptoms and skin problems can occur. Nurses frequently care for clients with cancer who are receiving anticancer drugs. These drugs represent a significant hazard for nurses (Foley, 2004).

There are other conditions that are not necessarily work-related but that warrant periodic screening evaluation to prevent development of disease process. These include, but are not limited to, such conditions as hypertension, hyperlipidemia, colon cancer, breast cancer, cervical cancer, prostate cancer, and testicular cancer. In those with risk factors, a regular screening by a dermatologist for mole changes or skin lesions is prudent. Some conditions are more age specific, such as birth control or the need to consider taking hormone replacement therapy after menopause. Birth control methods include regular use of condoms, which protects from pregnancy and many sexually transmitted diseases, including Acquired Immunodeficiency Syndrome (AIDS).

Despite the fact that smoking has a well-documented negative impact on health, the use of nicotine continues to increase in younger populations, particularly young White females. This is of concern to the nursing profession whose workforce consists largely of White females. Recognizing that smoking is an unhealthy behavior can often be the first step in seeking help to stop. The next step is to seek help for eliminating the behavior. Alcohol and other drug abuse also have serious health consequences that need expert treatment. Perhaps, because of the stresses encountered in their work, health care professionals have been noted to have a propensity for drinking excessively and for abusing drugs. Professionals who are aware of this predisposition to alcoholism and drug addiction will prevent the associated physical consequences or seek professional care early.

Unfortunately, many of the choices made in youth, such as whether to exercise, take drugs, use alcohol, diet, or smoke, have lifelong physiological effects. The immediate results of such choices on a young person's health may not be seen and this in itself can create a false sense of security and a continuation of the detrimental behaviors. Good nutrition, including the five to seven fruits and vegetables per day, and regular exercise increasingly show up in research as being essential to good health. Knowledgeable health care professionals have the responsibility to make healthy choices, particularly in view of their potential to serve as possible role models.

Psychological Domain

Values and expectations impact emotional health. The ways in which people cope with stress impacts everyone. **Hardiness,** or resilience to stress, and perceptions are significant influences on psychological well-being. Burnout can be the natural consequence of not caring, resulting from an extended period of stress. There are many sources of stress in the workplace. For example, one significant source is nurse/supervisor conflict and staff/physician conflict. There are, of course, other areas that can cause turmoil and psychological stress in the work area (Ekstedt & Fagerbert, 2005). Excessive stress leading to burnout may be related to an inadequate fit between the employee's assigned job and the institution's work policies. A restrictive work environment or one that stifles autonomy will have a devastating effect on employee well-being. Stress and burnout are common occurrences in the nursing profession. Tinsley and France (2004) found that nurses repeatedly expressed symptoms of stress and burnout as reasons for exiting the profession. They also found that the workplace is oppressive and creates work dissatisfaction among nurses. In assessing stress in the health care professional and in determining strategies that promote psychological health, it is wiser to look beyond individual responses to the broader picture of the work setting and work team.

It has been pointed out that burnout is associated with anxiety, frequency of illness, and negative job attitudes, as well as with lack of collegial support (Lindike & Sieckert, 2005). A positive collegial and supportive network is also associated with feelings of job satisfaction.

Student Stress

Students have unique areas of stress. Grades can be a demonstration of pushing for perfection. When only A's are acceptable, anything less can produce anxiety and discontent. Some students argue for hours over a grade of 98 percent. Procrastination, on the other hand, is another student-related demon that can cause major psychological distress.

These results indicate that strategies that facilitate positive peer relationships increase positive job attitudes and, perhaps, even job satisfaction. Professionals who seek out or create positive work settings will enjoy better psychological health and experience fewer episodes of psychological crisis.

Congruence between personal values and the values held by the employing institution also plays an important role in increasing job satisfaction, decreasing job turnover, and improving the psychological health of the employed professional. Individuals who experience personal conflict between their values and those of their employer are at risk for experiencing low self-esteem and burnout. Feelings of autonomy and of control are also important to preventing psychological distress. Buerhaus et al. (2005) found that nurses with advanced degrees were significantly more likely to be very satisfied with their present job. They also found that RNs who reported that their organization emphasized client

care and that management recognized the importance of their personal lives, and who had positive relationships with their colleagues were also more satisfied with their chosen profession. Decreases in job satisfaction were predicted in those feeling a sense of burnout and stress related to too many nonnursing tasks.

Individuals most susceptible to burnout are usually bright, perfectionistic, hardworking, and idealistic. Hardiness is related to four C's: control, communication, challenge, and commitment. Four behaviors drain a health care professional's energy: perfectionism, complaining, resisting reality, and judging others. There are many positive strategies that reduce stress and decrease the energy drain. These may include seeking support from psychologically positive individuals, exercising, eating right, and resting when needed. Adopting healthy coping practices is also essential to prevent psychological distress. Table 19-1 illustrates one way to evaluate individual coping strategies.

Spiritual Domain

A spiritual life is a large part of what makes us different from other species. It is a defining characteristic of human nature (Maslow, 1970). **Spirituality** has been identified as an integral component of nursing practice (Miklancie, 2001). The concept has been defined in many ways, but most definitions include concepts related to religion and states of awareness. Spirituality is concerned with the whole personality and emotional sharing. The word *spirituality* is derived from the Latin *spiritus*, meaning "breath," and also relates to the Greek word *pneuma*, meaning "breath" or "the vital spirit of the soul" (Dossey, Keegan, and Guzetta, 2000). A belief in the sacredness of

TABLE 19-1 Coping Practices

Healthy Coping Practices			Unhealthy Coping Practices	
Listen to music			Avoid social contact	
Express emotions: cry, talk			Drink or use drugs	
Exercise: walk, jog, bike, swim		1 = Often	Smoke or overeat	
Pray, meditate, read		2 = Sometimes	Blame others for your problems	
Go outdoors, enjoy nature			Yell or curse at others	
Practice deep breathing		3 = Rarely	Drive fast or recklessly	
Attend concerts, plays, events		4 = Never	Anticipate worst possible outcome	
See a counselor or minister			Ignore the problem	
Total Points			**Total Points**	

Add scores for each column. Do you score higher on healthy or unhealthy coping practices? How can you minimize unhealthy coping?

every person and of every living thing can be included in the definition of spirituality.

The concept of wellness is multidimensional and includes the spiritual domain in addition to all of the other domains. A spiritually well person seeks a harmony between that which lies within the individual and the forces that come from outside the individual. A health promotion approach to care, whether for the client or the health care professional, incorporates spirituality. It is recognized that spirituality can provide personal comfort and is a source of major support for clients. What is not always as obvious is that the spiritual dimension can also be a resource for the health care professional.

Health care professionals come into contact with the spiritual dimension of life in their everyday practice. It is important for them to have some understanding of this spiritual dimension, not only for themselves but also for assessment of others. Professionals, such as the nurses who provide for the most intimate care of an individual, must be comfortable in recognizing the spiritual needs of clients and providing spiritual care. Most importantly, they must recognize that spirituality can be a personal strength for themselves in the role of caregiver (Ackley, 2000).

The research literature reveals studies describing measurable indicators of spirituality. Nurses, in particular, are expected to be familiar with these indicators in order to make accurate nursing diagnoses. The North American Nursing Diagnosis Association (2007) has identified Risk for Spiritual Distress as a diagnosis that refers to the impaired ability to experience and integrate meaning and purpose in life through a person's connectedness with self, other persons, art, music, literature, nature, and a power greater than oneself (p. 210). Some specific indicators of spiritual distress include lack of hope, loss of meaning and purpose in life, and a refusal to interact with others. When understanding how these apply to individuals, especially to those who are enduring a physical or mental illness, the professional nurse is able to identify issues that may be blocks to spirituality. For example, persons who have no belief in God or a Higher Power may feel they are completely on their own to combat the fear and anxiety of a poor health state or acute health problem. These individuals may believe that no outside power is available to help support or direct them in their current crisis. Isolation and lack of significant relationships in one's life may be indicators of poor self-esteem, inability to give or receive love, and subsequent behavior patterns based on the belief that one must earn another's love and respect by being perfect.

Although health care professionals are aware of the importance of the spiritual dimension from the client's point of view, most do not stop to assess their own spirituality. Tending to their own spiritual needs can be a source of comfort that adds focus to life and provides a sense of fulfillment. Frankl (1978) describes lack of purpose in life as existential vacuum, a sense of emptiness and boredom that leads to a state of unhappiness with

one's life. Often this spiritual boredom is compounded by the stresses that occur in the professional workplace. People have a tendency to make their work their life's priority and do not take time to renew their spiritual life. Many caregivers are uncomfortable with their own spiritual dimension and choose to ignore this aspect of life until they are faced with a crisis. By performing a personal spiritual assessment, knowing themselves spiritually, and taking the time to renew their spirituality, health care professionals will become more comfortable with the spiritual care that they are expected to provide. Box 19-2 provides a spiritual assessment guide for the health care professional.

Sociocultural Domain

Working as a health care professional in today's society is a major challenge that takes some special skills. The changes that are impacting society today also have an impact on health care. Social issues such as the ethnic minority population influx, economic challenges, workforce supply, and technological changes

BOX 19-2 Spiritual Assessment Guide

1. What gives your life meaning?
2. Do you have a sense of purpose in your life?
3. What is the most important or powerful force in your life?
4. What brings you joy and peace in your life?
5. What are your personal beliefs?
6. Do you pray?
7. How do you show love to yourself?
8. Who are the significant people in your life?
9. Do you have close friends or family you can call for help when you need it?
10. Is it easy for you to forgive yourself and others?

have the potential to overburden workers. Unless they respond to demands through personal changes, today's health care professionals will be stressed and will ultimately experience burnout.

In our constantly changing society, job security is a thing of the past. Instead, wise health care professionals place their loyalty in their profession and in their clients. Today's nurses, for example, can best view themselves almost as independent contractors. In the movement from traditional security to working for self, old values and assumptions must be reevaluated. This change requires a major shift in perception. Institutional loyalty and commitment, an attitude frequently displayed in the past, has evolved to a commitment to the clients and loyalty to the practice discipline. This shift is harder for health care workers who have practiced for a while and less of a problem for beginning practitioners.

Many providers of health care would prefer to not view health care as a business, but it is, and the more that they know about the business end, the better off they will be. In this business, the client, and often the family, is the customer. The nurse's documentation, for example, directly leads to the bottom line and to the viability of the organization and therefore to the nurse's job. What nurses do and know affects their salaries and the economics of the employing institution. It is important to recognize that nurses and health care professionals are power brokers who often form partnerships and important bonds with their clients. It is not unusual for clients to follow their nurses or other health care practitioners to their new jobs, such as in home health. This client preference for a specific practitioner is common in other professions but is sometimes viewed with skepticism in health care disciplines other than medicine.

Many of the health care professions are still in transition. Take the nursing culture, for example. Agencies and hospitals want the nurse to be loyal or to be independent as it suits the employer, usually related to client census or other bottom lines of economics. But nurses, like other professionals employed in health care fields, must assume responsibility for themselves, not in an angry defiant way but in a mature responsible manner. Communicating in clear and respectful ways and being well informed on insurance and reimbursement changes as well as other pertinent data helps employees be equal partners in health care. Using effective communication skills, taking ownership for solving problems, and cultivating positive work relationships will go a long way in furthering a career. Taking risks, letting go, and embracing change are powerful attitudes for the health care professional to cultivate.

Environmental Domain

Another significant area of possible stress is the physical environment of the workplace. An unsafe work environment can place nursing's future at risk. Unsafe environ-

ments can have adverse effects on recruitment and retention of nurses. Nursing cannot afford to have an image of necessitating work in an unsafe environment during a time of acute nursing shortage and demand. The environment can affect client safety as well as the nurses themselves. It is critically important that nurses maintain their own health and safety (Foley, 2004). The crowded, noisy areas where many professionals work impact job satisfaction and self-care. If there is little control over the environment, stress and dissatisfaction will increase. The elimination of negative factors in the environment is essential to the achievement of job satisfaction in the health care employee.

Nursing can enhance its environment through increased personal control, contact with nature, and creation of aesthetically pleasing spaces. Surrounding ourselves with positive people rather than those who whine or complain is important. Being around complainers drains energy and can decrease morale and productivity.

There are also many other environmental issues that are potentially serious for the health care professional. Workplace violence, for instance, has been recognized as a peril for health care workers. Workplace violence is one of the most complex and dangerous hazards facing nurses who work in our health care environment. Dangers arise from the exposure to violent individuals and from the fact that violence prevention programs and protective regulations are sorely lacking (McPhaul & Lipscomb, 2004). It is not uncommon to hear about a nurse who was punched in the eye or slammed to the floor. Agitated clients in health care facilities and the emergency room as well as clients with dementia or a history of assault can pose a great risk to the nurse caring for them. Demanding the right to a safe environment is one step in curbing violence in the workplace. The next is becoming aware of the employing institution's policies on violence and how incidents have been dealt with in the past.

Other environmental issues most frequently identified are needlestick injuries, latex allergy, and exposure to physical hazards such as radiation. Needlestick injuries to the health care professional can transmit hepatitis B and C viruses if the injected client was infected. The hepatitis viruses and human immunodeficiency virus (HIV) affect thousands of health care workers annually, most often through needlesticks (Bain, 2000; Foley, 2004).

Latex allergies are also a source of concern to the health care profession. Allergy to the latex in gloves and other medical products occurs in workers in health care institutions. Latex sensitization is most commonly caused by using powdered latex gloves, which allows the latex to become airborne and gain access to the respiratory system. This allergic response can cause minor symptoms such as skin irritation or flushing, but unfortunately, latex allergy can also cause shock, laryngeal spasms, and cardiac arrest.

Physical hazards are all around the health care worker's environment. It is essential for the health care professional to recognize the risks in the environment and to formulate a plan that addresses them. It is also essential that the professional become cognizant of the roles of the employee health and risk management departments. Appropriate protection from potentially damaging environmental hazards is a priority.

Technological Domain

Technology has transformed the traditional health care industry as well as the delivery of client care. While technology has brought better and more advanced care to our client populations, it has also been a source of stress for nurses and health care workers who recognize the need to update their skills in order to remain competent in the health care setting. Registered nurses (RNs) are the primary information managers in clinical settings. They collect data, transform data to usable formats, integrate information from many diverse sources, analyze information, make data-based nursing care decisions, and communicate information to others as appropriate (Shinn et al., 2002). The skills employed and the technology-related activities undertaken by RNs make RNs the consummate knowledge workers of today. Nurses are expected to upload and monitor complex data such as data from computerized monitors and medical records. Along with cognitive nursing skills that are needed for such critical thinking activities, nurses are expected to use information technologies to arrive at critical decision making. They must be able to deal with various complexities that require the application of technology in the clinical setting.

Some recent technological developments that have been a source of assistance as well as stress for today's nurses include computerized automated medication delivery systems, bedside computerized charting, and other equipment such as the new intravenous pumps with preset alerts that notify nurses of mistakes in administration amounts. Nurses must be able to keep up with the latest technologies and, through the Internet, have the ability to find information from all over the world quickly and without difficulty. The Internet has provided opportunities for nurses to learn about interventions and programs that other countries have established to provide better care. Technological advances can also assist nurses in assessing their own health and wellness. Digital technology provides nurses with information at their fingertips such as data on their own blood pressure readings, glucose monitoring, fat analysis, and so forth. This information can be used to make wise lifestyle choices.

NURSING PROCESS AND HEALTH PROMOTION PLANNING

Previous chapters have established that the nursing process is a problem-solving method useful in gathering and interpreting data in order to formulate a plan of care. This same process can be applied in determining a plan of action to address health promotion problems or potential health promotion problems affecting the health care professional. The domains covered throughout the text are useful as the organizing structure for assessing problems and planning interventions for the health care professional at risk. For example, an assessment of the biological domain may reveal physical problems such as peptic ulcers and high blood pressure. Further assessment may also reveal that the professional has been experiencing major work-related stress, exhibits angry behavior, and is having difficulty communicating with coworkers. The nursing process action plan can then address healthy coping skills, anger management, and communication skills.

The nursing process is useful in assessing personal needs and values and helps in the making of decisions that affect long-term career planning. Career planning is not an accident. Having an idea of what is happening on a personal level and in the health care arena is necessary in planning for the future. Identification of strategies that are useful in preventing career-related health problems is essential in promoting healthy behaviors among the health professional workforce. Table 19-2 provides an example of a nursing process plan addressing problem areas that affect health promotion in the health professional.

SUMMARY

Health care professionals are faced with many issues that impact their professional lives. In addition to being confronted with life and death issues in their daily work,

TABLE 19-2 Nursing Process Plan for the Health Professional

Assessment: Lucia is a 49-year-old Mexican American nurse working on an oncology floor. She is constantly stressed out due to the heavy client load. Most days she is responsible for caring for eight seriously ill clients. She is overweight and is always complaining of fatigue and backache.

Nursing Diagnosis(es)	Goals/Outcomes	Interventions
Ineffective coping related to inability to manage work-related stress	Will identify three social support networks	Identify social support networks such as friends, colleagues, organizations. Increase awareness of personal coping skills through use of assessment tools. List alternate ways of coping.
	Will learn how to manage time effectively	Invest in time management course. Engage in exercise. Establish work, play, sleep schedules.
Ineffective coping related to increased food consumption	Increase awareness of unsatisfactory behavior	Maintain journal on thoughts and behavior. Use positive self-talk.
	Identify stressors that increase eating behavior	Examine personal coping skills. Maintain food diary. Reward self for positive outcomes. Increase activity. Use friends for support in weight loss. Do not rationalize.
Risk for injury related to lack of knowledge	Will verbalize physical risks associated with caring for clients	Become aware of physical risks in moving heavy clients. Maintain proper positioning and good posture. Minimize back sprain.

they must adapt to a phenomenal amount of technological change. Health care professionals are impacted by heavy workloads, managed care, and an increasing focus on cost containment and outcomes measurement. Some health care disciplines seem to have bigger demands than other disciplines. The nursing profession, for example, must deal with severe nursing shortages in addition to all the issues confronting health care professionals today. Unless plans are made to focus on personal health promotion, occupational stress, burnout, and job turnover are the consequences that health care professionals will face.

A positive professional life begins in school. Students can take advantage of the many opportunities that will help them have a more satisfying professional future. Being proactive and in charge of one's career is vital. Health care professionals should know the risks

involved in their line of work. Education should include information on work-related risks that affect personal health promotion, finances, retirement benefits, and health insurance. Being professionally healthy means taking responsibility for it, staying open to new opportunities, and seeking these out. Key strategies include having positive relationships and networking with others. The investment on a personal level as well as in terms of career planning is worthwhile. Individuals engaging in careers in the health care professions should know that these careers are both rigorous and demanding. Those who choose these careers have countless opportunities to meet the needs of clients, from womb to tomb. As they respond to the call of those whom they serve, health care professionals must remember to put themselves as the priority. Modeling health and wholeness to others requires personal health promotion skills.

CASE STUDY David Fuentes: Sleep Deprivation; Ineffective Health Maintenance; At Risk for Latex Allergy Response; Imbalanced Nutrition: More Than Body Requirements

Objectives/Goals: Through participation in discussion of this case study, participants will have the opportunity to:

1. Identify specific factors or issues or both that may affect a nursing student.
2. Describe how a nursing student's health promotion practices influence curricular activities and outcomes.
3. Identify strategies for positive health promotion.

Health Promotion Concern, History and Physical, Present Health Status, Past Health Status, Family History, and Social History

David Fuentes is a 40-year-old male from Haiti returning to school for a second career. He is married and has three children, age 12, 14, and 16. He has a degree in business but is returning to attain a BSN and eventually an MSN so that he can assume an administrative role in a health care institution. David is employed at United Parcel Service (UPS) and works evenings, full-time, Monday through Thursday. He is also attending school on all days of the week. On those days that he has clinical lab, he spends eight hours there and then hurries to his evening job. On the other days, he leaves school at 2:00 PM and clocks in to work at 4:00 PM. He returns home at 12:00 midnight and studies until 2:00 every morning. He sleeps approximately 5½ hours each night. David is overweight but states that he rarely sits down for a full meal. His health history is nonremarkable.

Review of Pertinent Domains

Biological Domain

Physical exam reveals a 5'8" male who weighs 200 pounds.

Gastrointestinal: He drinks at least four cola drinks and eats a fast lunch every day. He dislikes vegetables but will eat fruit occasionally. He eats supper whenever he gets home.

Genitourinary: David reports no problems in this area. He has regular bowel movements and urinates with no discomfort.

Integumentary: David has been experiencing a rash on his hands which seems to be getting worse. He is allergic to bananas and some tropical fruits and has a history of a skin reaction to balloons.

Psychological Domain

David is a very intelligent person, but he is making average grades because of his tight schedule, which allows limited time for study. David appears to be exhausted most of the time. His wife reports that he has been slightly depressed. David has trouble staying awake during lectures. He drinks alcohol only during the weekends and not to excess.

Social Domain

David has not been getting along with his family. He becomes very exasperated anytime that he is asked to join in social activities. In addition, even though David is working, he is making considerably less money than he did at his previous job, and he is having problems making ends meet. His wife is having difficulty supporting David emotionally because she is not sure that he should be pursuing a BSN.

Environmental Domain

David has been experiencing a rash on his hands that causes redness and swelling. He thinks that his rash is getting worse. He did not have this problem when he was at his previous job. David thinks that his rash may be stress-related.

Questions for Discussion

1. Describe specific factors that might affect David's school performance.
2. Identify three of David's health behavior patterns that are affecting his health status.
3. Identify strategies that David can use to achieve positive health promotion.

Key Concepts

1. There are many stress-provoking factors that impact the health of those who provide health care to others.

2. Technological change is forcing many health care professionals to return to the academic setting for additional preparation.

3. Job-related stress, burnout, and job turnover are consequences of the enormous responsibility assumed by health care professionals.

4. Students enrolled in health career courses are not immune to some of the same work-related stresses experienced by the health care professional.

5. Nursing supply and demand factors impact professional nursing delivery.

6. Health care professionals are not immune to health problems and must apply their special knowledge and principles to themselves.

7. Back injuries, psychological stress, spiritual distress, needlestick injuries, and latex allergies are health risks associated with the health care disciplines.

8. The nursing process can address health promotion problems and risks affecting health care professionals.

9. Technological changes can affect stress levels in nurses but can also be used to assess negative lifestyle behaviors.

Learning Activities

1. What are some specific factors that impact nursing students?

2. Describe the difference between occupational stress and burnout. Are these two synonymous?

3. List two health risks that confront health care professionals according to domain.

4. Draw your family genogram. Include age, causes of death, any cancer, cardiac conditions, hypertension, overweight, substance abuse, mental illness, chronic illnesses, and other pertinent findings. Refer to Figure 19-3 as a reference. Ask your family for information. There may be issues that your family members may not want to discuss.

5. After completing the genogram, consider the following:
   a. What health changes might be personally necessary?
   b. What new information did you learn?
   c. Did you discover any risk factors for diseases?

6. Read a professional nursing journal (current). Identify technological advances in nursing.

True/False Questions

1. T or F Nurses are more at risk for burnout than are other health care professionals.

2. T or F Occupational stress can lead to physical and emotional symptoms.

3. T or F The nursing shortage is predicted to be more resistant to short-term economic strategies that have worked in the past.

4. T or F The field of ergonomics is of interest to the health care disciplines

5. T or F Latex allergies occur infrequently and are of little concern to health care professionals.

6. T or F Nurses are exposed to chemical risks in the work environment on a daily basis.

Multiple Choice Questions

1. Environmental hazards for nurses in the workplace include:
   a. Ergonomics
   b. Dementia
   c. Musculoskeletal injury
   d. Autonomy

2. All of the following are factors affecting nursing students and the profession accept:
   a. Age
   b. Ethnicity
   c. Genetics
   d. Stress

Websites

http://nursingworld.org ANA Nursing World. Provides information on preventing needlestick injury in practice. This website provides a guide to the types of work-related injuries that occur in the workplace.

References

Ackley, N. L. (2000). Spirituality and the nurse. *Texas Nursing, 74*(1), 6.

Allender, J. A., & Spradley, B. W. (2001). *Community health nursing: Concepts and practice* (5th ed.). Philadelphia: Lippincott.

American Association of Colleges of Nursing (AACN). (2000). The baccalaureate degree in nursing as minimal preparation for professional practice. Retrieved October 26, 2005, from http://www.aacn.nche.edu/Publications/positions/baccmin.htm

American Association of Colleges of Nursing (AACN). (February, 2004a). Nursing fact sheet. Retrieved October 26, 2005, from http://www.aacn.nche.edu/Media/shortageresource

American Association of Colleges of Nursing (AACN). (March, 2004b). Your nursing career: Look at the facts. Retrieved October 26, 2005, from http://www.aacn.nche.edu/Education/nurse_ed/career.htm

American Association of Colleges of Nursing (AACN). (2005). Nursing shortage. Retrieved October 26, 2005, from http://www.aacn.nche.edu/Media/Factsheets/Nursingshortage.htm

American Nurses Association. (2003). Position statement on elimination of manual patient handling to prevent work-related musculoskeletal disorders. Retrieved October 26, 2005, from http://www.nursingworld.org/readroom/position/workplace.htm

Bain, E. I. (2000). Assessing for occupational hazards. *American Journal of Nursing, 100*(1), 96.

Black, J. M., & Hawks, J. H. (2005). Medical-surgical nursing: Clinical management for positive outcomes. St Louis: Elsevier-Saunders.

Buerhaus, P. I. (2005). Six-part series on the state of the RN workforce in the United States. *Nursing Economics, 23*(2), 58–60.

Buerhaus, P. I., Donelan, K., Ulrich, B. T., Kirby, L., Norman, L., & Dittus, R. (2005). Registered nurses' perceptions of nursing. *Nursing Economics, 23*(3), 110–118.

Chang, E., & Hancock, K. (2003). Role stress and role ambiguity in new nursing graduates in Australia. *Nursing and Health Sciences, 5,* 155–163.

Christman, L. (1998). Who is a nurse? *Image: The Journal of Nursing Scholarship, 30*(3), 211–214.

Cohen-Katz, J., Wiley, S. D., Capuano, T., Baker, D., & Shapiro, S. (2004). The effects of mindfulness-based stress reduction on nurse stress and burnout. *Holistic Nursing Practice, 18*(6), 302–308.

Dossey, B., Keegan, L., & Guzetta, C. (2000). *Holistic nursing: A handbook for practice* (3rd ed.). Gaithersburg, MD: Aspen Publications.

Egglefield-Beaudoin, L, & Edgar, L. (2003). Hassles: Their importance to quality of nurses' work life. *Nursing Economics, 2*(3), 106–113.

Ekstedt, M., & Fagerbert, I. (2005). Lived experiences of the time preceding burnout. *Journal of Advanced Nursing, 49*(1), 59–67.

Foley, M. (2004). Caring for those who care: A tribute to nurses and their safety. *Online Journal of Issues in Nursing, 9*(3), Manuscript 1. Retrieved January 4, 2007, from http://www.nursingworld.org/ojin

Frankl, V. (1978). *Man's search for meaning.* New York: Beacon Press.

Friese, C. R. (2005). Nurse practice environments and outcomes: Implications for oncology nursing. *Oncology Nursing Forum, 32*(4), 765–772.

Gillespie, M., & Melby, V. (2003). Burnout among nursing staff in accident and emergency and acute medicine: A comparative study. *Journal of Clinical Nursing, 12,* 842–851.

Greenwood, J. (2000). Critique of the graduate nurse: An international perspective. *Nursing Education Today, 20,* 17–23.

Health Resources and Services Administration. (2001). *The registered nurse population: March 2000 findings from the national sample survey of registered nurses.* Rockville, MD: U.S. Department of Health and Human Services.

Heller, B. R., Oros, M. T., & Durney-Crowley, J. (2000). The future of nursing education: Ten trends to watch. *Nursing and Health Care Perspectives, 21*(1), 9–13.

Hess, A. K. (2005). Health and safety: Ensure a long and safe career. *American Journal of Nursing, 105*(6), 96.

Huerta, C. (1990). *The relationship between life change events and academic achievement in registered nursing education students.* Unpublished doctoral dissertation, Texas A&M University.

Layne, C. M., Hohenshil, T. H., & Singh, K. (2004). The relationship of occupational stress, psychological strain, and coping resources to the turnover intentions of rehabilitation counselors. *Rehabilitation Counseling Bulletin, 48*(1): 19–30, 59–60.

Lindike, L., & Sieckert, A. (2005). Nurse-physician workplace collaboration. *Online Journal of Issues in Nursing, 10*(1). Retrieved March 9, 2006, from http://nursingworld.org/ojin

Maslow, A. (1970). *Motivation and personality.* New York: Harper & Row.

McPhaul, K. M., & Lipscomb, J. A. (2004). Workplace violence in health care: Recognized but not regulated. *Online Journal of Issues in Nursing, 9*(3). Retrieved September 12, 2005, from http://nursingworld.org/ojin

McVicar, A. (2003). Workplace stress in nursing: A literature review. *Journal of Advanced Nursing, 44*(6), 633–642.

Miklancie, M. (2001). *The spiritual lived experience of nurse educators within the context of their teaching practice.* Unpublished doctoral dissertation, George Mason University.

Milstein, J. M., Gerstenberger, A. E., & Barton, S. (2002). Healing the caregiver. *Journal of Alternative and Complementary Medicine, 8*(6), 917–920.

Nawar, M. (2000). Back me up! Stop injuries now! *The American Nurse.* January/February, 32(1), 22.

Nicholls, H., & Timmins, F. (2005). Programme-related stressors among part-time undergraduate nursing students. *Journal of Advanced Nursing, 50*(1), 93–100.

NANDA (2007). *Nursing diagnoses: Definitions and classifications, 2007–2008.* Philadelphia: NANDA International.

Reineck, C., & Furino, A. (2005). Nursing career fulfillment: Statistics and statements from registered nurses. *Nursing Economics, 23*(1), 25–30.

Rosenstein, A. H. (2005). Disruptive behavior and clinical outcomes: Perceptions of nurses and physicians. *Nursing Management, 36*(1), 18–29.

Shinn, L. J., Milholland, K., Ballard, K., Gould, E. J., Brunt, B. A, & Schaag, H. A. (2002). *The nursing risk management series.* ANA Continuing Education. Retrieved March 9, 2006, from http://nursingworld.org

Stacciarini, J. R., & Tróccoli, B. T. (2004). Occupational stress and constructive thinking: Health and job satisfaction. *Journal of Advanced Nursing, 46*(5), 480–487.

Sullivan Commission. (2004). *Missing persons: Minorities in the health professions.* A Report of the Sullivan Commission on Diversity in the Healthcare Workforce. Retrieved October 31, 2005, from http://www.aacn.nche.edu/Media/pdf/SullivanReport.pdf

Tinsley, C., & France, N. E. (2004). The trajectory of the registered nurse's exodus from the profession: A phenomenological study of the lived experience of oppression. *International Journal for Human Caring, 8*(1), 8–12.

U.S. Department of Health and Human Services (USDHHS). (2000). *The Registered Nurse Population.* Retrieved January 4, 2007, from http://bhpr.hrsa.gov/healthworkforce/reports/rnsurvey/default.htm

Bibliography

AbuAlRub, R. F. (2004). Job stress, job performance, and social support among hospital nurses. *Journal of Nursing Scholarship, 36*(1), 73–78.

Blais, K. K., Hayes, J. S., & Kozier, B. (2005). *Professional nursing practice: Concepts and perspectives* (5th ed.). Upper Saddle River, NJ: Pearson Prentice Hall.

Institute of Medicine. (2004). Crossing the quality chasm: A new health system for the 21st century. Retrieved from http://iom.edu

Jenkins, R., & Elliott, P. (2004). Stressors, burnout, and social support: Nurses in acute mental health settings. *Journal of Advanced Nursing, 48*(6), 622–631.

Leddy, S. K. (2006). *Health promotion: Mobilizing strengths to enhance health, wellness, and well-being.* Philadelphia: F. A. Davis.

Pinikahana, J., & Happell, B. (2004). Stress burnout and job satisfaction in rural psychiatric nurses: A Victorian study. *Austrian Journal of Rural Health, 12*(3): 120.

Chapter 20

ECONOMIC AND QUALITY CONCERNS

Diane Frazor, EdD, MSN, RN
Debra Otto, DM, RNP

KEY TERMS

capitation

diagnosis-related groups (DRGs)

exclusive provider organization (EPO)

health maintenance organization (HMO)

managed care

managed care organization

preferred provider organization (PPO)

primary care providers

prospective payment system (PPS)

OBJECTIVES

Upon completion of this chapter, the reader should be able to:

- Describe the changes that affect the cost and quality of health care today.
- Describe the factors influencing increases in health care costs.
- Describe efforts made by health-care–conscious organizations, the government, and consumers to control health care costs.
- Define managed care.
- Define the different types of managed care organizations.
- Discuss the nurse's role in managed care.
- Identify measures indicative of a quality managed care organization.
- Describe some of the functions of the National Committee for Quality Assurance.
- Describe how national standards and nursing quality issues are affected by managed care.
- Describe how the concept of health promotion relates to managed care and health care costs.

INTRODUCTION

Over the last several years the health care system in the United States has seen some dramatic changes in the way reimbursement for delivery of services occurs. In the past, health care costs were reimbursed to providers as fee for service through the client's Medicare or Medicaid service, indemnity insurance plan, or other pay-ment options as arranged by the client and provider. Traditional fee-for-service health care has gradually become less prevalent as cost-saving health care options such as managed care have become the norm. Managed care health insurance has become the most common type of health insurance coverage in the United States. With health care costs almost constantly on the rise, managed care health insurance has offered a more affordable option to traditional fee-for-service plans (Health Insurance In-depth, 2005).

Chapters 1 and 3 defined and described the concept of health promotion. This chapter will focus on how health promotion and health care costs relate to economic as well as quality issues. Factors that have driven health care costs upward will also be described. Managed care will be introduced as a method to curtail health care costs.

FACTORS DRIVING COSTS UP

Many factors are contributing to an increase in health care costs. Box 20-1 presents an overview of factors affecting health care costs. One of the greatest factors contributing to the rise in health care costs is hospital spending. This is attributable in part to higher prices being paid for hospital services and a recent surge in hospital wage rates. Hospital organizations have regained a sizable amount of negotiating leverage over health plans and have used this leverage to demand large rate increases. Spending on hospital services increased by 12 percent in 2001, reflecting increases in both hospital payment rates and use of hospital services. Hospital spending accounted for more than half of the total increase, making it the key driver of overall cost growth (Strunk, Ginsburg, & Gabel, 2002).

Changing economic conditions are also contributing to the rise in health care costs. Softer labor markets, increasing unemployment rates, and lower profit margins spur employers to control their company's rising health insurance premium expenses through insurance buy-down programs that reduce employee benefits and increase employee cost sharing. "The large benefit buy-down in 2002 was driven by two cost-sharing changes in particular: a large increase in in-network Preferred Provider Organization (PPO) deductibles, and increases in drug co-payment amounts" (Strunk, Ginsburg, & Gabel, 2002, p. 307).

Third, the health insurance industry continues to contribute to the rise in health care costs through unprecedented profits. Though cyclical in nature, this phase of the underwriting cycle reflects the restoration and solidification of the industry's profitability rather than the gaining of market share. "During the past few years the health insurance underwriting cycle, along with underlying cost trends, has played an important role in premium increases. Strong profitability reflects insurers' continuing ability to raise prices more rapidly than their costs are rising" (Strunk, Ginsburg, & Gabel, 2002, p. 307).

Fourth, gatekeeping, the most important effect of the managed care revolution, is diminishing, thereby contributing to the rise in health care costs. The most recent health care cost data provide concrete evidence that managed care's ability to constrain payment rates for the use of hospital services has decreased. According to the most recent trends in private health care, costs are back to where they were before managed care began to dominate the health insurance landscape (Strunk, Ginsburg, & Gabel, 2002).

The role of the consumer continues to impact the cost of health care. "For the past three decades, cost containment, control, efficiency, and reduction efforts have remained at the forefront of health care policy, overshadowing innovation, quality, and safety concerns" (Robbins & Brill, 2005, p. 1). Despite such detours, there is a movement away from denial-based mentalities to consumer-driven health care (CDH). As consumers become more participative in their care, providers must be truly interested in cultivating CDH by providing the consumer with the knowledge and ability to make more discriminating choices (Robbins & Brill, 2005).

The sixth factor escalating health care costs is the medical care provided to those individuals who are uninsured. "With the number of uninsured people exceeding forty-one million in 2001, insuring the uninsured is again a major policy issue" (Hadley & Holahan, 2003, p. 1). According to recent estimates, people who were uninsured during the year 2001 received $98.9 billion in care, of which $34.5 billion was uncompensated. Funding sources such as Medicare and Medicaid make a substantial contribution to support hospitals that treat poor and uninsured clients. Such government spending

Ask Yourself

Consumer Utilization of Health Care Benefits

How many people do you know who because they carry health care insurance go see their health care provider for a minor ailment that requires no treatment? Do you have health care insurance? Do you see your provider for minor ailments too? Does overutilization of health care impact health care cost?

BOX 20-1 Factors Affecting Health Care Costs

- Rise in hospital spending
- Changing economic conditions
- Unprecedented health insurance industry profits
- Managed care's inability to constrain payment rates for hospital-based care
- The role of the consumer
- Individuals who are uninsured
- Lawsuits

Adapted from "Tracking Health Care Costs: Growth Accelerates Again in 2001," by B. C. Strunk, P. B. Ginsburg, and J. R. Gabel, 2002, Health Affairs Web Exclusive, 299–310; "Blending Ethics and Empowerment with Consumer-Driven Healthcare," by D. Robbins and J. Brill, 2005, Patient Safety and Quality Healthcare, May/June; and "How Much Medical Care Do the Uninsured Use, and Who Pays for It?" by J. Hadley and J. Holahan, 2003, Health Affairs Web Executive, 66–81.

estimates are between $6.2 billion and $6.9 billion a year (Hadley & Holahan, 2003).

The seventh and last factor is the increase in lawsuits, which has had a dramatic effect on the cost as well as the accessibility of health care. Every time health care professionals are sued, their liability insurance rates increase, which, in turn, requires them to charge higher rates for their services to cover that cost. Some physicians actually eliminate services for high-risk conditions, such as obstetrics or emergency care, to avoid being sued and having to pay higher insurance premiums or, even worse, losing their medical licenses. Any time an insurance company has to pay to defend its client, whether the client wins or loses, the company will pass the cost on to the client (physician) in the form of increased insurance premiums.

EFFORTS TO CONTROL COSTS

Several attempts to help control costs for health care have been implemented. The following sections will describe the effects of the Medicare/Medicaid programs and the prospective payment system on health care costs. Efforts by consumers of health care services and by nurses will be addressed as well.

Medicare and Medicaid

As described in Chapter 1, the U.S. government created the Medicare and Medicaid programs in an effort to assist in payment of health care costs for the elderly, the chronically ill, children, and the poor. The effects of the Medicaid and Medicare programs on health care costs and health care reforms, and their subsequent effects on the advancement of health promotion, are profound. For example, national health spending is projected to grow at an average annual rate of 7.3 percent, reaching $3.1 trillion by 2012. This increase would bring health care spending to approximately 17.7 percent of gross domestic product (GDP) by 2012, up from its 2001 share of 14.1 percent. Over the entire projection period, national health spending growth is still expected to outpace economic growth (Heffler, et al., 2003). Table 20-1 presents an overview of Medicare and Medicaid programs with a look at expenditures over the past 38 years. As can be seen in the table, the participant costs and state and federal costs continue to rise.

Access to Health Care

Although the Medicare and Medicaid programs were created by the U.S. government to assist children, the chronically ill, the poor, and the elderly with health care costs, there have been reductions in benefits, and this, coupled with the escalating costs of health care, has exacerbated the difficulties faced by these vulnerable populations in accessing care. The elderly, for example, have seen some of their health care benefits sharply reduced. Medicare, the nation's largest health insurer, does not cover all prescription drugs. The elderly frequently face problems with drug access due to affordability. Many elderly live on limited incomes, which may impact their health care. Research has found that some of the elderly tend to ration their medications, substitute

TABLE 20-1 Overview of Medicare and Medicaid

	Medicare	Medicaid
Provisions	Hospital (Part A) and medical insurance (Part B)	Shared federal and state funding to assist states in paying for health care services for the needy
Funded by	Federal government	Federal and state governments
Administered by	Federal government	State government
Eligibility	Over age 65, disabled receiving Social Security benefits, end stage renal disease patients	Poor, medically needy, aged, disabled, and their dependent children and families
1967 participant costs	Part A—$40 deductible Part B—$50/year, $3/month	None
2006 participant costs	Part A—$39.95/month, $952 deductible Part B—$88.50/month, $124 deductible Part D—$32/month, $250 deductible + payment schedule	Minimal to none depending on state
1967 state and federal costs	$5 billion	$2.3 billion

2006 baseline projections for Medicare/Medicaid			
2008	$361 billion	**2010**	$419 billion

From Center for Medicaid and Medicare Services, U.S. Department of Health and Human Services, 2006, retrieved May 31, 2006, from http://www.cms.hhs.gov.

medications, and sometimes postpone treatment (Xu, Scott, & Borders, 2003). Results of a recent study show that the average price of dozens of brand-name prescription drugs used by the elderly has risen more than twice as fast as general inflation. A study funded by the Kaiser Family Foundation and the Commonwealth Fund found that 25 percent of the elderly who responded to a survey stated that they were forgoing taking any medications because of cost (http://www.therubins.com). Health care cost must obviously be taken into consideration when determining a health promotion plan for the elderly.

Children, however, have fared better when it comes to accessing adequate health care. Legislation passed by Congress in 1997 builds on the Medicaid program that started covering children over four decades ago. The Child Health Insurance Program (CHIP) is a Medicaid program designed to cover health care costs of children living in poverty. Under federal law, all states must cover children up to the age of 6 if their family earns up to 133 percent of the federal poverty level (FPL) and children 6 and older born after September 30, 1983, with family incomes at or under 100 percent of FPL (U.S. Department of Health and Human Services, 2006). Although there have been recent attempts by the federal government to cut CHIPs, every state in the nation now has a health insurance program for infants, children, and teens. Even individuals with a variety of immigration statuses are eligible. For little or no cost, the CHIP pays for doctor visits, prescription drugs, and hospitalizations. Most states also cover the cost of dental care, eye care, and medical equipment (USDHHS, 2006).

Prospective Payment System

In the early 1980s, health care costs were speeding out of control despite past containment efforts. As a result, Congress responded with a Social Security Amendment that, beginning in October 1983, changed Medicare's cost-based, or retrospective, method of paying for hospital health care to a **prospective payment system (PPS).**

The PPS was a method of payment to hospitals based on the concept that similar medical diagnoses result in the same hospitalization costs. Consequently, a fixed predetermined payment was allowed according to the classification of the client's diagnosis (American Hospital Directory, 2005). The diagnosis classification system used with the PPS was identified as **diagnosis-related groups (DRGs)** and contained 468 diagnoses. Hospitals were forced to control client costs in order to remain within the reimbursement allowance according to DRGs. Reimbursement to physicians was, in turn, affected as hospital administrators scrambled to curb costs at every angle, including human resources, procedures, equipment, supplies, and construction.

The PPS helped somewhat to contain health care costs for the Medicare client because administrators began to cut costs by decreasing the length of time a client

Spotlight On

Cost Containment with the Prospective Payment System

With the PPS, a client is admitted to the hospital and treated for a diagnosis of pneumonia. According to the PPS, the hospital would be reimbursed for that client based on a preset fee for that diagnosis, regardless of how much money the hospital spent on the client. If the hospital spent more than the reimbursement amount, then the hospital would lose that money. How could this have been avoided? What role does the nurse have in controlling costs in the hospital? If this were a recurrent problem, how do you think the hospital would respond to it?

stayed in the hospital so that they would not exceed their reimbursement according to the prospective payment. Many private-pay insurers followed in the government's footsteps and began by reimbursing care providers more on the diagnosis of the client, thus developing a standard reimbursement for different types of health care services.

Even with these changes in reimbursement, health care costs have continued to rise. For this very reason the United States has seen some remarkable changes in the health care system, from how it is organized to how it is financed (Bazzoli, Dyanan, Burns, & Yap, 2004). Some of these changes include the development of health maintenance organizations and managed care organizations, discussed later in the chapter.

CONSUMER EFFORTS IN COST CONTAINMENT

Because the rising cost of health care has created a major problem that affects many major facets of our society, it is essential that the consumer as well as the health care professional become involved in efforts to contain cost. Solutions to the rising costs of health care are not easy, but there are several factors that consumers can control. One of these is to investigate or shop around for quality health care at the lowest cost. Health care providers are involved in the business of making people well and like any other major business, competition exists among the providers. For example, eye examination cost varies depending on whether the eye care provider is self-employed or works for a major discount store. The difference in cost may be significant.

Frivolous lawsuits drive up the costs of health care, since even unmerited lawsuits require that the health care provider employ a defense team. The defense costs

Ask Yourself

Nurses and the Consumer

Do you think that nurses should play an active role in encouraging health care consumers to investigate the costs of different health care services prior to choosing them? Or is it not our place to interfere with consumer health care unless it directly involves delivery of nursing care? Do you as a consumer of health care "shop around" for your health care plan?

are passed on to the consumers through increased health care costs and insurance premiums. After all, someone has to pay for the time and effort required to settle the lawsuit. Thus consumers must become educated about frivolous lawsuits.

Although the concepts of health promotion and disease prevention are not new and certainly have been discussed in this textbook, many times health promotion efforts are overlooked as potential solutions to decreasing the cost of health care. Health-promoting behaviors must be encouraged in order for individuals to avoid entry into the health care delivery system where treatment of a disease or illness can become costly.

MANAGED CARE

In 1973 the Health Maintenance Organization Act was passed providing federal funding for health maintenance organizations (HMOs) that followed the federal regulations, which were stricter than the state regulations. The HMO Act also required large organizations to provide an HMO for their employees as a health care option. The establishment of HMOs led to the development of the concept called managed care. **Managed care** is a method of delivering health care that integrates and coordinates the delivery of health care with the costs of that service (Strunk, Ginsburg, & Gabel, 2002). A **managed care organization** is a health plan that provides consumers access to quality health care at what is considered a reasonable cost by determined health care cost standards. These types of health plans usually rely on **primary care providers,** who are health care providers that the client sees first for health care services. Primary care providers are physicians, predominantly family practice physicians. The primary care provider acts as a gatekeeper for the consumer's health care and prevents the use of unnecessary or inappropriate health care services, thus resulting in less expensive treatments or interventions (Health Insurance In-depth, 2005).

Managed care's focus is to provide the consumer with services that will emphasize health promotion and prevention through the primary care provider (American

Nurses Association, 2005). By encouraging participants in the health plan to participate in health promotion and prevention activities, the organization saves monies that would have been spent to treat preventable illnesses. An example of this would be encouraging clients to exercise regularly because they will decrease their weight and cholesterol level and, therefore, decrease their chances of developing heart disease later in life. This, in turn, will save the consumer's health plan from spending large amounts of money treating its client who has developed heart disease.

There are several types of organizations that deliver managed care. The major ones are the health maintenance organization, the preferred provider organization, and the exclusive provider organization. These types of managed care organizations are described in Table 20-2 and are briefly discussed in the following sections.

Health Maintenance Organization

A **health maintenance organization (HMO)** is one type of managed care service that provides health care to members for a fixed, usually monthly, payment (Health Insurance In-depth, 2005). HMO organizations can be either nonprofit or for profit. They have a fixed monthly payment that may or may not be part of a benefit package offered by employers. HMOs are very active on the prevention side of medicine. Because of their emphasis on disease prevention, disease risk reduction, and self-care by the client, HMOs fit in nicely with the concept of health promotion as described in previous chapters.

Preferred Provider Organization

Another type of managed care service is the **preferred provider organization (PPO),** which uses provider networks to deliver health care to its members (Health Insurance In-depth, 2005). A PPO plan includes preferred health care institutions such as hospitals, preferred provider physicians, insurers, and employers. Individuals enrolled in a PPO may only use providers within the network. PPOs do not require going through a primary care physician as a gatekeeper to obtain services from specialists or other caregivers. The health care providers who meet the qualifications of the PPO are paid discounted fees for being part of that PPO. Charges to the consumer cannot exceed those set by the PPO (Health Insurance In-depth, 2005).

Exclusive Provider Organization

The **exclusive provider organization (EPO)** is a plan that requires its members to get their services within that particular network only (Health Insurance In-depth, 2005). The participants usually must select a primary care physician and a hospital that they will use exclusively. The primary incentive is that little or no copayment is required when the exclusive provider network is

TABLE 20-2 Types of Managed Care Organizations

Health Maintenance Organization (HMO)	Preferred Provider Organization (PPO)	Exclusive Provider Organization (EPO)	Capitation
Has a fixed, usually monthly payment	Members may only use providers within the network	Members must get all services within the network	Fixed payment to provide all reasonable and necessary medical services required by plan members
Can be for profit or nonprofit	Providers are paid discounted fees	Participants must choose a primary care physician	Fixed payment per member per month charged to employer or insurance carrier
Is active in the prevention side of health care	Usually does not have a primary care physician as a gatekeeper	Primary care physician may refer to other physicians in the network	Health care organization must maintain some control of physician-generated utilization
Promotes wellness		Only care allowed outside of the network is emergency care	Primary care provider is gatekeeper

used (Health Insurance In-depth, 2005). The primary care physician may refer to other physicians in the network if deemed necessary. The only care allowed outside of the network is emergency care.

Capitation

Capitation is another, and relatively new, type of health care plan that is becoming popular. With capitation, the employer or insurer will pay a provider a set fee for all the medical expenses necessary for each member covered under that plan. This provider may be a hospital that provides all the health care services to the insured. In order to be profitable the hospital needs to provide care for less than the set fee. Otherwise the hospital will lose money (Health Insurance In-depth, 2005).

The hospital and health care providers must work cooperatively to keep health care costs down or the capitation plan will not work. This requires less hospitalization for the plan members. The hospital's goal will no longer be to fill beds, but to keep them empty. The hospital must also develop practice guidelines for the physician to follow so that the physicians maintain controlled utilization. Again, the primary care physician will operate as a gatekeeper in keeping these costs down and ensuring that the care given is quality care. Capitation hospitals succeed more often if the physicians profit by cutting costs. This may involve having the physician be a partner in the capitation plan.

NURSING'S ROLE IN MANAGED CARE

In today's world of changing health care delivery, managed care, and capitation, the nursing profession will need to change its way of delivering services just as have hospitals and health care providers. Nursing needs to start thinking of health care delivery from a business perspective just as hospitals and health care providers have had to do. The nursing profession needs to understand the concepts of managed care and be able to learn new tasks and procedures to make it successful (Burns, 2005).

Nurses need to be involved in decision making about how to cut costs and still deliver quality client care and ensure client satisfaction (Burns, 2005). Critical thinking and decision-making skills will be increasingly important in the delivery of quality managed care. As illustrated in Figure 20-1, health care reform measures to control costs and meet the health care needs of the nation have implications for both consumers and the profession of nursing.

Because these measures affect the health care provider's financial gains, there is considerable competition for consumers. Consumers, in most cases the employers of the consumers, thus are in a better position to choose the managed care plan that is most reasonable cost-wise but yet provides the assurance of quality health care. Expanded primary care services reduce health care costs and increase quality of care.

The effects of managed care and health care reforms affect nursing practice in a very fundamental manner. The nursing profession's philosophy has changed over time in response to some of the health care reform measures. For example, nursing has evolved from a profession focused on treating illness to one that emphasizes disease prevention, holistic care, and health promotion through client empowerment.

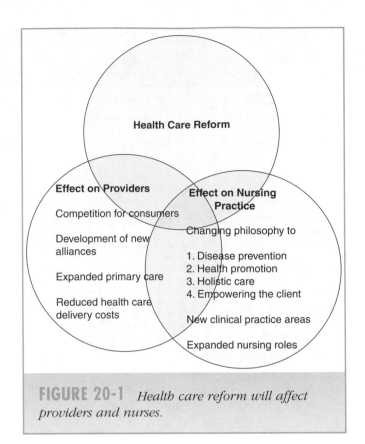

FIGURE 20-1 *Health care reform will affect providers and nurses.*

QUALITY MEASURES AND MANAGED CARE

Providers who are delivering health care today are practicing in a time when quality health care must be delivered at a reasonable cost. Controlling costs has resulted in decreased resources, both technical and human. With such reductions, a way of measuring the quality of care being delivered needed to be implemented. It was determined that utilizing an accreditation process was an appropriate way to determine whether the managed care organization was abiding by a set of quality standards. (Agency for Healthcare Research and Quality, 2005). Two regulatory agencies were selected as being responsible for measuring the quality of health care in managed care organizations. They are the National Committee for Quality Assurance (NCQA) and the Joint Commission (JC), formerly known as the Joint Commission on Accreditation of Healthcare Organizations (JCAHO).

National Committee for Quality Assurance (NCQA)

The NCQA is a private, not-for-profit organization dedicated to assessing and reporting on the quality of managed care plans. The NCQA provides information to purchasers and consumers of managed health care that enables them to distinguish among plans based on quality, thereby allowing them to make more informed health care purchasing decisions. Accreditation by the NCQA is required by most businesses and organizations

that purchase managed care plans (National Committee for Quality Assurance, 2005).

Some of the areas evaluated by the NCQA include quality improvement programs, clinical practice guidelines, clinical measurement activities, and intervention and follow-up for clinical issues. Data are collected through a set of standardized performance indicators led by the Health Plan Employer Data and Information Set and also through employer and business mandates (National Committee for Quality Assurance, 2005).

The Joint Commission (JC)

The Joint Commission (JC) is an independent, not-for-profit organization, established more than 50 years ago. The JC is governed by a board that includes physicians, nurses, and consumers. The JC sets the standards by which health care quality is measured in America and around the world. The JC evaluates the quality and safety of care for more than 15,000 health care organizations. To earn and maintain accreditation, organizations must have an extensive on-site review by a team of JC health care professionals at least once every three years. The purpose of the review is to evaluate the organization's performance in areas that affect client care. Accreditation may then be awarded based on how well the organization meets JC standards. During the evaluation phase, the JC is measuring the organization's improvement in areas such as rights and responsibilities of clients, continuum of care, education, communication, health promotion and disease prevention, leadership and management, management of information, and improving network performance (Joint Commission on Accreditation of Healthcare Organizations, 2005).

NATIONAL STANDARDS AND MANAGED CARE

In the past, consumer groups and HMOs have requested that the federal government develop national standards to guide managed care plans. Ideally these standards would replace the individual states' regulations, which have not provided the structure desired by the American health care consumer. Rather than incur the cost and time constraints required in developing national standards, not-for-profit organizations such as the NCQA have been encouraged to develop nationally recognized standards called the Health Plan Employer Data and Information Set (HEDIS). HEDIS is a set of standardized performance measures designed to ensure that purchasers and consumers have the information they need to reliably compare the performance of managed health care plans. The performance measures in HEDIS are related to many significant public health issues such as cancer, heart disease, smoking, asthma, and diabetes. HEDIS also includes a standardized survey of consumers' experiences that evaluates plan performance in areas such as customer service, access to care, and claims processing (National Committee for Quality Assurance, 2005).

Nursing Quality Issues

The nursing profession continues to express concern over the state of health care reform and quality of care. The American Nurses Association's (ANA) Health Care Agenda 2005 states that the U.S. health care system remains in a state of crisis. At this time, the number of uninsured continues to increase, the cost of care continues to rise, and the safety and quality of care continue to be questioned. The ANA remains committed to the following five basic principles:

1. Health care is a basic right, and universal access should be assured to a standard package of health care services for all citizens and residents.

2. The ANA believes the development and implementation of health policies that reflect safe and effective, patient-centered, timely, efficient, and equitable service that is based on outcomes research will ultimately save health care dollars.

3. The current health care system must be redirected away from the overuse of expensive acute hospital-based services to one in which a balance is achieved between high-cost treatments and community-based preventive services.

4. The ANA supports a single payer model as the most desirable option to reform health care at this time.

5. For health care delivery to be safe, effective, fair, and affordable, there must be an adequate supply of well-educated, well-distributed, and well utilized registered nurses (American Nurses Association, 2005).

Research Note

Relationship Between Knowledge of Insurance Coverage and Compliance

Study Problem/Purpose: To determine if gaps in knowledge regarding drug coverage and medication costs exist in older adults and whether this lack of knowledge leads to medication noncompliance. Lack of knowledge regarding health care insurance coverage may be a cause for older adults to be noncompliant with their medications and health care follow-up.

Methods: This study was conducted via the Internet. A nationwide cross-sectional survey was sent to adults age 50 and over who had prescription drug coverage and at least one chronic illness. A total of 3,118 adults responded to questions regarding features of their drug benefits and whether they had experienced problems due to medication costs in the prior year.

Findings: Twenty-five percent of respondents reported not knowing their usual prescription insurance co-payments and 41 percent did not know if there were cost caps on their drug coverage. Lack of knowledge regarding insurance coverage was associated with a greater likelihood of cutting back on medication use and forgoing basic health care needs.

Implications: Many older adults with prescription coverage do not know the important features of their insurance benefits. Racial minorities and those with low incomes have greater difficulty understanding insurance coverage. Efforts to educate older adults regarding health insurance coverage will improve compliance.

Piette, J. D., and Heisler, M. (2006). The relationship between older adults' knowledge of their drug coverage and medication cost problems. *Journal of the American Geriatrics Society, 54*(1), 91-96.

HEALTH PROMOTION, HEALTH CARE COST, AND MANAGED CARE

Because the U.S. health care system continues to be in such a state of crisis, the overwhelming problems require significant attention on the part of health professionals, policy makers, and the public (American Nurses Association, 2005). Nurses hold the pivotal role of health care advocate for individuals and families. They are on the forefront of health care through their ability to help clients learn health promotion and prevention of disease through education, leadership, and example. By utilizing health promotion concepts, nurses empower their clients to adopt healthier lifestyles that may also focus on cost containment from the client's point of view.

SUMMARY

This chapter has focused on how the delivery of health care is in a constant and rapid state of change. It is hoped that these changes will positively affect our rising health care costs in the United States. Many factors are contributing to an increase in health care costs. These factors include the rise in hospital spending, changing economic conditions, unprecedented health insurance industry profits, managed care's inability to constrain payment rates for hospital-based care, the role of the consumer, and individuals who are uninsured. These factors continue to drain limited health care resource dollars.

Efforts to control escalating costs have evolved to the current concept of managed care by managed care organizations. Some types of managed care systems such as health maintenance organizations emphasize health promotion and wellness in an effort to contain costs. Health promotion and disease prevention are very important measures that consumers of health care can use to affect rising costs. Even those individuals who already have illnesses can learn how to promote the optimal health attainable for them and prevent disease progression or development of related illnesses.

The nursing profession has experienced many changes with the implementation of managed care systems. Nurses have expressed dissatisfaction with the current system of client care. It is the nursing profession's responsibility to ensure quality client care. One way is for nurses to empower clients to take control of their own care and adopt health-promoting behaviors. Learning health promotion concepts and principles through nursing education is as important to clients as any other skill.

Key Concepts

1. Health care costs in the United States have continued to spiral and changes are occurring to stop this trend.

2. The rise in hospital spending, changing economic conditions, unprecedented health insurance industry profits, managed care's inability to constrain payment rates for hospital-based care, the role of the consumer, and individuals who are uninsured are all factors that contribute to the increases in healthcare costs.

3. Managed care is a method of delivering health care that integrates and coordinates the delivery of service and the costs to the consumer.

4. HMOs, PPOs, and EPOs are types of managed care organizations.

5. The regulatory agencies responsible for measuring quality in managed care organizations are the NCQA and the JC.

6. Some of the areas evaluated by the NCQA include quality improvement programs, clinical practice guidelines, clinical measurement activities, and intervention and follow-up for clinical issues.

7. The five basic principles of the 2005 ANA Health Care Agenda are: (1) health care is a basic right; (2) the development and implementation of health policies that reflect safe and effective patient-centered care will ultimately save health care dollars; (3) a balance must be achieved between high-cost treatments and community-based preventive services; (4) a single payer model is desirable for current health care reform; and (5) in order for health care delivery to be safe, effective, fair, and affordable, there must be

an adequate supply of well-educated, well-distributed, and well-utilized registered nurses.

8. By empowering clients to adopt health promotion lifestyles, nurses can focus on cost containment from the client's perspective.

Learning Activities

1. List the factors that contribute to the increase in health care costs.

2. Define the three types of managed care organizations: HMOs, PPOs, and EPOs.

3. List the five basic principles of the 2005 ANA Health Care Agenda.

True/False Questions

1. T or F   The prospective payment system was developed by the federal government.

2. T or F   Nursing cannot affect the increase in health care cost.

3. T or F   Managed care organizations usually rely on a primary care physician to be the gatekeeper.

4. T or F   Managed care has just begun developing in the last couple of years.

5. T or F   There are federal guidelines regulating managed care organizations.

Multiple Choice

1. Factors affecting health care costs include all of the following except:
   a. Changing economic conditions
   b. Increased number of insured individuals
   c. Increased hospital expenditures
   d. Lawsuits

2. A managed care organization:
   a. Emphasizes treatment, not prevention
   b. Increases health care costs by the consumer
   c. Is maintained through federal funding
   d. Provides consumers with access to quality care

3. The Joint Commission is an independent, not-for-profit organization that:
   a. Evaluates the quality of care provided by all public health agencies in the United States and the world
   b. Exclusively focuses on the rights and responsibilities of health care professionals

c. Provides leadership training for professionals in the health care arena

d. sets standards by which health care quality is measured

Websites

http://www.nln.org National League for Nursing. Provides information that prepares the nursing workforce to meet the needs of diverse populations in an ever-changing health care environment.

http://www.uhcan.org/ Universal Health Care Action Network. Provides information on the national campaign for affordable health care for all.

http://www.iccr.org/ Interfaith Center on Corporate Responsibility. Includes information on access to health and wellness for all.

Organizations

Administration On Aging (AOA)
One Massachusetts Avenue
Suites 4100 and 5100
Washington, DC 20201
Tel: (202) 619-0724

Agency in the U.S. Department of Health and Human Services that is one of the nation's largest providers of home- and community-based care for older persons and their caregivers. AOA's mission is to develop a comprehensive, coordinated, and cost-effective system of long-term care that helps elderly individuals to maintain their dignity in their homes and communities.

U.S. Department of Health and Human Services
200 Independence Avenue SW
Washington, DC 20201
Tel: (202) 619-0257; (877) 696-6775

The principal government agency for protecting the health of all Americans and for providing essential human services, especially for those least able to help themselves. The department includes more than 300 programs, covering a wide spectrum of activities.

The Joint Commission
601 13th Street, NW
Suite 1150N
Washington, DC 20005
Tel: (202) 783-6655
Fax: (202) 783-6888

JC's mission is to continuously improve the safety and quality of care provided to the public through the provision of health care accreditation and related services that support performance improvement in health care organizations.

References

Agency for Healthcare Research and Quality. (2005). Effective health care. Retrieved December 21, 2005, from http://www.ahrq.gov/

American Hospital Directory. (2005). Medicare prospective payment system. Retrieved December 13, 2005, from http://www.ahd.com

American Nurses Association. (2005). ANA's health care agenda 2005. Retrieved December 20, 2005, from http://nursingworld.org/

Bazzoli, G. J., Dynan, L., Burns, L. R., & Yap, C. (2004). Two decades of organizational change in health care: What have we learned? *Medical Care Research and Review, 61*(3).

Burns, A. (2005). Mentoring toward autonomy in the ambulatory care environment. *American Academy of Ambulatory Care Nursing*, Retrieved December 21, 2005, from *AAACN viewpoint*, http://www.findarticles.com

Hadley, J., & Holahan, J. (2003). How much medical care do the uninsured use, and who pays for it? *Health Affairs Web Exclusive*, 66–81.

Health Insurance In-depth. (2005). Is a managed care network the right choice for you? Retrieved December 18, 2005, from http://www.healthinsuranceindepth.com

Heffler, S., Smith, S., Keehan, S., Clemens, M. K., Won, G., & Zezza, M. (2003). Health spending projections for 2002–2012. *Health Affairs Web Exclusive*, 54–65.

http://www.therubins.com. (2005). Prescription drugs and the elderly.

The Joint Commission. (2006). Facts about the Joint Commission. Retrieved January 9, 2006, from http://www.jointcommission.org

National Committee for Quality Assurance. (2005). Common ground, common goals: Improving quality and value together. *2005 Annual Report*. Retrieved December 18, 2005 from http://www.ncqa.org. Retrieved December 21, 2005, from http://hprc.ncqa.org

Piette, J. D., & Heisler, M. (2006). The relationship between older adults' knowledge of their drug coverage and medication cost problems. *Journal of the American Geriatrics Society, 54*(1), 91–96.

Robbins, D., and Brill, J. (May/June 2005). Blending ethics and empowerment with consumer-driven healthcare. *Patient Safety and Quality Healthcare*. Retrieved December 18, 2005, from http://www.psqh.com

Strunk, B. C., Ginsburg, P. B., & Gabel, J. R. (2002). Tracking health care costs: Growth accelerates again in 2001. *Health Affairs Web Exclusive*, 299–310.

U.S. Department of Health and Human Services. (2006). Center for Medicaid and Medicare services. Retrieved May 31, 2006, from http://www.cms.hhs.gov/

Xu, K. T., Smith, S. R., & Borders, T. F. (2003). Access to prescription drugs among noninstitutionalized elderly people in west Texas. *American Journal of Health-System Pharm, 60*, 675–682.

Bibliography

Gresenz, C. R., Rogowski, J., & Escarce, J. (2006). Dimensions of the local health care environment and use of care by uninsured children in rural and urban areas. *Pediatrics, 117*(3), 509–517.

Marrelli, T. M. (2001). Prospective payment in home care: An interview. *Geriatric Nursing, 22*, 217–218.

Miller, C. A. (2004). *Nursing for wellness in older adults*. Philadelphia: Lippincott Williams & Wilkins.

Wellstood, K., Wilson, K., & Eyeles, J. (2006). "Reasonable access" to primary care: Assessing the role of individual and system characteristics. *Health and Place, 12*(2), 121–130.

Chapter 21

ETHICAL, LEGAL, AND POLITICAL CONCERNS

Carolina G. Huerta, EdD, MSN, RN

Betty Johnson, MSN, RN

KEY TERMS

accreditation	credentialing	introspection	respect for others
advance directives	crime	justice	standard of best
assault	deontology	law	interest
autonomy	Equal Protection	multistate licensure	teleology
battery	ethical principles	negligence	tort
beneficence	ethics	nonmaleficence	values
breach of duty	fidelity	paternalism	values clarification
certification	informed consent	registration	veracity

OBJECTIVES

Upon completion of this chapter, the reader should be able to:

- Recognize ethical, legal, and political issues that can influence the health promotion goals of professional nursing.

- Identify basic principles of ethics.

- Discuss values clarification.

- Describe legal concerns affecting the delivery of health care.

- Explain the concepts of licensure and professional standards of care and their impact on the delivery of nursing care.

- Describe how nurses can apply ethical-legal concepts in decision making for health promotion.

INTRODUCTION

Complex personal, interpersonal, professional, institutional, and social issues constantly challenge nurses. These issues are rarely confined to caring for the client in the health care institution. Since nursing's goals are health promotion and the provision of holistic client care, these constant challenges must be addressed. Responses depend upon such variables as contextual factors, client and family values, relationships, moral development, religious beliefs, spiritual perspectives, cultural orientation, and legal constraints. Historically, nursing has been involved in most aspects of health care delivery and in all aspects of health promotion. Such intimate involvement in the delivery of care has provided nurses with the opportunity to witness countless situations that pose ethical as well as legal dilemmas. In order to provide quality client care, nurses must develop an awareness of the ethical and legal considerations pertaining to nursing practice.

Ethical and legal dilemmas are common in the nursing profession. Nurses are frequently called upon to treat clients who may be considered a detriment to society and are expected to treat them as they would any other client. For example, a nurse might be called to treat a prison inmate who has been convicted of committing a heinous crime. The attending nurse may be tempted to provide substandard care because of her or his personal feelings toward the client. This, of course, creates both an ethical and a legal dilemma, since under U.S. law, all similarly situated individuals are entitled to be treated similarly under the **equal protection** guarantee (Monarch, 2002). Substandard care to this prison inmate involves such basic issues as determining who has the right to receive care and determining what constitutes legal equality in relation to health care. Nurses are called upon daily in their practice to make decisions affecting the client's care. Frequently, these decisions may pertain to what is right or wrong, and no clear answers are evident. Decisions, however, should be made on sound ethical principles as well as professional and legal standards.

The previous chapter discussed health care cost, health care financing, and quality issues associated with the delivery of care. This chapter also focuses on issues related to health care cost, access to health care, and the government's involvement in the delivery of health care but from the standpoint of ethical and legal concerns affecting the delivery of quality nursing care. Issues regarding a client's choice of treatment and rationing of health care as they relate to health promotion efforts will also be explored. In order for the reader to fully understand the effect of ethical and legal issues on a client's health promotion status, basic principles of ethics and legal concerns will be described.

ETHICAL AND LEGAL ISSUES INFLUENCING NURSING CARE

Nurses are expected to provide quality care to all of their clients. In providing this quality care, the nurse assumes the role of a client advocate who speaks up about poor, inadequate, or incompetent care. Because of nursing's advocacy role and since nurses provide the majority of direct client care, they are frequently expected to make decisions that involve ethical or legal issues. When nurses make decisions involving ethical or legal issues, these decisions must always be rooted in the professional standards as set forth in the American Nurses Association's (ANA) *Code of Ethics for Nurses with Interpretive Statements* (2001), *Scope and Standards of Practice* (2004), and *Standards of Clinical Nursing Practice* (1998). (See Chapter 2 for related information.) Nursing decisions must also always be made with an awareness of the client's rights to receive care. These rights entitle the client to receive safe and effective care at all times regardless of where the health care is delivered. In fact, several health care organizations have established a bill of rights for clients. The American Hospital Association (AHA) is one of the primary organizations that have established a bill of rights for clients. AHA's *Patient's Bill of Rights* was last revised in 1992 (AHA, 1992). Other entities, such as the U.S. Advisory Commission on Consumer Protection and Quality in the Health Care Industry, have adopted their own bills of rights for clients. Many health plans have adopted these principles, which include the right to information disclosure, choice of provider and plans, access to emergency services, participation in treatment decisions, respect and nondiscrimination, and confidentiality as well as the right to complain about a health plan, a hospital, health care personnel, or a doctor. A client is also given the right to appeal a decision related to health care plans (American Cancer Society, 2004). The federal government recognizes the need for a client's bill of rights and has introduced legislation that facilitates client access to care.

In addition to the professional standards, decisions regarding client care must abide by legal statutes. The state legislative body sets forth legal rules governing licensure of nursing practice. These provisions that govern nursing can be found in the rules and regulations mandated by the administrative agencies where legislative authority is vested. These regulations are compiled and published by the state board of nursing as the Nursing Practice Act.

ETHICAL ISSUES

Ethical issues have arisen over time as a result of technological and scientific advances. Ethical dilemmas are perplexing to nurses and other health care workers because most of the time there are no clearly right or wrong courses of action (Monarch, 2002). Occasionally professional decisions are clear cut and all the health care providers agree with the course of action (Guido, 2006). This, unfortunately, happens quite infrequently. Interspersed with the dilemmas of ethics are concerns dealing with legalities and concerns of cost and access to health care for all, young or old, rich or poor. The concept of health as a goal of society as described by health promotion models is both an ethical and legal issue since it questions whether health promotion behaviors can be imposed on society.

Ethics is the branch of philosophy that is related to moral values and actions. It deals with the rules or principles that distinguish right from wrong or good behavior from bad behavior. Ethical individuals make decisions based on acceptable standards of conduct and moral judgment. Ethical nurses conduct themselves according to fundamental ethical principles and moral reasoning. It is thus important for nurses to study ethics in order to care fully for their clients and provide quality care. Nurses care for critically ill people and face more difficult and immediate ethical conflicts than do people in other jobs. The clients are ill and less able to fend for themselves, and they need nurses who can make ethical decisions regarding their care and provide them with the information that is needed to make decisions, frequently involving life and death. There are ethical theories and basic principles of ethics that are helpful to the nurse involved in an ethical dilemma.

ETHICAL THEORIES

There are several theories that are important to a discussion of ethical issues. Ethical theories guide by providing the context in which a situation should be viewed. They also provide an integrated view of what values, like pieces in a puzzle, logically fit in and should be considered when dealing with ethical issues. Although there may be more theories related to ethics, teleology and deontology are the more familiar ethical theories.

Teleology is an ethical theory that justifies actions based on the results attained by those actions. This theory can easily be summarized by the old adage, the end justifies the means. For example, consider the near-fatal side effects of certain potentially life-saving experimental treatments or the wholesale slaughter of animals for research. This theory lends itself to the judgment that the greatest good is for the greatest number of people. Consequently, if teleology theory is used in decision making in the preceding example, it is logical to have some clients become ill when undergoing experimental treatment or to kill many animals if a cure for diabetes or cancer is found. The problem associated with using teleology to rectify or resolve ethical dilemmas is that there are no rules to determine the rightness or wrongness of a particular action (Monarch, 2002).

Deontology is a theory of moral or professional obligation. The morality of the ethical decision is completely separate from its consequences. For example, health care providers could universally limit organ transplant on the basis of age or gender, with the hypothetical assumption that because there are more female donors, there would be more female recipients. Another example is the belief that alcoholism is a self-inflicted disease with increased chances of progression to liver failure. Thus available organs for transplant should be allocated to those recipients deemed more worthy and without a history of self-inflicted disease. These are examples mixed with justice and veracity, two ethical principles to be discussed later in this chapter. Deontology's strength is in its emphasis on the dignity of human beings (Guido, 2001).

BASIC PRINCIPLES OF ETHICS

Ethical decision making involves an understanding of the basic principles of ethics. **Ethical principles** are basic concepts and rules to guide and give direction to nursing practice. If ethical principles are not used, a decision will rest solely on personal emotions and values (Guido, 2006). Table 21-1 lists nine basic principles of ethics.

Principle of Autonomy

Nurses are expected to understand the concept of autonomy and be advocates for all clients. **Autonomy** involves independence and freedom and is based on the right to self-determination. The root of the word is *auto*, mean-

ing "self," and *nomy*, which refers to control (Ellis & Hartley, 2004). Autonomy is the right to choose what will happen to one's own person and gives the client the right to determine personal care and who will give it. Situations that involve consideration of this principle include those related to a client's right to die, receive treatment, or refuse treatment. Informed consent to allow a surgeon to do a procedure on an individual is a legal doctrine reflecting autonomy. It is important to note, however, that autonomy does not give the client absolute rights. Restrictions may be placed on the rights of the client if those rights interfere with another's safety. For example, a person with a communicable disease may be quarantined, even if he or she does not want to be, if not

TABLE 21-1 Basic Principles of Ethics

Principle	Meaning
Autonomy	Freedom to make choices
Beneficence	Promote good
Nonmaleficence	Invokes obligation not to harm others
Veracity	Practice of telling the truth
Confidentiality	An individual's right to privacy
Justice	Fair, equitable, and appropriate treatment
Fidelity	Faithfulness to another's cause
Standard of best interest	Assists client in making decisions about own health care
Respect for others	Acknowledges right of person to make decisions and live or die by those decisions

doing so will expose others to the danger of the communicable disease (Guido, 2006). Occasionally, a client's capacity for autonomy is brought into question, and a legal opinion must be sought. The courts may then assume the role of surrogate decision maker regarding situations involving the principle of autonomy. Situations that may require legal intervention when client autonomy is in question frequently involve religious tenets prohibiting treatment or refusal of treatment due to mental illness.

Principle of Beneficence

Beneficence is a principle that requires nurses to act in ways that benefit clients. Beneficence provides the groundwork for the trust that society and individuals place in nurses. The primary goal of beneficence is to do good for clients under the care of a health care worker. This principle indicates that in caring for clients, the nurse should always take action to promote "good," or what is best for the client. This principle also maintains that nurses must prevent harm or evil. Although this principle seems very simplistic, the problem with this principle is determining what constitutes "good" (Guido, 2006). The *Code of Ethic for Nurses with Interpretive Statements* (ANA, 2001) is quite clear in addressing the nurse's role in promoting the principle of beneficence. The code stresses that the nurse has an obligation to the client and that this obligation includes protection of the client from incompetent, unethical, or illegal practice (ANA, 2001). Situations that involve the nurse and the principle of beneficence may include decisions regarding the benefits and risks of certain treatments or procedures that determine who will live and who will die when only one individual can be saved. Nurses in their practice must always function with knowledge of the beneficence principle and will often encounter situations in which opposing values play against one another (Ellis & Hartley, 2004).

Principle of Nonmaleficence

Nonmaleficence requires nurses to act in such a way as to avoid causing harm to clients. The nonmaleficence and beneficence principles are very similar. The primary difference lies in the fact that the beneficence principle strives to achieve what is good while the nonmaleficence principle seeks to do no harm in situations requiring nursing actions. Included in the nonmaleficence principle are actions that produce deliberate harm, risk of harm, or even harm that occurs during the performance of beneficial acts. Prohibited by this principle are procedures performed for monetary gain, or experimental research that assumes negative outcomes for the participants. Individual state nursing practice acts address issues related to the nurse's responsibility to do no harm. For example, the Texas Nursing Practice Act specifically addresses a nurse's responsibility in promoting a safe environment for clients and others. It is the nurse's responsibility to report unsafe nursing practice by another RN if there is reasonable cause to suspect unnecessary exposure of a client to risk of harm as a result of failure to conform to the minimum standards of care (Will Mann, 2002).

Principle of Veracity

The principle of **veracity** is simply the practice of telling the truth. It is a universally accepted virtue, and most of us were taught as children to always tell the truth. Telling the truth is promoted in all professional codes of ethics and can certainly be found in nursing's code of ethics. Veracity engenders respect, open communication, trust, and shared responsibility. Not telling the truth is deception, and nurses are not supposed to conceal the truth from clients. Violation of the veracity principle in dealing with clients has serious consequences for nurses. Everyone who knows the truth will remember this deception and be inclined to believe that health professionals cannot be relied on (Ellis & Hartley, 2004). The intimate dealings with clients and their family members usually place the nurse in a position of trust. Questions are asked of the nurse that may deal with delicate issues or that are related to the client's condition. Although the nurse is taught to uphold the principle of veracity, at times telling the truth may result in awkward or confusing situations because family members have kept important information from the client. It is expected that the physician or primary health care giver share with the client the truth about the diagnosed illness. This may not always be the case so it may be incumbent upon the nurse to provide the client with the truth.

Principle of Confidentiality

Although most textbooks do not list confidentiality as a principle of ethics, it is not possible to care for clients appropriately without recognizing that all people have a right to privacy. Nurses are privy to information that cannot be made public knowledge without a state or federal court ruling. Again, the *Code of Ethics for Nurses with Interpretive Statements* (ANA, 2001) has a very clear position on the issue of confidentiality. The code asserts that it is the nurse's responsibility to safeguard a client's right to privacy by protecting information of a confidential nature. A major area of concern related to confidentiality involves the issue of who might have access to medical records. The Federal Health Insurance Portability and Accountability Act of 1996, known as HIPAA, was passed to establish a national framework for security standards and protection of confidentiality with regard to health care data and information. Nurses are expected to comply with HIPAA regulations in protecting the client's confidentiality regarding health or personal matters. The implications of this federal regulation on the health care community are considerable. For example, some health care institutions are no longer placing a client's name on the hospital room door so that the client's name is not visible to others. While this may ensure a client's right to confidentiality, this policy may also cause more hospital-related safety infractions to occur.

There are only a few times when confidentiality may be broken. This can occur only if the nurse knows that the client is a danger to self or others. Then it is the nurse's legal duty to warn significant others of the impending danger. For example, this is clearly evident in any case involving violent behavior.

Principle of Justice

Justice is fair, equitable, and appropriate treatment according to what is due or owed to persons, with the understanding that giving to some will deny receipt to

Nursing Alert

Institutional Ethics Committees

Most health care institutions have an active Ethics Committee that deals with client ethical issues. Whenever a nursing situation occurs that involves ethics and requires decision making, the nurse should refer the case to the Ethics Committee.

others who might otherwise have received those things. It may be agreed that in this great nation, excellent health care is available. However, it is not available to all for various reasons. Nurses are well aware that need is sometimes not the basic factor involved in determining who receives care and who does not. The concept of justice is often expanded to include what is called distributive justice, which states that all people are entitled to be treated equally regardless of gender, marital status, medical diagnosis, social standing, economic level, or religious beliefs (Catalano, 2006). Distributive justice, thus, includes the idea that all people should have access to health care. Unfortunately what is not described through this principle is who will incur the costs. For that reason, the principle of justice, specifically distributive justice, is often challenged in health care.

Principle of Fidelity

Fidelity is often related to the concept of faithfulness and the practice of keeping promises. Nurses have been granted the right to practice nursing by licensure and certification. As described in ANA's *Code of Ethics for Nurses* (2001), it is the nurse's responsibility to provide services to clients and safeguard their rights to health care. This is considered fundamental to quality nursing practice and addresses the principle of fidelity. The promise to care for the client is primary. Nurses fulfill that promise in many ways—verbally, mutually contracting or interacting, and a host of other ways. Fidelity relates closely to the concept of accountability

Standard of Best Interest

The **standard of best interest** is one that allows individuals to share in decision making. This principle is used to assist clients in making choices regarding health care. In using this principle, nurses can assist clients in decision making when they lack the expertise or knowledge and data to make decisions. If the entire decision is taken away from the client, this principle is obviously avoided (Guido, 2006). The nurse who does not take the client's wishes into consideration in determining a plan of nursing care is using the concept of **paternalism.** Paternalism encourages individuals to make decisions for others. Obviously, paternalism is an undesirable principle.

Principle of Respect for Others

Respect for others is seen as the highest ethical principle. It incorporates the concepts found in all the other principles previously described. Respect for others acknowledges that individuals are capable of making decisions for themselves in all areas of their lives, including decisions relating to life or death (Guido, 2006). Nurses are crucial in upholding this principle since they can positively reinforce this principle on a daily basis in their actions with peers, clients, the health care team, and family members. Utilization by nurses of the principle of respect for others includes recognition of the client's culture, gender issues, religion, ethnicity, and race.

NURSING AND ETHICS

Nurses providing client care need to constantly be cognizant of the nine ethical principles set forth above. They must recognize that there are rarely any black or white answers to dilemmas dealing with the variability in human nature. For this reason, each nurse should develop a philosophically consistent framework on which to base contemplation, decision, and action. Ethical and moral principles provide the background for the development of a rational decision-making framework.

ETHICAL DECISION MAKING AND PERSONAL VALUES

In determining solutions for ethical dilemmas, the values with which the nurse was brought up, the values the nurse holds dear, or both of these will provide needed direction. Clarification of these values is essential if the nurse is to assist clients in decision making. An awareness of personal values empowers both the nurse and the client and fosters the achievement of their mutual goal, which is to promote the client's personal health status. **Values** make up a set of personal beliefs and attitudes about such things as truth, beauty, justice, and the worth of any thought, object, or behavior. In developing values, a person acquires direction and gives meaning to life. Values reflect how people live or have been brought up and are derived from personal life experiences. They affect the disposition one has toward a person, object, or idea. Values are usually not isolated but are interwoven with each other and with specific life events. In addition, values influence each other and are always changing. In sorting through decisions that need to be made, individuals use their own process for clarifying personal values. This **values clarification** is the process

of becoming more conscious of and naming what one values or considers worthy. This process sheds light on a person's personal perspectives.

Steps in Values Clarification

There are several steps identified in the values clarification process. These steps provide a systematic approach to obtaining a more comprehensive understanding of how a value is acquired. Although the steps identified in the literature are not always identical, the same concepts are included and considered inherent to the process. By using the steps involved in values clarification, nurses as well as nursing students can understand their own value system as well as that of their clients. Box 21-1 lists several steps that are helpful in clarifying personal values.

The steps involved in values clarification are useful in gaining perspective on personal values. The first step in the process is essential if the nurse wants to deal appropriately with ethical dilemmas. This step involves the mental activity called introspection. **Introspection** refers to the ability to look inside oneself and examine thoughts and personal meaning for identified values. Without this activity it is almost impossible to determine whether certain situations are wrong or whether they are in conflict with personal values. The act of clarifying values also necessitates recognition that personal freedom

---

BOX 21-1   Steps in Values Clarification

1. Engage in personal introspection.
2. Recognize individual freedom to choose personal values.
3. Evaluate personal meaning of value choices.
4. Understand that there are many other individual values.
5. Develop commitment to values.
6. Determine congruence of actions with values choices.

does not allow any one value to be dictated and that everyone makes decisions regarding values based on personal meaning and individual situations. The final steps in values clarification are also essential. These require a commitment to the values that are chosen and demand congruence between value choices and personal actions and behaviors.

It is important to note that values can either be tangible or intangible and are often measured by behavior. Therefore, values are considered to be internal controls for behavior. Many issues facing the practice of nursing today are emotionally charged, and if they were not they would not be considered important. Only by considering all aspects of an issue can a nurse hope to seek understanding of the issue and move into decision making that is beneficial for everyone.

Value Conflicts

There are times when personal values are at odds with the values of the client or of the institution. This can create friction between the nurse and the employing institution as well as result in poor quality of client care. The negative outcomes in such a situation can be prevented by becoming more aware of personal values and what actions are acceptable or not acceptable. It is important to deal with values conflict in an effective way, acquiring a conscious awareness of one's own values as well as the perceived values of others. Differences in values do arise, and a choice can be made to respond to the other's viewpoint by seeking understanding and common ground.

LEGAL ISSUES

Nursing decisions should reflect adherence to standards of nursing practice and recognition of the associated legal implications as well as ethical ones. There are many instances when the nurse involved in clinical practice may be faced with a legal situation. Clinical practice, for instance, can involve legal situations such as disconnection of clients from life support, restraint or medicating of clients against their will, and omission or lack of care, to name a few. Legal issues may also arise in situations where **informed consent** (see Figure 21-1), or a clear explanation of procedures to be had along with associated risks and benefits, is not provided to the client. Legal situations may also arise when the nurse or a health care professional is thought to have provided inadequate or incompetent care. Clients may then take legal action and attempt to highlight incompetence through the legal system. It is thus important for nurses to know that the profession is held to the same legal standards as the average citizen as well as to those relating to nursing. It is also important to note that as the nursing profession's scope of practice increases, the laws applicable to nursing will continue to evolve.

LAW AND NURSING PRACTICE

Law has been defined in a variety of ways. Law, very simply, can be defined as the sum total of rules and regulations by which a society is governed. Law includes rules and regulations established and enforced by a given community, state, or nation. Laws are created by people and are used to regulate behavior in all persons (Guido, 2006). Laws provide society with rules or standards of conduct that have been determined through legislative bodies and then tested in courts around the world. The ultimate goal of law is to protect and safeguard the public. Likewise, nursing's ultimate goal is to protect the public by providing safe, quality client care.

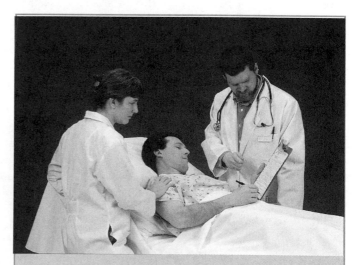

FIGURE 21-1 *The nurse is ethically and legally accountable when engaging in clinical practice. The witnessing of informed consent is one of many nursing responsibilities making the nurse ethically and legally responsible.*

Nurses are not exempt from state or constitutional law and must adhere to all civil and criminal statutes. They must adhere to all aspects of the Nursing Practice Act (NPA) and are legally accountable for all actions in their nursing practice, including those that have been delegated to others. This accountability arises from the fact that nurses are licensed to practice through a legal regulatory mechanism (ANA, 2003). The NPA regulates the practice of nursing in both the United States and Canada. At the same time, each state in the United States and each province in Canada has its own nursing practice act, enacted by individual state or province law.

Nurses in their role as promoters of health act as client advocates. As client advocates, nurses are expected to protect clients from unsafe procedures and see that their legal rights to safe and equitable health care are not violated. The standards of nursing practice also guarantee that clients receive quality nursing care and assure that all clients are provided with the information needed to make decisions about health promotion, maintenance, and restoration (ANA, 2004). These standards are used as measurable expectations in a court of law, and nurses are expected to adhere to the standards of practice as well as to the NPA. The registered nurse must also practice within the rules of the Board of Nurse Examiners (BNE) for the state where the nurse is practicing, and within laws relating to the specific practice setting. The rules provided by the BNE provide more detailed guidance to the registered nurse than does the NPA.

COMPETENCY INDICATORS

Although it may seem unusual to describe competency indicators as being important to the nurse's role as a promoter of health, the truth is that these competency indicators are essential to the practice role of the professional nurse. These indicators demonstrate that standards of nursing practice are being maintained and that safe,

competent care is being delivered. Several measures can be used as indicators of nursing competency and accountability. Table 21-2 lists several indicators of nursing accountability along with their meaning.

Licensure

A nurse must attain licensure to practice professional nursing in the United States. This licensure is mandatory and provides a measure of accountability to the general public indicating that the nurse meets minimal competency to provide safe nursing care. Once licensure is attained, the nurse becomes a registered nurse. **Registration** is the listing of an individual's name and other information on the official roster of a governmental or nongovernmental agency. Nurses who are registered are permitted to use the title Registered Nurse or RN. To be registered, the nurse must complete a basic course of nursing studies in an approved, accredited program and pass the national qualifying examination with an acceptable grade.

Individual states in the United States have their own licensure policies. For example, in the state of Texas, applicants may take the licensing examination every 45 days and within four years of completion of graduation requirements. If the exam is not passed within four years, applicants must complete a board-approved nursing program (Board of Nurse Examiners for the State of Texas, 2006). This is not true of all states. New graduates of accredited nursing programs in the United States and Canada who are applying for initial licensure will be issued a temporary permit after they have been determined eligible. States may vary in these procedures.

Temporary permits differ from temporary licenses. A holder of a temporary license has the same authority to practice professional nursing as does a permanent license holder. This is considered licensure by endorsement without examination and is only for nurses who are licensed as registered nurses in a territory or possession of the United States or foreign country and who demon-

TABLE 21-2 Accountability Indicators

Indicator	Meaning
Licensure	Indication of the minimum degree of competency to practice safely
Credentialing	Recognition of competence through specialty knowledge, education, registration, certification, licensure, and accreditation
Certification	Judgment of competency by practicing nurses in specialty practice
Accreditation	Recognition of demonstrated compliance with established criteria, usually a symbol of excellence
Standards of care	Guideposts ensuring competent practice

strate the same degree of fitness required by the state to which they apply. Licensure by endorsement also applies to nurses who are licensed to practice professional nursing in other states. These are licenses issued after meeting requirements as set forth by each state board.

Multistate Licensure

The concept of licensure as previously described may soon be a thing of the past. As a result of increased nursing mobility between states, the United States is moving toward the concept of multistate licensure. **Multistate licensure** refers to the recognition of a single license allowing registered nurses to practice nursing throughout the country. Although not all states in the United States have adopted this type of licensure, compact legislation has been enacted among several states recognizing a single nursing license. This multistate licensure compact provides a process through which states agree to mutually recognize each other's licensees and thus discontinues the process of requiring duplicate licenses. The compact requires that nurses be licensed in their home states and comply with the state practice laws of the state in which they practice (RN Update, 2000).

Credentialing

The nursing profession is becoming increasingly more accountable as the general public is becoming more knowledgeable about its right to receive safe and competent care. Like other professions, nursing uses the credentialing process as an indicator of competency and demonstrated accountability. **Credentialing** is a process that recognizes professional achievements such as specialty practice knowledge, educational accomplishments, certification, licensure, and accreditation. The credentialing process is one way in which the nursing profession maintains standards of practice and demonstrates accountability for the educational preparation of its members. The credentialing process is also a means of recognizing technical competence in areas requiring special-level expertise (Ellis & Hartley, 2004). The most highly visible nursing credentialing board is the American Nurses Credentialing Center, which is an independent agency of the ANA and offers various advance practice nursing certifications.

Certification

Certification is the process by which an individual registered nurse who has met certain established criteria or qualifications is granted recognition for competency. These criteria may include a judgment of competence by nurses who are themselves practicing in the area of specialization and the completion of certain educational courses and clinical practice. A crucial component of certification is successful completion of an examination that tests knowledge in the specialty area (ANA, 2003).

In many instances, certification is required for entrance into specialty practice such as nurse practitioners, nurse midwives, or certified registered nurse anesthetists.

Accreditation

Accreditation is a form of certification or licensure that recognizes demonstrated compliance with established criteria. This certification or licensure is given to agencies or institutions rather than to individuals. Universities, schools of nursing, and hospitals seek accreditation according to the type of business they conduct or service that they provide. For example, The Joint Commission (JC) formerly the Joint Commission on the Accreditation of Healthcare Organizations (JCAHO) is an accrediting body that is very important to health care organizations. The JC's mission is to evaluate a health care institution's performance in all areas that affect health care, with specific focus on the quality and safety of care. To earn and maintain accreditation, an extensive on-site review by a team of Joint Commission health care professionals is conducted at least once every three years. Accreditation is awarded based on how well the organization meets the Joint Commission standards (The Joint Commission, 2006). Organizations such as hospitals must seek the accreditation process and demonstrate compliance with specific, published criteria. Schools of nursing must meet accreditation standards set by the Board of Nurse Examiners for the state. They may also choose to be recognized as an accredited school by the National League for Nursing (NLN) or the Commission on Collegiate Nursing Education (CCNE), which accredits baccalaureate and graduate nursing education programs. Entry into the armed forces as a commissioned officer requires evidence of having graduated from an NLN- or a CCNE-accredited nursing program. Admission into graduate school usually requires the same evidence.

Standards of Care

Throughout this chapter, there have been multiple references to standards of nursing care. These standards ensure safe practice to the public and serve as guidelines established by the profession for nursing practice. They also serve as parameters and reminders to nurses regarding the boundaries of practice. Standards of care have been referred to as safety checklists. The ANA has established general standards of care as well as standards for such specialty areas as acute care, college health, oncology, pediatric clinical, maternal-child, medical-surgical, geriatric, and surgical nursing. Box 21-2 provides a list of some of the standards of practice developed by the ANA.

A nurse is expected to provide safe and competent care, abide by clinical principles and legal statutes, and do no harm. Within this environment, the nurse contracts with the client either in an expressed or implied manner. As soon as the client-nurse relationship is established, the nurse has a legal and binding duty to the client. The *Lunsford v. Board of Nurse Examiners* (1983) case made it very clear that duty is owed to a client when a client-nurse relationship is established. By virtue of licensure, this relationship automatically exists whenever a client seeks care and is met by a nurse (Guido, 2006). The nursing care plan, which is developed by the nurse and the client or family or both collaboratively, also serves as a contract of an explicit or expressed nature. The responsibility for nursing actions rests solely with the nurse. If the nurse believes an action will be harmful to the client, the nurse must refuse to carry out the action. The validity of the action as well as the potential consequences of the action must be documented. In the event that a questionable action has been performed that might be harmful to the client, it is always best to inform the supervising nurse, document succinctly in writing, and keep a personal copy of the report.

TORTS, NEGLIGENCE, AND BREACHES IN LEGAL DUTY

A **tort,** which is a legal wrong committed against a person or property, is settled in civil court and involves some type of compensation, usually money. A tort differs from a **crime,** which is also a legal wrong committed against a person or property. A crime involves a wide range of malfeasance from minor citations to murder and is punishable by the government at the county, state, or federal level (Ellis & Hartley, 2004). Torts may result from a breach of a legal duty and may be intentional, quasi-intentional, or nonintentional acts, and the courts provide a remedy in the form of an action for damages.

Negligent torts are the most frequent basis for liability of nurses, physicians, and hospitals. **Negligence** involves failure to provide the care that a reasonable person would provide in similar circumstances and is considered a civil or personal wrong, to distinguish it from criminal conduct. It denotes conduct lacking in due care and equates with carelessness. Negligence can also include doing something that a reasonably prudent person would *not* do. According to this definition, anyone can be liable for negligence (Guido, 2006). Negligence alone is not enough to establish liability; there must also be an injury caused by the negligence. Four elements must be present in order to establish liability negligence. Table 21-3 lists these elements along with the concepts necessary to understand their meaning.

The first element that must be proven in any action for negligence to occur relates to duty. There are two

---

BOX 21-2 Selected ANA Standards of Practice

Scope and Standards of Practice in:

- Addictions Nursing
- College Health Nursing
- Diabetes Nursing
- Gerontological Nursing
- Home Health Nursing
- Hospice and Palliative Care Nursing
- Neonatal Nursing
- Neuroscience Nursing
- Nursing Administration
- Nursing Informatics
- Nursing Professional Development
- Pain Management Nursing
- Pediatric Nursing
- Pediatric Oncology
- Plastic Surgery Nursing
- Psychiatric Mental Health Nursing
- Public Health Nursing
- School Nursing
- Vascular Nursing

TABLE 21-3 Elements in Liability Negligence

Element	Concept
Duty	Duty is owed to a client. Nurse fails to meet standard of care. Scope of duty is within professional nursing boundaries.
Breach of duty	Deviation from standard of care is established.
Injury	Financial, physical, emotional harm is established.
Causation	Direct cause for failure to meet standard of care clearly established.

aspects of duty. It must first be proved that a duty was owed to the person harmed, and second, it must be affirmed that the scope of that duty is within the boundaries of the profession, usually called the standards of care. The second element refers to the idea that a **breach of duty** has occurred. That is, there must be a deviation in some manner from the standard of care, which is established on showing that something was done by the nurse that should not have been done, or something was not done that should have been done. Proof of this hinges on showing that the care of the client was substandard. The third element that must be proven involves the establishment of actual injury. Some type of physical, financial, or emotional injury or any combination must be incurred. The actual injury must be demonstrated in order for negligence to be established. The last element refers to causation. This final element is probably the most important in establishing negligence. To prove that negligence has occurred as a result of breach of duty, it is essential to establish that the breach of duty without a doubt caused the injury.

RIGHT TO REFUSE TREATMENT

At the core of health promotion is the concept that the client is the expert in his or her own treatment and care. Thus, in utilizing a health promotion framework in planning for the client's care, the nurse must be cognizant of the client's right to refuse treatment. The law also recognizes that a person has the right to refuse treatment. Additionally, it recognizes that a client possesses the right to be free from aggression and the threats of actual aggression. If the client refuses treatment and a nurse provides treatment anyway, charges of assault or battery or both may be filed by the client. **Battery** actually involves physically touching the person and is considered a physical violation. **Assault** is an infringement upon the mental security or tranquility or both of another. Assault involves an attempt or threat to touch another person. If a client refuses a procedure or has certain procedures done without consent, these actions can lead to a civil claim of assault or battery or both (Zerwekh & Claborn, 2006).

Clients cannot be restrained unless they are in danger. Restraints, especially for an extended period, require the order of a physician. Restraining a client may result in charges of assault, battery, or false imprisonment being filed against the nurse, physician, and the medical establishment. Liability for restraints usually involves a client fall or escape that might cause injury to self or others. Courts are more critical when they believe the nurse left the client unattended in order to do something less important. Failure to provide a restrained client with a signaling device, failure to restrain a client properly, and failure to provide attendance when the restraints are removed from a client are all reasons that the courts can find the nurse liable.

STUDENT NURSE LIABILITY

Student nurses are held liable for their own acts of negligence committed in the course of clinical experiences. If students are performing duties that are within the scope of professional nursing, they will be held to the same standard of skill and competence as a registered professional nurse. A lower standard of care will not be applied to the action of nursing students. To fulfill their client responsibilities and to minimize exposure to liability, nursing students should make sure that they are prepared to care properly for assigned clients and should ask for additional help or supervision if they feel inadequately prepared for an assignment (Guido, 2001). Student nurses are expected to carry personal liability insurance.

ETHICAL, LEGAL, AND POLITICAL CONCERNS RELATED TO HEALTH CARE COST AND ACCESS

There have been many changes in the last decades that have affected the delivery of care, impacted the finances of health care institutions, escalated health care costs, and made health care literally inaccessible for hundreds of thousands of people nationwide. Although a national health policy was hinted at when the Colonies were first established as far back as the seventeenth century, a national health policy that provides care for all people has not become reality. It is a sad testimony that a nation as rich as the United States still has citizens who are unable to access health care.

Although the nursing profession expects health promotion, restoration, support, and maintenance to be integral components of the nurse's responsibility, ethical and legal concerns still arise over questions of who can receive health care delivery services, who can afford health care services, and who has the right to access health care. Nurses, in their attempt to address these questions, have established that in addition to health care access, health promotion strategies and preventive health care programs should be accessible to all citizens.

Health Care Delivery and Health Care Costs

Rapidly rising health care costs along with unsuccessful attempts to deal with them in the context of the increasingly worrisome federal deficit have had the greatest influence in shaping today's health care system. The high cost of health care has given rise to managed care plans, combining insurance and provider functions, horizontal integration of health care facilities into larger organizations, and hospital expansion into ambulatory surgery, home care, and other centers such as substance abuse treatment centers. The result of all of these measures is that the current health care delivery system is fragmented, delivers poor-quality services, and at times provides inadequate care.

There has emerged a major restructuring of the hospital workforce and an implementation of cost-cutting diagnostic-related systems that dictate reimbursement rates. All kinds of institutional and alternative delivery systems have been established over the last decade. These have grown as an incentive to provide care at a lower cost. Physicians, for example, are moving toward group practice, and it is expected that the greatest growth in physician group practice will be in either individual practice associations or preferred provider organizations (PPOs), associated with a health maintenance organization (HMO) or primary case management model. The origination of PPOs and IPAs helps a group of providers negotiate fee schedules with hospitals and third-party reimbursers. The financial shift has gone from the health plans to the physicians. Today, HMOs view themselves as managed care organizations that offer an array of managed care plans. It is important to ask who is responsible for charges for health care services. The availability of private insurance, Medicaid, Medicare, or private pay does not constitute a solution to the delivery of health care in an ethical and cost-effective manner. Sufficient funds must be available to pay for any of these so-called solutions.

Ask Yourself

The Right to Health Care: An Ethical or a Legal Concern?

Do you think health care is a right or a privilege? Should all people have access to the same health care services regardless of ability to pay? How should ability to pay influence access to health care services? If you believe health care is a right, how much health care is each person entitled to? As a taxpayer, are you willing to fund taxes that provide health care to all?

Health Care Access

The decline in access to health care is most evident in the very young, the very old, and the poor and in minority populations. This decline in accessibility can only be partially attributed to a lack of insurance. Actually, lack of health insurance at most explains only a small percentage. Researchers have identified many barriers that delay or prevent access to care, but there has been no one specific factor that prevents health care access. One of the better ways, perhaps, to investigate why individuals do not access either preventive or treatment health services is through exploring the sociological and cultural domains.

Sociological Domain

There are many sociological reasons why people do not access care or preventive services or both. One overwhelming reason relates to lack of resources. This lack of resources may be material such as in lack of money or living in poverty. The poor and the elderly are very vulnerable to problems with access to care (Allender & Spradley, 2004). Coupled with a lack of financial resources may be fear due to an illegal immigrant status. For example, there are many undocumented illegal immigrants living in California, New York, and Texas who may not seek health care for fear of being deported to their country of origin.

Lack of resources in accessing health care is a major problem related to the cycle of poverty. Many U.S. residents are without access to health care because they are poor and without health services coverage (Allender & Spradley, 2004). This cycle of poverty extends to poor intellectual ability and even to ignorance of where to seek assistance. Inability to communicate in English or the language identified as the predominant language may also pose a sociological barrier to access to health care.

Cultural Domain

The value that an individual gives to activities involving health care access and health promotion activities frequently reflects cultural or religious beliefs or both. For example, many people may not access modern health care services; yet, they see folk healers or traditional culturally sensitive healers when they are ill. Members of the various ethnic and cultural groups manifest beliefs concerning health, disease prevention, and health promotion. These beliefs play a major part in terms of which health delivery services will be sought. Nursing professionals should be sensitive to the fact that certain ethnic groups may first seek help outside the modern health care system. Nursing's code of ethics specifies that nurses are to provide services that recognize human dignity and the uniqueness of the client. If nurses do not recognize human diversity and the beliefs that are important in accessing care, they are unethical in their nursing performance and are probably guilty of a legal infraction as well.

Research Note

A Comparative Study on Perceptions of Ethical Role

Study Problem/Purpose: To understand nursing ethics in the context of multiple role relationships and in the context of cultural settings. Culture may impact perceptions of the ethical role responsibilities relevant to nursing practice.

Methods: The Role Responsibilities Questionnaire (RRQ) was administered to a sample of nurses in China, the United States, and Japan. A total of 1,096 nurses were administered the RRQ.

Findings: Multidimensional preference analysis showed the patterns of rankings given by the different ethnicities to the statements that they considered important ethical responsibilities. The study findings revealed that the Chinese nurses were more virtue-based in their perception of ethical responsibilities, the American nurses were more principle-based, and the Japanese nurses were more care-based.

Implications: The findings indicate that cultural differences must be taken into account in outlining ethical responsibilities pertaining to nursing practice. This study is important in fostering international partnerships.

Pang, S. M., et al. (2003). A comparative study of Chinese, American, and Japanese nurses' perceptions of ethical role responsibilities. *Nursing Ethics, 10*(3), 295-311.

ETHICAL-LEGAL CONCEPTS AND HEALTH PROMOTION

According to the *Scope and Standards of Practice* (ANA, 2004) and *Nursing's Social Policy Statement* (ANA, 2003), professional nurses are expected to provide for client participation in all aspects of health promotion. The nurse is to keep the client and family informed regarding client status, collaborate with them in developing a nursing care plan, and provide them with information needed to make decisions and choices regarding care.

In assuming the responsibility for client participation in health promotion activities, the nurse is also expected to abide by the profession's code of ethics and the NPA. These documents spell out nursing's commitment to the caring and nurturing of clients and nursing's clear responsibility to advocate for the client, communicate with the client, family, and members of the health care team, and support health actions that restore health.

Many ethical and legal issues arise in nursing practice and in the activities associated with health promotion. Nurses may be expected to participate in decision making surrounding some of these issues. As a member of the profession, the nurse will be held ethically and legally accountable. Table 21-4 illustrates examples of potential nurse role/practice conflicts that may be encountered and their ethical and legal implications.

It is important to remember that as health promotion agents, nurses have a duty to advocate quality health care for clients not only at the bedside but also in the community and at the licensing board level (Creasia & Parker, 2001). The profession's accountability and ethical standards thus bind the nurse in the role of health care promoter. It is important to note, however, that several ethical and legal questions concerning health promotion remain. For example, does nursing have the right to determine what constitutes health? If so, does the profession set health agendas for people and decide on uniform health promotion strategies applicable to everyone?

NURSING AND HEALTH PROMOTION

In responding to the issue of whether nursing has the right to determine what health is and what health-promoting strategies must be espoused by nurses to achieve their clients' health, differentiation of health promotion from disease prevention becomes important. Integral to the concept of health promotion is concern for the problems that compromise health and well-being. Early development of positive health habits can result in a decrease of social problems (Pender, Murdaugh, & Parsons, 2006). Although nursing is concerned with the concept of illness and disease prevention, nursing also

Nurse Role	Potential Practice Conflict Examples	Ethical (E) and Legal (L) Implications
Nurturer	A nurse providing home care to a mother suspects child abuse after observing the mother's reaction to her child. The nurse must decide whether to report the situation to authorities and risk having the child placed in foster care.	**E** Nursing is committed to caring for and nurturing clients. In this example, the nurse must decide who the client is and how the concept of nurturing applies to the child. **L** The nurse must find out if reporting the abuse is within the scope of professional nursing. State laws governing reporting abuse must be determined.
Client advocate	A homeless person without any insurance is being provided substandard care by the medical team.	**E** Nursing's code indicates that the nurse act to safeguard the client at all times. As a client advocate, the nurse must assist the client in receiving the care deserved. **L** The NPA requires that the nurse advocate on the client's behalf and report unsafe care.
Health promotion agent	A nurse provides unsolicited dietary counseling to an extremely obese client being treated for a minor injury.	**E** The nurse must decide whether nursing professionals have the right to regulate a person's eating habits, even when such advice is unsolicited. **L** Legally the nurse owes a duty directly to the client. A client has the right to refuse counseling.
Communicator	A community health nurse is informed by a client that he has been diagnosed with diabetes and requests that no information regarding his illness be shared with his wife.	**E** Nursing's code of ethics asserts that a client's right to privacy should be maintained through the protection of confidential information. **L** The nurse should know that the practice act protects client confidentiality and that a client's family or significant other does not automatically have a right to confidential information.
Restorer and supporter of health	A client who is paralyzed is considering physician-assisted suicide and asks the nurse for help in locating a physician.	**E** The nurse must review personal feelings about nursing's multiple roles as client advocate and restorer and supporter of health. **L** The nurse must investigate whether physician-assisted suicide is legal in the state where he or she is practicing. The NPA should be reviewed to determine if a nurse can help in physician-assisted suicide.

focuses on those activities that promote social well-being. Accordingly, nursing promotes practices that foster positive health through healthy living and personal as well as family development. Nursing does not prescribe or dictate health promotion strategies nor set health agendas. Nursing, instead, clarifies client goals and encourages their achievement. People choose to do what they please. Nurses can only empower their clients; they cannot mandate behavior that promotes health.

From an ethical viewpoint, it is important to recognize that nursing views health and health promotion from the perspective of supporting self-defined goals whether of individual clients, their families, or the community in which they reside. Through support of their clients' self-defined goals, nurses empower them. Ethically, clients are empowered by being allowed to make choices that determine their physical well-being. Nurses support health promotion by providing education regarding choices that can be made and serving as a professional resource.

Legally, nursing is bound by the profession's standards of care and the NPA, both of which demand professional accountability. Health promotion is addressed in these documents in terms of advocating for clients in their pursuit of health and in assuring that a safe environment exists for them. Although nursing's goal is the achievement of positive health and well-being for all, from a legal standpoint a mentally competent client can refuse all nursing interventions. In the event that there is a possibility of harm to self or others, nursing can intervene through the legal court system, thus indirectly determining health promotion strategies for clients.

SUMMARY

Nurses are called upon regularly to make decisions that critically affect their clients' lives and well-being. Ethical and legal concerns are closely related and usually interwoven into the decision-making process. When nurses make decisions that have ethical and legal implications, these decisions must be rooted in the professional standards as set forth by the ANA. Decisions related to client care must also be made with an awareness of legal statutes, particularly those that relate to licensure laws and nursing practice. Ethical theories and principles guide nursing decision making by providing the context in which individual situations should be viewed. A process called values clarification can help the nurse become more conscious of personal values, which is important in developing insight.

As client advocates, nurses are expected to protect clients from unsafe procedures or situations and to see that their legal rights to safe and equitable health care are not violated. Registered nurses, by way of being licensed and belonging to the profession, are legally accountable for their actions. The nursing profession is becoming progressively more accountable as the role of the nurse evolves. Student nurses are not exempt from being accountable. There are several indicators of nursing's accountability and competency.

There is an apparent decline in access to health care. This decline is related to more than just lack of insurance. Nursing is concerned with a client's access to quality health care. It focuses also on activities that promote the social well-being and health of clients. Nursing does not prescribe or dictate health promotion strategies but clarifies client goals and their achievement. Through support of self-identified client goals, nurses empower clients. Although nursing's goal is the achievement of positive health, from a legal standpoint a mentally competent client can refuse all nursing interventions.

Key Concepts

1. Nursing decisions regarding ethical or legal issues must be rooted in the profession's standards and must abide by legal statutes.

2. Ethical principles and ethical theories, such as teleology and deontology, guide nursing decision making by providing a context in which a situation can be viewed.

3. Basic principles of ethics include autonomy, beneficence, nonmaleficence, veracity, confidentiality, justice, fidelity, standard of best interest, and respect for others.

4. The values clarification process, a process critical in decision making, assists nurses in the understanding of their own value systems and those of their clients.

5. Indicators of nursing's accountability and competency include licensure, credentialing, certification, accreditation, and an adherence to standards of care.

6. To prove negligence, the most frequent basis for nursing liability, the nurse's action causing harm must be within the nurse's professional scope, a breach of duty must have occurred, and this breach of duty must have caused the injury or harm.

7. Ethical and legal questions still arise over who can receive health care, who can afford health care services, and who has the right to access health care.

8. The high cost of health care has given rise to extreme cost-cutting measures that result in fragmentation and inadequacy of the care.

9. Nursing promotes practices that foster positive health through healthy living and personal as well as family development.

10. Through support of clients' self-defined health promotion goals, nurses empower clients.

Learning Activities

1. Look in your favorite nursing journal and find two clinical situations that can potentially require ethical decision making by the nurse.

2. As a nurse you will be expected to communicate pertinent information to your clients concerning their diagnosis, prognosis, procedures, and treatments. Think of a clinical situation in which you have provided client care. Determine which of the ethical principles listed in Table 21-1 were important to your communication with the client. Provide a rationale for your choice of principles.

3. In your own words, describe why licensure is important to the nursing profession.

4. Describe a situation that you encountered that required values clarification. What steps did you take in the process?

True/False Questions

1. T or F Ethics is a branch of philosophy dealing with moral values and actions.

2. T or F The principle of confidentiality regarding clients should never be broken.

3. T or F The nursing practice act makes nurses legally accountable for their actions.

4. T or F Assault can occur without battery.

Multiple Choice Questions

1. Ethical dilemmas are defined as which of the following?
   a. A problem that can be solved through the use of research data
   b. Clearly identified needed information
   c. Decisions requiring choices between undesirable alternatives
   d. Decisions requiring legal consultation

2. Which of the following is a legal guide for nursing?
   a. American Nurses Code of Ethics
   b. Hippocratic Oath
   c. Nightingale Pledge
   d. State Nursing Practice Act

3. Which of the following indicates that the client has given informed consent?
   a. Accepts the plan of care
   b. Gets a second opinion
   c. Is knowledgeable regarding the choices given
   d. Participates in an experimental procedure

4. The nurse assesses, explores, and determines personal values through the process of:
   a. Enrolling in an ethics class
   b. Personal meditation
   c. Reviewing the ANA Code of Ethics
   d. Values clarification

5. Which ethical principle is reflected when a nurse acts in the best interest of a client?
   a. Autonomy
   b. Beneficence
   c. Justice
   d. Nonmaleficence

Websites

http://www.counseling.org/ American Counseling Association. Provides information on general ethics issues, including ethical issues revolving around health-related problems.

http://www.ethics.org Ethics Resource Center. Includes information on organizational ethics as well as a question-and-answer section dealing with issues related to ethics.

Organizations

American Counseling Association
5999 Stevenson Avenue
Alexandria, VA 22304
Tel: (800) 347-6647; (800) 473-2329
Fax: (703) 823-6862
http://www.counseling.org
Agency that represents professional counselors in various practice settings.

Defense Research Institute (DRI)
150 North Michigan Avenue, Suite 300
Chicago, IL 60601
Tel: (312) 795-1101
Fax: (312) 795-0747
Espouses the defense viewpoint on cutting-edge issues in state and federal legislatures and courts.

Ethics Resource Center
1747 Pennsylvania Avenue NW, Suite 400
Washington, DC 20006
Tel: (202) 737-2258
Fax: (202) 737-2227
http://www.ethics.org

The oldest nonprofit in the United States devoted to organizational ethics; ERC advances understanding of the practices that promote ethical conduct through research, measurement of ethics and compliance program effectiveness in individual organizations, and the development of white papers and educational resources based on overall findings.

References

Aiken, T. D. (2004). *Legal, ethical, and political issues in nursing*. Philadelphia: F. A. Davis.

Allender, J. A., & Spradley, B. W. (2004). *Community health nursing: Concepts and practice* (6th ed.). Philadelphia: Lippincott Williams & Wilkins.

American Cancer Society. (2004). *The patient's bill of rights*. Retrieved January 25, 2006, from http://www.cancer.org

American Hospital Association (AHA). (1992). *A patient's bill of rights*. Chicago, IL: American Hospital Association.

American Nurses Association (ANA). (1998). *Standards of clinical nursing practice*. Washington, DC: American Nurses Publishing.

American Nurses Association (ANA). (2000). *American nurses credentialing center*. Retrieved May 30, 2006, from http://www.ana.org/ancc

American Nurses Association (ANA). (2001). *Code of ethics for nurses with interpretive statements*. Washington, DC: American Nurses Publishing.

American Nurses Association (ANA). (2003). *Nursing's social policy statement* (2nd ed.). Washington, DC: American Nurses Publishing.

American Nurses Association (ANA). (2004). *Scope and standards of practice*. Washington, DC: The Publishing Program of ANA.

Board of Nurse Examiners for the State of Texas. (2006). *Frequently asked questions about taking the NCLEX-RN examination*. Retrieved May 30, 2006, from http://www.bne.state.tx.us

Catalano, J. T. (2006). *Nursing now! Today's issues, tomorrow's trends* (4th ed.). Philadelphia: F. A. Davis.

Creasia, J., & Parker, B. (2001). *Conceptual foundations: The bridge to professional nursing practice*. St. Louis: Mosby.

Ellis, J. R., & Hartley, C. L. (2004). *Nursing in today's world: Trends, issues and challenges*. (8th ed.). Philadelphia: Lippincott Williams & Wilkins.

Guido, G. W. (2006). *Legal and ethical issues in nursing* (4th ed.). Upper Saddle River, NJ: Prentice Hall.

The Joint Commission. (2006). Retrieved May 30, 2006, from http://www.jcrinc.com

Lunsford v. Board of Nurse Examiners, 648 S.W.2d 391 (Tex. Ct. App.1983).

Monarch, K. (2002). *Nursing and the law: Trends and issues*. Washington, DC: American Nurses Publishing.

Pang, S. M., Sawada, A., Konishi, E., Olsen, D. P., Yu, P. L. H., Chan, M., & Mayumi, N. (2003). A comparative study of Chinese, American, and Japanese nurses' perceptions of ethical role responsibility. *Nursing Ethics, 10*(3), 295–311.

Pender, N. J., Murdaugh, C. L., & Parsons, M. A. (2006). *Health promotion in nursing practice* (5th ed.). Upper Saddle River, NJ: Pearson Prentice Hall.

RN Update. (April, 2000). *Return response required from all Texas registered nurses, 31*(2), 1.

Willmann, J. H. (2002). *Annotated guide to the Texas Nursing Practice Act*. Austin: Texas Nurses Association.

Zerwekh, J., & Claborn, J. C. (2006). *Nursing today: Transition and trends*. St. Louis: Saunders Elsevier.

Bibliography

Berntsen, K. (2005). Looking beyond tort reform toward safer healthcare systems. *Journal of Nursing Care Quality, 20*(1), 9–12.

Erlen, J. (2004). HIPAA: Clinical and ethical considerations for nurses. *Orthopedic Nursing, 23*(6), 410–413.

Leininger, M. (1990). *Ethical and moral dimensions of care*. (Ed.). Detroit, MI: Wayne State University Press.

Milston, C. (2005). Ethical issues: The ethics of respect in nursing. *Nursing Science Quarterly, 18*(1), 20–23.

Glossary

Abuse Physical, emotional, or sexual maltreatment.

Acanthosis Nigricans (AN) A skin condition associated with insulin resistance and type 2 diabetes.

Accreditation A form of certification or licensure that recognizes demonstrated compliance with established criteria.

Acculturation The process of adapting to, adopting, or taking on aspects of another culture; although something may be gained, something is also usually lost in the process; sometimes used interchangeably with *assimilation*.

Acne An inflammatory process of the sebaceous follicles of the skin, characterized by papules, comedones, and pustules.

Active Listening The act of perceiving what is communicated verbally as well as nonverbally.

Adaptation The process of changing behavior in response to external or internal stimuli or surroundings.

Addiction A gradual process that occurs when a person has developed both a biological and a psychosocial dependence on the substance of use.

Advance Directives Written instructions regarding specific procedures to be followed if the client becomes incapacitated.

Advocate One who takes the client's side and provides complete information to allow him or her to make decisions concerning individual health care.

Ageism Prejudice against the elderly.

Agraphia In a literate person, the inability to coordinate hand muscles sufficiently to produce handwriting.

Alogia An inability to speak in a person who has the ability to think.

Alpha Brain Waves Rhythmical brain waves associated with a quiet, resting state in the brain and body.

Amniocentesis Sampling of the amniotic fluid through a transabdominal puncture with ultrasound guidance.

Andragogy The education of adults.

Andropause The male climacteric caused by diminished levels of the androgen hormone, testosterone.

Anorexia Nervosa An eating disorder in which the individual voluntarily refuses to eat because of excessive concern over body shape or weight; the relentless pursuit of thinness or a prolonged refusal to eat or maintain body weight for age or height.

Anosmia Absence of the sense of smell.

Aphemesthesia In a literate person, the inability to understand the spoken or the written word.

Assault Infringement upon the mental security or the tranquility or both of another.

Assisted Living Facility (ALF) A facility designed to provide a special combination of personalized care, supportive services, and health-related services for care of the elderly.

Ataxic Aphasia See 'motor aphasia.'

Atrophy Muscle wastage.

Attachment Unique, specific, and enduring relationship involving mutual trust, responsiveness, and caring between the infant and the mother.

Attention-Deficit/Hyperactivity Disorder Neurobehavioral disorder characterized by increased impulsivity, inability to concentrate, hyperactivity, and difficulties in school and family relationships.

Auditory Amnesia *See* Auditory Aphasia.

Auditory Aphasia (Auditory Amnesia, Word Deafness) Ability to think and hear without the ability to understand the spoken word heard.

Authenticity Being real and genuine, as opposed to hiding behind a mask of professionalism.

Autonomy Principle based on the right to self-determination; gives an individual the right to choose what will happen to his or her own person.

Ayurveda Form of healing originating in India that focuses on physical health and spiritual growth, using meditation, sound, massage, herbs, the breath, and types of food specific to the individual to help balance the body and its energy field.

Baby Boomers Adults born between 1945 and 1964.

Balance This term implies that the total energy intake into the body in the form of nutrient calories does not exceed the body's expenditure of energy.

Ballistic Stretching Repeated bouncing.

Basal Metabolic Rate The amount of energy required to carry out involuntary bodily activities at rest; the rate at which the body uses energy to support its involuntary activities that are necessary for life.

Battery Involves physically touching a person; a physical violation.

Beneficence A principle that requires nurses to act in ways that benefit the client.

Body Composition The relative amount of fat in the body compared to fat-free weight such as muscle, bone, and other elements in the body.

Body Image Disturbance A distorted image that a person has of himself or herself.

Body Language The use of nonverbal communication behaviors that include personal presentation, proxemics, kinesics, and touch.

Body Mass Index (BMI) A number that shows body weight adjusted for height and that can be calculated using inches and pounds or meters and kilograms; a convenient tool that relates height and weight to determine whether the individual is considered overweight or obese.

Breach of Duty Deviation in some manner from the standard of care.

Bruising Leakage of blood into skin tissue damaged by a direct blow or a crushing injury.

Building-Related Illness A diagnosable illness that can be directly linked to airborne building contaminants.

Bulimia Nervosa An eating disorder characterized by binge eating followed by purging through self-induced vomiting, laxatives, diuretics, or excessive exercise.

Burnout The state of physical and emotional exhaustion that occurs when health care givers deplete their adaptive energy sources.

CAM Complementary and alternative medicine viewed as a group of diverse medical and health care systems, practices, and products that are not currently considered conventional medicine or that which is practiced by medical doctors or other health professionals, such as physical therapists, psychologists, and registered nurses. Complementary modalities are used as an adjunct to conventional medicine, while alternative modalities are used instead of conventional medicine.

Capacity Building A developmental process that results in independence and self-confidence.

Capitation Type of health care plan in which insurer or employer will pay a provider a set fee for all medical expenses necessary for each member covered under the plan.

Carcinogen A substance that can cause or promote the growth of cancer.

Cardiovascular Fitness Synonymous with cardiorespiratory fitness, aerobic fitness, or cardiorespiratory endurance, terms that refer to the circulatory system and respiratory system and how effectively and efficiently they function to transport oxygenated blood to working muscles for an extended period of time.

Career Ladder A degree completion program focusing on transitioning from one educational level to the next.

Caring Having a personal interest in the client; *feeling* for the client; involves an investment of the self.

Centenarian Person who lives past his or her 100th birthday.

Central Obesity A pattern of obesity in which a high proportion of fat is localized around the abdomen and upper body.

Certification Process by which an individual registered nurse who has met certain established criteria or qualifications is granted recognition for competency.

Chakras Spinning wheels of energy that help move healing energy from the universal field through the layers of the individual field (spiritual, mental, emotional, etheric) to the human body, and back to the universal field.

Chemical Sensitivity The physiological response to a toxic substance following long-term exposure to low-level chemicals that were not recognized as harmful in the past.

Chi An Asian concept referring to invisible energy and vitality by which all living things, earth, and sky are interrelated cosmically.

Chromotherapy The use of color in therapeutic ways.

Chronic Illness Type of disease or disorder that causes limitation of activity for a prolonged period.

Climacteric Change of life.

Code of Hammurabi The earliest written reference to health; established standards and practices of living for the ancient civilization of Babylonia.

Cohabitation Two unrelated adults of the opposite sex living together without a binding social or institutional contract.

Communication The process of conveying ideas, thoughts, opinions, or facts from one person to another.

Community Refers to a collection of people who interact with each other and who have common interests that form a sense of unity or belonging.

Community-Level Intervention Activity that occurs at the community level, rather than the individual or family level, to promote health or reduce illness or injury. For example, fluoridation of the water supply is a preventive community-level intervention. Mandating seat belt use is a community-level intervention to reduce the incidence of injury.

Comorbidity Another disability is present in addition to the substance use/abuse/addiction.

Concept A generalized notion or idea useful in describing facts or occurrences.

Conceptual Framework Concepts, facts, and/or propositions that are useful for defining nursing and provide a way to shape nursing and nursing practice into a meaningful configuration.

Constipation Difficult or infrequent passage of hard, dry fecal material.

Consumer Information Processing Model (CIP) Model that incorporates concepts related to the use of information and the motivational effect of using this information in making choices.

Context Conditions under which communication occurs.

Cool Down Refers to a warm down that is gradual and should be the last 5 to 10 minutes of the completed workout.

Coordinator of Care Assures the appropriate sequence of events in the client's plan of care.

Coping Strategies Techniques used by an individual to deal with situations that are perceived as stressful.

Couvade Medical term for sympathetic pregnancy experienced by the father.

Credentialing A process that recognizes professional achievements such as specialty practice knowledge, educational accomplishments, certification, licensure, and accreditation.

Crime A legal wrong committed against a person or property, punishable by the state and involving jail time.

Crisis Situation of severe disorganization resulting when an individual's coping mechanisms are not effective, or when usual resources are lacking, or a combination of both.

Cross Tolerance Drugs that are similar to each other and produce similar effects on the body and brain.

Cultural Competence Incorporating *emic* and *etic* cultural knowledge into holistic and cultural congruent client care.

Cultural Congruent Care Care that is provided to fit with the values, beliefs, and lifeways of an individual, a group, or an institution.

Cultural Tapestry The appreciation of the beauty that multiple cultures offer, weaving the unique and beautiful strands of each together in a rich array; AKA cultural mosaic.

Culture Dynamic adaptation; a learned way of life that includes interrelated attitudes, morals, beliefs, values, ideals, knowledge, symbols, artifacts, customs, traditions, and norms of a particular group that are transmitted intergenerationally, guide behavior, and make life meaningful.

Culture Broker A go-between who advocates on behalf of individuals, families, or communities, providing an effective approach to community engagement.

Decoder The person who receives and is able to interpret an encoded message in order to understand the sender's original idea, thought, opinion, or fact.

Dementia A progressive, organic mental disorder resulting in changes in personality, confusion, and impaired function, memory, and judgment.

Dental Caries Progressive decalcifications of the enamel of a tooth.

Deontology A theory of moral or professional obligation.

Desirable Body Weight Entails achieving a balance between adequate nutrition, proper body fat, and physical activity.

Detoxification Taking an individual who is using drugs off the drug.

Diagnosis-Related Groups (DRGs) The classification system created in 1983 that contained 468 diagnoses to be used with the prospective payment system for Medicare to pay hospital costs.

Diarrhea Frequent passage of watery, unformed fecal material.

Dietary Guidelines Recommendations for healthy Americans 2 years and over regarding food choices.

Dietary Reference Intakes (DRIs) A new system that replaces the Recommended Dietary Allowances and that focuses on the role of certain nutrients in reducing the risk for chronic diseases.

Diffusion of Innovations Model Model that addresses how new ideas, products, and social practices spread within a society or from one society to another.

Disease Cluster A group of individuals experiencing the same disease in greater numbers than would happen by chance.

Disease Prevention Measures taken to reduce the occurrence and severity of disease.

Domains Areas of concern affecting optimal health.

Drug Abuse The use of a drug or drugs inconsistent with social norms for purposes other than those for which they were intended, usually to alter feelings or mood, and without relation to medical or health reasons.

Drug Misuse The use of a drug or drugs inconsistent with social norms for purposes other than those for which they were intended, usually to alter feelings or mood, and without relation to medical or health reasons.

Dual Diagnosis Identification of those with both substance abuse and mental or physical health concerns.

Dysomnia Inadequate or dysfunctional sleep patterns.

Egocentric Concentrating upon self with little or no regard to others or the external world.

Elder Abuse Any knowing, intended, or careless act that causes harm or serious risk of harm to an older person, whether physically, mentally, emotionally, or financially.

Embryo The product of pregnancy from conception to eight weeks.

Emic **Knowledge** Subjective view; an insider's perspective; understanding the *emic* perspective is considered a prerequisite for cultural competence.

Empathy State-of-being experienced by identifying closely with your client because you are able to imagine yourself in the client's situation and able to feel the client's feelings as if they were yours.

Empowerment Process of helping others to help themselves; to enable or give power to your client.

Encoder The person who initiates communication by placing a message in a form that is understandable to the person meant to receive it.

Encopresis Fecal incontinence in a child 9 years of age or older who has no physical abnormality causing the incontinence.

Energy A dynamic quality or power that has the capacity for doing work.

Energy Field A field of energy that is composed of constantly changing vibrational frequencies and that surrounds and connects all matter. All living things are energy fields that affect and are affected by all other forms of energy, creating health and disease.

Enuresis Involuntary urinary incontinence in a child 5 years of age or older who has no physical abnormality causing the incontinence.

Environmental Health Hazard A substance or agent that has the ability to cause any type of adverse health effect. The effect can range from a minor illness to a serious illness to death.

Environmental Health Risk The probability that there will be actual consequences from the potential danger of an environmental hazard.

Environmental Tobacco Smoke (ETS) Tobacco smoke in the air; also known as involuntary, sidestream, or second-hand smoke.

Epidemiology A field of study that examines the relationships among disease, the environment, the individual, and the community; concerned with the time, place, and person components of disease, defect, disability, or death.

Equal Protection A guarantee under U.S. law that all similarly situated individuals are entitled to be treated similarly.

Ergonomics The science of relationships of furniture and tools to the human body; the study and analysis of human work as it relates to an individual's anatomy and other human characteristics.

ESADDI The *e*stimated *s*afe and *a*dequate *d*aily *d*ietary *i*ntake.

Essential Nutrients A nutrient is considered essential when the body requires it for growth and maintenance but does not manufacture it in sufficient amounts to meet the body's needs.

Ethical Principles Basic concepts and rules to guide and give direction to nursing practice.

Ethics The branch of philosophy that is related to moral values and actions.

Ethnicity A large group of people classified according to common national, tribal, linguistic, or cultural origin or background *and* who feel a sense of shared identity.

Ethnocentrism Literally, a belief that one's ethnic group is better than or superior to someone else's (inherent is the belief that someone else's ethnicity is inferior); the term's usage has been broadened to refer to a belief that one's particular cultural beliefs, worldview, and way of life are better than someone else's.

Etic **Knowledge** Objective view; an outsider's perspective.

Eustress A positive form of stress that mobilizes us to action.

Exchange System A system for classifying foods into numerous lists based on their macronutrient composition and for establishing serving sizes so that one serving of each food on a list contains the same amount of carbohydrate, protein, fat, and energy (calories).

Exclusive Provider Organization (EPO) Type of managed care service that requires its members to get their services within the network only.

Expected Outcomes Measurable goals set by the nurse and the client for the client and derived from the nursing diagnosis.

Expressive Aphasia The ability to think without the ability to speak.

Feedback The process by which effectiveness of communication is determined. This is the encoding and sending of a message from the receiver back to the original sender in order to let the original sender know how the message was received.

Feng Shui An ancient Chinese practice of configuring one's environment to promote a healthy flow of chi, or vital energy, for health, happiness, and prosperity.

Fetus The product of pregnancy from the eighth week until delivery.

Fidelity The concept of faithfulness and the practice of keeping promises.

Flexibility The ability of a joint or group of joints to move freely through a range of motion.

Folk Health Sector The health arena comprised of unlicensed, nonprofessional specialists who are usually members of the local community; "folk" is sometimes used to incorporate "lay/popular," although it is best to differentiate the terms; "indigenous," "generic," and "traditional" sometimes are used interchangeably with both "lay/popular" and "folk" and usually refer to people's nonprofessional, tried-and-true health practices.

Food Guide Pyramid A guide to the amounts and kinds of foods that we should eat daily to maintain health and to reduce risks of developing diet-related diseases.

General Adaptation Syndrome (GAS) An adaptational response to stress consisting of three phases, including an alarm reaction, a resistance or adaptation phase, and an exhaustion phase.

General Systems Theory Focuses on the exchange of energy between the individual and the environment and has as a central concept that a person is whole and more than a sum of parts.

Genogram A tool that diagrams and depicts family relationships over a period of several generations, usually at least three.

Geriatrics Specialized branch of medicine that focuses on the diagnosis and treatment of diseases affecting the elderly.

Gerontology The study of all aspects of aging, including all domains and their impacts on the elderly and society.

Gestational Diabetes Diabetes that occurs during pregnancy as a result of hormonal changes.

Global Aphasia The inability to express or receive verbal messages in any form in a person who can think.

Gonads Generic terms for the female sex glands (the ovaries) and the male sex glands (the testes).

Grounding Using thought and breath to connect to the Earth as a source of stable, steady energy and to the universal source of healing energy.

Gynecomastia Enlargement of breast tissue in the male.

Half-life Half the time it takes for a drug to be metabolized out of the system.

Hardiness Resilience to stress.

Health Encompasses the total functioning of an individual and includes effective physical, psychological, social, cultural, environmental, and technological functioning.

Health Behavior Patterns Health habits that may relate to physical functioning or to the person's psychological, spiritual, and/or professional lives.

Health Belief Model Model developed by four social psychologists, Hochbaum, Kegeles, Leventhal, and Rosenstock; suggests that a person's susceptibility to a health threat and its seriousness influence his or her decision to engage in a preventive health behavior.

Health Education A tool or mechanism for health-related learning resulting in increased knowledge, skill development, and change in behavior.

Health Maintenance Organization (HMO) Type of managed care service that provides health care to members for a fixed usually monthly payment.

Health Promotion Any process directed at enhancing the quality of health and well-being of individuals, families, groups, communities, and/or nations through strategies involving supportive environments, coordination of resources, and respect for personal choice and values.

Health Promotion Plan A plan that focuses on achieving wellness and that, along with the client, determines the activities that are necessary to achieve optimal health. The plan examines the client's vulnerability to health imbalance, assesses client weaknesses and strengths, and determines potential for illness.

Health Protection Frequently used interchangeably with disease prevention and reflects a disease-related focus that is consistent with the medical model supported by the discipline of medicine.

Healthy People 2000 A document developed by the United States Surgeon General, in conjunction with health care constituents across the nation, that delineates 22 priority areas with 300 specific measurable objectives for health promotion, health protection, and surveillance and data systems for the United States to be achieved by the year 2000.

Healthy People 2010 A national health promotion and disease prevention initiative that brings together national, state, and local government agencies; nonprofit, voluntary, and professional organizations; businesses; communities; and individuals to improve the health of all Americans, eliminate disparities in health, and improve years and quality of healthy life. It is designed to serve as a roadmap for improving the health of all Americans through two major goals and 467 objectives in 28 focus areas.

Heart Rate Reserve The difference between the resting heart rate and the maximum heart rate.

Heliotherapy The use of sunlight for healing.

Heterogeneity The quality or state of not being the same throughout; diversity.

High-Level Wellness Describes a step above health that is the dynamic state of wellness which occurs at the individual, environmental, cultural, and social levels; keys to achieving this step are the capability and potential of the individual.

Holistic Refers to a view of people in their complex entirety or totality.

Holistic Care Care in which the client is viewed as an integrated whole whereby the physical, mental, social, emotional, and spiritual needs are considered. The whole is considered to be greater than the sum of the parts. The total inner and outer environments of the client are considered when looking for causes for the imbalances in health and life, and how to correct them.

Holistic Healing Assisting the establishment and maintenance of balance and wholeness in mind, body, and spirit of client and nurse.

Holistic Medicine An approach to health care that uses social, psychological, and spiritual aspects to bring about wellness.

Holistic Nursing A view of nursing in which the whole is defined as equal to the sum of the parts.

Homeostasis A state of equilibrium within the body.

Homosexuality The sexual orientation of a person who is sexually attracted to a person of the same sex.

Human Ecological Model Model developed by nurse researcher Joan Shaver that considers all factors that influence human health, whether they act alone or in combinations.

Hypnosis An induced, trance-like state of altered perception and memory resulting in heightened suggestiveness whereby the person often will follow instructions given.

Hypothalamus The gland in the brain responsible for control of metabolic activities, regulation of body temperature, integration of sympathetic and parasympathetic activities, and secretion of releasing (stimulating) and inhibiting hormones.

Ideal Body Weight What a person should reasonably weigh as compared to height.

Imagery Creating and holding a mental picture of what we want to happen in life using all five senses. It is the communication mechanism between perception, emotion, and bodily change. Using imagery regularly can bring about changes in the body, mind, energy field, and spirit.

Immune Modulation A factor, either physical, emotional, or treatment variable, that alters the degree of immune functioning.

Immunoenhancement A factor that can bring about increased immune function, prevention of disease, and recovery from illness in an individual.

Incest Sexual contact with a child or adolescent by any member of the family or household.

Incontinence Inability to retain urine or feces.

Infant Live-born individual from the moment of birth until one year of life.

Informed Consent A clear explanation of procedures to be had along with associated risks and benefits.

Intensity Refers to how hard a person must work to improve physical fitness.

Interventions Nursing actions that enable the client to achieve the desired goal.

Intimate Partner Violence A pattern of assault or coercion to force a partner to comply with the other partner's wishes.

Introspection The ability to look inside oneself and examine thoughts and personal meaning for identified values.

Isoimmunization Rh-negative mothers sensitized by exposure to Rh-positive blood, its involuntary activities which are necessary to life.

Justice Fair, equitable, and appropriate treatment according to what is due or owed to persons.

Kinesics How we move our bodies or body parts, including conscious and unconscious changes in body posture, facial expressions, and gestures.

LaLonde Report A classic document, created by the Canadian Minister of National Health in 1974, which was the first to publicly acclaim health promotion as a major disease prevention strategy.

Law The sum total of rules and regulations by which a society is governed.

Lay/Popular Health Sector Same as popular health sector; the nonprofessional, nonspecialist health care arena consisting of the individual along with family and friends; "folk" is sometimes used to incorporate "lay/popular," although it is best to differentiate the terms; "indigenous," "generic," and "traditional" sometimes are used interchangeably with both "lay/popular" and "folk" and usually refer to people's nonprofessional, tried-and-true health practices.

Learned Helplessness A phenomenon that has negative physical and psychological consequences and that occurs when an individual believes he or she has no control over an experience, whether a negative or positive experience. The individual becomes helpless or quits trying to affect or change the experience. It can be reversed if control is regained.

Managed Care Method of delivering health care that integrates and coordinates the delivery of health care with the costs of that service.

Managed Care Organization: A health plan that provides consumers access to quality health care at a reasonable price.

Masturbation Self-manipulation of the genitals for the purpose of sexual pleasure.

Maximum Heart Rate The fastest rate the heart can attain under maximal exercise conditions and still receive benefit.

Medicaid Program A 1965 amendment to the Social Security Act designed to provide a share of payments made by state welfare to health care agencies caring for the poor, medically needy, aged, disabled, and their dependent children and families.

Medicare Program A 1965 amendment to the Social Security Act designed to provide hospital insurance and supplement medical insurance for people over age 65, disabled people receiving Social Security benefits, and patients in end-stage renal disease.

Medicocentrism The belief that professional health care practices are better than lay/popular or folk health care practices, reflecting ethnocentrism by members of the professional health care system.

Meditation The intentional focusing of attention on a singular activity, thought, or object such as one's own breathing,

a visual image, a religious symbol, or a phrase repeated silently to oneself; a technique (there are many) to interrupt unconscious, rampant thoughts of the mind. This is often done by noticing and observing what we are thinking or replacing thoughts with more beneficial ones. The body and mind become more relaxed, the stress response ceases, and healing is enhanced.

Melanoma A malignant, darkly pigmented skin lesion which develops from repeated exposure to the sun.

Menarche The initiation of menstruation.

Menopause The cessation of menses; usually considered complete after a year of amenorrhea.

Message The content (idea, thought, opinion, or fact) one person wishes another person to receive in the process of communication.

Metabolic Syndrome An association of obesity, insulin resistance, glucose intolerance, hypertension, and dyslipidemia that predisposes the individual to diabetes and cardiovascular disease.

Metaparadigm Used by an individual discipline to provide a global perspective of the field; e.g., nursing's metaparadigm describes the concepts specific to nursing.

Mind-Body Dualism A philosophy of the separateness of the mind and body, which has existed in medicine at least since 1619, and has allowed investigation and treatment to focus on the illness of the body, with only a few diseases being thought to have a primary cause related to the mind.

Model A visual representation of the concepts that work together to become a theory.

Modeling and Role Modeling A nursing theory developed by Helen Erickson, RN, Ph.D., which says that for people to heal, their needs must be met; to meet their needs, they can look at the stressors in their life and their resources for coping with those stressors.

Morbidity Illness rate.

Mortality Death rate.

Mosaic Code Regulations for society developed by ancient Hebrews that included an organized system for disease prevention.

Motor Aphasia (Ataxic Aphasia) An ability to think with an inability to coordinate the muscles responsible for speech (alogia) or writing (agraphia).

Multistate Licensure Recognition of a single license allowing registered nurses to practice nursing throughout the country.

Muscular Endurance The ability of a muscle or group of muscles to perform or sustain a muscle contraction over an extended period of time.

Muscular Strength The ability or capacity to exert force with a muscle against resistance, under maximal conditions in a single effort.

Mutagen A substance that can change genetic material found in chromosomes.

MyPyramid Replaces the Food Guide Pyramid and is used as a food guidance system.

Nationality In general, refers to country of origin or birth.

Needs Theory Theory that describes people as whole with many complex needs that motivate behavior.

Negative Energy Balance A state that occurs when a person's energy needs exceed that produced by the foods consumed.

Negligence Involves failure to provide the care that a reasonable person would provide in similar circumstances.

Nightmare An anxiety dream to which the child responds by awakening.

Night Terror Form of a nightmare in which the child screams out, cries, and does not respond by awakening.

Noise Any loud, discordant, or disagreeable sound or sounds that can decrease body energy or cause auditory damage.

Nonessential Nutrients Nutrients that the body can make.

Nonmaleficence A principle that requires nurses to act in such a way as to avoid causing harm to clients.

Nonverbal Communication The conveyance of messages without the use of words. It consists of body language and paralanguage.

Nonverbal Vocalizations Sounds such as grunts, groans, sighs, and sobs that make up one type of paralanguage.

Nurse Healer A nurse who helps others to heal or remember their inherent state of wholeness by cherishing, nurturing, and promoting their growth and development. Nurse healers are aware that personal presence with the client is a factor in healing.

Nursing: A Social Policy Statement The first document, prepared by leaders in the profession, to describe nursing and the profession's responsibility to society.

Nursing Diagnosis Consists of the actual identification of a client's need.

Nursing Process Method for developing an appropriate plan of care and wellness outcomes for clients that includes four phases: assessing and establishing a nursing diagnosis, planning, implementing, and evaluating.

Nutrients Substances found in foods that the body can use for the maintenance of body functions throughout life.

Nutrition Study of food substances or nutrients and their processes essential for health.

Obesity The condition of being overweight or of being more than 20 percent over the ideal body weight.

Occupational Stress Stress that is job related and leads to extreme tension, anxiety, and possibly even physical symptoms.

O'Donnell Model of Health Promotion Behavior Developed by health care administrator Michael O'Donnell, this model is a composite of Ajzen's Theory of Planned Behavior, the Theory of Social Behavior, the Health Belief Model, and the Pender Health Promotion Model.

Optimal Body Composition The proper balance between body fat, muscle mass, and bone.

Outcomes The results of nursing intervention with clients, stated in client-centered, measurable terms.

Outgassing The production of a toxic gas from the breakdown of formaldehyde in synthetic products.

Overload Principle Overload means the body is being forced to do more than it normally does.

Over-the-Counter (OTC) Drugs Those drugs that can be purchased from pharmacies or supermarkets for use when symptoms are of a minor nature.

Overweight Being at or above the 95th percentile for age/sex-specific BMI.

Papanicolaou (Pap) Test A laboratory test for cancer in which cells are collected from areas that shed cells and are microscopically examined for early changes which may be related to the development of cancer.

Paradigm An example that serves as a pattern or model for something.

Paralanguage The use of nonverbal components of spoken language.

Particulate Matter Small particles or liquid droplets that can be suspended in the air.

Paternalism A system that encourages individuals to make decisions for others.

Pedagogy The education of children.

Peer Individual of the same age with an equal standing in age, class, or rank.

Pender Health Promotion Model Developed by nurse researcher Nola Pender, this model integrates concepts from the expectancy-value model of human motivation and social cognitive theory with self-efficacy as a predominant concept. It is unique to nursing because of its holistic perspective.

Perceptions The process of recognizing and interpreting an illness, a sensation, or an experience in order to gain understanding or give it meaning.

Perimenopause A time of transition from normal menstrual periods to cessation of menses occurring gradually over 2 to 15 years.

Personal Presentation How we show ourselves to the world, including how we dress, groom ourselves, and use cosmetics, perfumes, and deodorants to create an identity by which we choose to be known.

Physical Fitness The ability to be physically active on a regular basis.

Phytochemicals Herbs or plants used to promote and maintain health and cure disease; bioactive compounds of plant origin that can provide protection against heart disease, arthritis, and some types of cancer.

Pica Ingestion of substances that have no food value.

Plantar Fasciitis Arch pain commonly occurring in walkers and runners.

Polypharmacy The use of many drugs at one time; the use of multiple medications without the knowledge of a supervising physician or nurse practitioner.

Positive Energy Balance A state that occurs when the amount of food consumed exceeds the energy used by the body.

Postpartum The time between delivery and the return of a woman's reproductive organs to the nonpregnant state.

Posttraumatic Stress Disorder (PTSD) The constellation of continuing, long-term detrimental effects resulting from exposure to trauma.

PRECEDE-PROCEED Model A model to guide the development of health promotion programs for groups and communities. It is multidimensional, multi-leveled, and broad-based and is focused on outcomes rather than inputs.

Preferred Provider Organization (PPO) Type of managed care service that uses provider networks to deliver health care to its members.

Premenstrual Syndrome (PMS) The cyclic recurrence of distressing physical, psychological, and/or behavioral changes related to the menstrual cycle.

Prescription Drugs Medications prescribed by a physician or nurse practitioner that contain substances that aid in the prevention of disease, the diagnosis of a condition, or the alleviation of symptoms, or help in the recovery from a disease or disorder.

Presence Being with another in a meaningful way, giving of one's self in the current moment, listening, and providing unconditional acceptance. Presence involves giving of one's self and being open to the experience of another through an interpersonal relationship that is reciprocal.

Primary Care Provider A health care provider that the client sees first for health care services. The primary care provider is usually a family practice physician.

Primary Disease Prevention Level of prevention that includes activities and lifestyle factors that can be changed or maximized with high-level wellness as the goal.

Primary Prevention Prevention for those who have not used tobacco, alcohol, or other drugs, with the goal of preventing exposure to and experimentation with drugs.

Principle of Progression Implies that gradually the overload stimulus is increased as adaptations to the existing workload occur.

Principle of Specificity Applies to all types of training and states that one must overload the body systems or the specific fitness component to achieve a specific outcome.

Professional Health Sector The formally organized, modern, scientific health community; much more than only medical care; encompasses professional nursing, medicine, pharmacy, dietetics, etc.

Prospective Payment System (PPS) A fixed predetermined method of payment to hospitals based on the concept that similar medical diagnoses result in the same hospitalization costs.

Prospective Studies Research studies that follow subjects without the disease or outcome of interest forward in time. Animal subjects are followed for enough person-years to establish incidence, morbidity, or mortality rates.

Protection Motivation Theory A fear-driven model proposing that a perceived threat to health activates thought processes regarding the severity of the threatened event, the probability of its occurrence, and coping mechanisms.

Protective Factors Factors that build resiliency against substance abuse and increase the likelihood that an individual will resist substance abuse.

Proxemics How we use the personal space around us, including conscious and unconscious changes in the distances we maintain from others and the manner in which we touch and are touched by others.

Psychoneuroimmunology (PNI) Study of the interrelationship of the mind and body.

Psychotropic Drugs Drugs that modify mental activity and affect psychic function, behavior, or experience and are normally used to treat mental disorders.

Puberty The period in life during which members of both genders become capable of reproduction.

Race A category of humankind that shares certain distinctive physical traits.

Rate of Perceived Exertion A feeling for the amount of intensity or exertion being attained.

RDA *R*ecommended *d*ietary *a*llowance; daily dietary intake that is sufficient to meet the nutrient requirements of 97 to 98 percent of all healthy individuals.

Reflexology A touch therapy using the pad of the thumb to apply pressure to specific points on the feet and hands that correspond to areas of the torso. This technique can enhance relaxation of, stimulate circulation to, and aid healing of the corresponding areas.

Registration Listing of an individual's name and other information on the official roster of a governmental or nongovernmental agency.

Regular Physical Exercise The act of engaging in exercise behaviors that involve large muscle groups in dynamic movement at least three or more times a week for 20 minutes or more each time and that is performed at an intensity requiring 60 to 80 percent of a person's cardiovascular capacity.

Relapse Prevention Prevention of the return to substance use. Relationships among variables and are useful in describing, explaining, predicting, and controlling.

Relaxation Response A technique developed by Herbert Benson, M.D., that uses focus on a chosen repetition, such as the breath or a word, to interrupt the stress response and promote relaxation.

Relaxation Techniques A group of strategies involving breathing or mind control used to decrease stress and tension. Relaxation techniques can be used as an active coping strategy and actually result in changes in heart rate, respiratory rate, and metabolism.

Respect for Others Seen as the highest ethical principle and incorporates all the other ethical principles; acknowledges that individuals are capable of making decisions for themselves.

Retrospective Studies Research studies that identify subjects with the illness or outcome of interest and evaluate their past experiences for postulated causal factors.

RICE A good modality to use with muscle sprains or strains or other minor discomforts. Refers to *r*est, *i*ce, *c*ompression, and *e*levation.

Risk Factor A characteristic associated with increased likelihood of disease or injury.

SAD Syndrome Seasonal affective disorder believed to be related to increased melatonin levels. Symptoms associated with SAD syndrome include fatigue, increased craving for carbohydrates in the diet, weight gain, lethargy, and severe clinical depression. Physiological problems such as infertility, alterations in menstrual cycles, and premenstrual syndrome may also occur.

Sandwich Generation The middle adult period in which people are "sandwiched" between their children who need nurturance and support and their aging parents, who also need care.

Scoliosis Abnormal curvature of the spine, usually consisting of an abnormal lateral curvature and a compensatory curve.

Screening The use of a diagnostic procedure such as a laboratory test or an evaluation tool to determine the presence of a particular disease or risk factors known to be associated with a health problem.

Secondary Prevention Level of prevention that involves health screenings that identify abnormalities within a population; strategies aimed at preventing substance abuse by individuals at risk for developing problems and those who are already using substances.

Self-efficacy Self-conviction or belief that one can be successful in achieving the desired behavior.

Sensitivity of a Screening Test Ability of a screening test to correctly give a positive result when the individual has the disease or condition being tested for.

Sensory Channel Means by which a message is sent. The three primary routes are the visual (sight), auditory (hearing), and kinesthetic (touch) channels.

Set Point of Weight Control Theory States that all individuals have a unique, stable, adult body weight that is the result of several biological factors.

Severe Obesity The state of being 100 pounds or more over normal body weight.

Sexuality Broad term that includes not only the dimensions of sexual desire and sexual response but also the individual's view of self and presentation of self.

Sha An Asian concept that refers to bad chi, which is believed to bring bad luck and poor health as well as family and business difficulties.

Sick Building Syndrome The cluster of vague symptoms that are traced to pollutants in sealed buildings.

Simultaneous Perception A system used to experience our environment by combining the responses of all our senses.

Sleep Apnea A sleep disorder characterized by recurrent periods of absence of breathing for 10 seconds or longer, occurring at least five times per hour.

Social Security Act Legislation enacted by the U.S. government in 1935 to provide eligible citizens with public aid, social services, and aid to the elderly.

Social Support The presence of a group of interconnected, cooperating significant others who provide assistance and help strengthen the individual.

Specificity of a Screening Test Ability of a screening the test to correctly give a negative result when the individual being screened does not have the disease.

Spiritual Health A balance between self and others.

Spiritual Well-being The affirmation of life in a relationship with God or a higher power, self, community, and environment that nurtures and celebrates wholeness.

Spirituality Concepts that refer to experiences traditionally considered religious as well as to all states of awareness.

Sprain Injury to a ligament.

Standard of Best Interest Standard that allows individuals to share in decision making regarding health care.

Static Stretching Slow and deliberate stretching.

Strain Injury to a muscle.

Stress An emotional and physiological response to a stressor.

Stress Response An adaptive response by the individual to a stressor in which the pituitary gland and the sympathetic branch of the autonomic nervous system are activated, sending a message to the central nervous system via epinephrine or norepinephrine that elicits the fight-or-flight reaction, otherwise known as the stress response, to the stressor.

Stressor An event, a situation, or a life change perceived as a threat to an individual's physical or psychological well-being; stress-provoking factor that can impact the health of those who provide health care to others.

Substance Abuse The habitual use of alcohol and/or illegal substances such as marijuana, cocaine, methamphetamine, and numerous others.

Tao A concept of Asian life that means to be connected.

Target Heart Rate The level or zone one should attain during aerobic activity to obtain training benefit.

Taxonomy A common classification structure that links nursing diagnoses, interventions, and outcomes.

Teleology An ethical theory that explains phenomena and justifies actions by results, or the doctrine of final causes.

Teratogen A substance that can cause birth defects or abnormal development in embryonic structures.

Terrorism The unlawful use of force and violence against persons or property to intimidate or coerce a government, the civilian population, or any segment thereof, in furtherance of political or social objectives.

Tertiary Prevention Seeks to address the situation once symptoms have occurred and is directed toward minimizing disease or disability; prevention of death and disability of individuals in long-term treatment.

Theory A set or group of interrelated concepts, facts, definitions, and propositions that specify relationships among variables and are useful in describing, explaining, predicting, and controlling.

Theory of Planned Behavior Developed by Icek Ajzen to explain behavior as on a control continuum with total control at one end and absence of control at the other end. Control is viewed as being influenced by resources, support, skills, and self-efficacy needed for a certain behavior.

Theory of Social Behavior Developed by sociologist Henry Triandis, this theory distinguishes behavior under the individual's control from behavior that has become automatic or habit.

Therapeutic Communication The use of verbal and nonverbal techniques focused on client needs and with the avoidance of unhelpful or nontherapeutic techniques.

Therapeutic Touch A technique developed by Dolores Krieger, RN, Ph.D., and Dora Kunz that uses the hands to perceive and balance the energy field to enhance relaxation, pain relief, and healing.

Tolerance Occurs when more of a drug is required to obtain the desired effects.

Tort Legal wrong committed against a person or property and settled in civil court.

Touch Manner in which we come into bodily contact with others.

Transcultural Theory Theory that focuses on the individual and describes how culture influences and provides meaning to everything a person does, thinks, feels, or hears.

Transtheoretical Model (TTM) A theoretical model explaining behavior change though five distinct stages that contain elements of thought, action, and time along with nine processes of change related to experiential (what the individual is experiencing in relation to self, the environment, and others), and behavioral (the processes that enhance success for change).

Triad Diagnosis Presence of a mental health issue, a physical health issue, and a substance abuse issue simultaneously.

Unconditional Positive Regard Demonstrating acceptance and respect for the client as a fellow human being, without imposing any conditions for that acceptance.

Urinary Incontinence The involuntary leakage of urine.

Utter Watchfulness The ability to pay equal attention to everything in the environment at once, emphasizing nothing and omitting nothing.

Values A set of personal beliefs and attitudes.

Values Clarification The process of becoming more conscious of and naming what one values or considers worthy.

Veracity The practice of telling the truth.

Verbal Communication Use of words to convey messages. Most often these words are written or spoken, but they may be formed in other ways, such as by the use of sign language.

Visual Aphasia (Word Blindness) Inability of a literate person to decode the written word.

Volatile Organic Compounds (VOCs) Gases released from certain solids or liquids.

Warm-up Consists of stretching and mild exercise to gradually increase the heart rate, circulation, and body temperature.

Weapons of Mass Destruction (WMDs) Chemical, biological, and radiological weapons or devices intended to cause death or serious bodily harm to a significant number of people.

Weapons of Mass Effect (WMEs) Term that denotes the motives of terrorists to cause widespread chaos and despair by whatever method used.

Weight Control The change, acquisition, and maintenance of a desirable body weight.

Weight Cycling The losing and regaining of weight seen in yo-yo dieting or the repeated practice of dieting.

Word Blindness *See* Visual Aphasia.

Word Deafness *See* Auditory Aphasia.

Worldview (also **World View**) Reflects values, norms, expressions, taboos, myths, rituals, rites, and so forth; refers to the way people perceive the world, including health, wellness, illness, sickness, death, human nature, etc.

Yang A principal power of Chinese philosophy that works in opposition to yin to regulate the universe and balance the mind, body, and spirit; yang is the male element associated with positive energy, action, generativity, the sun, light, and the creativity of life.

Yin A principal power of Chinese philosophy that works in opposition to yang to regulate the universe and balance the mind, body, and spirit; yin is the female element associated with negative energy, passiveness, destruction, the moon, darkness, and death.

Index

Page numbers in italics indicate figures and tables

A

AACN. *See* American Association of Colleges of Nursing

AARP. *See* American Association of Retired Persons

Abortion, 181

Abuse
adolescents, 228–229, *229*
child abuse and neglect, 191–192
defined, 228
domestic violence during pregnancy, 178–179, *179*
drug abuse, 369–370
elder abuse, 279–280, *281*
intimate partner violence, 240, *240*
substance abuse, 366–382

Acanthosis nigricans, 205, *205, 209*

Accidents, adolescents, 230, *231*

Accreditation, 455

Acculturation, 108–109

Acetylcholine, 151

Acid rain, 121–122

Acne, 220, *220*

Acquired immune deficiency syndrome (AIDS), impact of depression on, 161

ACTH. *See* Adrenocorticotropin hormone

Active listening, 88

Activity
adolescents, 222
infants and toddlers, 187
preschool and school-age children, 204

Acupressure, 406–407

Adaptation Model (Roy), 30

Adaptation theory, 30

Addiction
biological basis of, 370, *371*
defined, 370
psychosocial basis of, 370–371, *371*

ADHD. *See* Attention-deficit/hyperactivity disorder

Administration On Aging (AOA), 290, 445

Adolescents, 218–233
abuse, 228–229, *229*
accidents, 230, *231*
acne, 220, *220*
activity, 222
biological domain, 218–226
blood pressure, 222
body image, 226
cognitive development, 226–227
cultural influences, 229
dental caries and gum disease, 222–223
depression, 227, *227*
eating disorders, *221,* 221–222, *222*
emotional development, 227–228
environmental domain, 230–231, *231*
family life, 228
invulnerability, 226
moral development, 226–227
nutrition, 221–222
obesity, 222, 347
peers, 228
political domain, 229–230
pregnancy, 170, 173, 232
psychological domain, 226–228
puberty, 218–221, *219*
safety, 230–231, *231*
screening, 222–226
sexuality, 231–232
smoking, 377
social domain, 228–229
spiritual domain, 232–233
substance abuse, *222–225,* 223–225
substance abuse and, 376–377
suicide, 227–228, *228*
violence, 230–231

Adrenal gland, *152*

Adrenocorticotropin hormone (ACTH), 151–152

Adult learning, 91–92

Adults. *See* Middle-aged adults; Motherhood; Older adults; Young adults

Advocate, 63

Age
in cultural assessment, 104
nursing supply and, 423
substance abuse and, 376–377

Ageism, 279

Aging, theories of, 271, *272*

AHNA. *See* American Holistic Nurses Association

AIDS. *See* Acquired immune deficiency syndrome

Air pollution, 115–124
health promotion and nursing interventions for, 122–123, *122–125*
indoor air, 115–119, *116–125*
outdoor air, 120–122
Sick building syndrome, 115, *116*
smog, 121
worksite air quality, 119, *121*

Ajzen, Icek, 42–43

Alcohol use. *See also* Substance abuse
addiction, 375–376
adolescents, *222–225,* 223–225
central nervous system, 376
osteoporosis, 375
physical effects of, 375, *375*
preconception, 172
pregnancy, 174
risk factors and health promotion for middle-aged adults, 259–260, *260*

ALF. *See* Assisted living facility

Alpha brain waves, 234

American Academy of Pediatrics, 186

American Association of Colleges of Nursing (AACN), 38

American Association of Retired Persons (AARP), 290

American Diabetes Association, 311

American Dietetic Association, 311, 319

American Holistic Medical Association, 389

American Holistic Nurses Association (AHNA), 166, 389

American Hospital Association, *Patient's Bill of Rights,* 448

American Medical Association, 7

American Nurses Association (ANA)
changes in nursing policy, 12–13
Code for Nurses, 12
Code of Ethics for Nurses, 20, *20, 21,* 448, 450, 451
contact information for, 38
Health Care Agenda 2005, 443
Nursing: A Social Policy Statement, 12, *21,* 22
Nursing's Social Policy Statement, 12, 459
Scope & Standards of Practice, 20, *21,* 459
Standards of Clinical Nursing Practice, 20, *21*

American Obesity Association, 319, 364

American Pediatrics Association, 212

American Sleep Apnea Association, 364

American Speech-Language-Hearing Association (ASHA), 95

Amniocentesis, 174

Amygdala, 151

Ancient health promotion, 3–5

Andragogy, 91–92, *92*

Andropause, 251

Anemia, 254
screening for, 188

ANA. *See* American Nurses Association

Anorexia nervosa
incidence of, 304
overview of, 221–222, 306
risk factors for, *222*
sign and symptoms of, *221*

Anosmia, 132

AOA. *See* Administration On Aging

Aromatherapy, 410, *410*

Asbestos, 118
health promotion guide, *124–125*

ASHA. *See* American Speech-Language-Hearing Association

Assault, 457

Assessment, in nursing process, 65
nutrition health, 313
physical fitness program, 334, *335*
weight control, 352–357, *354–357*

Assisted living facility (ALF), 284, 286, *286*

Atrophy, 275

Attachment, 190

Attention-deficit/hyperactivity disorder (ADHD), 209–210, *210*

Authenticity, 88
Autonomic nervous system, 150, *151*
Autonomy principle, *449*, 449–450
Ayurveda, 388
Ayurvedic Institute, 414–415

B

Baby boomers, 268
Babylonia, health promotion in, 4
Back injuries, 426
    preventing, 133, *134*
Balance, weight control and, 345
Ballistic stretching, 326
Basal metabolic rate, 302, 347
Battery, 457
Behavior, models for health promotion, 44–53
Beneficence principle, *449*, 450
Benson, Herbert, 399
Bereavement, 158–159
Bioaerosols, health promotion guide, *124–125*
Biological contaminants, 118
Biological domain
    adolescents, 218–226
    communication and, *91*
    health professionals, 426–427
    infants and toddlers, 183–189
    middle-aged adults, 249–251, *250–251*
    nutrition, 299, 302–303
    older adults, 271–278
    overview of, 58
    pregnancy, 171–178
    preschool and school-age children,
        199–209
    weight control, 347–349
    young adults, 233–236
Birth control, 171, *172*, 180–181
Birthdate, 104
Birthplace, 104
Blood pressure, adolescents, 222
B lymphocytes, 152–153
BMI. *See* Body mass index
Body composition, 324, 326, *326*
    assessment methods, *357*
    optimal, 354
Body image, adolescents, 226
Body image disturbance, 350
Body language
    defined, 83
    kinesics, 85
    personal presentation, 83–84
    proxemics, *84*, 84–85
Body mass index (BMI)
    assessment for weight control, 356–357
    calculating, 326, *326*
    preschool and school-age children,
        200, *200*
Brain
    parts and function of, 368, *369*
    stress response, *155*
Breach of duty, 457
Breast feeding, 183–184, *184*, *185*
Breast self-examination, 235, *236*
Breath, *397*, 397–398
Bruising, 192
Building-related illness, 115, *116*
Bulimia nervosa
    overview of, 221–222, 306

risk factors for, *222*
signs and symptoms of, *221*
Burnout, 419, 427–428

C

Caffeine, 372
    average amounts in beverages, 173
CAH. *See* Department of Child and Adolescent Health and Development
CAM. *See* Complementary and alternative medicine
Canada, influence on health promotion, 10
Cancer
    middle-aged adults, 263
    screening for young adults, 235–236, *236*
    skin cancer prevention, 234, *234*
Capacity building, 387
Capitation, 441, *441*
Carbon monoxide, health promotion and
        nursing interventions for, *122–123*
Carcinogens, 113
Cardiovascular fitness, 323–324, 325
Career ladder, 26
Caring
    communication, 88
    defined, 88
    values, belief and norms, 108
Car safety
    adolescents, 229, 230, *231*
    car seats, 192–193, *193*
    older adults and driving, *282*, 282–283
CDC. *See* Centers for Disease Control and
        Prevention
Centenarians, 272
Center for Cross-Cultural Health, 111
Center for the Study of Complementary and
        Alternative Therapies (CSCAT), 414
Centers for Disease Control and Prevention
        (CDC), 384
    contact information, 245
    tracking hazardous agents, 113
Central nervous system, 150, *151*
    alcohol use and, 376
Central obesity, 344
Centre for Health Promotion, 17
Certification, 455
Cervical cancer, risk factors, 236, *236*
Chakras, 394–396, *395*
Channel, in communication, 80
Chemical sensitivity, 114, *125*
Chi, 135
Child abuse, 191–192
Child Health Insurance Program (CHIP), 439
Children. *See* Adolescents; Infants and toddlers;
        Preschool and school-age children
Children's Safety Network (CNS) National Injury and Violence Prevention Resource Center, 217
China, ancient, health promotion in, 5
CHIP. *See* Child Health Insurance Program
CHP. *See* ILSI Center for Health Promotion
Chromotherapy, 132
Chronic illnesses, 248
CIP. *See* Consumer Information Processing Model
Climacteric, 249–251
CNS. *See* Children's Safety Network
Code for Nurses (ANA), 12

Code for Nurses (INC), 12–13
Codeine, 371–372
Code of Ethics for Nurses (ANA), 20, *20*, 21,
        448, 450, 451
Code of Hammurabi, 4
Cognitive development
    adolescents, 226–227
    infants and toddlers, 189, *190*
    older adults, 270–271, *271*
    young adults, 236–237, *237*
Cohabitation, 239
Color
    health and, 131–132
    holistic care and, 401–402, *402*
Communication, 78–94
    active listening, 88
    as assumption in health promotion, 29
    authenticity, 88
    barriers to, *90*
    caring, 88
    channel, 80
    context, 81
    cultural competence, *102*
    decoding, 80
    defined, 78
    elements of, 78–81
    empathy, 87–88
    empowerment through, 91–93
    encoding, 78–79
    feedback, 80–81
    Health Promotion Model, 90–91
    Healthy People 2010, 88, 90
    holistic care, 408
    impairments in, *82*, 82–83
    kinesics, 85
    message, 79
    nonverbal, 83–86
    nursing theory and, 86–87, *87*
    paralanguage, 85–86
    personal presentation, 83–84
    proxemics, *84*, 84–85
    technology and, 93
    therapeutic communication techniques,
        88, *89*
    in therapeutic relationship, 86–88
    touch, 85, *85*
    unconditional positive regard, 87
    verbal, 81–83
Community
    defined, 65
    nursing process and, *69*, 70
Community-level interventions, 255
Complementary and alternative medicine
        (CAM), 389, *389*
Comorbidity, 367
    substance abuse, 378–379
Competency indicators, 454–456
Concept, defined, 20–21
Conceptual framework, 22
Condom, *226*
Confidentiality principle, *449*, 451
Constipation, 185, *186*
Consultant, 63
Consumer Information Processing Model
        (CIP), 48
Context, in communication process, 81
Contraception, 171, *172*, 178, 180–181
Cooldown, 331

Coordinator of care, 63
Coping strategies, 150
Corticotropin releasing factor, 151–152
Cost containment
    changes in nursing practices and, 12
    consumer efforts in, 439–440
    ethical and legal concerns, 458
    factors driving costs up, 436–437, 437
    managed care, 440–444
    Medicare and Medicaid, 438, 438–439
    prospective payment system (PPS), 439
Couvade, 179
CPSC. See U.S. Consumer Product Safety
    Commission
Credentialing, 455
Crime, 456
Crisis, 160, 161
Cross tolerance, 370
CSCAT. See Center for the Study of
    Complementary and Alternative
    Therapies
Cultural assessment, 102–105
    age, 104
    birthplace, 104
    education, 105
    ethnicity, 104
    gender, 103
    generations in U.S., 104
    languages spoken, 104–105
    marital status, 104
    name, 103
    occupation, 105
    race, 104
    religion/spiritual faith, 103–104
    tools for, 102, 103
    years in U.S., 104
Cultural competence
    communicating, 102
    components of, 101–102
    importance of, 109
Cultural congruent care, 32
Cultural domain, 105–109
    acculturation, 108–109
    adolescents, 229
    caring behavior, 108
    diversity and similarities, 108
    health care access, 459
    infants and toddlers, 192
    lay, folk and professional wellness-
        illness cultural systems, 107,
        107–108
    lifestyle, 105
    middle-aged adults, 254–255
    older adults, 282
    preschool and school-age children, 211
    risk factors, 72
    rituals and rites of passage, 106–107
    taboos and myths, 106
    values, norms, expressions, 105–106
    worldviews, 106
Cultural pride, 101
Culture, 96–102
    attributes of, 97
    defined, 96–97, 97
    ethnicity, 99–100
    labels, 100–101
    nationality, 100
    race, 98–99, 99

religion, 100
    worldviews, 97
Culture broker, 72
Curie, Marie, 7
Curie, Pierre, 7

D

DASH. See Dietary Approaches to Stop
    Hypertension Eating Plan
Day care, 191
Deaths
    causes of, historical perspective, 6, 6
    infant mortality, 182
    pregnancy complications, 173
    unhealthy lifestyles, 41–42
Decoding, 80
Dementia, 276
Demographics, in cultural assessment, 102
Dental caries, 222–223
Dental health, middle-aged adults, 258–259
Deontology, 449
Department of Child and Adolescent Health
    and Development (CAH), 217
Depression
    adolescents, 227, 227
    affect on disease, 161
    major depressive disorder, 252–253
    middle-aged adults, 252–253
    older adults, 279
    postpartum, 179–180, 180
    pregnancy, 178, 179
Desirable body weight, 345
Detoxification, 370
Developmental delay screening, infants and
    toddlers, 189
Diabetes
    acanthosis nigricans, 205, 205, 209
    gestational diabetes, 176
    middle-aged adults, 263
Diagnosis, in nursing process, 65–66
Diagnosis-related groups (DRGs), 439
Diarrhea, 185
Dietary Approaches to Stop Hypertension
    (DASH), Eating Plan, 308
Dietary Guidelines for Americans 2005,
    307–309, 308
Dietary Reference Intakes (DRIs), 296
Diffusion of Innovations Model, 48–49
Disease cluster, 113
Disease prevention, defined, 41
Domains, 57–61, 58. See also specific
        domains
    biological, 58
    defined, 58
    environmental, 59–60
    intellectual, 61
    overview, 57–58, 58
    political, 60
    psychological, 58–59
    risk appraisal according to domains, 71
    sexual, 61
    sociological, 59
    spiritual, 60–61
    technological, 61
Domestic violence
    pregnancy, 178–179, 179
    screening for, 179

Dossey, Larry, 400
DRGs. See Diagnosis-related groups
DRIs. See Dietary Reference Intakes
Drug abuse, 369–370
Drug misuse, 369
Drug use. See also Substance abuse
    adolescents, 222–225, 223–225
    commonly abused psychotropic drugs,
        371–372
    drug abuse, 369–370
    drug defined, 367
    drug mechanics, 368, 368, 369
    pregnancy, 174
    routes for drug administration, 367
    sources and categories of drugs, 367–368
    withdrawal, 370
Dual diagnosis, 378
Dysomnia, 276

E

Earthquakes, 137–138
Eating disorders, 304, 306
    adolescents and, 221, 221–222, 222
Echinacea, 409, 409
Ecstasy, 372
Education
    in cultural assessment, 105
    levels of, and nursing, 26, 28
    nurse role in, 63
    nursing supply, 424
    older adults, 278
    risk factors, 70, 72
Egocentric, 209
Ego development, 237, 237
Egypt, ancient, health promotion in, 4
Elder abuse, 279–280, 281
Elderly. See Older adults
Electromagnetic radiation, 122
Elimination
    infants and toddlers, 185–186
    preschool and school-age children,
        202–203
Embryo, 173
Emergency contraception, 180–181
Emic knowledge, 101–102
Emotional development
    adolescents, 227–228
    infants and toddlers, 189–190, 191
    preschool and school-age children, 209
    young adults, 238, 238
Emotions
    eating behavior and, 350
    neuropeptides and, 151
Empathy, 87–88
Empowerment, 267
    defined, 91
    role of nurse in, 63
    through communication, 91–93
Encoding, 78–79
Encopresis, 203
Endocrine system, 151–152
    function, 153
    interaction with immune system, 154
    structure, 152
Energy, 393
Energy field, 393–396, 394, 395
Enuresis, 202–203

Environmental disasters, 137–144
  health promotion and nursing
    interventions, *142*, 142–143
  natural disasters, 137–138
  posttraumatic stress disorder, 140–142,
    141
  preparation for disasters, 143, *144*
  technological disasters, 138–139
  terror-related disasters, 139–140, *140*
Environmental domain
  adolescents, 230–231, *231*
  communication and, *91*
  health professionals, 430–431
  infants and toddlers, 193, *194*
  middle-aged adults, 253–254
  nutrition, 304–305
  older adults, 282–287, *282–287*
  overview of, 59–60
  pregnancy, 181
  preschool and school-age children, 212
  weight control, 349–350
  young adults, 241
Environmental factors
  air pollution, 115–124
  body's response to, 113–114, *114*
  environmental disasters, 137–144
  general systems theory, 31–32
  holistic care, 407–408, *408*
  light, 129–130
  in metaparadigm, 24
  nursing theory and, 32
  problem identification, 112–113
  risk factors, 70
  soil pollution, 124–126
  sound pollution, 126–129, *128*
  space and health, 130–137
  water pollution, 124–126
Environmental health hazard, 113
Environmental health risk, defined, 113
Environmental Protection Agency (EPA)
  disease cluster and risk assessment, 113
  role of, 113
Environmental tobacco smoke (ETS), 118
  health promotion and nursing
    interventions for, *122–123*
  health risk for children, 373, *373*
EPA. *See* Environmental Protection Agency
Epidemiology
  development of, 5
  historical perspective on causes of
    death, 6, *6*
Epinephrine, 150, 368
EPO. *See* Exclusive provider organization
Equal protection, 447
Equilibrium set-point theory, 348
Ergonomics, 133–134, 426
Erickson, Helen, 391
Erikson, Erik, 189–190, *191*, 209, 227, 238,
    252, 270, *271*
ESADDI. *See* Estimated safe and adequate
    daily dietary intake
Essential nutrients, 295
Estimated safe and adequate daily dietary
    intake (ESADDI), 296
Ethical principles, *449*, 449–452
Ethics/ethical issues, 447–453
    autonomy principle, *449*, 449–450
    beneficence principle, *449*, 450

Code for Nurses, 12–13
Code of Ethics for Nurses (ANA), 20, *20*,
    21
  confidentiality principle, *449*, 451
  defined, 448
  deontology, 449
  ethical decision making and personal
    values, 452–453
  fidelity principle, *449*, 451
  health care cost and access, 457–459
  health promotion and, 459–461, *460*
  Justice principle, *449*, 451
  nonmaleficence principle, *449*, 450
  overview, 447–448
  respect for others principle, *449*, 452
  standard of best interest principle, *449*,
    451–452
  teleology, 448–449
  veracity principle, *449*, 450–451
Ethnicity
  compared to race, 99
  in cultural assessment, 104
  defined, 99
  as element of culture, 99–100
  nursing supply, 423–424
  substance abuse, 377
Ethnocentrism, 106
Etic knowledge, 101–102
ETS. *See* Environmental tobacco smoke
Eustress, 279
Evaluation, in nursing process, 67
  nutritional health, 316
  physical fitness program, 336
  weight control, 360–361
Examination stress, 158
Exchange system, 311
Exclusive provider organization (EPO),
    440–441, *441*
Exercise. *See also* Physical fitness
  health benefits of, 322
  holistic care, 408
  middle-aged adults, 255, 257
  myths and facts about, 333, *333*
  older adults, 275–276
  postpartum, 177
  pregnancy, 176
  young adults, 233–234
Expected outcome, 66
Eyes, stress response, *155*

F

Fabiola, 388
Fad diets, 307
Families, nursing process and, 67, 69
Family Leave Act, 181
Family life
  adolescents, 228
  infants and toddlers, 190–191
  preschool and school-age children,
    210
Feedback, in communication, 80–81
Feng shui, 134–137, *136*
Fetus, 173
FDA. *See* U.S. Food and Drug Administration
Fidelity principle, *449*, 451
Field, Tiffany, 406
Fifty Plus Fitness Association, 290

Fight-or-flight response, 150, 154
Fitness, older adults, 275–276
FITT. *See* Frequency, intensity, time, type
    of training
Fitzgerald, William, 405
Five a Day program, 312
Flexibility, 324, 325–326
Folk health sector, *107*, 107–108
Food Guide Pyramid, 309
Food labels, 311, *311*
Formaldehyde, 119
Freeze Frame, 396
Frequency, intensity, time, type of training
    (FITT), 328–329

G

Galen, 5, 149
Garlic, 409, *409*
Gaseous pollutants, 118–119, *119*
Gender
  in cultural assessment, 103
  nursing supply, 422–423
  risk factors, 72
  substance abuse, 376
General adaptation syndrome, 154
General systems theory, 30, 388
Genogram, 424, *425*
Geriatrics, 267. *See also* Older adults
Gerontology, 267
Gestational diabetes, 176
Gilligan, Carol, 227
Ginkgo biloba, 409, *409*
Ginseng, 409, *409*
Glucocorticoids, 151–152, *154*
Gonads, 219
Greece, ancient, health promotion in, 4
Growth hormone, *154*
  response to stress, 156
Guide to Clinical Preventive Services, 255
Gum disease, 222–223
Gynecomastia, 220

H

Half-life, 370
Hallucinogens, 372
Hardiness, 427
Havighurst, R. J., 270, *271*
Healing
  defined, 387
  love and, 410–411
  nurse's attitude toward, 390
Healing molecule, 151
Healing Touch, 404
Healing Touch International Inc., 414
Health
  defined, 25, 40
  in metaparadigm, 24–26
  nursing theory and, 32–33
  view of, 25
Health Aging Project, 269
Health behavior patterns, 424–425, *425*
Health Belief Model, 44–45, *46*
  physical fitness, 333–334
Health care
  ethical and legal concerns related to cost
    and access, 457–459

lay, folk and professional wellness-
    illness cultural systems, *107*, 107–108
nursing role and changes in, 72
Health care costs
    consumer efforts in cost containment,
        439–440
    containment efforts and changes in
        nursing practices, 12
    establishment of Medicare/Medicaid
        programs and, 9
    ethical and legal concerns, 458
    factors driving costs up, 436–437, *437*
    historical perspective on, 8–9, *9*
    managed care, 440–444
    Medicare and Medicaid, *438*, 438–439
    older adults and, 279
    prospective payment system (PPS), 439
Health care reform, 8–9
    federal government involvement in
        health care, 8–9
    Medicaid and Medicare, 9
Health education, 3
Health insurance, preschool and school-age
    children, 211–212
Health maintenance organization (HMO),
    440, *441*
*Healthy People: Surgeon General's Report on
    Health Promotion and Disease Pre-
    vention,* 10
Health Plan Employer Data and Information
    Set (HEDIS), 443
Health professionals, 418–432
    biological domain, 426–427
    burnout, 427–428
    changes in health care and, 419
    environmental domain, 430–431
    health behavior patterns, 424–425, *425*
    issues impacting, 419–420
    nursing process, 431, *432*
    nursing student characteristics, 421
    nursing student stress, 421–422
    nursing supply, 422–424
    occupational stress, 419
    psychological domain, 427–428
    sociocultural domain, 429–430
    spiritual domain, 428–429
    technological domain, 431
Health promotion
    assumptions of, *27*, 27–29
    Canada's role in, 10
    defined, 2–3, 42
    future of, 13–15
    government initiatives for, 9–12
    historical perspective on, 3–7
    models for, 44–53
    social mandate for, 6–7
    sociopolitical influences, 8–9
Health Promotion Model. *See* Pender's Health
    Promotion model
Health promotion plan
    assessment and data collection, 53
    for community, 54
    defined, 54
    developing, 53–54
    evaluation, 53
    planning and implementation, 53
    sample, *54*
Health protection, defined, 41

HealthRecord.com, 73
Healthy People 2000, 3, 10
    obesity and overweight, 345
Healthy People 2010, 3, 60
    communication and, 88, 90
    focus areas, *298*
    focus areas and health indicators, 10–12, *11*
    goals of, 12
    nutrition and overweight objectives,
        297, *297*
    obesity and overweight, 345
    objectives related to middle-aged
        adults, *248*
    physical activity, 322
    substance abuse, 366
Hearing
    middle-aged adults, 261–262
    screening for deficits in infants and
        toddlers, 188
Heart rate
    resting, 329
    target, 329–330
Heart rate reserve, 329
HEDIS. *See* Health Plan Employer Data and
    Information Set
Heliotherapy, 400
Henchey, Norman, 14
Henderson, Virginia, 32, *34–35*
Henry Street Settlement, 8
Herbs, 408–409, *409*
Heroin, 371–372
Heterogeneity, 268
Hierarchy of needs, *23*, 23–24, *24*
High-level wellness, 41
Hippocampus, 151
Hippocrates, 4, 5
Hispanic, as ethnicity, 99
Historical perspective on health promotion, 3–7
    ancient times, 3–5
    first movement, 7
    holistic care, 388–390
    middle ages, 5–6
    Renaissance and Early America, 6
    second movement, 7
    social mandate for health promotion,
        6–7
    third movement, 7
HIV/AIDS. *See* Human immunodeficiency
    virus
HMO. *See* Health maintenance organization
Holistic care, 386–411
    acupressure, 406–407
    aromatherapy, 410, *410*
    as assumption in health promotion, 27, *27*
    breath, *397*, 397–398
    categories of practice overview, *393*
    color, 401–402, *402*
    communication, 408
    defined, 386–387
    energy field, 393–396, *394, 395*
    environment and, 407–408, *408*
    exercise, 408
    healing, 387
    Healing Touch, 404
    herbs, 408–409, *409*
    Hippocrates and, 4
    history of, 388–390
    imagery, 398–399

light, 400–401, *401, 402*
love and healing, 410–411
massage, 405–406
meditation, 399, *399*
nurse-client relationship, 390–392,
    391–392
nurse healer, 387–388
nurse's attitude toward healing, 390
nurse's attitude toward self, 390
nursing practice and, 62
nurturing self, 407–411
nutrition, 408
overview of, 61–62
prayer, 400
reflexology, 405, *405*
sleep, 408
sound, 402–404, *403*
teaching and learning techniques,
    392–393
therapeutic touch, 394, *394,* 404
thoughts and feelings, 396–397, *397*
Holistic healing, 386–387
Holistic medicine, defined, 149
Holistic nursing, 387
Homeostasis, 26
Homosexuality, 232, 239
    older adults, 277
Hormone replacement therapy, 250–251
Hormones, effect on immune system, *154*
Household drugs, 372
Human becoming theory, 31
Human care theory, 31
Human immunodeficiency virus (HIV/AIDS),
    older adults, 278
Hurricanes, 138
Hydrostatic weighing, 326
Hypnosis, 158
Hypothalamic-pituitary-adrenal axis, 151
Hypothalamus, 151, *152*
    eating behavior and, 348
    puberty, 219, *219*

I

IAQ INFO. *See* Indoor Air Quality Information
    Clearinghouse
Ideal body weight, 346, 355–356
*Illuminations: The Human Becoming Theory
    in Practice and Research* (Parse), 31
ILSI Center for Health Promotion (CHP), 75
Immune modulation, 154
Immune system
    chemical effects of hormones on, *154*
    examination stress, 158
    interaction with neuroendocrine
        system, 154
    measuring immune response, 153–154
    overview of, 152–153
    response to stress, 156
    role of, 152
Immunization
    infants and toddlers, 187–188
    middle-aged adults, 257–258
    preconception, 171–172
    pregnancy and, 174–175
    preschool and school-age children,
        204–205, *206–208*
Immunoenhancement, 158

Immunoglobulins, 152–153
Implementation, in nursing process, 67
    nutritional health, 314–316
    physical fitness program, 335–336
    weight control, 358–360
Incest, 229
Incontinence, 202
Individuals with Disabilities Education
    Act, 212
Indoor air pollution, 115–119, *116–125*
    biological contaminants, 118
    gases, 118–119, *119*
    particulate matter, 117–118
    risk assessment for, *120*
    sick building syndrome, 115, *116*
Indoor Air Quality Information Clearinghouse
    (IAQ INFO), 145
Industrial Revolution, 6
Infants and toddlers
    biological domain, 183–189
    breast feeding, 183–184, *184, 185*
    child abuse and neglect, 191–192
    cognitive development, 189, *190*
    cultural influences, 192
    day care, 191
    defined, 173
    elimination, 185–186
    emotional development, 189–190, *191*
    environmental domain, 193, *194*
    family life, 190–191
    immunization, 187–188
    mortality rate, 182
    nutrition, 183–185, *184, 185*
    overview of health promotion during, *195*
    pacifiers, 186
    political domain, 192–193
    psychological domain, 189–190
    safety, 192–193, *193, 194*
    screening, 188–189
    sexual domain, 193
    sleep and activity, 186–187
    social domain, 190–192
    spiritual domain, 193–194
    Sudden Infant Death Syndrome
      (SIDS), 186
    WIC program, 192
Influenza, 187
    vaccine, 257
Informed consent, 453, *453*
Insulin resistance, acanthosis nigricans, 205,
    205, 209
Intellectual domain, overview of, 61
Intensity, fitness program, 328
International Food Information Council, 364
Interventions
    defined, 67
    in nursing process, 67
Intimate partner violence, 240, *240*
Introspection, 452
Invulnerability, 226
Isoimmunization, 175–176

J

JC. *See* Joint Commission
Jenny, Hans, 402
Joint Commission (JC), 442–443, 445
Justice principle, *449,* 451

K

Kava, 409, *409*
Kinesics, 85
King, Imogene, 32, *34–35,* 86
Knowles, Malcolm, 91
Koch, Robert, 7
Kohlberg, Lawrence, 226–227
Krieger, Dolores, 389, 394, 404

L

Labels, 100–101
LaLonde Report, 10
Language
    in cultural assessment, 104–105
    primary and preferred, 105
Lay/popular health sector, *107,* 107–108
Lead
    health promotion guide, *124–125*
    pregnancy and, 181
Lead Poisoning Prevention Branch, 146
Learned helplessness, 396
Learning, adult learners, 91–92
Legal issues, 453–461
    breach of duty, 457
    competency indicators, 454–456
    health care cost and access, 457–459
    health promotion and, 459–461, *460*
    informed consent, 453, *453*
    integrative therapy, *407*
    law and nursing practices, 453–454
    negligence, 456–457
    overview, 447–448
    pregnancy and discrimination, 181
    right to refuse treatment, 457
    student nurse liability, 457
    torts, 456
Leininger, Madeleine, 31, 32, *36–37*
Levinson, Daniel, 238
Licensure, 454–455
Life expectancy, *268,* 268–269
Light, 400–401, *401, 402*
    health and, 129–130
Listening, active, 88
Lister, Joseph, 7
Liver, stress response, *155*
LSD. *See* Lysergic acid diethylamide
Lysergic acid diethylamide (LSD), 372

M

Managed care, 440–444
    capitation, 441, *441*
    defined, 440
    exclusive provider organization,
      440–441, *441*
    health maintenance organization,
      440, *441*
    impact on nursing, 424
    national standards, 443
    nursing's role in, 441–442
    preferred provider organization,
      440, *441*
    quality measures, 442–443
Managed care organization, 440
Manners, Peter, 402
Maslow's hierarchy of needs, *23,* 23–24, *24*

Massage, 405–406
Masturbation, 231
Maximum heart rate, 329
McGuire, Charlotte, 389
MDMA. *See* Methylenedioxymethamphetamine
Medicaid
    cost containment, *438,* 438–439
    establishment of, 9
    preschool and school-age children,
      211–212
Medicare
    cost containment, *438,* 438–439
    establishment of, 9
Medicocentrism, 106
Meditation, 234, 399, *399*
Melanoma, 234, *234*
Men
    couvade, 179
    postpartum depression, 180
Menarche, 220
Menopause, 250–251
Mentgen, Janet, 404
Message, in communication, 79
Metabolic Syndrome, 201–202, *202*
Metabolism, screening for defects of, 188
Metaparadigm, 21
    defined, 21–22
    environment, 24
    health, 24–26
    nursing profession, 26
    nursing theory and, 32–33
    overview of, *34–37*
    person, 22–24
Methylenedioxymethamphetamine
    (MDMA), 372
Middle-aged adults, 247–263
    biological domain, 249–251, *250–251*
    body changes during, *250–251*
    cancer, 263
    climacteric, 249–251
    culturally competent care, 254–255
    demographics of, *248, 249*
    dental health, 258–259
    depression, 252–253
    diabetes mellitus, 263
    educating about risk reduction and
      health promotion, 259–261
    environmental domain, 253–254
    exercise, 255, 257
    guidelines for health
      promotion/screening, *255*
    immunizations, 257–258
    importance of health promotion during,
      247–248
    nutrition, 255
    occupational safety, 259
    osteoporosis, 263
    psychological domain, *252,* 252–253
    risk assessment, *256*
    sandwich generation, 247
    screening, 261–263, *262*
    sexuality, 254
    sleep, 258
    smoking, 253–254
    sociological domain, 253
    spiritual domain, 254
    tobacco avoidance, 257
    vision and hearing, 261–262

Middle Ages, health promotion in, 5–6
Mind-body connection. See Psychoneuroim-
    munology (PNI)
Mind-body dualism, 149
Minerals, 295–296, *295–296, 298–303*
Modeling, 391
Models
    Consumer Information Processing Model
        (CIP), 48
    defined, 42
    Diffusion of Innovations Model, 48–49
    Health Belief Model, 44–45, *46*
    O'Donnell Model of Health Promotion
        Behavior, *52, 52*–53
    Pender Health Promotion model, 50, *51*
    PRECEDE-PROCEED, *49,* 49–50
    Protection Motivation Theory, 45, *47*
    Transtheoretical Model of Behavior
        Change, 45–46, *48*
Modern Practice of Adult Education:
    Andragogy versus Pedagogy, The
    (Knowles), 91
Moral development, adolescents, 226–227
Morbidity, 170
Morphine, 371–372
Mortality, 170
Mosaic Code, 4–5
Motherhood
    biological domain, 171–178
    environmental domain, 181
    political domain, 180–181
    psychological domain, 178–180
    rate of planned/unplanned, 170
    sexual domain, 181–182
    sociological domain, 178–180
Multistate licensure, 455
Muscles
    muscular endurance, 324, 325
    muscular strength, 324, 325
    soreness, 331
    stress response, *155*
Music, 128
    holistic care and, 402–403
Mutagens, 113
MyPyramid, 309–311, *310*
Myths, 106

N

Names, in cultural assessment, 103
NANDA. See North American Nursing Diagnosis
    Association
NANDA International, 75
NASSO. See North American Association for
    the Study of Obesity
National Association of Anorexia Nervosa and
    Associated Disorders, 319
National Cancer Institute, 161–162, 319
National Center for Complementary and Alter-
    native Medicine (NCCAM), 162, 389
National Center for Cultural Healing, 111
National Committee for Quality Assurance
    (NCQA), 442
National Epidemiologic Survey of Alcoholism
    and Related Conditions (NESARC), 252
National Institute for Clinical Applications of
    Behavioral Medicine, 166, 414
National Institute on Aging, 290

National Institute on Drug Abuse (NIDA), 385
National Institutes of Health (NIH), 370, 385
Nationality, as element of culture, 100
National Lead Information Center, 145
National Pesticide Information Center
    (NPIC), 145
National Radon Hotline, 146
National School Lunch Program, 212
Native language, 105
Natural disasters, 137–138
Natural killer cells, 153
NCCAM. See National Center for Complemen-
    tary and Alternative Medicine
NCCAM Clearinghouse, 414
NCQA. See National Committee for Quality
    Assurance
Needs, hierarchy of, *23,* 23–24, *24*
Needs theory, 31
Negative energy balance, 347
Negligence, 456–457
Nervous system
    interaction with immune system, 154
    overview of, 150, *151*
NESARC. See National Epidemiologic Survey
    of Alcoholism and Related Conditions
Neuropeptides, 150–151
New Perspective on Health of Canadians,
    A, 10
NH-PAL, Inc. See Nurse Healers-Professional
    Associates International
Nicotine, 373–374
NIDA. See National Institute on Drug Abuse
Nightingale, Florence
    accomplishments of, 7
    environmental factors, 24
    environment for healing, 163
    holistic nursing, 388
    overview of theories of, *34–35*
Nightmares, 203–204
Night terror, 203
NIH. See National Institutes of Health
Nitrogen oxide, health promotion and nursing
    interventions for, *122–123*
NNN Taxonomy of Nursing Practice, The, 66
Noise, 127
Nonessential nutrients, 295
Nonmaleficence principle, *449,* 450
Nonverbal communication, 83–86
    defined, 81
    kinesics, 85
    paralanguage, 85–86
    personal presentation, 83–84
    proxemics, *84,* 84–85
    tough, 85, *85*
Nonverbal vocalizations, 85–86
Norepinephrine, 150, 151, *154*
Norms, 105–106
North American Association for the Study
    of Obesity (NASSO), 319
North American Nursing Diagnosis Associa-
    tion (NANDA), 396
    contact information, 75
    nursing diagnosis, 66
Notes on Nursing (Nightingale), 7, 24
NPIC. See National Pesticide Information
    Center
Nurse-client relationship, 390–392, *391–392*
Nurse healer, 387–388

Nurse Healers-Professional Associates
    International (NH-PAL, Inc.), 415
Nurse practitioner, 72
Nurses/nursing. *See also* Health professionals
    burnout, 419, 427–428
    changes in policy, 12–13
    competency indicators, 454–456
    cost containment and changes in
        practice, 12
    defined, 22
    educational levels and health promotion,
        26, *28*
    evolution into profession, 7
    factors affecting profession, 420–424
    health behavior patterns, 424–425, *425*
    health promotion practices by domains,
        426–431
    impact of managed care on, 424
    metaparadigm, 20–26
    nursing student characteristics, 421
    nursing student stress, 421–422
    nursing supply, 422–424
    as profession, 26
    professional practices, and health
        promotion, 19–20
    shortage of, 420–421, 422
    substance abuse, 377–378
Nursing: A Social Policy Statement (ANA),
    12–13, *21,* 22, 459
Nursing diagnosis
    across lifespan, *68*
    defined, 65
    for individual, family, community, 67,
        69, 70
    nutrition health, 313
    physical fitness program, 334, *336*
    weight control, 357
Nursing Metropolitan Life Insurance
    Company, 8
Nursing Practice Act, 454
Nursing process
    assessment, 65
    community and, *69,* 70
    defined, 62
    evaluation, 67
    families and, 67, *69*
    health professionals, 431, *432*
    holistic approach, 62
    implementation, 67
    individuals and, 67, *69*
    nursing diagnosis, 65–66
    nutritional health promotion, 313–316,
        314–316
    overview, 64–65
    physical fitness program, 334–336
    planning, 66–67
    weight control, 351–361
Nursing roles
    communication and, 86, *87*
    current factors affecting, 72–73
    in managed care, 441–442
    overview of, 62–64, *63*
Nursing's Social Policy Statement (ANA), 12
Nursing theory
    adaptation, 30
    communication and, 86–87, *87*
    human becoming, 31
    human care, 31

Nursing theory, *continued*
   metaparadigm and, 32–33
   needs, 31
   overview of, *34–37*
   systems, 30
   transcultural, 31–32
Nutrients, 295
Nutrition, 294–316
   adolescents, 221–222
   anorexia nervosa, 306
   biological domain, 299, 302–303
   bulimia, 306
   defined, 294
   Dietary Guidelines for Americans 2005,
     307–309, *308*
   environmental domain, 304–305
   essential nutrients, 295
   exchange system, 311
   fad diets, 307
   Five a Day program, 312
   food labels, 311, *311*
   Healthy People 2010, 297, *297–298*
   holistic care, 408
   importance of, 294–296
   infants and toddlers, 183–185, *184, 185*
   middle-aged adults, 255
   MyPyramid, 309–311, *310*
   National School Lunch Program, 212
   nonessential nutrients, 295
   nursing process and, 313–316, *314–316*
   older adults, 273, 275
   overnutrition, 305–306
   preconception, 171
   pregnancy, 173–174
   preschool and school-age children, *200,*
     200–202, *202*
   psychological domain, 303–304
   sociocultural, religious and spiritual
     domain, 304
   strategies promoting healthful, 307–312
   technical domain, 305
   undernutrition, 306
   vitamins, nutrients and minerals,
     295–296, *295–296, 298–303*
   young adults, 233

O

Obesity. *See also* Weight control
   adolescents, 222, 347
   central obesity, 344
   childhood, 201–202, *202,* 347
   consequences of, 343–345
   defined, 343–344
   diseases associated with, 305
   incidence of, 324, 343
   percentage of adults, 255, *257*
   severe, 344
Occupation, in cultural assessment, 105
Occupational Safety and Health Administration (OSHA), 146
Occupational stress, 419
O'Donnell, Michael, 50
O'Donnell Model of Health Promotion Behavior, *52,* 52–53
ODPHP. *See* Office of Disease Prevention and
   Health Promotion
Office of Disease Prevention and Health Promotion (ODPHP), 9–10, 17, 291

Office on Smoking and Health, 146
Older adults, 267–287
   assisted living facility (ALF), 284,
     286, *286*
   biological domain, 271–278
   cultural domain, 282
   demographics, 268, *269*
   depression, 279
   developmental tasks of aging,
     270–271, *271*
   driving safety, *282,* 282–283
   education, 278
   elder abuse, 279–280, *281*
   environmental domain, 282–287,
     282–287
   fitness and exercise, 275–276
   health care expenditures, 279
   medication and, 284, *284, 285*
   nutrition, 273, 275
   population trends, 268–269, *269, 270*
   poverty, 278
   psychological domain, 279–280
   risk assessment, *287*
   safety at home, *283,* 283–284
   sex, 276–278
   sleep, 276
   socioeconomic domain, 278–279
   spiritual domain, 280–281
   stress, 279
   substance abuse, 377
   theories of aging, 271, *272*
Opiates, 371–372
Opium, 371–372
Orem, Dorothea, 31, *34–35,* 86–87
OSHA. *See* Occupational Safety and Health
   Administration
Osler, William, 149
Osteoporosis
   alcohol use and, 375
   middle-aged adults, 263
OTC. *See* Over-the-counter drugs
Ott, John, 400
Outcomes, 259
Outgassing, 119
Overload principle, 327
Overnutrition, 305–306
Over-the-counter (OTC) drugs, 368
Overweight
   defined, 201
   preschool and school-age children,
     201–202, *202*

P

Pacifiers, 186
Palestine, ancient, health promotion in, 4–5
Pancreas, *152*
   stress response, *155*
Pap test. *See* Papanicolaou test
Papanicolaou (Pap) test, 235–236
Paradigm, 20
Paralanguage, 85–86
Parasympathetic nervous system, 150, *151*
Parathyroid, *152*
Parse, Rosemarie, 31, *36–37*
Particulate matter, 117–118
Partnership for Children's Health and the
   Environment, 217
Pasteur, Louis, 7

Paternalism, 452
PCP. *See* Phencyclidine
Pedagogy, 91–92, *92*
Peers
   adolescents, 228
   preschool and school-age children, 210
Pender, Nola, 50
Pender's Health Promotion model, 50, *51,* 259
   communication and, 90–91
   nutritional status, 315–316
   physical fitness program, 333–334
   weight control, 359
Peplau, Hildegard, 86, *87*
Perceptions, stress and, 156
Performance-related fitness, 323
Perimenopause, 249–250
Peripheral nervous system, 150, *151*
Person, in metaparadigm, 22–24
Personal presentation, 83–84
Phencyclidine (PCP), 372
Physical fitness, 321–338
   assessing, 324–326
   balanced program, 330
   benefits of, 322
   body composition, 324, 326, *326*
   cardiovascular fitness, 323–324, 325
   defined, 321, 322–323
   flexibility, 324, 325–326
   Health Belief Model, 333–334
   muscular strength and endurance,
     324, 325
   myths and facts about exercise, 333, *333*
   nursing process and, 334–336
   overload principle, 327
   performance-related fitness, 323
   planning program, 328–329
   problems related to exercise, 331–332
   progression principle, 327–328
   resting heart rate, 329
   result expectations, 330
   RICE method, 332–333
   specificity principle, 327
   starting training program, 326–327
   target heart rate, 329–330
   training elements, 330–331
   training tips, *338*
Phytochemicals, 312, 408–409, *409*
Piaget, Jean, 189, *190,* 209, 226, 236–237
Pica, 174
Picky Eater, 200, *200*
Pineal gland, *152*
Pituitary gland, *152*
Planned behavior, Theory of, 42–43, *42–43*
Planning, in nursing process, 66–67
   nutritional health, 313–314
   physical fitness program, 334–335
   weight control, 357–358
Plantar fasciitis, 331
PMS. *See* Premenstrual syndrome
PNI. *See* Psychoneuroimmunology
Political domain
   adolescents, 229–230
   health care cost and access, 457–459
   infants and toddlers, 192–193
   overview of, 60
   pregnancy, 180–181
   preschool and school-age children,
     211–212
   young adults, 240

Pollution
    acute exposure, 114
    air, 115–124
    body's response to, 113–114, *114*
    chronic exposure, 114
    connecting pollutants with symptoms, *115*
    exercise and, 332
    health promotion and nursing
        interventions for, 122–123, *122–125*
    soil, 124–126
    sound pollution, 126–129, *128*
    water, 124–126
Polypharmacy, 284, *284,* 370
Positive energy balance, 347
Postpartum. *See also* Pregnancy
    biological domain, 176–178
    defined, 176
    depression, 179–180, *180*
    psychological domain, 179–180
    sociological domain, 179–180
Posttraumatic stress disorder (PTSD),
    140–142, *141*
Poverty, older adults, 278
PPS. *See* Prospective payment system
Prayer, 400
PRECEDE-PROCEED model, *49,* 49–50
Preconception. *See* Pregnancy
Preferred language, 105
Preferred provider organization, 440, *441*
Pregnancy
    adolescent, 232
    adolescents, 170, 173
    biological domain, 171–178
    common complaints/recommendations
        for, *175*
    common complications of, *173*
    counseling issues during, *177*
    couvade, 179
    depression and, 178, *179*
    domestic violence, 178–179, *179*
    environmental domain, 181
    exercise, activity and sleep, 176
    gestational diabetes, 176
    immunization during, 174–175
    isoimmunization, 175–176
    middle-aged adults, 253
    nutrition, 173–174
    overview of health promotion
        during, 183
    pica, 174
    political domain, 180–181
    postpartum depression, 179–180, *180*
    psychological domain, 178–180
    rate of planned/unplanned, 170
    screening, 174–176
    sexual domain, 181–182
    sociological domain, 178–180
    stress and, 178
    substance abuse, 174
    urinary incontinence, 178
Premenstrual syndrome (PMS), 242, *242*
Preschool and school-age children, 199–214
    attention-deficit/hyperactivity disorder,
        209–210, *210*
    biological domain, 199–209
    cultural influences, 211
    elimination, 202–203
    environmental domain, 212
    immunization, 204–205, *206–208*

Individuals with Disabilities Education
    Act, 212
Medicaid/SCHIP, 211–212
National School Lunch Program, 212
nutrition, *200,* 200–202, *202*
obesity, 201–202, 347
overview of health promotion during,
    214
political domain, 211–212
psychological domain, 209–210
relationships, 210
safety, 212, *213*
screening, 205, *205,* 209
sexual domain, 212–213
sleep and activity, 203–204, *204*
social domain, 210–211
spiritual domain, 213–214
television, 210–211, *211*
weight control, *200,* 200–202, *202,* 347
Prescription drugs, 368
Presence, 387–388
President's Council on Physical Fitness and
    Sports, 245
Prevention
    primary, 380–381
    relapse prevention, 382
    secondary, 381
    substance abuse, 379–382, *380*
    tertiary, 381–382
Primary care providers, 440
Primary disease prevention, 67
Primary language, 105
Primary prevention, 380–381
Professional health sector, *107,* 107–108
Progression principle, 327–328
Prospective payment system (PPS), 439
Prospective studies, 157
Protection Motivation Theory, 45, *47*
Protective factors, 379–380
Provider of care, 64
Proxemics, *84,* 84–85
Psychocutaneous disease, stress and, 161
Psychological domain
    adolescents, 226–228
    communication and, *91*
    health professionals, 427–428
    infants and toddlers, 189–190
    middle-aged adults, *252,* 252–253
    nutrition, 303–304
    older adults, 279–280
    overview of, 58–59
    pregnancy, 178–180
    preschool and school-age children,
        209–210
    weight control, 350
    young adults, 236–238
Psychoneuroimmunology (PNI)
    bereavement, 158–159
    cancer and, 161–162
    chronic stress, 159, *160*
    controversy over, 162–163
    crisis, 160, *161*
    defined, 150
    depression factors, 161
    effect of stress on disease, 160–162
    examination stress, 158
    nursing implications, 163
    overview of, 150
    physiological basis, 150–154

psychocutaneous disease, 161
research focus areas, *157,* 157–158
role of stress, 154, *155, 156, 156*
spirituality and, 162
thoughts and feelings, 396–397, *397*
Psychotropic drugs, 368
    commonly abused, 371–372
PTSD. *See* Posttraumatic stress disorder
Puberty, 218–221, *219*
Pulmonary system, stress response, *155*

Q

Qi Gong, 399

R

Race
    compared to ethnicity, 99
    in cultural assessment, 104
    defined, 98
    demographic profile of U.S., *99*
    as element of culture, 98–99
Radon, *118,* 118–119
    health promotion guide, *124–125*
Rate of perceived exertion, 329–330
Recommended daily allowance, 296
Reflexology, 405, *405*
Registration, 454
Relapse prevention, 382
Relationships
    nurse-client relationship, 390–392,
        391–392
    preschool and school-age children, 210
    young adults, 238–240
Relaxation Response, 399, *399*
Relaxation techniques, 158
Religious domain
    communication and, *91*
    in cultural assessment, 103–104
    as element of culture, 100
    nutrition, 304
Renaissance, health promotion in, 6
Resources for Cross Cultural Health Care, 111
Respect for others principle, *449,* 452
Rest, ice, compression, and elevation (RICE)
    method, 332–333
Resting heart rate, 329
Retrospective studies, 157
Rhogam, 176
RICE. *See* Rest, ice, compression,
    and elevation method
Right to refuse treatment, 457
Riley, Joe, 405
Risk assessment
    indoor air pollution, *120*
    older adults, *287*
    risk appraisal according to domains, *71*
Risk factors
    cultural and spiritual influences, 72
    education, 70, 72
    environment, 70
    gender, 72
    middle-aged adults, 255
    risk appraisal according to domains, *71*
    socioeconomic level, 70
    substance abuse, 379
    work, 70
Rites of passage, 106–107

Rituals, 106–107
Röentgen, 7
Rogers, Martha, 31, 32, *34–35*, 388–389, 393
Role modeling, 391
Roles. *See* Nursing roles
Rome, ancient, health promotion in, 5
Roy, Callista, 30, 32, *36–37*

S

SAD. *See* Seasonal affective disorder
Safe Drinking Water Hotline, 146
Safety
    adolescents, 230–231, *231*
    infants and toddlers, 192–193, *193, 194*
    older adults, 282–286, *282–287*
    preschool and school-age children, 212,
        213
St. John's wort, 409, *409*
Sandwich generation, 247
Saw palmetto, 409, *409*
Scent
    aromatherapy, 410, *410*
    health and, 132
SCHIP. *See* State Children's Health Insurance
    Program
Science of Unitary Human Beings Theory
    (Rogers), 31, 32
Scoliosis, 205
Scope & Standards of Practice (ANA), 20,
    21, 459
Screening
    adolescents, 222–226
    defined, 188
    infants and toddlers, 188–189
    middle-aged adults, 261–263, *262*
    pregnancy, 174–176
    preschool and school-age children, 205,
        205, 209
    sensitivity of screening test, 261
    specificity of screening test, 261
    young adults, 234–236, *235, 236*
Seasonal affective disorder (SAD), 129, 401
Secondary prevention, 67, 381
Secondhand tobacco smoke, 118, 212
Self-Care Deficit Theory (Orem), 31
Self-efficacy, defined, 43
Selye, Hans, 154
Sensitivity of screening test, 261
Serotonin, 151, 368, 401
Set-point of weight control theory, 348
Severe obesity, 344
Sex, older adults, 276–278
Sexual domain
    adolescents, 231–232
    infants and toddlers, 193
    middle-aged adults, 254
    overview of, 61
    pregnancy, 181–182
    preschool and school-age children,
        212–213
    young adults, 241–242
Sexuality, defined, 181
Sexuality Information and Education Council
    of the United States, 290–291
Sexually transmitted infections, 225–226
    middle-aged adults, 254
    young adults, 235

Sha, 135
Shaping behavior, weight control and, 360
Shattuck, Lemuel, 7
Shattuck Report, 7
Shealy, Norm, 389
Sheehy, Gail, 238
Sheppard-Towner Act, 8
Sick building syndrome, 115, *116*
Side stitch, 331
SIDS. *See* Sudden infant death syndrome
Simultaneous perception, 130
Skin
    acanthosis nigricans, 205, *205,* 209
    skin cancer prevention, 234, *234*
    stress affect on dermatologic
        conditions, 161
    stress response, *155*
Skinfold calipers, 326, *326*
Sleep
    holistic care, 408
    infants and toddlers, 186
    middle-aged adults, 258
    older adults, 276
    postpartum, 177
    pregnancy, 176
    preschool and school-age children,
        203–204, *204*
    young adults, 234
Sleep apnea, 344
Smallpox, 187
Smog, 121
Smoking. *See also* Substance abuse; Tobacco
        use
    adolescents, *222–225*, 223–225, 377
    cessation, 45–46, *48*, 235, *235*
    deaths and conditions linked to, 373, *373*
    early studies on, 9–10
    middle-aged adults, 253–254
    nicotine, 373–374
    preconception, 172–173
    pregnancy, 174
    profile of tobacco user, *376*
    quitting and middle-aged adults, 257
    secondhand tobacco smoke, 118,
        373, *373*
Smoking cessation, 235, *235*
    Transtheoretical Model of Behavior
        Change, 45–46, *48*
Social domain
    adolescents, 228–229
    infants and toddlers, 190–192
    overview of, 59
    pregnancy, 178–180
    preschool and school-age children,
        210–211
    young adults, 238–240
Social mandate for health promotion, 6–7
Social Security Act, 8
Social support, 150
Sociocultural domain
    communication and, *91*
    health professionals, 429–430
    nutrition, 304
    weight control, 350–351
Socioeconomic domain
    older adults, 278–279
    risk factors, 70
Sociological domain

health care access, 458
    middle-aged adults, 253
Soil pollution, 124–126
Somatic nervous system, 150, *151*
Sound, holistic care, 402–404, *403*
Sound pollution, 126–129, *128*
Space
    color, 131–132
    Feng shui, 134–137, *136*
    health and, 130–131
    scent, 132
    workplace safety and, 132–134
Specificity of screening test, 261
Specificity principle, 327
Spiritual domain
    adolescents, 232–233
    communication and, *91*
    health professionals, 428–429
    infants and toddlers, 193–194
    middle-aged adults, 254
    nutrition, 304
    older adults, 280–281
    overview of, 60–61
    preschool and school-age children,
        213–214
    young adults, 242
Spiritual health, defined, 60
Spirituality, 428
    assessment guide, *429*
    in cultural assessment, 103–104
    psychoneuroimmunology and, 162
    risk factors, 72
Spiritual well-being, 281
Sprains, 331
Standard of best interest principle, *449,* 451–452
Standards of care, 455–456
Standards of Clinical Nursing Practice (ANA),
    20, *21*
Stanford Prevention Research Center, 75
State Children's Health Insurance Program
    (SCHIP), 211–212
Static stretching, 326
Stimulants, 372
Stomach, stress response, *155*
Strains, 331
Stress
    affect of, on disease, 160–162
    bereavement, 158–159
    cancer and, 157, 161–162
    categories of stressors, 156, *156*
    chronic stress, 159, *160*
    crisis, 160, *161*
    defined, 154
    depression and, 161
    eustress, 279
    examination stress, 158
    general adaptation syndrome, 154
    hardiness, 427
    immune system response, 156
    massage and, 406
    nursing implications, 163
    nursing student stress, 421–422
    occupational, 419
    occupational stress and health
        professional, 419–420
    older adults, 279
    perceptions and, 156
    pregnancy and, 178

psychocutaneous disease, 161
research on, *157*, 157–158
stress response, 154, *155*, 156
tips for easing mental stress, *158*
Stressors
categories of, *156*
defined, 154, 418
Stress response
defined, 154
effect on body, 154, *155*, 156
Substance abuse, 366–382
addiction, 370–371, *371*
adolescents, *222–225*, 223–225
age and, 376–377
alcohol use and addiction, *375*, 375–376
commonly abused psychotropic drugs, 371–372
comorbidity, 378–379
in control, 382
defined, 224
detoxification, 370
drug defined, 367
drug mechanics, 368, *368, 369*
drug misuse and abuse, 370–371
ethnicity, 377
gender and, 376
hallucinogens, 372
health promotion strategies, 379–382
household drugs, 372
incidence of, 367
mental health issues, 378
nurses and, 377–378
opiates, 371–372
out of control, 382
overview of, 366–367
physical health issues, 378
pregnancy, 174
prevention, 379–382, *380*
primary prevention, 380–381
protective factors, 379
risk factors, 379
routes for drug administration, *367*
secondary prevention, 381
sources and categories of drugs, 367–368
spiritual health issues, 378–379
stimulants, 372
tertiary prevention, 381–382
tobacco use and addiction, 373–374, *373–374*
tolerance, 370
withdrawal, 370
Sudden Infant Death Syndrome (SIDS), 186
Sunlight, 400–401, *401, 402*
health and, 129–130
Superstition, 106
Surgeon General's Call to Action to Prevent and Decrease Overweight and Obesity, The, 322
Sweat glands, stress response, *155*
Sympathetic nervous system, 150, *151*
Systems theory, 30

T

Taboos, 106
T'ai Chi, 399
Tannahill, Andrew, 50
Tannahill Model of Health Promotion, 50

Tao, 135
Target heart rate, 329–330
Taxonomy, 66
Taylor, George, 406
Technical domain, nutrition, 305
Technological disasters, 138–139
Technological domain
communication and, *91*
health professionals, 431
overview of, 61
Technology
communication and, 93
increases in, and nursing role, 72–73
Teleology, 448–449
Television, preschool and school-age children, 210–211, *211*
Teratogens, 113, 170
Terrorism, 14, 139–140, *140*
Terror-related disasters, 139–140, *140*
Tertiary prevention, 67, 381–382
Testicular cancer, self-examination, 236, *236*
Thalamus, 152
Theories
adaptation, 30
of aging, 271, *272*
defined, 22
goal attainment, 32
human becoming, 31
human care, 31
needs, 31
of planned behavior, 42–43, *42–43*
protection motivation theory, 45, *47*
of social behavior, 44, *44*
systems, 30
transcultural, 31–32
Theory of Goal Attainment, 32
Theory of Modeling and Role Modeling, 391
Therapeutic communication techniques, 88, *89*
Therapeutic relationship, communication in, 86–88
Therapeutic touch, 389, 394, *394*, 404
Thermogenesis, 347–348
Thyroid, *152*
Thyroxin, *154*
T lymphocytes, 152, 153
Tobacco use, 373–374, *373–374. See also* Smoking; Substance abuse
environmental tobacco smoke, 373, *373*
nicotine, 373–374
prevention, 380
profile of tobacco user, *376*
Toddlers. *See* Infants and toddlers
Tolerance, 370
Tornadoes, 138, *139, 140*
Torts, 456
Touch
acupressure, 406–407
guidelines for, 404
massage, 405–406
in nonverbal communication, 85, *85*
reflexology, 405, *405*
Toxic Substance Control Act (TSCA) Assistance Information Service, 146
Transcultural nursing theory, 31–32
Transtheoretical Model of Behavior Change, 45–46, *48*

Travelbee, Joyce, communication and, 86
Trephining, 3
Triad diagnosis, 378
Triandis, Henry, 44
TSCA. *See* Toxic Substance Control Act Assistance Information Service
Tsunami, 138

U

UCLA/RAND Center for Adolescent Health Promotion, 245
Unconditional positive regard, 87
Undernutrition, 306
United Nations, health promotion, 10
United States
health promotion during, early America, 6
national goals for health, 10–12
Urinary incontinence, pregnancy and, 178
U.S. Army Center for Health Promotion & Preventive Medicine, 17
U.S. Census Bureau, 291
U.S. Consumer Product Safety Commission (CPSC), 146
U.S. Department of Health and Human Services, 16–17, 445
U.S. Food and Drug Administration (FDA), 384
U.S. Public Health Service, 146
Utter watchfulness, 130

V

Values
defined, 105, 452
ethical decision making and personal values, 452–453
steps in values clarification, *452*, 452–453
Values clarification, *452*, 452–453
Veracity principle, *449*, 450–451
Verbal communication, defined, 81
Viagra, 277
Violence
adolescents, 230–231
domestic violence during pregnancy, 178–179, *179*
intimate partner violence, 240, *240*
Vision, middle-aged adults, 261–262
Vision screening, 205, *205*
Vitamins, 295, *295–296, 298–303*
VOCs. *See* Volatile organic compounds
Volatile organic compounds (VOCs), 119, *119*
health promotion and nursing interventions for, *122–123*

W

Wald, Lillian, 8
Warm-up, 330
Warning labels, 119, *119*
Water pollution, 124–126
Watson, Jean, 31, *36–37*
Watson's Theory of Transpersonal Caring (Watson), 31
Weapons of mass destruction, 139

Weapons of mass effect, 139
WebMD, 73
Weight control, 343–361
    assessment, 352–357, *354–357*
    behavior and attitude, 359–360
    biochemical influences and eating
        behavior, 348–349
    biological domain, 347–349
    body image disturbance, 350
    defined, 345
    desirable body weight, 345
    environmental domain, 349–350
    equilibrium set-point theory, 348
    health promotion and, 345
    Health Promotion Model, 359
    ideal body weight, 346, 355–356
    issues related to, 351
    maintenance suggestions, *351*
    myths, *352,* 352–353
    nursing process, 351–361
    obesity consequences, 343–345
    obesity defined, 343–344
    obstacles to, 345–347
    optimal body composition, 354
    preschool and school-age children, *200,*
        200–202, *202*
    psychological domain, 350
    shaping and guided practice, 360
    sociocultural domain, 350–351
    thermogenesis, 347–348
Weight cycling, 348
Weight management, *Healthy People 2010,*
    297, *297*
Wellness, 41
Wellness-illness continuum, 7
WIC program. *See* Women, infants,
    and children program
Withdrawal, 370
Women, infants, and children program
    (WIC program), 192
Workplace
    adolescents and safety, 230
    in cultural assessment, 105
    ergonomics, 133–134
    pregnancy and, 181
    risk factors, 70
    workplace safety, 132–134, 259
    worksite air quality, 119, *121*
    young adults and occupational hazards,
        241, *241*
World Health Organization, health promotion,
    3, 10

Worldviews
    cultural domains, 106
    defined, 97

Y

Yin/Yang, 5, 135, *136*
Yoga, 399
Young adults, 233–242
    biological domain, 233–236
    cognitive development, 236–237, *237*
    emotional development, 238, *238*
    environmental domain, 241
    exercise, 233–234
    nutrition, 233
    political domain, 240
    psychological domain, 236–238
    relationships, 238–240
    screening, 234–236, *235, 236*
    sexuality, 241–242
    skin cancer prevention, 234, *234*
    sleep, 234
    social domain, 238–240
    spiritual domain, 242
    workplace safety, 241, *241*